AF699248

Differential Diagnosis of Eye Diseases

Differential Diagnosis of Eye Diseases

By Hans Pau

Translated by Gerhard Cibis

390 figures
184 illustrations in color
14 tables

1978

W. B. Saunders Company
Philadelphia · London · Toronto

Georg Thieme Publishers
Stuttgart

Author

Professor Dr. med. H. Pau
Director of the Ophthalmologic Clinic of Düsseldorf University

Translator

Dr. Gerhard W. Cibis
Formerly: Instructor, Department of Ophthalmology, University of Iowa
Currently: Clinical Assistant Professor of Ophthalmology, Children's Mercy Hospital
University of Missouri — Kansas City

Original German Edition: Differentialdiagnose der Augenkrankheiten
© 1974 by Georg Thieme Verlag, Stuttgart

Authorized English edition co-published 1978
by W. B. Saunders Company, Philadelphia, London, Toronto
and Georg Thieme Verlag, Stuttgart

© 1978 Georg Thieme Publishers, Herdweg 63, P.O.B. 732, D-7000 Stuttgart 1
Printed in Germany by C. Maurer, Geislingen/Steige

Some of the product names, patents and registered designs referred to are in fact registered trademarks or proprietary names even though specific reference to this fact is not always made in the text. Therefore, the appearance of a name without designation as proprietary is not to be construed as a representation by the publisher that it is in the public domain.

All rights, including the rights of publication, distribution and sales, as well as the right to translation, are reserved. No part of this work covered by the copyrights hereon may be reproduced or copied in any form or by any means — graphic, electronic or mechanical including photocopying, recording, taping, or information and retrieval systems — without written permission of the publisher.

ISBN 3-13-546301-X
ISBN 0-7216-7117-9
LCCCN 76-1240

To my dear wife
Dr. Margret Pau
with gratitude

Foreword

What is the most difficult of all?
That which seems the easiest:
To see with your eyes what lies
directly in front of you.

J. W. v. Goethe, *Xenien*

The difficulty experienced in rapid orientation to some of the most important clinical pictures in ophthalmology is observed almost daily by the clinical instructor during teaching rounds and in discussion of differential diagnosis. Detailed information is available in the excellent, expansive systems and handbooks of ophthalmology and the less extensive but excellent textbooks. These are only rarely used, however, for rapid establishment of a differential diagnosis.

For this reason I have fulfilled the request of many colleagues and the Georg Thieme publishing house, in attempting to write a short text of differential diagnosis. The scope of the book is directed entirely to the discussion of differential diagnosis on an everyday basis. Its plan is completely subjective and will therefore appear too specialized to some readers and too generalized to others. Its orientation is directed totally to differential diagnosis in the office and clinic and is not intended as a forum for scientific papers. If this book provides some pleasure to a young (or old) colleague in the intellectual exercise of differential diagnosis, its purpose will have been fulfilled.

Hans Pau

Düsseldorf, Autumn 1977

Table of Contents

5 Dazzle, Photophobia, Night Blindness, Day Blindness

6 Hyperemia of the Eye or Its Surroundings

7 Swelling Around the Eye and Its Environs

8 Oculomotor and Sensory Anomalies

9 Pain and Symptoms Arising from or Localized in the Eye

10 Lids

11 Lacrimal System

12 Conjunctiva

13 Cornea

14 Sclera

15 Anterior Chamber

16 Iris

17 Ciliary Body

18 Choroid

19 Intraocular Pressure

20 Vitreous Body

21 Lens

22 Retina

23 Optic Nerve

24 Pupil

25 Orbit and Globe

26 Damage from Light and Ionizing Radiation

Hint for the Reader

As some disease manifestations are discussed in the context of several different syndromes, it will be helpful to consult the index.

1 Loss of Vision, Chromatopsia, Scintillations, Photopsias

Sudden Deterioration of Vision

Visual Deterioration without Redness or Ocular Complaints

Unilateral blindness — Unilateral loss of vision — Unilateral loss of visual field — Bilateral loss of vision (with homonymous hemianopia, vertical hemianopia) — Transient loss of vision.

Unilateral Blindness

It seems as if the light was suddenly turned off: central retinal artery embolus (Plate XXIV, Fig. 4, page 224 h), traumatic damage to the optic nerve, for example, fracture of the bony optic canal and laceration of the optic nerve in the bony optic canal. Blindness may be longstanding and only suddenly noticed when the other eye is covered.

Unilateral Decrease in Vision

The light in one eye suddenly seems dimmer: central retinal vein thrombosis (Plate XXII, Fig. 6, page 224 f), vitreous hemorrhage, acute keratoconus (Fig. 13. 4).

Unilateral Visual Field Loss

Portions of the visual field are suddenly lost in one eye only: branch artery embolus (Fig. 22.12, page 269) or branch vein thrombosis (Plate XXIII, Fig. 1, page 224 g) in the retina, retinal detachment.

Bilateral Visual Deterioration

Vision has suddenly declined bilaterally with *homonymous hemianopia:* stroke, hemorrhage, aneurysm, trauma (in the optic radiations, optic tract), acute elevation of intracranial pressure, potential carbon monoxide poisoning (central damage). Inferior altitudinal hemianopia can occur with recurrent severe blood loss (metrorrhagia, gastric bleeding, etc.). Optic atrophy develops 2 to 3 weeks later (see page 23).

Transient Loss of Vision

Darkening of vision is transient on fainting, with vasomotor collapse, heart failure, essential hypotension, and circulatory disturbances when stooping over or straining. Transient hypotension also occurs with fatigue, hunger, vitamin deficiency, *chronic hypotension,* hormonal disorders, and arteriosclerosis.

Complaints: Dizziness, ringing in the ears, fainting, flimmering vision and palpitations.

Transient darkening of vision also occurs with elevated intracranial pressure, in eclamptic uremia caused by vascular spasm, in toxemia of pregnancy and in diabetic coma. Carbon monoxide poisoning may cause cortical blindness or hemianopia. Transient amaurosis or hemianopia is also seen with caisson disease (rapid atmospheric decompression). Cerebral ischemia with transient blindness can occur with increasing gravitational force due to acceleration in an airplane or by a centrifuge device. Pre-emboli (see page 270) can lead to transient vision loss.

Visual Deterioration with Redness or Other Ocular Symptoms

Glaucoma attacks can cause sudden visual loss with severe pain in the eye and the head (Fig. 19.1).

Progressive Visual Loss

Visual Loss Without a Red Eye or Ocular Symptoms

Cloudy vision — Mobile opacities — Central scotoma (positive, negative) — Distorted vision — Central and peripheral visual field loss — Temporary visual loss.

Progressive Permanent Cloudy Vision

Everything is cloudy or becomes cloudy: corneal opacities, corneal dystrophy, opacification of the lens (all acquired cataracts), vitreous opacities.

Mobile Opacities

Opacities which move with the eyes: The more or less normal vitreous floaters (muscae volitantes), inflammatory vitreal opacities (as in cyclitis) or with hemorrhage. With retinal detachment light flashes may be followed by a "dark curtain" or "gray veil" over the eye.

Central Scotoma

There is a central visual field defect.
Positive (subjective) central scotoma: A gray or brown opacification covers the object of regard. Pathology at the retinal center (macular hemorrhage, macular detachment, central serous retinopathy) (Figs. 3.1–3.3, pages 11–12).
Negative (objective) central scotoma: Centrally there is an area of missing vision. Pathology is in the papillomacular bundle of the optic nerve (retrobulbar neuritis) due to central retinal scars, central chorioretinal damage (myopic degeneration, macular degeneration without exudate or hemorrhage), and suppression scotoma with strabismus. Pain, particularly with movement of the eyes, occurs early in the course of optic or retrobulbar neuritis. In these cases an amblyopic or amaurotic iridoplegia is present.

Distorted Vision (Metamorphopsia)

A distortion of vision may accompany visual deterioration. Straight lines appear crooked and objects vary abnormally in size and shape. This is caused by retinal scars of any etiology: disciform macular degeneration (Fig. 22.27, page 281); protracted, specifically recurrent forms of retinitis (central serous retinopathy [Plate XXVI, Fig. 5, page 288 b], retinitis proliferans); retinal hemorrhages; and retinal detachment.

Central Scotoma with Peripheral Field Loss

Visual loss from a central scotoma associated with other *field defects includes* various forms of retinal, neural and choroidal inflammation; optic atrophy; degenerative retinal and choroidal processes; glaucoma; and intraocular as well as orbital and brain tumors.

Temporary Visual Loss

Causes of temporary visual loss include migrainous scintillating scotomata, blackouts with brain tumors, blindness in pseudouremia and functional blindness (hysteria, malingering).
Transient central blindness with maintained pupillary reaction can be seen in pseudouremia and chronic lead poisoning (leaded gasoline – tetraethyl lead, "anti-knock" compounds).

Visual Loss with Hyperemia or Ocular Complaints

Visual loss with hyperemia and ocular complaints — Foggy vision with eye pain and headaches — Visual loss with hyperemia and hypotony — Visual loss with hyperemia and exophthalmos.

Visual Loss with Hyperemia and Ocular Complaints

Everything is or becomes cloudy; associated with hyperemia and ocular complaints: keratitis, iritis, cyclitis.

Cloudy or Foggy Vision with Ocular Pain and Headaches

Visual loss, specifically cloudy vision with ocular pain and headaches of varying degrees: chronic angle closure glaucoma; secondary glaucoma (as in iritis, scleritis, cyclitis, rubeosis iridis, anterior or posterior subluxation of the lens, intraocular tumor, etc.); optic neuritis; retrobulbar neuritis; endophthalmitis; and panophthalmitis.

Visual Loss, Hyperemia, Hypotony

Visual loss associated with redness and marked hypotony of the globe: choroidal detachment (Fig. 18.1 b) associated with a flat anterior chamber; choroidal detachment associated with a deep anterior chamber; and phthisis bulbi following inflammation or perforating injury.

Visual Loss with Hyperemia and Exophthalmos

Exophthalmos in conjunction with visual loss

and hyperemia: orbital cellulitis (Plate XXXII, Fig. 3, page 288 h); panophthalmitis (Fig. 16.20, page 203); pulsating exophthalmos (caput medusae [Plate XXXI, Fig. 6, page 288 g]); and cavernous sinus thrombosis.

Functional Visual Loss and Malingering

Hysterical Visual Loss

In spite of allegedly total visual field loss or with maintenance of only a small central island of vision, the hysterically blind patient is able to move about freely in his environment. The pupillary reaction is intact. The hysteric is not feigning his illness. Often children come home from school claiming sudden onset of unilateral blindness or bilateral decrease in acuity. If the visual field shows marked contraction of all isopters or "spiraling" while spatial orientation and pupillary reaction remain intact, this is highly suggestive of a functional etiology. The ophthalmologist should quickly be able to point out the functional nature of such cases and direct them for psychotherapy. Failure at school or an excessive need for attention is frequently an underlying cause.

Malingering and Aggravating

In cases where the claimed *uniocular* visual loss is questionable, it is useful not to let the patient know which eye is being tested or to reveal the true size of the optotypes being used; for example, with Gratama tubes, the subject sees the right picture with the left eye and the left picture with the right eye.

Visual acuity testing is done binocularly with a plus lens in front of one eye, while the other remains unencumbered. Through rapid switching of fogging lenses between the healthy and "blind" eye, one hopes to trick the malingerer into reading out of the allegedly blind eye while the good eye is fogged.

If the test letters are projected via several mirrors, it is easy to become confused as to their actual size. The malingerer may then admit to considerably better vision.

When binocular vision is present, the introduction of small amounts of prism will produce a shift in fixation. In cases of simulated uniocular blindness, a 10 diopter prism introduced base out in front of the allegedly blind eye will produce an immediate inward shift of the eye.

After covering the seeing eye, one asks the patient to look up, down and to either side. At the same time the examiner points in the appropriate direction. If, however, during this maneuver the examiner suddenly points in a direction other than the one verbally indicated, the malingerer will usually follow the motion of the hand.

With the healthy eye covered, a sudden threatening motion is made with an object or bright light in front of the allegedly blind eye. A blink reflex is often elicited but it can be suppressed. Paramount to the success of each of these "tricks" is that the patient be unaware they are being used. The approximate visual acuity can be measured objectively using the optokinetic response (nystagmometer of Goldmann, Günter, Ohm-Romberg, etc.). The optokinetic response can voluntarily be suppressed by the patient.

Only rarely will a patient simulate *bilateral* blindness. Compared to the truly blind person, the malingerer feigning bilateral blindness will markedly overplay his disability.

The *differential diagnosis* includes amblyopia and retrobulbar neuritis. To diagnose amblyopia consider the history, angle of deviation, parafoveal fixation, eccentric fixation, anisometropia with the more hyperopic eye being the weaker, nystagmus, pseudopapilledema, lack of fusion (Worth four-dot, Titmus, vectograph), and maintained pupillary reaction (Schapero 1971).

In addition to decreased visual acuity, hallmarks of retrobulbar neuritis are central scotoma, pain on pressing or moving the eye, and temporal pallor of the disk after two to three weeks. In such cases there is an afferent pupillary defect.

Congenital Dyslexia, Visual Agnosia

Congenital dyslexia or alexia should be considered when a properly educated patient is unable to read. Minimal brain damage may be an etiology (Goldberg et al. 1960, Hartstein 1971).

Visual agnosia occurs in various forms as a result of disturbances in *cortical integration.*

Hemialexia occurs when the interconnection between area 18 of the two hemispheres is disturbed.

Letter, word, and numeral alexia can be congenital or acquired. When acquired, it is usually due to central nervous system damage, resulting from stroke, trauma, or carbon monoxide poisoning.

Dyslexia results from a failure of connection between perception and psychovisual interpretation.

Visual agnosia can occur when the patient suffers from a major disturbance in orientation. This is most frequently seen in cases of marked visual field loss leaving a residual "tunnel" or "key-hole" visual field. The most severe psychovisual defect is occipital blindness. These patients may deny that they are blind (Anton's syndrome).

Visual Loss or Blindness in Childhood

In children, particularly infants, it is usually impossible to elicit subjective evidence as to the type of visual loss. Nonetheless, all known forms of decreased vision occur in the child.

Anophthalmos and, with exceptions, microphthalmos imply blindness or markedly reduced vision. Individuals with rubella microphthalmos may have surprisingly good vision, especially if amblyopia treatment is instituted early.

Corneal causes include hereditary dystrophies (see page 164) and inflammations such as varicella, rubeola, vaccinia, and gonorrhea.

Congenital cataracts have a myriad of causes (see page 244). All processes in the *vitreous* leading to pseudoglioma (see page 234) result in blindness or marked visual loss.

Primary *retinal causes* of visual loss are: infantile macular degeneration (page 278), tapetoretinal degeneration (page 286) and pseudoretinitis pigmentosa (page 291), embryopathies (page 244), retinoschisis, Coat's disease, retrolental fibroplasia, retinal detachment, high myopia, albinism, achromatopsia and retinoblastoma.

Optic nerve aplasia and atrophy can be hereditary (page 305) or secondary such as with: various dystrophies (page 314); hydrocephalus; tumors – astrocytoma, craniopharyngioma, glioblastoma, meningioma, angioma, metastatic tumor; inflammatory damage – encephalitis (tuberculous meningitis), encephalomyelitis, etc.; trauma-fracture at the orbital canal, subdural hematoma, cerebral hemorrhage. It may be associated with major brain damage – idiocy, epilepsy, cortical paresis, deafness.

Even prior to birth the *uveal* tract can be damaged as with chorioretinitis, pseudoglioma, or iridocyclitis. Congenital coloboma of the choroid is a cause of poor visual acuity.

Hydrophthalmos or buphthalmos (see page 225) accompanies *glaucoma* in the first year of life. This can be congenital, primary infantile, or secondary.

True psychic blindness is very rare, and includes agnosia (see page 4), alexia (see page 4).

Chromatopsia

Xanthopsia occurs in santonin poisoning and is sometimes preceded by the sensation that everything is violet. It may also be seen with digitalis intoxication, streptomycin, sulfonamides, barbiturates, phenacetin, salicylic acid, Atabrine, amyl nitrite, DDT poisoning, extractum filicis maris, picric acid, chromic acid and chromates as well as with certain snake venoms (Cloetta 1928).

Cyanopsia is observed with digitalis intoxication or allergy, post-cataract surgery, with carbon monoxide poisoning, picric acid and mushroom poisoning, as well as after the ingestion of mescaline or Atabrine.

Erythropia occurs in snow glare, aphakia, iris colobomata, albinism, pupillary dilatation, acrobatic flying (forward looping, flying upside down), iodine, cyanide and tobacco intoxication. The sensation of seeing red may occur in bright sunlight due to the oblique entry of light into the eye through the sclera. Vitreous hemorrhages can lead to the sensation of erythropia.

The sensation of seeing everything as *green* can occur with use of digitalis, barbiturates and Atabrine (Cloetta 1928).

Visual sensations such as a bright cloud or the illusion that everything is covered with snow occur after injuries as with CS^2 (Duke-Elder 1954), asterol-dihydrochloride (fungicide), or with the use of antiepileptic drugs such as trimethadione, paramethadione and oxazolidine. The effect is supposed to originate in the retina (Dekking 1950, Heydenreich 1966).

The use of **hallucinogenic** or **psychomimetic drugs** can lead to psychopathic alterations of visual impressions. In such situations the surroundings in which the experiment takes place, as well as the expectations and orientation of the subject play an important role. Listening to music, for example, may lead to a wild splash of colors; everything is one thousand times more vivid than before. This can progress to synesthesia where music is "seen" as well as heard and colors elicit sound. Cosmic consciousness supervenes where the "self" seems to leave the body and observe itself without any relationship to time or place. The feeling of self is then totally lost, and is subsumed in a pulsating mass.

These sensations are particularly strong with LSD (lysergic acid diethylamide). They are also obtained with peyote, a cactus root; the agent is mescaline. Another natural hallucinogen is psilocybin found in the mushroom *Psilocybe mexicana*.

Cannabis (marijuana, hashish) can act as hallucinogen in certain persons. Paintings become more vivid and musical impressions increase in intensity. The same is true for alcohol. Hallucinations occur in delirium tremens (DT's). Cocaine abuse rarely leads to hallucinations.

Hallucinations caused by irritation of certain areas of the cerebral cortex also belong in the category of **psychovisual disturbances.** Stimulation of the cortex in area 17 results in scintillating scotomata such as seen in migraine. Stimulation of area 19 evokes more complex hallucinations, specifically size distortions resulting in macropsia or micropsia. Irritation of the frontal cortex leads to delirium. Parietal, temporal and occipital processes can evoke true (psychotic) hallucinations.

Scintillations, Light Flashes, Photopsy

Scintillations Not Associated with Organic Diseases

Scintillations prior to fainting — Scintillations with migraine.

Scintillations Prior to Fainting

The patient complains that he sees silvery or colored sparks and lights, or that "everything goes black." This may occur with circulatory collapse, hypotensive episodes, strenuous physical exertion when circulation is inadequate, and in debilitating diseases and emotionally labile persons. These symptoms, associated with orthostasis, occur predominantly in young people.

Scintillations with Migraine

A relatively frequent occurrence related to disturbances in the visual cortex and optic pathways is the so-called scintillating scotoma of migraine. The scotoma, associated with flickering sparks and zigzag lines, lasts about 15 minutes and may move from the center of the visual field to the periphery or vice versa. Ten minutes to hours later, the scotoma may be followed by a severe headache which can be hemicranial, and associated with nausea and vomiting. A scotoma exists when the patient sees nothing in the scintillating area. It may be concentric or hemianopic in character. Heredity is one of the possible etiologic factors.

Attacks can be triggered by lack of sleep, alcohol or emotional stress. In rare cases arteriosclerosis or brain tumor may be the underlying cause. Stars and lightning flashes occur in the early stages of delirium tremens.

Scintillations Associated with Organic Ocular Disease

Retinal detachment — Choroiditis and chorioretinitis — Acute vitreous detachment — Iridodonesis.

Scintillations associated with organic disease last longer and can usually be elicited at will.

Retinal Detachment

A retinal detachment or retinal tear must always be excluded with scintillations.
Light flashes, especially in association with "floaters", may occur with retinal detachment. Such light flashes may be due to vitreous traction on the retina and precede a retinal tear. With persisting retinal detachment the mechanical irritation of the retina producing light flashes may disturb the patient to such a degree that he requests enucleation.

Choroiditis and Chorioretinitis

Any acute choroiditis or chorioretinitis (Plate XV, Fig. 5, page 192 g) can lead to a "flickering image" or light flashes.

Acute Vitreal Detachment

Acute detachment of the vitreous is frequently associated with light flashes.

Iridodonesis

Hypercritical patients may find the wobbling of the iris following cataract extraction to be disturbing.

Trauma

Trauma to the globe elicits photopsy in the following forms: lightning flashes, sparks or "stars", or dark or bright circles or spots. Cerebral contusion can also produce the sensation of colors.

References

Cloetta, M.: Vergiftungen durch Schlafmittel. Die Vergiftungen durch Alkaloide und Pflanzenstoffe, ed. by F. Flury, H. Zangger, in: Lehrbuch der Toxikologie, Springer, Berlin (1928) S. 273–314

Dekking, H. M.: Acta XVI int. Kongr. Ophthalm. London Vol. I (1950) 465

Duke-Elder, St.: Textbook of Ophthalmology, Vol. IV. Injuries, London 1954

Goldberg, H. K., C. Marshall, E. Sims: The role of brain damage in congenital dyslexia. Amer. J. Ophthal. 50 (1960) 586–590

Hartstein, J.: Current concepts in Dyslexia. Mosby, St. Louis 1971

Heydenreich, A.: Chemisch-toxische Schäden der Augen. Klin. Mbl. Augenheilk. 149 (1966) 145–165

Schapero, M.: Amblyopia. Chilton Book Comp., Philadelphia, New York, London 1971

2 Deficiencies of Color Vision

Congenital Deficiencies of Color Vision

Total Color Blindness and Complete Cone Deficiency

Total color blindness of the cones *(monochromatism)* has good visual acuity and is therefore different from complete cone blindness *(achromatopsia).* Achromatopsia is associated with low visual acuity (20/200 to 20/400), central scotomata, pendular nystagmus and photophobia. Loss of inhibitory influences of cones on rods leads to an altered adaptation in achromatopia. Marked photophobia and day blindness *(hemeralopia)* result. The photophobia diminishes as the patient grows older.
Both forms of total color blindness are extremely rare (between 1:40,000 and 1:100,000). Achromatopsia is primarily inherited as autosomal recessive (François and Verriest 1960, François et al. 1955). The electroretinogram (ERG) can show purely photopic or mixed photopic/scotopic changes in achromatopsia (Pinckers 1972).

Dichromatopia

In dichromatopia only two colors in addition to black and white are perceived.
In congenital color blindness, *protanopia* (red blindness) is differentiated from *deuteranopia* (green blindness). In both cases colors in the middle of the spectrum seem more and more colorless until, at a certain point in the spectrum, only gray is perceived – the so-called "neutral point".

Protanopia

In red deficiency (protanopia) red seems five times as dark as in deuteranopia. The long-wave end of the spectrum is correspondingly shortened.

Deuteranopia

With a deficiency for green (deuteranopia), the color spectrum is normal in length but sensitivity is reduced by 50 percent.

Tritanopia

In tritanopia or blue-yellow blindness, red and green are seen. The short-wave end of the spectrum is reduced. Congenital tritanopia is extremely rare.

Anomalous Color Vision

In anomalous color vision, there is no total lack of perception of certain colors, but there is a weakness. Again, one must differentiate between **protanomaly,** a deficiency in the perception of red; **deuteranomaly,** deficiency in green; and the rare **tritanomaly,** partial deficiency in blue.
With anomalous color vision, greater *saturation* and *intensity* of the deficient color is needed for recognition. The *area* seen (visual angle) must be *greater* than for normal individuals. The *time* needed to recognize *colors* is *greater* and *adaptation* or *fatigue* for colored stimuli occurs earlier than in normal individuals. Color contrast is enhanced (successive and simultaneous contrast).

Frequency of Congenital Color Defects

Congenital dichromatopia and trichronomaly are common; they occur in 8.0 percent of all men and 0.4 percent of women. Heredity is sex-linked recessive. Trichronomaly: protanomaly (1.6 percent), deuteranomaly (4.2 percent).
Dichromatopia: protanopia (0.7 percent), deuteranopia (1.5 percent). Only red-green blindness is of practical significance. Tritano-

pia, specifically tritanomaly (i.e., congenital blue-yellow defects), are purely of academic interest.

Color Vision Asthenopia

Color asthenopia occurs when there is normal color perception in the rested state but the range of color matches increases after prolonged presentation (15 seconds).

Color Vision Amblyopia

The term color vision amblyopia is used when an increase in the range of color matches is present; uncertainty in color matching on the anomaloscope results (Grützner 1971).

Acquired Color Vision Defects

In deciding whether an acquired color vision defect is being dealt with *numerous factors* must be considered (Jaeger and Grützner, 1963). Factors in addition to color perception such as acuity, visual field, or light perception play a role. Frequently, the color vision defect occurs unilaterally or only in part of the visual field. Unless the color vision defect was acquired early, the patient will name colors as he sees them and not as he thinks a normal person would describe them.

For the differential diagnosis of acquired color vision defects, it is important to remember that one is dealing with a disturbed form of normal color vision. At times this affects the red-green mechanism more than the blue or vice versa. In the end, however, all color perception is impaired.

In acquired color vision defects (Jaeger and Grützner 1963, François and Verriest 1960), a disturbance of the red-green mechanism is associated with optic nerve disease while defects in blue perception indicate retinal disease.

Acquired Red-Green Disturbances with Normal Brightness Perception

Cases of acquired red-green disturbances with normal perception of brightness almost exclusively denote optic nerve disease. These include *tobacco-alcohol amblyopia, thallium poisoning, retrobulbar neuritis* and *Leber's optic atrophy.*

Acquired Red-Green Deficiencies with Shortening of the Red End of the Spectrum

Acquired red-green color vision disturbances with loss of perception of the long-wave end of the spectrum occur almost exclusively in the *hereditary maculopathies.*

Acquired Blue Defect with Normal Brightness Perception

Acquired defects for blue perception with normal brightness perception occur in *retinal detachment, tapetoretinal degeneration, tapetochorioretinal degeneration* (choroideremia), and in dominant hereditary optic atrophy.

Acquired Blue Defect with Shortening of the Red End of the Spectrum

An acquired loss for blue with shortening of the red end of the spectrum is seen with *central serous retinopathy* and in the *macular form of diffuse tapetoretinal degeneration.*

Color Vision Testing

Various testing modalities are available to aid in the differential diagnosis of color vision defects (Heydenreich 1969, Cruz-Coke 1970).

Comparison testing: In this test two similar colors have to be selected from a variety of choices.

Color plates *(pseudoisochromatopsia,* pseudoanisochromatopsia, increased color contrast, decreased color contrast with unsaturated colors = florcontrast). The best known pseudoisochromatic plates are those of Ishihara and Stilling-Hertel-Velhagen.

Color mixing device: The most useful spectrometer to test color vision is the *Nagel anomaloscope* (Fig. 2.1). The patient fixates on a round test object, the lower half of which consists of sodium yellow of varying intensity. In the upper half of the target, lithium red may be mixed with mercury or thallium green until the upper and lower halves appear equal. This mixture corresponding to the lower half is called color equation (Rayleigh equation). Matches made on the anomaloscope in various color deficiencies are shown in Fig. 2.1 (Grützner and Jaeger).

Individual color matching: This method is best represented by the Farnsworth panel (100 and the smaller 15 color test). Even the smaller Farnsworth test allows for a separation of protan, deuteran, and tritan disturbances. In this simplified examination, 15 colored disks 5 mm in diameter must be arranged in relationship to a given reference color. The order in which mistakes are made permits a quick differentiation of protan, deuteran and, most important, tritan color-vision defects (Grützner and Jaeger).

Chromatopsia (see page 4).

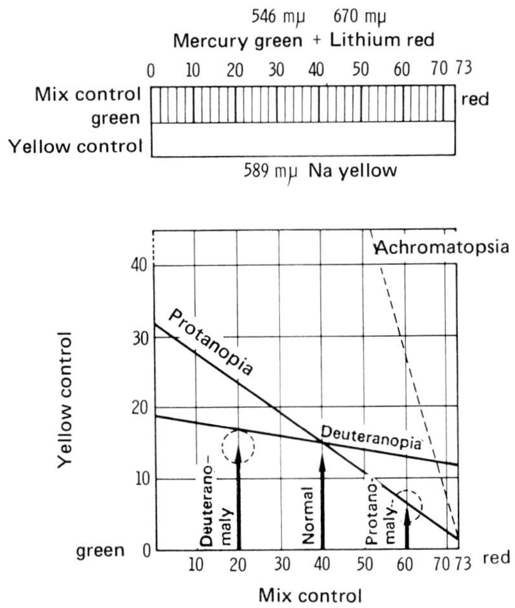

Fig. 2.1 Settings on the anomaloscope in various color vision deficiencies (normal mean 40/15 = mix control/yellow control) (after Grützner and Jaeger)

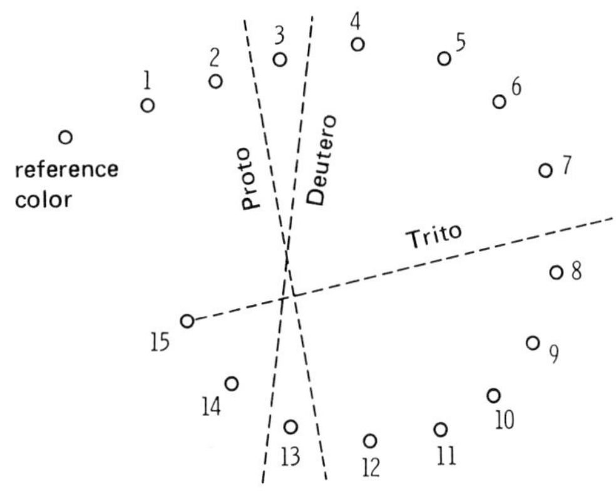

Fig. 2.2 Farnsworth panel D-15 test. The 15 different hues are arrayed sequentially in relationship to the given reference hue (after Grützner and Jaeger)

References

Cruz-Coke, R.: Color blindness. Charles C. Thomas, Springfield, Illinois 1970

François, J., G. Verriest: Les dyschromatopsies acquises. Ann. Oculist. (Paris) 190 (1957) 713–746, 812–859, 893–943

François, J., G. Verriest: Contribution à l'étude des dyschromatopsies congénitales à symptomes intermédiaires entre ceux des systèmes dichromatiques classiques et ceux de l'achromatopsie typique: Observation personelle et revue de la littérature. Ann. Oculist. (Paris) 192 (1959) 81–120

François, J., G. Verriest: Trois nouvelles observations d'achromatopsie congénitale atypique. Ann. Oculist. (Paris) 193 (1960) 123–137

François, J., G. Verriest, A. de Rouck: L'achromatopsie congénitale. Docum. ophthal. 9 (1955) 338–424

Grützner, P.: Über Farbenanomalien, Farbenamblyopie und Farbenasthenopie. Klin. Mbl. Augenheilk. 158 (1971) 89–96

Grützner, P., W. Jaeger: Anleitung zur Untersuchung des Farbsinnes. In: Entwicklung und Fortschritt in der Augenheilkunde. Enke, Stuttgart (1963), 683–689.

Handbook of Sensory Physiology VII/4. Visual Psychophysics. Springer, Berlin, Heidelberg, New York 1972

Heydenreich, A.: Untersuchungsmethoden des Farbsinnes. In: Der Augenarzt, ed. by K. Velhagen, VEB Thieme, Leipzig (1969) 773

Jaeger, W., P. Grützner: Entwicklung und Fortschritt in der Augenheilkunde. Enke, Stuttgart (1963) 591–614

Pinckers, A.: Achromatopie congenitale. Ann. d'oculist 205 (1972) 821–834

3 Visual Field Loss

A variety of visual field defects may be distinguished from one another. Each carries its own diagnostic implications (Harrington 1971).

Central scotoma — Concentric contraction of isopters — Ring scotoma — Eccentric visual field loss — Enlargement of the blind spot — Hemianopia: heteronymous hemianopia — Homonymous hemianopia — Functional field loss.

Central Scotoma

A central scotoma (Figs. 3.1, 3.2, 3.3) may be *objective* = *negative* (central defect) or *subjective* = *positive* (gray, black or brown central spot). The scotoma may be *absolute* or *relative*. A positive scotoma implies that the damage is in the eye itself (hemorrhage, exudative retinopathy, retinal detachment, etc.). Metamorphopsia may be associated with a positive scotoma. A negative scotoma occurs with damage to the visual pathways (neuritis, retrobulbar neuritis, optic tract), central retinal and choroidal scars, longstanding macular degeneration, myopic degeneration, suppression scotoma, etc. Contrary to central scotomata, which are immediately obvious, peripheral scotomata such as in chorioretinitis are frequently not noted at all. In new cases they may be associated with light flashes.

Concentric Constriction of Visual Field

Concentric constriction of the visual field occurs with tapetoretinal degeneration (retinitis pigmentosa [Fig. 3.4]) and toxic retinopathy (chloroquine, phenothiazine, quinine, opto-

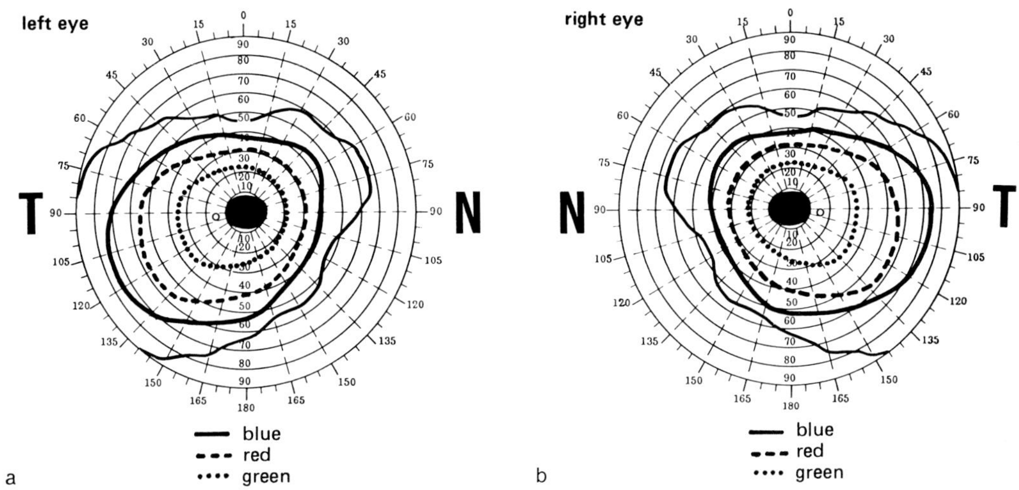

Fig. 3.1 Bilateral central scotomata in toxic neuritis

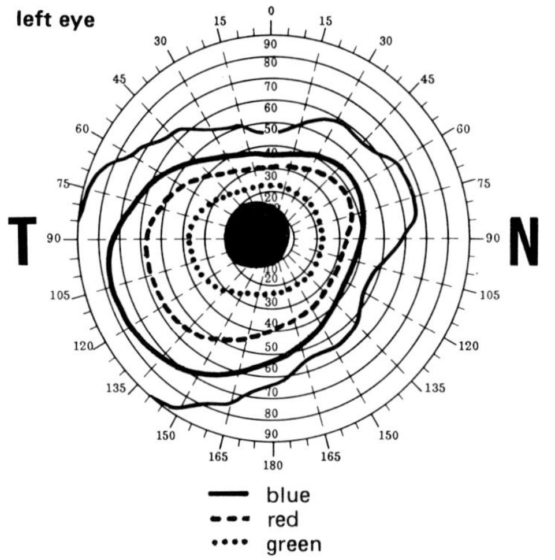

Fig. 3.2 Central scotoma in retrobulbar neuritis

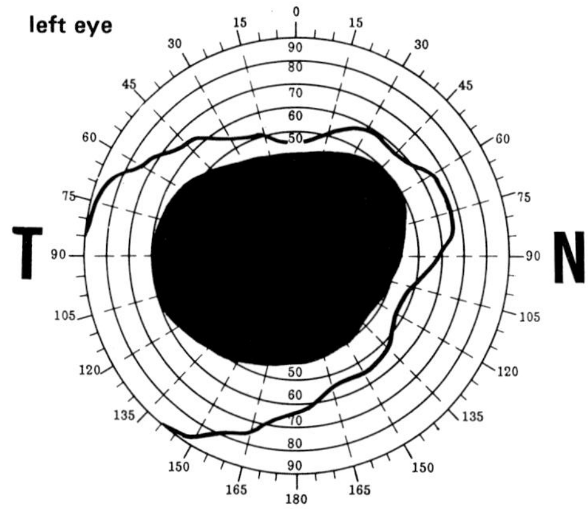

Fig. 3.3 Large central scotoma in retrobulbar neuritis

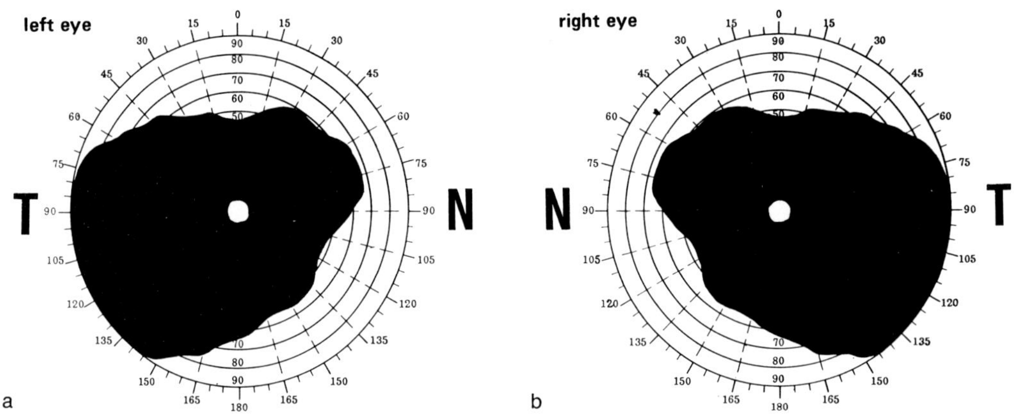

Fig. 3.4 Concentric constriction of the visual field in tapetoretinal degeneration

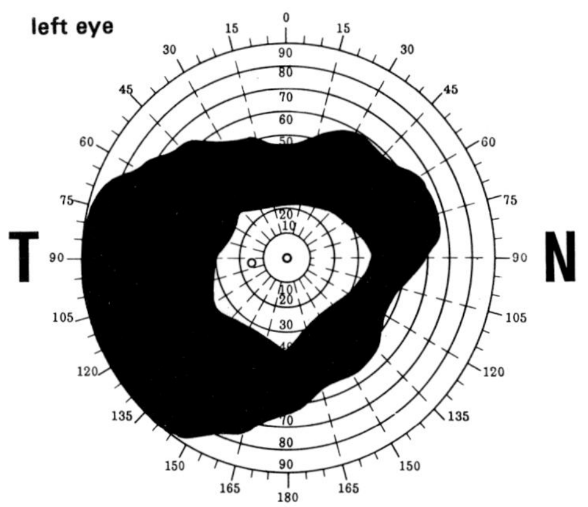

Fig. 3.5 Concentric visual field loss in long-standing papilledema leading to optic atrophy

chin, arsenic and salicylates) as well as with mechanical injury to the retina (pseudoretinitis pigmentosa). Optic atrophy secondary to long standing papilledema (Fig. 3.5), luetic optic atrophy, perineuritis and possibly glaucoma (Figs. 3.9, 3.10) can also lead to concentric constriction of the visual field. Hysterics will show a concentrically constricted visual field but retain normal spatial orientation in their environment. A functional etiology (hysteria) must be considered when a patient with marked concentric visual field loss moves about freely (does not bump into objects, etc.).

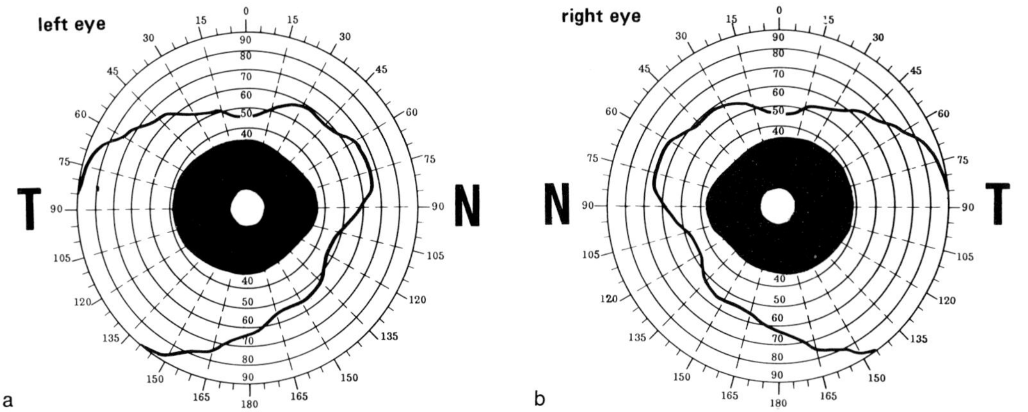

Fig. 3.6 Ring scotoma in tapetoretinal degeneration

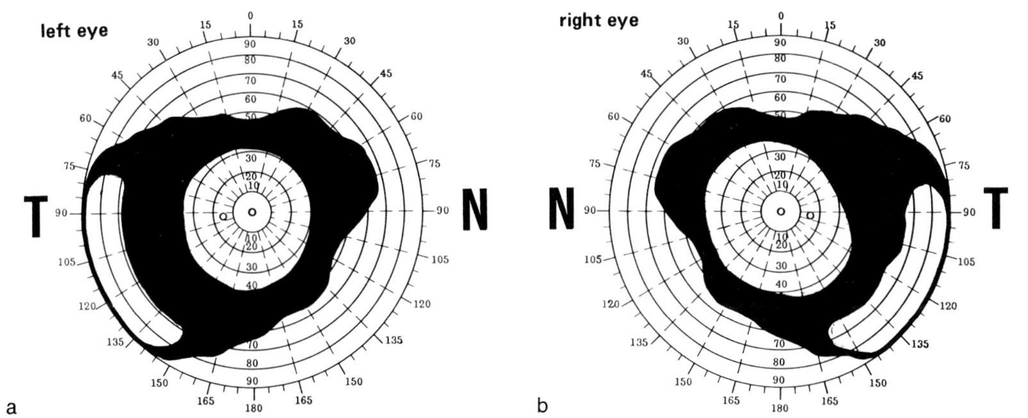

Fig. 3.7 Refraction, ring scotoma, caused by strong convex lenses in aphakia

Ring Scotomata

Ring scotomata occur in tapetoretinal degeneration (Fig. 3.6) and precede the concentric visual field loss. Ring scotomata can also be caused by strong plus lenses (see page 14 [Fig. 3.7]).

Eccentric Visual Field Loss

Diseases of the Retina, Choroid and Optic Nerve

With eccentric visual field loss, the first thought should be a disease of the retina, choroid or optic nerve: vascular occlusion (branch vessel embolus, branch vessel occlusion), glaucoma (Figs. 3.8, 3.9, 3.10), retinal detachment (Fig. 3.11), large chorioretinal scars, juxtapapillary chorioretinitis (Fig. 3.12), choroidal coloboma.

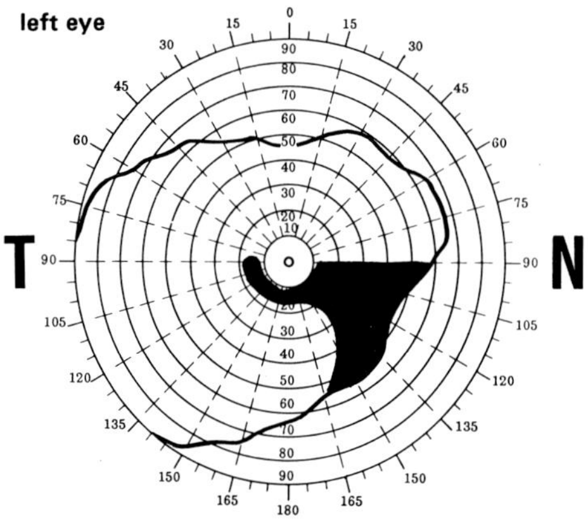

Fig. 3.8 Glaucoma, Bjerrum scotoma, nasal step

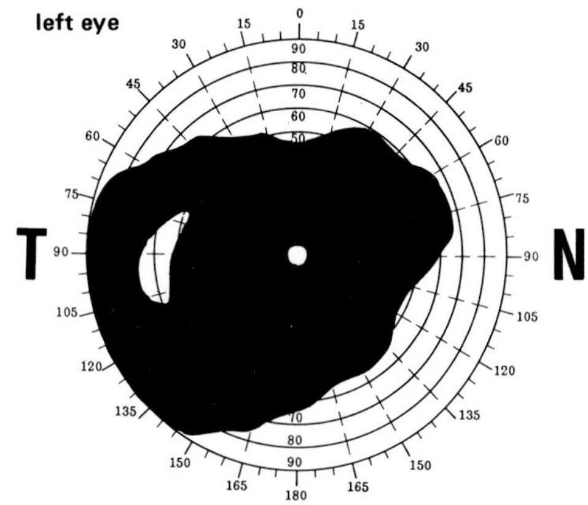

Fig. 3.10 Glaucoma, central and peripheral islands of vision

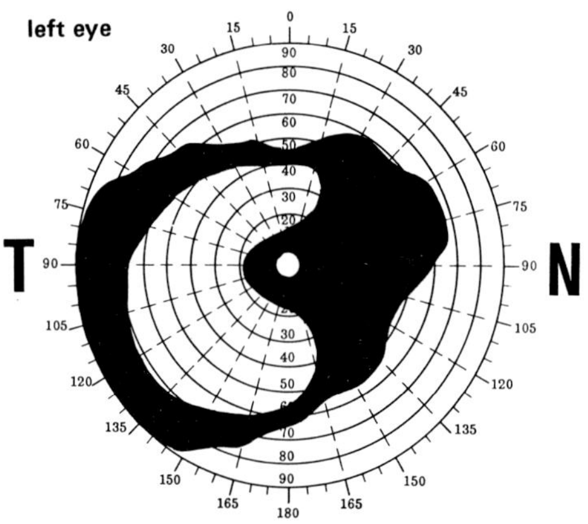

Fig. 3.9 Glaucoma, nasal step and Bjerrum scotoma both inferiorly and superiorly

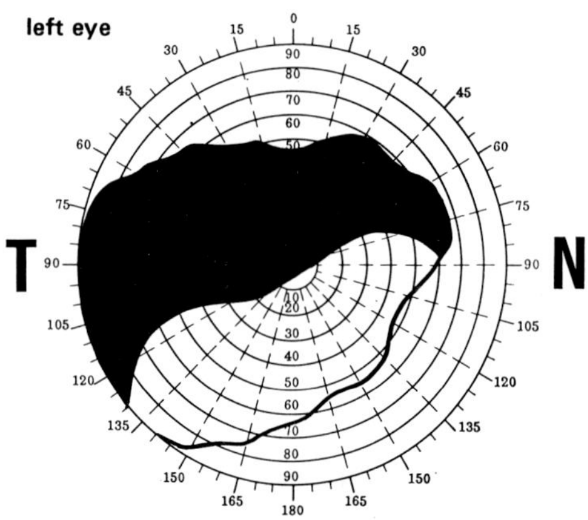

Fig. 3.11 Inferior retinal detachment

Sharply delineated visual field loss, usually in the horizontal meridian, is seen with vascular lesions such as branch emboli, thromboses, temporal arteritis, and recurrent general hemorrhages (page 23). Loss of nerve fibers leads to curved, scimitar-shaped field defects. This occurs with juxtapapillary chorioretinitis, glaucoma, and drusen of the optic nerve head. In high myopes, field defects of various shapes can be seen. These are caused by *myopic fundus changes* and refraction scotomata (Blatt 1964): concentric constriction, temporal sector defects, quadrant defects, homonymous or heteronymous defects, central scotoma, paracentral scotoma.

Refraction Scotoma

Scotomata which disappear with change in the refraction may occur whenever the corrective lens used is inappropriate for the retinal area being tested. This is particularly common with posterior staphylomas where the macular refraction differs significantly from that of peripapillary retina.

Visual Field Loss Caused by Spectacles

The *rim of glasses* or frames may cause a scotoma, as does the prismatic jump induced by *high plus lenses* in aphakia (Fig. 3.7). In such cases a contact lens should be used.

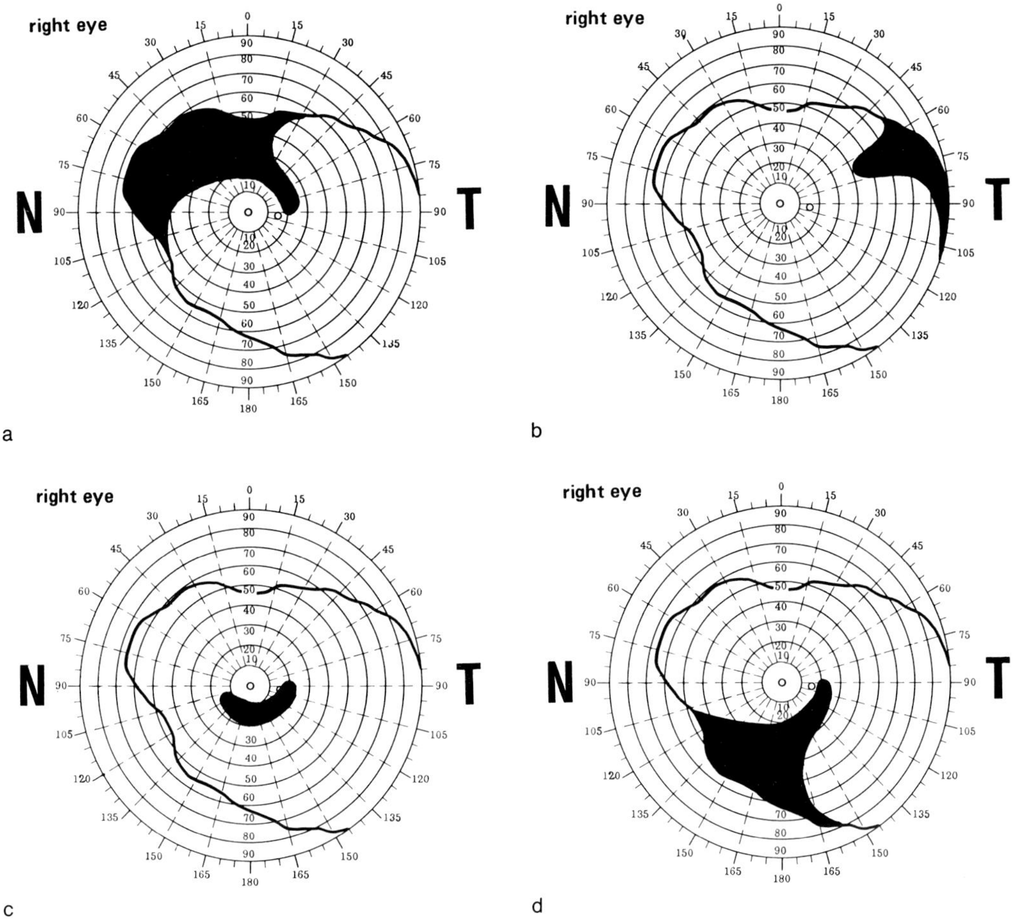

Fig. 3.12 Crescent-shaped visual field loss in juxtapapillary chorioretinitis
a) Lesion inferior temporal to the disk, b) lesion inferior nasal and peripheral to the disk, c) lesion superior temporal to the disk, d) lesion superior temporal to the disk

Enlargement of the Blind Spot

Enlargement of the blind spot occurs with myopic conus, age-dependent senile halo of the disk, nasal conus, coloboma of the optic disk, medullated nerve fibers, drusen of the optic disk, papilledema (Fig. 3.13), and juxtapapillary chorioretinitis. When it occurs in glaucoma, it is usually a partial Bjerrum scotoma. Enlargement of the blind spot occurs normally as a function of test conditions. It is, therefore, not a good test parameter in glaucoma.

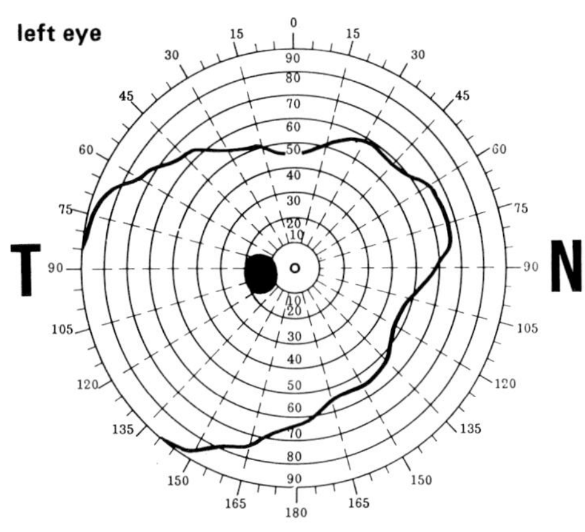

Fig. 3.13 Enlarged blind spot in papilledema

Heteronymous Hemianopia

Bitemporal hemianopia (chiasmatic lesion, refraction scotoma, toxic amblyopia) – Binasal hemianopia (hysteria, retinal damage, glaucoma, chiasmatic lesions).

Bitemporal Hemianopia

Chiasmatic Lesion (see Fig. 8.18)

Chiasmatic lesions produce unilateral temporal field loss, bitemporal field loss or temporal field loss with total loss of vision in the other eye (Figs. 3.14, 3.15, 3.16).

Two thirds of the cases result from *pituitary tumors* (primarily chromophobe adenomas, less frequently eosinophilic, least often basophilic adenomata). About one fifth result from *brainstem tumors* or *tumors of the floor of the cranium* (especially meningiomas). Elevated intracranial pressure may present as a *pseudochiasmic syndrome* where one would expect to see papilledema. Internal hydrocephalus may also cause bitemporal hemianopia. *Bilateral central scotomata* (Fig. 3.17) indicate a lesion at the anterior chiasm. *Paracentral bitemporal* scotomata (Fig. 3.18) imply a lesion at the posterior chiasm. *Bitemporal inferior quadrantanopia* indicates that the lesion is pressing down from above (Fig. 3.19). *Bitemporal superior quadrantanopia* (Fig. 3.20) implies that the lesion is pressing up from below.

After pituitary tumors, the most common cause for the chiasmic syndrome in children is craniopharyngioma. The field loss is typically asymmetric and, because of rapid growth of the tumor in children, elevated intra-cranial pressure with papilledema and secondary optic atrophy is often seen.

In such cases one frequently sees thalamic and psychic disturbances. In about thirty percent of such children, the adiposogenital syndrome (infantilism, diabetes insipidus, hypogonadism) occurs. Roentgenologic findings include supra-sellar calcification, spreading of sutures, changes in the sella.

Classic bitemporal hemianopia or less characteristic field loss can occur in association with optic atrophy caused by *various parasellar tumors*, as well as *glioma, aneurysms, luetic* or *tuberculous meningitis* and *opticochiasmatic arachnoiditis*.

The causes of opticochiasmatic arachnoiditis are primarily trauma, sinusitis, encephalitis, tuberculosis and syphilis. Opticochiasmatic arachnoiditis can occur in children. Feld and Auvert (1947) described 64 percent male and 36 percent female patients with this disease. The youngest patient was five years of age.

Optic atrophy occurs four to six weeks after damage to the chiasm.

Refraction Scotoma

A common cause for *bitemporal* relative *field loss* is a refraction scotoma. Retesting with the appropriate lenses (usually more minus due to staphyloma) improves the defect.

Toxic Amblyopia

In toxic amblyopia *cecocentral scotomata* occur temporally.

Migraine

True migraine can lead to bitemporal scotomata. These are usually transient and scintillating.

Demyelinating Disease

This is sometimes a cause of a bitemporal defect which is usually highly incongruous.

Binasal Hemianopia

Retinal Damage

Binasal field loss is generally due to retinal disease when the defects are incongruous and do not bisect the fixation point. Causes include retinitis, vascular occlusion, extensive temporal retinoschisis, and glaucoma. Bilateral optic neuritis occasionally presents with binasal field defects; the same is true for drusen of the optic disk.

Glaucoma

One should always think of glaucoma when binasal hemianopia is present (bilateral nasal step) (Fig. 3.9).

Damage to the Chiasm

Pressure on each side of the chiasm from *sclerotic* or *aneurysmal carotid arteries* or a *tumor*

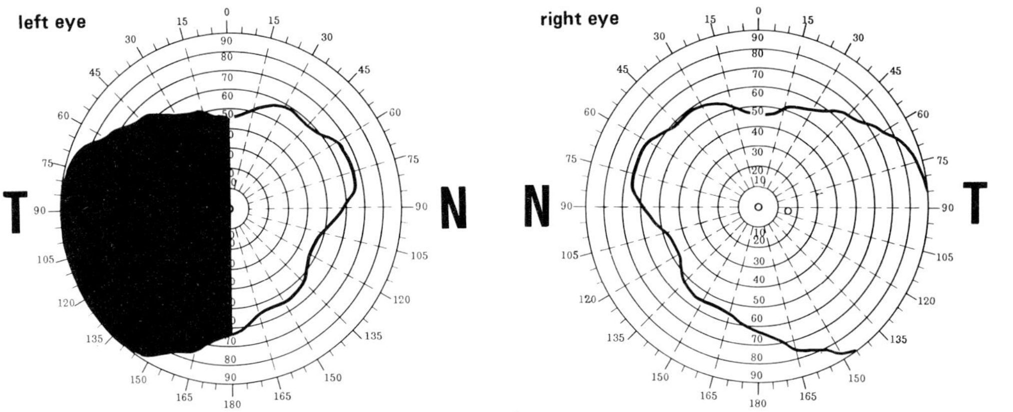

a b

Fig. 3.14 Temporal field loss, left eye only, from damage to crossing fibers from the nasal retina in the region of the chiasm

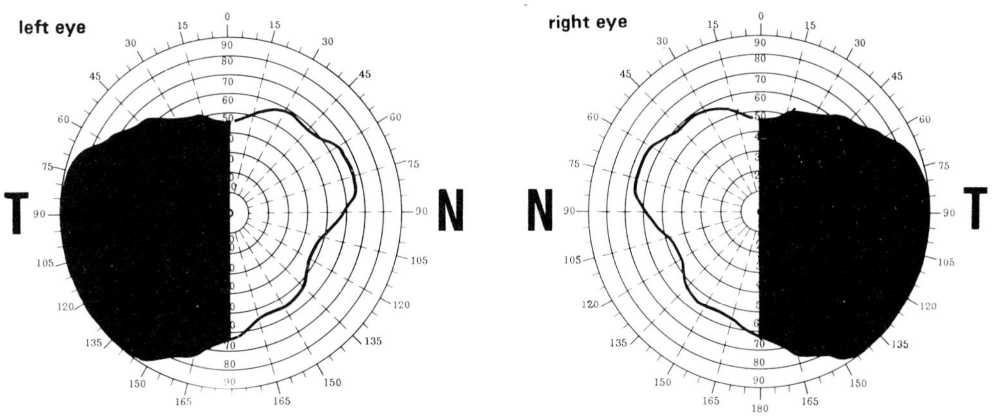

a b

Fig. 3.15 Heteronymous-bitemporal hemianopia due to a pituitary tumor

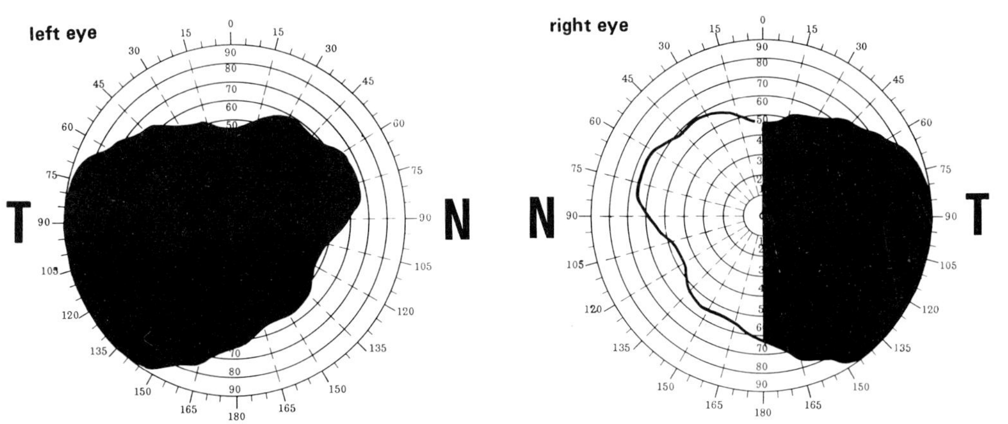

a b

Fig. 3.16 Chiasmatic lesion with destruction of crossed and uncrossed fibers from the left eye: amauroses left, and temporal hemianopia right

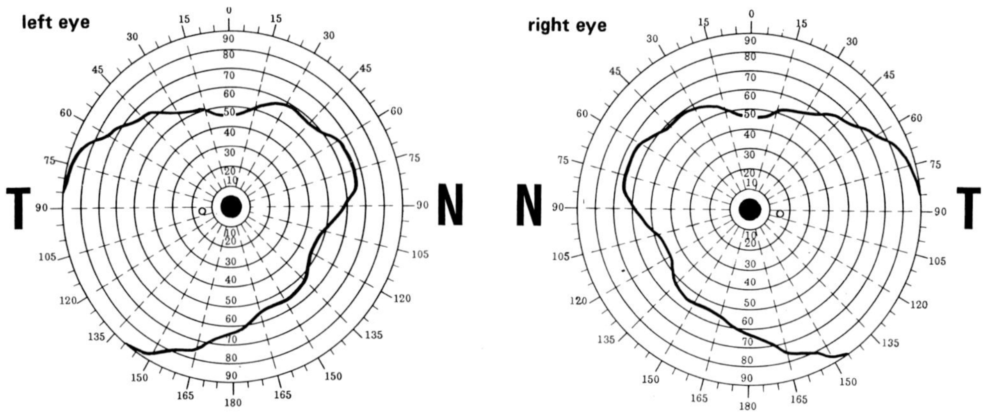

a b

Fig. 3.17 Lesion pressing on the anterior angle of the chiasm = anterior = bitemporal central scotoma

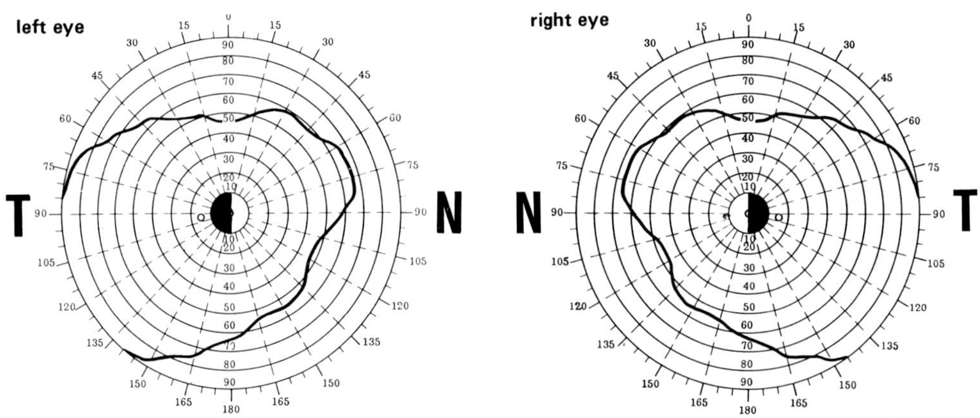

a b

Fig. 3.18 Lesion pressing on the posterior angle of the chiasm = posterior = bitemporal, paracentral scotoma

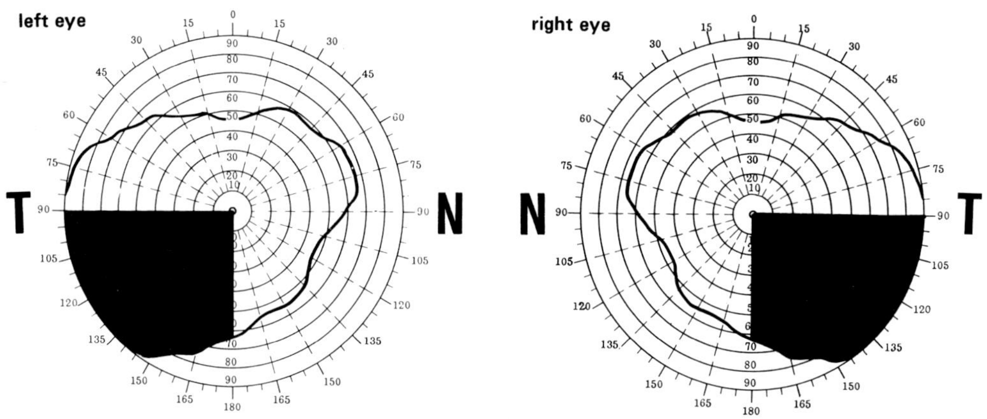

a b

Fig. 3.19 Pressure on the chiasm from above = superior = bitemporal inferior quadrantanopsia

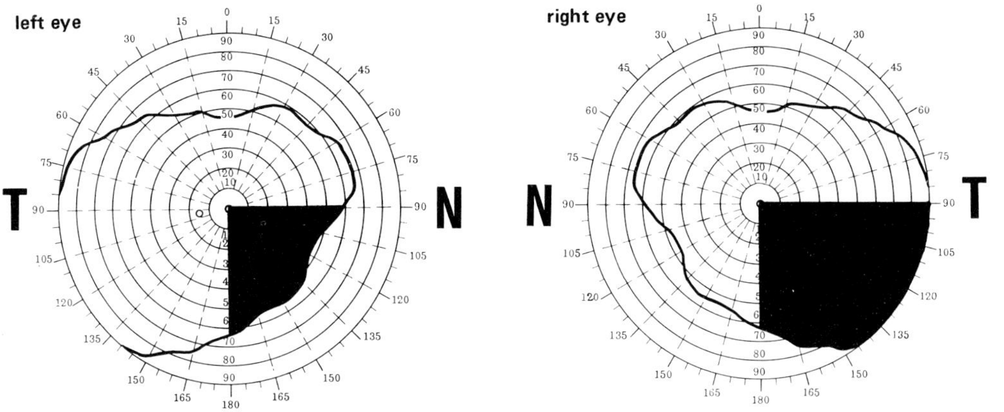

a b

Fig. 3.24 Damage to the inner portion of the optic radiations = contralateral homonymous inferior quadrantanopsia

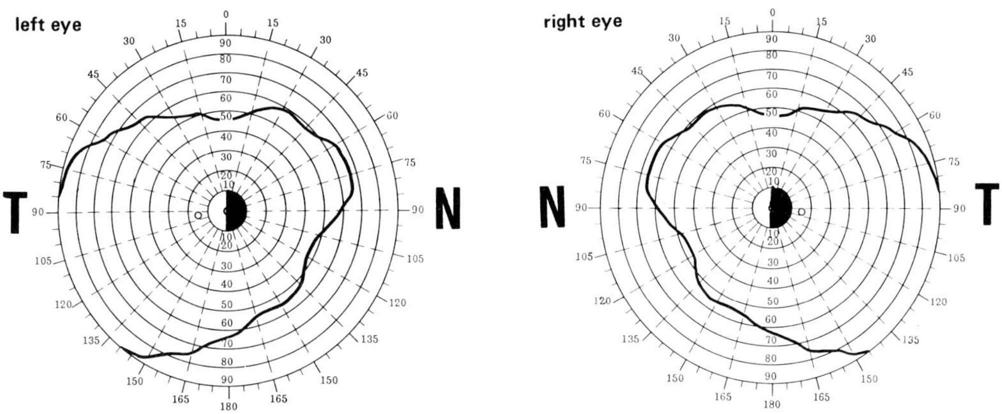

a b

Fig. 3.25 Damage to the macular portion of the occipital cortex of one hemisphere = contralateral macular homonymous hemianopia

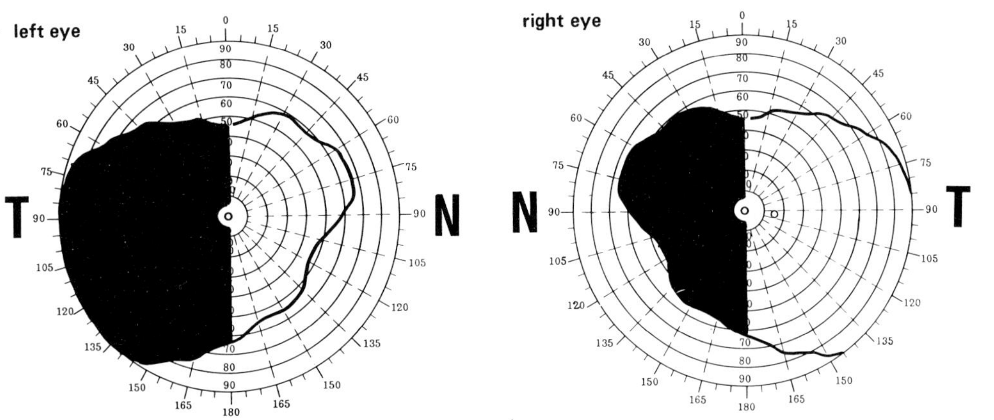

a b

Fig. 3.26 Left homonymous hemianopsia with macular sparing

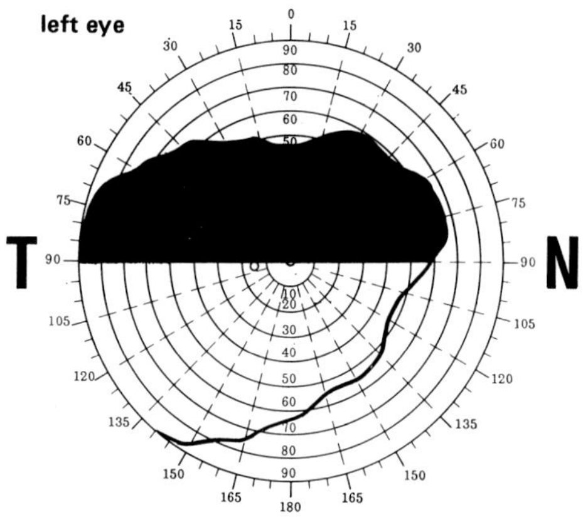

Fig. 3.27 Altitudinal hemianopia with superior field loss due to occlusion of the inferior branch of the central retinal artery

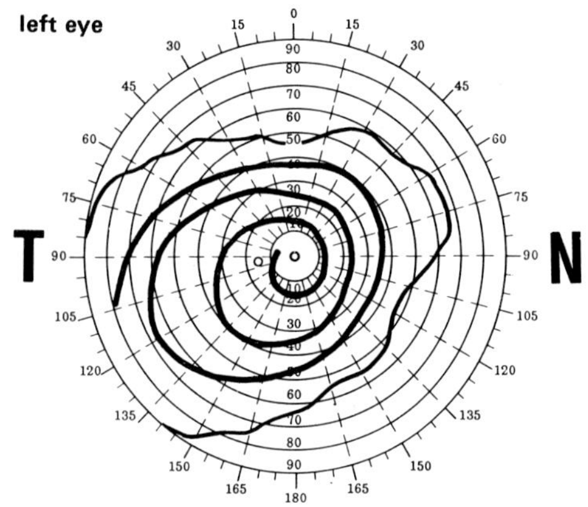

Fig. 3.29 Spiraling on a functional basis

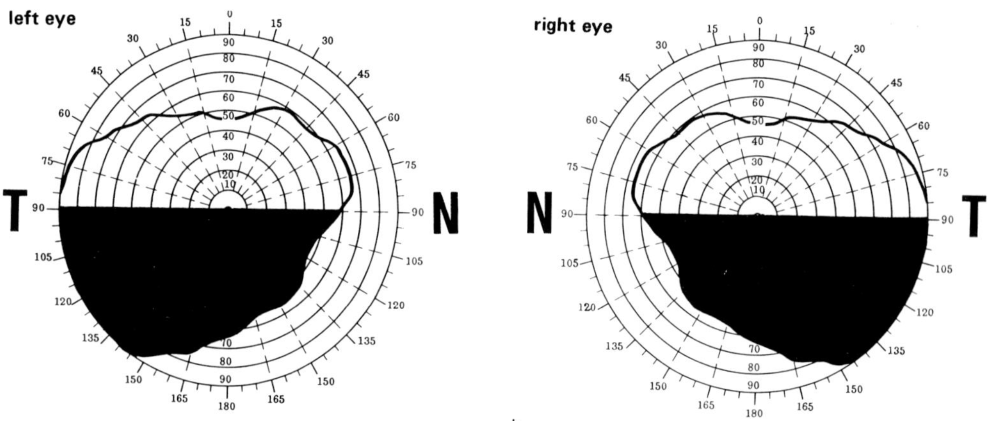

a b

Fig. 3.28 Inferior altitudinal homonymous hemianopia following repeated blood loss

tract lesions eventually causes partial optic atrophy and pupillary hemiakinesia (Wernicke's pupil, see page 323).

The hemianopia is vertical and tends to bisect fixation. The differential diagnosis in tract hemianopia includes:

Lesions at the base of the skull such as tumors (hypophyseal, craniopharyngioma, nasopharyngeal carcinoma, chordoma, rarely gliomas), aneurysm, basilar meningitis, demyelinating disorders, and trauma.

Lesions of the temporal lobe such as hemorrhages, subdural hematomas, vascular thrombosis, emboli, encephalopathy, demyelinating disorders, encephalitis, tumors, glioblastoma, astrocytoma, meningioma, and metastases.

Lesions of the Optic Radiations and Calcarine Fissure

Lesions in the optic radiations *(geniculocalcarine pathway)* and *calcarine fissure* are not associated with optic atrophy. Whether the pupillary reaction is normal or whether a hemianopic pupillary akinesia exists is not yet clear (see page 323). Macular sparing occurs frequently in lesions lying above the lateral geniculate.

Macular sparing occurs in about one-fourth of the cases of hemianopia due to cortical or subcortical lesions. Two-thirds of the cases with macular sparing are caused by an occipital process. These cases primarily result from apoplectic insults (encephalopathy, hemorrhage), tumors (glioblastoma, astrocytoma, meningioma, metastases), rarely encephalitis, demyelinating disease, aneurysms, and occipital trauma. Poisoning must also be considered (carbon monoxide, digitalis, opium).

Altitudinal Homonymous Hemianopia

Bilateral superior (Fig. 3.27) or *inferior* hemianopia (Fig. 3.28) is occasionally seen with gunshot wounds of the *calcarine cortex*. On rare occasions tumors, hemorrhages, brain abscess, meningitis, or encephalitis causes such a hemianopia.

If the altitudinal defect occurs only in one eye, the most likely cause is arterial (rarely venous) occlusion in the retina, retinal disease such as detachment, juxtapapillary chorioretinitis, inflammation, etc. Glaucoma may also be the cause. Vascular damage of the optic nerve such as in temporal arteritis, arteriosclerosis (ischemic optic neuropathy) as well as coloboma of the optic nerve causes unilateral altitudinal hemianopia.

Blood Loss

An inferior homonymous hemianopia may occur after repeated and severe blood loss (Fig. 3.28). If the optic nerve is damaged, blurring of the disk followed by partial optic atrophy can be seen.

Pseudo-Visual Field Loss and Functional Visual Field Loss

Pseudo or false constrictions of the visual field due to *anatomic causes* include sunken globes (age, dehydration, fracture of the orbit), ptosis, prominent bridge of the nose, protruding orbital rims, bushy eyebrows.

Other causes are: *aphakia* with or without correction (see page 14); *refraction scotoma* as with staphyloma (see page 14); *media opacities* (cornea, lens, vitreous); and *disoriented*, hysteric or mentally defective patients.

In cases of *functional field loss*, spiraling may be seen (Fig. 3.29). If the patient is moved farther from the test object, the scotoma will be smaller rather than larger. This occurs when the hysteric or malingering patient does not understand the principle of the examination. Concentric constriction of the visual field without loss of orientation is a hallmark of functional field loss. In functional, as opposed to organic, field loss, optokinetic nystagmus is present.

References

Blatt, N.: Gesichtsfeldveränderungen bei hochgradig Myopen. Klin. Mbl. Augenheilk. 145 (1964) 680–712

Feld, M., J. Auvert: Conclusions à l'étude d'une statistique de 148 cas d'arachnoidite opto-chiasmatique opérés. Rev. Oto-neuro-ophthal. 19 (1947) 315–320

Harrington, D. O.: The visual fields. Mosby, Saint Louis 1971

4 Refraction and Accommodation

Refraction

A *refractive error* may be at fault when a disparity between near and distance visual acuity occurs in an apparently normal eye with central fixation. If the visual loss does not seem to be caused by a refractive error or other discernible ocular pathology, the differential diagnosis primarily consists of amblyopia, hysteria or malingering (functional), and retrobulbar neuritis.

The patient with normal distance acuity without optical aids or use of accommodation is *emmetropic*.

When an apparently normal eye with central fixation has poor near and distance vision, astigmatism, amblyopia (see page 39) and, in older persons, hyperopia must be considered.

If a young patient has poorer visual acuity after cycloplegia than previously, he is probably *hyperopic*. Poor distance vision but good near acuity speaks for *myopia*.

Transient changes in refractive error can occur. The usual tendency is for more myopia (suggests diabetes mellitus) rather than hyperopia (suggests central serous retinopathy).

Anisometropia (significant difference in refractive error) must be suspected when an apparently normal eye with central fixation has poorer visual acuity than the other eye. Anisometropia is also the most common cause of aniseikonia (unequal image size).

One can measure the axial length of an eye in vivo with ultrasound (Gernet 1965, Jansson 1963).

Emmetropia

Emmetropia exists when an older or younger person with paralyzed accommodation (cycloplegia) has normal distance vision. This occurs when the refractive power of the eye in its resting nonaccommodating stage is such that a distant object is focused clearly on the fovea of the retina.

Astigmatism

In spite of central fixation and a normal-appearing eye, the regular astigmatic person sees poorly both near and at distance. The hyperopic astigmatic person will successively focus on one of the two focal lines and then on the other as long as he has the accommodative power to do so. This will refine his discriminatory ability and, in this sense, improve his acuity. Astigmatism occurs when the refractive surfaces are not symmetrical over 360 degrees and, therefore, do not focus light to a single point. Astigmatic individuals may eventually develop asthenopic symptoms (see page 69).

"Irregular" astigmatism is usually the result of distortions in the anterior corneal surface (scarring, ectasia, edema, ulcer, postinflammatory processes). This is correctable with hard contact lenses but not with glasses. When the astigmatism is severe enough, soft contact lenses will also fail to improve vision. In *"regular"* astigmatism the axes of greatest and least refractive power are at right angles. This regular astigmatism can be corrected with glasses. Compared to corneal astigmatism, lenticular astigmatism is usually insignificant. Astigmatism is corrected with cylindric lenses.

Astigmatism is myopic, hyperopic or mixed (one axis myopic, the other hyperopic). Power and axis of astigmatism may be hereditary (partial dominant). Rieger and Thums (1951) used astigmatism as biologic evidence of parenthood.

Hyperopia

Axial hyperopia — Refractive hyperopia — Transient hyperopia.

Hyperopia must be considered when a young person has accommodative asthenopia (blurring, headaches [see page 69]) following prolonged periods of close work. Blepharitis is also said to occur. Hyperopia is the probable cause when an older person has poor near vision with better distance acuity in a normal eye with central fixation. The same is true when a younger person has a worsening of his distance acuity after cycloplegia.

If the refractive power of an eye is too low for the length of the globe then rays of light from a distant object will focus behind the retina (hyperopia).

Axial Hyperopia

Most congenital *hyperopia* (high *hypermetropia*) is caused by too small an eye. Such eyes will generally have a flatter anterior chamber predisposing to angle closure glaucoma. This will occur only rarely in childhood. The hyperopic eye may have tortuous retinal vessels *(tortuositas vasorum)* (Fig. 22.1) and blurred disk margins (pseudopapilledema or pseudoneuritis) (Fig. 21.17).

Axial hyperopia also occurs when the globe is compressed from behind by an orbital tumor. Similarly, elevation of the retina by tumor or in central serous retinopathy causes axial hyperopia. Microphthalmia may be associated with excessively high hyperopia. High degrees of hyperopia (over 5 diopters) usually have some amount of associated amblyopia.

Because of their great range of accommodation (increase in refractive power of the lens due to ciliary muscle contraction), children will almost always have some part of their hyperopia uncorrected with refraction (latent hyperopia). They constantly accommodate to correct for this.

To discover the total hyperopia (manifest and latent) in children, one must completely paralyze the ciliary muscle by using a cycloplegic agent such as atropine, homatropine, Cyclogyl, etc. **Refractive hyperopia** differs from axial hyperopia in that it is caused by changes in the refractive media. It occurs in cornea plana, aphakia, posteriorly subluxated lenses, macular edema, ciliary muscle paralysis, etc.

For **transient hyperopia** see page 26.

In *hyperopia* the *strongest plus lenses* commensurate with good visual acuity are prescribed. Hyperopic individuals are prone to accommodative esotropia (see page 40 [Figs. 8.1, 8.2]) and asthenopic complaints (see page 69).

Myopia

Axial myopia — Refractive myopia — Night myopia — Transient myopia.

Myopia is probable when distance acuity is poor but near acuity is good. The refractive power of the optical system of the eye is too strong for the length of the globe. The image of distant objects is, therefore, focused in front of the retina.

Before the diagnosis of myopia can be made, the accommodative power of young persons must be paralyzed to rule out a functional or hysterical cause. The use of miotics will cause accommodative myopia (see page 319). Trauma may cause myopia through anterior dislocation of the lens, swelling of the lens or, more rarely, ciliary muscle spasm.

Refractive Myopia

Refractive myopia occurs with changes in the *radius of curvature* of the cornea: smaller corneal radius (stronger refractive power), microcornea (microphthalmia), and keratoglobus.

A frequent cause of acquired myopia is change in the refractive power of the lens. *Lens-induced myopia* occurs with any increase in the refractive index of the lens. This is particularly true with nuclear cataract (second sight). The change is less with brunescent than with gray nuclear cataracts. The degree of acquired myopia may reach 10 diopters. Lenses with nuclear cataract may develop two focal points (see page 239). Transient refractive changes (see page 26) and refractive changes due to alterations in the shape of the lens also occur: anterior or posterior lenticonus, microphakia and spherophakia usually have subluxated lenses, ectopia lentis. Colobomas of the lens generally cause irregular lenticular astigmatism.

Anterior or posterior lenticonus is easily seen with the slit lamp. Retinoscopy (skiascopy) reveals two focal points. *Monocular diplopia* occurs with refractive myopia: particularly keratoconus, nuclear cataract (where the lens has two focal points), subluxated lens, ectopia lentis, iridodialysis.

Axial Myopia

The most common cause of high myopia is an elongated globe.

In degenerative myopia, stretching of intraocular layers leads to progressive choroidal and pigment epithelial atrophy (see page 260). In highly myopic individuals, there is a sickle-shaped area temporal to the disk where choroid, Bruch's membrane and pigment epithelium are absent. The exposed sclera is seen as a pale crescent (conus myopicus or myopic crescent). Myopic degeneration is progressive. Children, if highly myopic, will not show major changes.

Marked myopic retinopathy (see page 260) includes: peripapillary and central stretch marks (lacquer cracks) (Plate XXI, Fig. 5, page 224 e), retinal atrophy, macular hemorrhages, macular pigmentation (Fuchs spot [see page 260]) (Plate XXII, Fig. 1, page 224 f), posterior staphyloma, nasal supervolution of the retina (mimics pseudo-optic neuritis), lattice degeneration of the retina, and liquefaction of vitreous, brunescent cataracts. These changes usually occur later in life. The vitreous liquefies early in myopic individuals; they are at greater risk for retinal detachment (see page 276). Congenital spondyloepiphyseal dysplasia includes high or malignant myopia as part of the syndrome. Congenital myopia is seen in the Pierre Robin syndrome. This is also associated with congenital glaucoma, bilateral retinal detachment, micrognathia, and cleft palate. Since myopia usually becomes manifest at puberty, it has been called "school myopia." It is no longer fashionable to attribute myopia to the prolonged convergence and accommodation accompanying school work. The relationship between body and eye growth is presently stressed as the origin of most myopia. Progressive, excessive myopia which worsens throughout life is probably hereditary.

Compared to progressive myopia, congenital myopia is more benign and less prone to progress or to lead to complications (Hiatt et al. 1965).

Night Myopia

In twilight or darkness, myopia worsens between 0.5 and 4.0 diopters. The average is 2.0 diopters. It is particularly prevalent in younger persons and less in older persons. According to Schober (1948, 1953), night myopia already begins at illumination levels which allow clear vision. In blue light the eye becomes more myopic. Increased pupillary diameter leads to spherical aberrations causing myopia. A certain amount of accommodation takes place (so-called accommodative myopia) whenever visual acuity decreases.

A 20 to 30 year old will have night myopia of 0.50 to 2.25 diopters compared to the 50 to 60 year old who has less, 0.50 to 1.75 diopters (Matthaeus 1965; Schober 1948, 1953). At rest, accommodation is between 0.5 and 2.0 diopters. When no visual target or fatigue is present, there is a "myopia of empty space" (Aust 1969).

Transient Changes in Refraction

Diabetes — Chemical agents and disease — Trauma — Post surgery.

Transient changes in refractive error are usually myopic, rarely hyperopic (see page 242).

Diabetes

The most common cause of transient refractive change is diabetes. Elevated blood sugar leads to transient myopia. Reduction of an elevated blood sugar may cause temporary hyperopia, which can last for days or weeks. This may be seen at the beginning of insulin therapy. Mylius et al. (1971) noted transient hyperopia in 68 of 941 patients started on oral hypoglycemic agents. The peak occurred on the fourth to fifth day of treatment with an average hyperopic change of 0.72 diopters.

Myopic changes will range from levels so minimal that the patient may not notice to minus 9 diopters (Loehlein 1939). Clinically, it is seen more often in adult diabetics (Waite and Beetham 1935).

There is general agreement that the cause of the refractive changes is in the lens. Exactly what the alterations consist of is more controversial.

Chemical Agents and Diseases

Transient myopia is observed with a variety of substances and diseases. With sulfa therapy

transient myopia can rapidly reach a maximum of minus 3 to minus 4 diopters or even minus 8 diopters (Lukomnik 1951). It decreases after four to five days. If transient myopia has occurred with large dosages of sulfa, it recurs when smaller non-toxic dosages are given (Mehlhose 1949).
Transient myopia with use of diuretics such as Diamox or Hygroton is attributed to changes in the electrolyte balance of the lens, ciliary muscle contraction, or allergy (Hermann 1963; Ericson 1969). Using ultrasound, Pallin and Ericson (1965) demonstrated a thickening of the lens in this situation.
Other insults can also cause transient refractive changes (Sachsenweger 1959 a). Myopia lasting 48 hours has been observed after injection of arsenicals. Occasional transient myopic changes have been reported with other medications: acetylsalicylic acid, ACTH, corticosteroids.
Various illnesses have also been linked to transient refractive changes: flu, viral respiratory infections, and debilitating disorders, especially marasmus, diarrhea, crash diets, malnutrition and the Sippy diet. Transient myopia may occur with iritis. Voisin (1963) observed transient myopia in the presence of Quincke's edema.

Trauma

Myopia can occur with trauma. When it is caused by temporary lens damage, the myopia will regress in one to four weeks. Frequently, there is damage to zonular fibers with subluxation of the lens, traumatic mydriasis, traumatic lens opacities, etc. In this situation the myopia may be permanent.

Post Surgery

Glaucoma operations to lower intraocular pressure, especially fistulizing procedures, are almost always accompanied by transient myopia. This may in part be due to forward displacement of the lens or temporary upset of lens metabolism. Such myopia usually disappears within days or weeks. There is always the danger of cataract formation. If a nuclear cataract develops, the myopia may increase steadily (sometimes as much as minus 15 diopters).

Complaints Associated with Changes in Refractive Errors

Hyperopia, overcorrected myopia, and astigmatism are the most common causes of *asthenopic complaints* (see page 69). The symptoms worsen with stress and prolonged close work. They include: headaches, eye pain, migraine-like headaches, dizziness, nausea, vomiting, photophobia, insomnia, fatigability, epiphora, lid twitch, burning, itching, pressure, claustrophobia, lack of concentration, and any other neurotic complaints.
Poor vision in one eye with central fixation, which is otherwise normal, should alert one to a difference in the refractive power of the two eyes.
Anisometropic correction with a *difference of 3 to 4 diopters between the two eyes* is usually the maximum which will be tolerated. Above 3 to 4 diopters, the disparity in image size between the two eyes *(aniseikonia)* and the prismatic effect on vertical and lateral gaze present a disturbance. Children tolerate greater differences in the dioptic power of the two lenses, often up to 6 to 10 diopters.

Aniseikonia

The most common cause of aniseikonia is a difference in the refractive power of the two eyes (anisometropia). There is a difference in the image size focused on the two retinas (Sachsenweger 1959 b; Bourdy 1961).
Aniseikonia can be the cause of asthenopic complaints (see page 69). In addition to corrected or uncorrected anisometropia, differences in pupillary diameter, accommodation, optical axis of the cornea, lens and pupil may all cause aniseikonia. Functional aniseikonia occurs with anomalous distribution of sensory cells in the retina. Asthenopic complaints caused by aniseikonia occur particularly when observing moving objects (riding in cars or trains, watching movies). Herzau (1956) showed that aniseikonia is a source of asthenopic symptoms. The occlusion of one eye resulted in the immediate relief of symptoms; a magnifying lens in front of the eye with the larger image aggravated the complaints. Binocular vision is no longer possible if the difference in image size exceeds 5 percent.

There are a number of eikonometers. Aniseikonia is readily diagnosed when the right and left halves of a circle or rectangle with a different polarization of light are viewed through polarized glasses. With aniseikonia the two halves appear to be different in size.

Accommodation – Changes in Range of Accommodation

Presbyopia — Paralysis of accommodation — Accommodative spasm — Tonic accommodation — Alterations in image size due to accommodation.

A decrease in the range of accommodation can only be diagnosed if *hyperopia* is absolutely ruled out and the possibility of *presbyopia* is considered. The range of accommodation decreases with increasing age (presbyopia), in accommodative paralysis, and with accommodative spasm. With tonic accommodation, accommodation is normal in range but occurs very slowly.
Changes in the accommodative impulses can lead to optical illusions of size (micropsia, macropsia).

Presbyopia

Accommodative ability declines progressively with age (at 10 years of age, it is 15 diopters; at 20 years of age, 10 diopters; at 40 years of age, 4 diopters; at 60 years of age, 0 diopters). In the *uncorrected hyperopic* individual, presbyopia manifests itself earlier, in the *uncorrected myopic* individual, later than normal.
Due to hardening of the lens, a complete loss of accommodative power is present after the age of 60.

Accommodative Paralysis

True accommodative paresis (rarely paralysis) may be diagnosed only after ruling out hyperopia through the use of parasympatholytic agents. Accommodative paresis leads to an inability to do close work (reading) because objects become blurred; micropsia occurs.
Underlying etiologies include: direct trauma to the eye, subluxation of the lens, ophthalmoplegia interna after use of scopolamine, atropine and belladonna derivatives (including systemic use).
With botulism, bilateral ophthalmoplegia occurs in association with gastroenteritis, dry mouth and throat and, rarely, gaze paralysis. First choice in the differential diagnosis of a true ophthalmoplegia interna would be tertiary or central nervous system lues (tabes, tabetic paralysis). Less frequently, other central nervous system diseases such as encephalitis, polioencephalitis, oculomotor paralysis, and tumors are responsible. Inflammation of the ciliary body such as in sympathetic ophthalmia or edema of the ciliary body such as with choroidal detachment can lead to accommodative paresis. Other causes include diabetes, chronic alcoholism, lead poisoning, and ergotism.
Isoniazid therapy (INH) frequently leads to a transient decrease in accommodative ability (usually in females) (Honegger and Genée 1969). In rare cases, extraocular muscle paralysis, mydriasis, nystagmus and optic neuritis occur. Other antitubercular agents such as para-aminosalicylic acid (PAS) or D-cycloserine can lead to transient loss of accommodation. Piperazine and anti-helminthines may cause accommodative paresis as well as nystagmus. Accommodative paresis without pupillary involvement may occur four to six weeks after an attack of diphtheria. In accommodative spasm it is the continuous accommodation by the patient which causes the loss of range of accommodation.

Accommodative Spasm

Accommodative spasm almost always has an underlying functional component (hysteria). The hyperopic individual must constantly accommodate for clear distance vision. This is not an accommodative spasm.
True accommodative spasm of organic etiology such as in brain damage is rare. More common is a psychotic reaction with marked accommodation and miosis (even convergence is possible) which causes a loss of acuity and acquired myopia. Voluntary (psychogenic)

nystagmus occurs (see page 65). Accommodative spasm is usually seen in children having problems in school or with their parents, or who are afraid of punishment, failure, etc. Accommodative spasms can be brought about by cholinergics (parasympathomimetics), morphine, alcohol, paresis of the sympathetic system, and pineal tumors.

Tonic Accommodation

In Adie's syndrome (tonic pupil) (see page 324), one finds a prolongation (3 to 15 seconds) of the time required for accommodation as well as for pupillary contraction on near gaze. There is an associated delay in disaccommodation and pupillary dilatation on far gaze.

Optical Illusions of Size (Dysmegalopsia)

Micropsia occurs with strong accommodative efforts (there is an associated convergence) without the appropriate results such as in presbyopia, accommodative paralysis, atropinization, use of scopolamine, botulism, and diphtheria.

Macropsia is seen when there is more accommodation than expected, as with use of miotics.

Dysmegalopsia consisting of macropsia, micropsia, teleopsia, or metamorphopsia can result from functional disturbances in cortical or subcortical regions. Causal agents include migraine, epilepsy, trauma, and intoxicants.

Central dysesthesia occurs when an appropriate accommodative impulse is interpreted incorrectly (Gramberg-Danielsen 1958).

References

Aust, W.: Refraktion und Akkommodation. Almanach für die Augenheilkunde. Lehmann, München (1969) 149–166

Bourdy, Cl.: L'aniséiconie. Ann. Oculist. (Paris) 194 (1961) 1048–1079

Ericson, L. A.: Hygroton-induced myopia and retinal edema. Acta ophthal. 41 (1963) 538–543

Duke-Elder, S.: Ophthalmic optics and refraction. System of ophthalmology V. Kimpton, London 1970

Gernet, H.: Ein Beitrag zur Frage der Emmetropisation. Ophthalmologica (Basel) 147 (1964) 235–243

Gernet, H.: Biometrie des Auges mit Ultraschall. Klin. Mbl. Augenheilk. 146 (1965) 863–874

Gramberg-Danielsen, B.: Über Lokalisation und Ursachen optischer Größentäuschungen. Klin. Mbl. Augenheilk. 132 (1958) 647–655

Hermann, P.: Myopie spasmodique au cours des traitements diurétique. Bull. Soc. Ophtal. (Paris) 63 (1963) 719–723

Herzau, W.: Erfahrungen bei Messung und Ausgleich von Aniseikonie. Ber. dtsch. ophthal. Ges., 60 (1956) 24–27

Hiatt, R. L., F. D. Costenbander, D. G. Albert: Clinical evaluation of congenital myopia. Arch. Ophthal. (Chicago) 74 (1965) 31–35

Honegger, H., E. Genée: Akkommodationsstörungen bei Behandlung mit Tuberkulostatika. Klin. Mbl. Augenheilk. 155 (1969) 371–380

Jansson, F.: Measurements of intraocular distances by ultrasound. Acta ophthal. (Kbh) Suppl., 74 (1963)

Löhlein, W.: Bericht über die Tagung der Ostpreuß. u. Danziger Augenärzte, Danzig v. 16. 10. 1938 s. R. Braun: Star und Refraktionsänderung beim Diabetiker. Klin. Mbl. Augenheilk. 102 (1939) 282

Lukomnik, S.: Die Verbindung von hoher transitorischer Myopie mit akutem Glaukomanfall bei Disulfanvergiftung. Vestn. Oftal. 30 (1951) 37–38 (Russian)

Matthäus, W.: Nachtmyopie und Straßenverkehr. Dtsch. Gesundh.-Wes. 20 (1965) 920–924

Mehlhose, F.: Zur Problematik der transitorischen Myopie nach Sulfamiden. Klin. Mbl. Augenheilk. 115 (1949) 217–227

Mylius, K., Stark, Salomon: Über ophthalmologische Untersuchungsergebnisse an mit den neuen oralen Diabetesmitteln behandelten Patienten. Dtsch. ophthal. Ges. (1957) 186–190

Pallin, O., R. Ericson: Ultrasound studies in a case of hygroton-induced myopia. Acta ophthal. (Kbh) 43 (1965) 692–696

Rieger, H., K. Thums: Augenärztliche Untersuchungen im Rahmen des anthropogisch-erbbiologischen Vaterschaftsnachweises. Wien. med. Wschr. 101 (1951) 594–601

Sachsenweger, R.: Untersuchungen über die Beeinflussung der Tiefenwahrnehmung durch Refraktionsanomalien. Albrecht v. Graefes Arch. klin. exp. Ophthal. 154 (1954) 617–636

Sachsenweger, R.: Pathologie und Klinik der Refraktionsanomalien. In: Der Augenarzt, Vol. II, ed. by Thieme, Stuttgart 1959a (pp. 217–420)

Sachsenweger, R.: Aniseikonie. In: Der Augenarzt, Vol. II, ed. by Thieme, Stuttgart 1959b (pp. 421–448)

Schober, H.: Die Nachtmyopie und ihre Ursachen. Albrecht v. Graefes Arch. klin. exp. Ophthal 148 (1948) 171–186

Schober, H.: Die Bedeutung der Nachtmyopie in der augenärztlichen Praxis. Ber. dtsch. ophth. Ges. 58 (1953) 36–40

Voisin, J.: Etat myopique transitoire au cours d'un oedème de Quincke à début palpébral. Bull. Soc. Ophthal. (Paris) 63 (1963) 497–500

Waite, J. H., W. P. Beetham: The visual mechanism in diabetes mellitus. New Engl. J. Med. 212 (1935) 367–379, 429–443

5 Dazzle, Photophobia, Night Blindness, Day Blindness

Dazzle

The more dark-adapted an eye, the more readily it is dazzled. In *physiologic dazzling*, visual ability is decreased. The ability to judge contrasts and see details diminishes. The speed with which an object of set luminance can be recognized is decreased. With physiologic dazzling there is a sense of dissatisfaction with the quality of vision due to a blinding light in the visual field even though visual acuity itself may not be decreased. Dazzling may be direct or indirect (snowfield, mirror, etc.). The lower retinal half appears to be less sensitive to dazzling than the upper half (Gramberg-Danielsen 1964).

The susceptibility to dazzle is determined by a variety of factors: pupillary diameter, light scattering at opacities in the optical media, transscleral light, and reflection of light at the retina. Increased dazzle occurs with age. This is partly caused by increased opacification of the optical media.

Photophobia

Photophobia occurs when too much light enters the eye, for example in mydriasis, (pharmacological, traumatic, iridoplegia), aniridia, iris coloboma, and albinism. Diffuse scattering of light by opacities in the optic media will also cause photophobia. As a result, nearly all inflammatory diseases (especially keratitis, conjunctivitis, iritis) have an associated photophobia. The photophobia associated with tuberculous (scrofulous) keratitis is particularly marked. Lenticular and vitreal opacities as well as inflammations at the posterior pole also cause photophobia. With increased illumination dazzle occurs in addition to the photophobia.

Photophobia may be seen with retrobulbar neuritis. Some infectious diseases such as measles are also associated with photophobia. It can occur without conjunctivitis (e.g., in epidemic typhus).

Photophobia is marked in total color blindness (achromatopsia).

Photophobia may occur without visible ocular disease: after severe cranial trauma, with brain tumors, meningitis, subarachnoid hemorrhage, trigeminal neuralgia, migraine and neurasthenia.

It is particularly marked with *rabies* (lyssa). A bright light can trigger attacks. Tearing, extraocular muscle palsies, and papilledema are also seen.

Night and Day Blindness

Correctly, nyctalopia means night blindness and hemeralopia means day blindness. Since the days of Galen and Hippocrates the two terms have been confused due to alternative etymologies of the Greek roots.

A) **Either**

nyx, nyktos = night; *alaos* = blind; *ōps* = eye:
nyctalopia = night blindness

or

nyx, nyktos = night; connecting *l*; *ōps* = eye:
nyctalopia = night seeing = day blindness

B) **Either**

hēmera = day; *alaos* = blind; *ōps* = eye:
hemeralopia = day blindness

or

hēmera = day; connecting *l*; *ōps* = eye:

hemeralopia = day seeing = night blindness

Night blindness (nyctalopia) occurs:

- congenitally (usually dominant inheritance), one variation of which is Oguchi's disease;

In **Oguchi's disease** (François et al. 1956), the fundus takes on a white-gray coloration especially around the optic disk and in the macular region after light exposure (one-half to one hour). Sometimes the color is more brown. After two to three hours in the dark, the posterior pole will appear almost normal (Mizuo phenomenon). Central visual acuity and the visual field are normal. Night blindness is always present. The scotopic components of the ERG are abnormal. Heredity is recessive since consanguinity is common. The disease is stationary and represents **one form of essential, congenital night blindness.**

- with degenerative myopia (rarefaction of receptors);
- nutritional night blindness following decreased vitamin A intake or uptake (xerophthalmia) and malnutrition (defects in absorption, gastritis, chronic liver disease, cachexia);
- with tapetoretinal degenerations (see page 286) and retinitis pigmentosa-like phenotypes (see page 287);
- with advanced glaucoma;
- with advanced optic atrophy and visual field loss (such as in tabes, post-papillitis atrophy [see page 313]);
- with retinal detachment;
- simulation by diffuse opacifications of the optic media (parenchymatous keratitis, corneal edema, premature nuclear cataracts, diffuse vitreal opacities or hemorrhages);
- prolongation of dark adaptation time and increased photosensitivity in the aged;
- rapid rarefaction of the atmosphere, specifically anoxia which can lead to hypoxia, causes disturbances in dark adaptation; the same occurs with circulatory insufficiency, anemia, and carbon monoxide poisoning;
- preadaptation with light influences the subsequent course of dark adaptation.

Testing for Light Sensitivity

Dark adaptation testing is done with an *adaptometer* (Engelking-Hartung, Goldmann-Weekers, etc.). Immediate adaptation and sensitivity to dazzling is tested with the *nyctometer* and *mesoptometer* (Aulhorn). Total adaptation means testing the entire retina as opposed to local adaptation of a circumscribed retinal area. Momentary adaptation is the reestablishment of the previous adaptative state following a short exposure to light. While 3 to 10 minutes of light adaptation suffice to break down most of the visual purple, 25 to 30 minutes of dark adaptation are required to reach optimal night vision. The major part of dark adaptation takes place in the first five minutes.

Day Blindness

Day blindness (hemeralopia) occurs with:

- central opacities of the cornea or lens and conditions producing photophobia and dazzling (pathologic mydriasis) (see page 321);
- total color blindness (allegedly caused by a loss of inhibitory influences of cones on the rods);
- albinism.

References

François, J., G. Verriest, A. de Rouck: La maladie d'oguchi. Ophthalmologica 131 (1956) 1–40

Gramberg-Danielsen, B.: Optische Funktionsleistungen und Verkehr. In: Der Augenarzt, Vol. VI, ed. by K. Velhagen. Thieme, Leipzig 1964 (pp. 579–713)

6 Hyperemia of the Eye or Its Surroundings

Redness Without Inflammation

Dilatation of conjunctival vessels with minimal subjective complaints — Dilatation of conjunctival vessels with symptoms — Subconjunctival or skin hemorrhages.

Dilatation of Conjunctival Vessels with Minimal or No Subjective Complaints

Dilatation occurs after rubbing the eyes, after trauma, with fatigue, in chronic congestive glaucoma (Plate XVI, Fig. 5, page 192 h), with miotics and other vasodilatory medications, with aneurysms and ectatic vessels, conjunctival tumors (hemangiomas, some melanomas). On rare occasions episcleral vessels will be dilated with intraocular tumors such as melanomas or metastatic carcinomas (Plate XIV, Fig. 6, page 192 f).

Dilatation of Conjunctival Vessels with Symptoms

Acute glaucoma attack (Fig. 19.1), intermittent exophthalmos from orbital varices, pulsating exophthalmos with rupture of the internal carotid artery in the cavernous sinus and cavernous sinus thrombosis are related phenomena.

Subconjunctival Hemorrhage (Hyposphagma [Plate IV, Fig. 6, page 128 d] *or Lid Hematomas* [Fig. 10.3])

These may occur with coughing, sneezing, squeezing, vomiting or any Valsalva maneuver which suddenly elevates venous pressure. In older persons recurrent hemorrhages, which are quite harmless, may occur in the same place. They clear within two to three weeks. The hemorrhage can be caused by injury, basilar skull fracture, childbirth, atherosclerosis, leukemia, hemorrhagic diathesis, Osler's disease, caisson disease, vicarious menstruation, etc.

Redness Associated with or Following Inflammation

Conjunctival injection — Ciliary injection — Mixed injection — Inflammatory redness with edema.

The most important differentiation in ocular inflammation is between conjunctival and ciliary injection (Plate I, Fig. 1, page 128 a).

Conjunctival Injèction

Conjunctival injection is bright red. Individual vessels are clearly visible, diminishing near the limbus and increasing toward the fornix.

Ciliary Injection

Ciliary injection is blue-red, in deeper layers.Individual vessels are less distinct and most marked in the perilimbal area, diminishing away from the limbus. All forms of keratitis, scleritis, iritis, iridocyclitis and acute glaucoma have an associated ciliary injection.

Mixed Injection

Combined conjunctival and ciliary injection: nearly every ciliary injection will, in time, lead to conjunctival injection through tearing and rubbing by the patient. *Chemosis* (edematous swelling of the conjunctiva [see page 120]), *orbital edema* (protrusion [see page 348]), or *lid edema* (see page 91) may occur.

7 Swelling Around the Eye and Its Environs

Noninflammatory or Minimally Inflammatory Swelling

Dermatochalasis — Traumatic (emphysema, hemorrhages) — Endocrine exophthalmos — Myxedema — Progressive scleroderma — Cardiac-renal diseases, (infectious) — generalized diseases — Elephantiasis, Melkersson-Rosenthal syndrome — Tumors and pseudotumors — Parasitic infestations — Trichinosis — Ascariasis — Onchocerciasis — Oculonasal reflex neurosis (Charlin syndrome) — Medications.

Dermatochalasis

Lax skin of the upper lid which hangs over the lid fissure simulating swelling (Fig. 10.12).

Trauma

Subcutaneous emphysema may occur with fracture of the sinuses (usually the lamina papyracea [Fig. 10.31]); there is crepitance on palpation. Hemorrhage occurs (Fig. 10.32) with basilar skull fractures, pertussis, injury, or surgery.

Endocrine Exophthalmos

(see page 339)

Myxedema (Fig. 25.11)

Finger pressure leaves no indentation as with true edema. Eye signs may include exophthalmos, strabismus, and papilledema. The skin is dry and tends to exfoliate.

Scleroderma

Progressive scleroderma can lead to chronic lid edema, decreased lacrimation, and eventually keratoconjunctivitis sicca.

Cardiac and Renal Diseases (Infectious Generalized Diseases

In all cases of noninflammatory swelling, cardiac and renal disease must be considered. Numerous infectious processes (scarlet fever, malaria, diphtheria, infectious mononucleosis, trypanosomiasis, etc.), as well as starvation, cachexia, and inflammation around the eye may lead to lid edema.

Elephantiasis, Melkersson-Rosenthal Syndrome

Elephantiasis implies a longstanding or permanent thickening of the lids due to hypertrophy of connective tissue. It is seen secondary to tumefaction (von Recklinghausen's disease, hemolymphangioma, etc.), following traumatic disruption of the lymph drainage system, after chronic eczema or infection (erysipelas, leprosy, lues, tuberculosis), and in the Melkersson-Rosenthal syndrome.

In the Melkersson-Rosenthal syndrome, recurrent swelling of the face, lips and tongue (lingua plicata) which becomes permanent is first seen. Later, recurrent facial paralysis and pain in the form of trigeminal neuralgia or migraine develops.

Tumors and Pseudotumors

Various tumors lead to a variety of different conjunctival, lid and facial swelling. These include hemangiomas (Fig. 25.13 b), neurofibromatosis (Fig. 10.58), benign and malignant ectodermal and mesodermal tumors (see page 103), pseudotumors (eosinophilic or basophilic granulomas, leukemic or amyloid degeneration, gumma, tuberculoma [Fig. 10.32], cysts, parasites, etc. [page 198]).

Parasitic Infestations

These represent a transitional form between obstructive and inflammatory edema. Lid edema is caused by nematodes (see page 198), tapeworms (see page 199), and myiasis (see page 199).

An early common symptom of *trichinosis* is marked lid and conjunctival edema (chemosis). Painful paresis of ocular muscles and exophthalmos is also common. Pupillary dilatation, accommodative paralysis, or isolated retinal hemorrhages occur less frequently.

Ascariasis may be associated with lid edema as well as blepharoconjunctivitis and keratitis, eczema or more rarely endophthalmitis, iridocyclitis, choroiditis, neuritis, and retinal neovascularization.

In *onchocerciasis* (filariasis) lymphedema of the lids may be present. The pseudotumor formed by the filaria can be situated in the area of the lids or orbits. Keratoconjunctivitis, iridocyclitis, chorioretinitis, and neuritis with optic atrophy occur.

Nasal Nerve Syndrome (Charlin Syndrome)

The nasociliary syndrome (Charlin syndrome [see page 79]) includes severe uniocular pain as well as lid and conjunctival edema associated with ipsilateral rhinorrhea. Keratitis and iritis occur. The syndrome is probably a migraine equivalent.

Medications

Strong vasodilating drugs such as Dionin (ethylmorphine) may cause chemosis.

Inflammatory Edema

Hordeolum, chalazion — Eczema, photodermatitis — Urticaria — Herpes simplex — Zoster ophthalmicus — Eczema vaccinatum — Erysipelas — Mycosis — Dacryoadenitis — Periostitis — Orbital phlegmon — Conjunctivitis — Keratitis — Scleritis — Anthrax — Chemical, heat, mechanical, radiation injuries.

Hordeolum, Chalazion

Acute hordeolum is a common cause of inflammatory edema of the lids (Plate I, Fig. 3, page 128 a). Hordeolosis can lead to lid abscess formation (Fig. 10.20, see page 91). Chalazion is a less inflammatory, more longstanding granulomatous swelling (Fig. 10.21, Plate II, Fig. 1, page 128 b).

Allergic Eczema (Contact Dermatitis), Photodermatitis

Allergic eczema is commonly seen with topical use of atropine (Plate II, Fig. 2, page 128 b), mercury, penicillin (Plate II, Fig. 3, page 128 b), anesthetics, iodine, Anthemis, etc. (see page 105). The eczema has particular diagnostic significance in scrofulous and eczematous keratoconjunctivitis (see page 106, 153).

Quincke's edema is also allergic in origin (Fig. 10.29). Photodermatitis causes lid edema (see page 157).

Urticaria

Urticaria, which burns or itches excessively, is usually allergic in origin. In addition to lid and conjunctival edema associated with hyperemia and vesicle formation, corneal edema, erosions, and iritis may be seen. Common causes are nettles, insect bites, food allergies, and drugs.

Herpes Simplex

This is a common cause of inflammatory lid edema (Fig. 10.26). It frequently recurs (with fever, menses, exhaustion, psychological stress, etc.).

Ophthalmic Zoster

Ophthalmic zoster (see page 95) leads to neuralgia, vesicle formation and edema in the distribution of the first branch of the trigeminal nerve. The involvement is unilateral and may include the ipsilateral side of the nose (nasociliary [Fig. 10.27]). Whenever the nose is affected, the eye is usually involved. Gray, subepithelial, nummular or, if deeper, disciform corneal infiltrates occur. Eventually, these may break down and ulcerate. Frequently, a hypocellular iritis with secondary glaucoma occurs. Rarely, one may see hyphemia, episcleritis, scleritis, scleral necrosis with intercalary staphyloma, retinal thrombosis, edema, and hemorrhages. Internal and external ophthalmoplegia occur (paresis of accommodation, pupil, extraocular muscles) (see page 54).

Vaccination, Variola

Four days to one and one-half weeks after vaccination, gray ulcerating lid-conjunctival lesions and marked lid edema may occur. Contact lesions can be present. The pre-auricular lymph nodes are swollen. The cornea may be involved (disciform keratitis); more rarely ocular paresis and sector iritis or atrophy of the iris occur; chorioretinitis, neuritis, retinal vessel emboli, or thrombosis are also seen.

Smallpox (variola vera) causes similar lesions (see page 96).

Erysipelas

Erysipelas can cause swollen, stiff lids that ultimately become gangrenous. This streptococcal infection is accompanied by fever. The globe itself is rarely affected (keratitis, iritis, neuritis). Other bacteria such as staphylococci may produce gangrene of the lid (see page 93).

Anthrax

Anthrax of the lids is rare. There is a two to three day incubation period after which a pruritic red papule progressing to a red-blue pustule arises. Preauricular adenopathy is present. The lid shows necrosis and eschar formation.

Mycoses

A variety of mycotic infections produce lid edema. Chronic nodules, blisters, and ulcers may occur (Fig. 10.22).

Dacryoadenitis

Acute dacryoadenitis (see page 113) causes erythema, edema, and pain in the superior temporal quadrant of the orbit (Fig. 11.1). Swollen preauricular lymph nodes are common. *Etiology:* mumps, staphylococcal infections, measles, etc. *Chronic dacryoadenitis* is basically pain free. *Etiology:* tuberculosis, syphilis (gumma), Mikulicz's syndrome (bilateral inflammation of lacrimal and salivary glands).

Other Causes of Lid Edema

Today lid edema caused by *periostitis* (gumma, tuberculoma) is rare (see page 94). *Orbital phlegmon* has marked edema and limitation of movement (see page 348). Lid edema occurs with certain *conjunctival inflammations* (diphtheria, ophthalmia neonatorum, scrofula, Parinaud's syndrome [see Chap. 12]), *keratitis* (scrofula, interstitial keratitis [see Chap. 13]), *scleritis* (scleromalacia perforans, posterior scleritis [Chap. 14]). Every *chemical, thermal, mechanical,* or *radiation injury* is accompanied by lid edema.

8 Oculomotor and Sensory Anomalies

(Hamburger and Hollwich 1966; Burian and v. Noorden 1974; Parks 1975)

Classification of Strabismus

(after Aust)

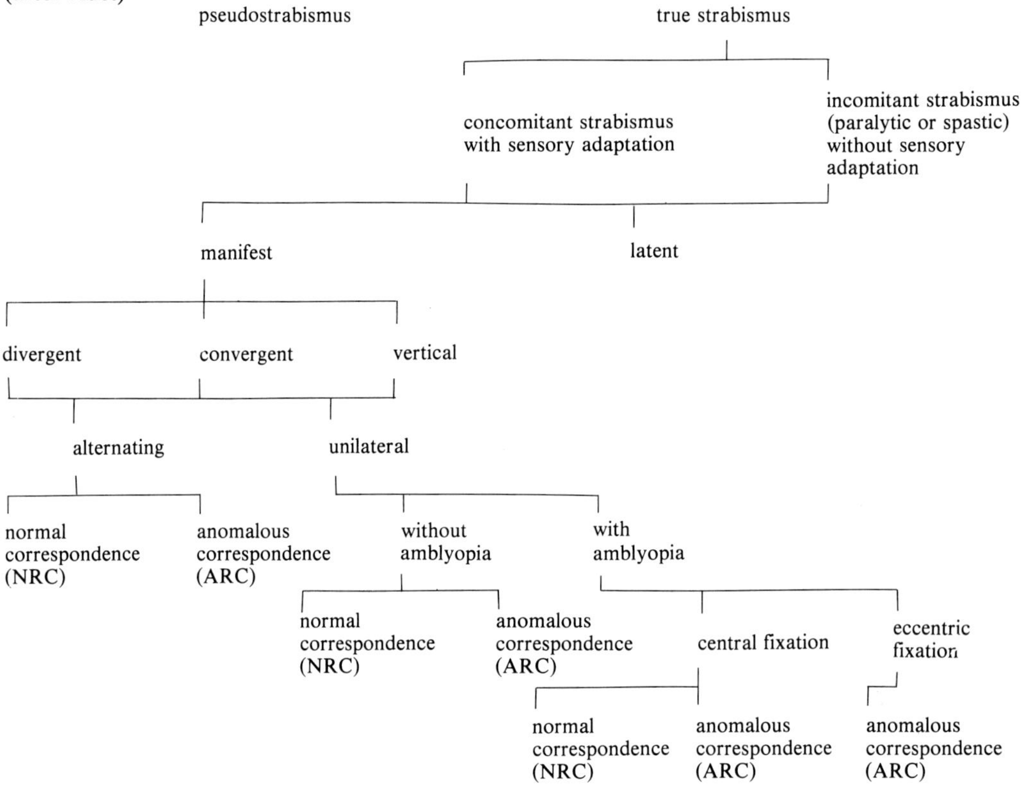

Screening Tests for Strabismus

Cover Test

Fixing a light or accommodative target (near 33 cm, distance 6 m)

1. Cover test (one eye is covered). The unilateral cover-uncover test must be done separately on each eye.

a) The uncovered eye moves to take up fixation: esotropic, exotropic, or vertical deviation; a manifest deviation (tropia) is present.

b) The uncovered eye fails to move: If *acuity is equal* in both eyes, the visual axes of the two eyes are parallel. If *acuity is decreased in one eye*, orthophoria with amblyopia and central fixation could be present. More likely, however, would be the presence of strabismus with amblyopia and eccentric fixation (objective angle = distance of foveola – eccentric fixation point). With deep amblyopia the target may not be seen and the eye does not move to pick up fixation. Usually an amblyopic eye will make searching movements.

When no tropia is present, a latent deviation (phoria) is determined by the cover-uncover test.

2. Cover-uncover test (one eye is covered, then uncovered).
The covered eye is observed for movement as the cover is removed.
a) No movement = no phoria.
b) Movement = phoria: esophoric, exophoric, vertical.
All cover tests must be done with the patient's optimum distance correction and a fixation target. To determine the accommodative component, the near test is repeated with a plus 3 diopter lens.
3. In addition to tropias and phorias, the unilateral cover-uncover test will also reveal *nonconcomitant deviations,* depending on which eye is fixing. If nonconcomitant deviation is present, it indicates a paralytic strabismus. Abnormal head position (tilt, turn, chin depression or lift) is a sign that binocular vision is or may have been present at some time, in some direction of gaze.
Latent nystagmus can be observed when one eye is covered.
Dissociated vertical deviation (alternating hyperphoria, occlusion hypertropia, dissociation hyperphoria or dissociated vertical divergence, alternating sursumduction) is present when the covered eye deviates upward. The eye returns to its original position when the cover is removed. Latent nystagmus is often also present. It may occur in only one eye or be present bilaterally.

Pupil Illumination Test

The pupil illumination test as described by Brückner (1962) is useful for diagnosing strabismus in early childhood. It consists of testing the Hirschberg corneal reflex, fundus reflex, and pupillary near response.
At a distance of about one meter, both eyes are illuminated simultaneously with a strong light source from a direct ophthalmoscope. If the position of the corneal reflex and the color of the pupils are
1. symmetric and similar, no strabismus is present;
2. asymmetric and varied, strabismus is present (the child must be looking directly at the light with at least one eye).
On rapidly illuminating first one and then the other eye,
1. if pupillary color, corneal reflex, and pupillary constriction are equal and there is no movement on the part of either eye to pick up fixation, there is no indication of strabismus;
2. asymmetry (variation in pupillary color, asymmetric corneal reflex) indicates strabismus. An asymmetric pupillary reaction indicates strabismus without amblyopia if the pupil of the newly fixing eye dilates at first but quickly constricts to equal the pupil of the other eye when it is fixing. Amblyopia must be suspected when the pupil of the newly fixing eye dilates and remains larger than that of the other eye when it is fixing, even though illumination is equal in both cases. Presumably the difference in pupillary size is due to a decreased accommodative-near pupillary constriction impulse with the amblyopic eye compared to the normal eye fixing. The amblyopic eye may make searching movements. When amblyopia is present, the child will usually resist having the healthy eye covered but is unconcerned when the amblyopic eye is covered.

Temporary Deviations of the Eyes

Heterophoria (Latent Squint, Relative Position of Rest)

The position of the globes is a function of numerous variables (course, insertion and tone of extraocular muscles, fascia, orbital fat, size of globe and orbit). With orthophoria the visual axes remain parallel even after fusion (see page 46) is disrupted. If they do not remain parallel, heterophoria is present. Heterophoria occurs in 75 percent of the population. Krümmel (1952) found esophoria in 43 percent, exophoria in 44.7 percent. Chajutin (1941) gives the values 32 percent and 30 percent respectively. Adults, especially myopic adults, tend to show convergence insufficiency and exophoria (latent divergence). Children, particularly in association with hyperopia, frequently demonstrate *esophoria* (latent convergence). *Hyperphoria* and *hypophoria* are latent vertical deviations, and *cyclophorias* are latent rotary deviations. Phorias are kept latent through fusion (integration of the two separate retinal images into a single binocular perception).

Heterophoria may lead to subjective asthenopic (muscular asthenopia [see page 69]) complaints consisting of a feeling of pressure or tension around the eyes, forehead, or occiput. The pressure may become persistent, may increase during the day, may be aggravated by close work and create an inability for concentrated effort. In labile, nervous, neurotic individuals, such asthenopic complaints may occur with minimal heterophorias (see page 69).

To *diagnose heterophoria* (Burian, v. Noorden 1974) fusion is interrupted. This is done by covering one eye or by placing a Maddox rod in front of one eye while both eyes are open and fixating a point light source. If heterophoria exists, the covered eye then assumes the appropriate deviation. The Maddox rod turns the point light source into a streak of light. With loss of fusion, the streak (seen by the eye with the Maddox rod) and point of light (seen by the other eye) separate in a manner and degree appropriate to the phoria. In orthophoria the light streak and point do not separate (light streak goes through the point). Heterophoria at close distances is most easily tested with the Maddox wing.

A phoria, especially when large, can be demonstrated whenever the ability to fuse is compromised (tropia). This may occur with any systemic illness where decreased acuity caused by ocular disease is present. General fatigue, narcotics, or excessive emotional strain may also lead to a permanent deviation.

Accommodation and convergence are linked. Esophoria, commonly present in children, may break down and lead to manifest strabismus whenever there is a weakening of fusional ability (e.g., monocular decrease in acuity or systemic illness), particulary when an uncorrected hyperopia is present. Adults are more commonly exophoric. Heterophoria is frequently *simulated* by *improperly centered glasses* which cause a *prismatic effect*.

Deviations at Close Distances

Convergence excess — Convergence insufficiency and convergence weakness — Divergence insufficiency and divergence excess.

Convergence Excess

Convergence excess can occur *voluntarily* in combination with *accommodative spasm* and sometimes, though rarely, in association with voluntary nystagmus (see page 65). A transition to hysteric spasm of convergence has then occurred.

A relative excess of convergence arises in *high uncorrected or undercorrected hyperopia* (accommodation and convergence are interrelated). When fusion is weakened, esotropia results. (The danger exists, especially in schoolchildren, that this artificial myopia resulting from accommodation is corrected by minus glasses.) In convergence excess the deviation is greater for close distances than for distances.

Convergence Insufficiency and Convergence Weakness

Convergence insufficiency or weakness is common. Not only convergence but also accommodation and pupillary near reaction are absent.

As possible etiology, wide interpupillary distance, esophoria of large degree, high myopia, and psychogenic reactions should be considered. Frequently, there is a history of psychological or physical trauma, difficulty at school, etc.

Divergence Insufficiency and Divergence Excess

These are usually the result of refractive errors or heterophoria. *Divergence paresis* is a different problem (see page 60).

Strabismus, Manifest Deviation

Esotropia; blocked nystagmus syndrome — Exotropia — Vertical deviations — Hypertropia, hypotropia — Elevation of the adducted eye (strabismus sursoadductorius) — Disassociation hypertropia — Pseudostrabismus

Manifest Strabismus (concomitant): Debilitating illnes can cause an existing fusional weakness to convert from a latent (heterophoria) to a manifest tropia. This may be intermittent or permanent. High degrees of heterophoria will become manifest when poor vision exists unilaterally. This may be congenital, acquired, organic, or refractive in nature. In such cases the need for single vision is decreased and manifest strabismus results. An inability to fuse may be purely congenital. In this case failure of the central nervous system to properly innervate and direct the sensory motor mechanism exists (Hamburger 1960).

Anatomic aspects rarely play a role in strabismus (asymmetry in position of the globes, anomalies in structure and position of orbital tissues, dysgenesis, etc.). Heredity is important. Strabismus is both recessive and dominant. Multiple factors, all leading to strabismus, have to be considered (Clausen and Brauer 1932; Harms 1938): refractive errors, relative position of rest, heterophoria, weak fusional reflex, monocular decrease in vision. Holland (1965) found inherited contributing factors in 41.5 percent of 967 strabismic children studied. Strabismus is frequently associated with congenital *syndromes* or inborn errors of metabolism (see page 245).

In the **Marinesco-Sjögren syndrome,** spinocerebellar ataxia, oligophrenia, cataracts and esotropia occur. Heredity is recessive, particularly with parental consanguinity. Constitutional infantilism and panmyelopathy **(Fanconi syndrome)** occur with multiple malformations such as microcephaly, microphthalmos, and strabismus.

Monocular and *alternating strabismus* must be differentiated. The deviation is monocular in 75 percent of untreated cases. The deviating eye in monocular strabismus is usually amblyopic and has the larger refractive error. In *alternating strabismus* the two eyes usually have equal vision.

Since both degree and direction of movement of the globes normally differ somewhat between the two eyes, the term **concomitant strabismus** is no longer used in its most literal sense. The current meaning is a nonparalytic strabismus but not necessarily perfectly concomitant.

Holland (1965) determined the onset of strabismus in 967 children:

Since birth	277 (28.6 percent)
1st year of life	226 (23.4 percent)
2nd year of life	210 (21.7 percent)
3rd year of life	130 (13.5 percent)
4th year of life	76 (7.9 percent)
5th year of life	27 (2.8 percent)
6th year of life	12 (1.2 percent)
7th year of life	6 (0.6 percent)
8th year of life	3 (0.3 percent)

Strabismus is socially important since about 4 percent of the total population are strabismic. Without treatment for amblyopia, it is safe to assume that 40 percent would suffer from deep amblyopia.

Esotropia (Figs. 8.1, 8.2)

Alternating and monocular esotropia — Blocked nystagmus syndrome.

The most common manifest deviation is esotropia (94 percent [Holland 1965]). Onset is usually in childhood and the patients are almost invariably hyperopic. For screening tests to establish the diagnosis, see cover test and pupil illumination test (page 37).

Alternating Esotropia

Uniocular or monocular esotropia should be differentiated from alternating esotropia. In alternating esotropia acuity is usually equal. Although fixation alternates, one eye may be dominant. Normal or anomalous correspondence may occur (see page 44).

Unilateral or Monocular Esotropia

The deviating eye usually shows some degree of amblyopia (on rare occasions, acuity may be normal). Amblyopia frequently occurs with anisometropia (the eye with the greater refractive error becomes amblyopic). A congenital defect is less often at fault (Schapero 1971).

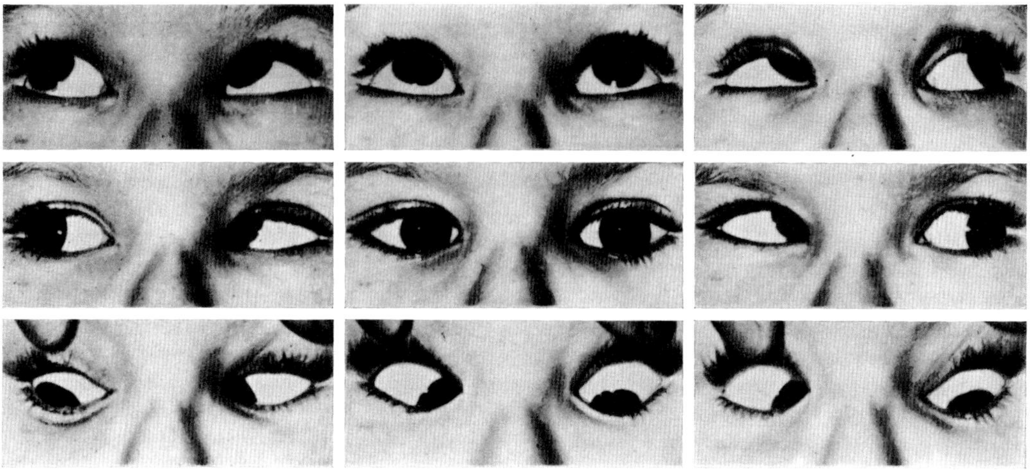

Fig. 8.1 Esotropia: V-pattern (hypertropia of the adducting eye — overaction of inferior obliques)

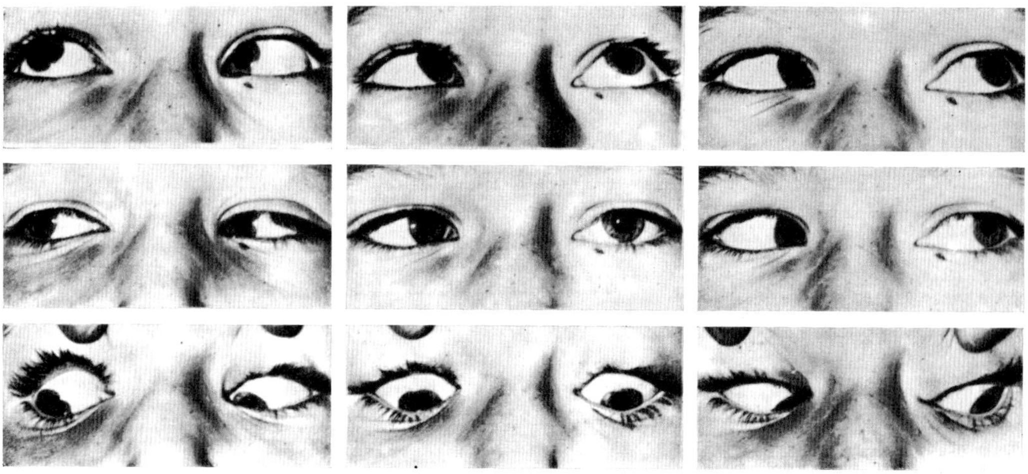

Fig. 8.2 Esotropia: A-pattern (hypotropia of the adducting eye — superior oblique overaction)

Retinal correspondence may be normal or anomalous (see page 44).

In order to see clearly at distance, the uncorrected hyperopic individual will accommodate automatically. Since accommodation and convergence are linked, the uncorrected hyperopic person with clear distance vision has to generate innervational impulses that compensate the tendency to converge. This is brought about by the desire for single binocular vision (fusion). Any systemic debilitating process (illness such as measles, scarlet fever, diphtheria, etc., or simply fatigue) can cause these compensatory mechanisms to break down, especially in the third and fourth year of life. Esotropia results.

The diagnosis *accommodative esotropia* is made "ex juvantibus", i.e., the deviation disappears when the appropriate glasses are worn. In pure accommodative esotropia, retinal correspondence is normal. In partially accommodative esotropia, correspondence is usually anomalous. Esotropia is often associated with overaction of the inferior obliques and *dissociated vertical deviation*.

There are a number of associated characteristics which assist in diagnosing *congenital* esotropia. Lang (1969) found a dissociated vertical deviation in 90 percent of patients with congenital esotropia. The nonfixing eye deviates upward. In 55 percent of the cases, latent nystagmus was present. In 65 percent cyclodeviation occurred. The vertically deviating eye extorts, the eye taking up fixation intorts. An abnormal head position was found in 70 percent of the patients.

In addition to *accommodation* other causative factors resulting in esotropia include *esophoria, weak fusional reflex, central nervous system disturbances, transient sixth nerve pareses* (Fig. 8.3), *nystagmus, anatomic-mechanical anomalies*, and *heredity*.

Anomalous retinal correspondence is an adaptive process to strabismus. Impulses reaching the macula lutea of the fixing eye fall on nasal retina in the esotropic one. This nasal area acquires a common visual direction (namely, straight ahead) with the fovea of the fixing eye. In this way, a weak form of binocular (not necessarily stereoscopic) vision is achieved.

Microstrabismus or small angle deviation is often referred to as fixation disparity in the English and American literature. "Fixation disparity" is an inappropriate term.

It has also been used to describe a physiologic disparity in heterophoria (Ogle 1950). Here the fixation point is imaged on imperfectly corresponding retinal elements, but it is still seen singly because the points are within Panum's fusional area.

A certain amount of binocularity is possible when small angle esotropia (less than 5 degrees) is present. The Worth four-dot test, especially at close distance, is positive. Microstrabismus occurs with NRC, ARC as well as foveal, central, and eccentric fixation.

Microstrabismus occurs primarily in congenital strabismus and only secondarily in residual deviations following corrective surgery or glasses (Lang 1973).

Blocked Nystagmus Syndrome

The blocked nystagmus syndrome (Adelstein and Cüppers 1966) consists of bilateral or monocular convergence where the adducted eye or eyes cannot be abducted to the midline. If monocular, it may alternate. The esotropia increases with prolonged fixation. An accompanying nystagmus is present which may be very fine in its excursions. Often, the nystagmus can be seen only with magnification (slit lamp, visuscope, etc.). Fixation is carried out in the adducted position. The patients usually have a head turn which is dependent on the fixing eye; with forced straight head position, however, both eyes are still adducted. Electromyography shows hyperactivity of both medial rectus muscles.

In the blocked nystagmus syndrome, the eyes will assume a parallel or even divergent position under anesthesia. This is true for any plane of anesthesia and is in contradistinction to what occurs with bilateral paresis of the sixth nerve. If forced ductions are positive, it becomes impossible to differentiate between strabismus fixus, bilateral abducens paresis with contraction of the recti mediales bulbi, and blocked nystagmus syndrome with secondary contractions (Haase 1970).

Exotropia

Children with congenital or acquired *impaired vision* tend toward *esotropia*. *After puberty* the tendency is toward *exotropia*. Frequently manifest *exotropia* (Fig. 8.4) develops from a decompensating exophoria associated with *convergence insufficiency, poor fusional amplitudes*, and anisometropia. *Intermittent* exotropia may precede constant exotropia. After puberty, *myopia*, especially if excessively high, tends toward exotropia.

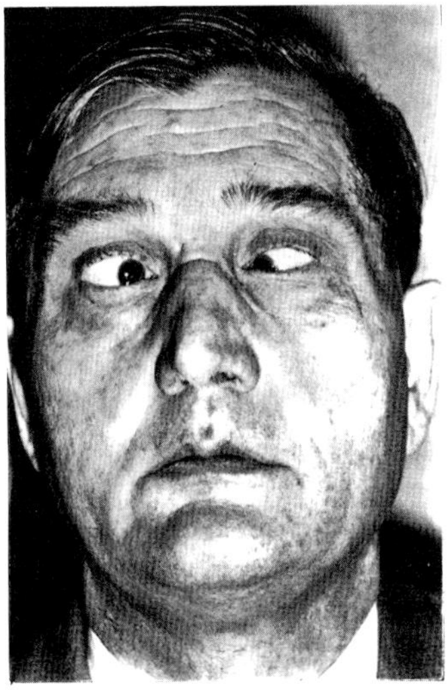

Fig. 8.3 Convergent strabismus fixus following bilateral abducens paresis (♂ 59 yrs.)

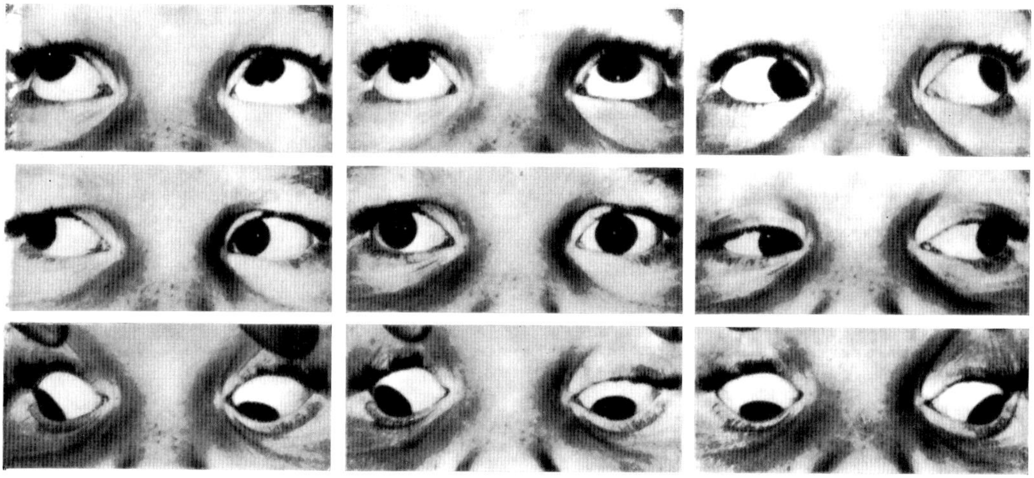

Fig. 8.4 Exotropia with an A-pattern

Exotropia may be *alternating* or *monocular*. Amblyopia is rarely found in exotropia.
In exotropia retinal correspondence is usually normal and rarely anomalous (see page 44). In congenital exotropia, correspondence is almost always normal. Only 5 to 15 percent of strabismic patients are exotropic. The average age at onset is 10 to 12.
Consecutive exotropia (following muscle surgery) is seen less frequently today.

Vertical Deviations

Manifest vertical deviations usually follow a hyperphoria or hypophoria. They almost always appear in combination with an esodeviation and rarely with an exodeviation. A true vertical deviation may be alternating or monocular.

Hypertropia of the Adducted Eye (Strabismus sursoadductorius)

On examination, the adducted eye deviates upward (overaction of the inferior oblique muscle), while the eyes are on the same level in primary position. This condition may be unilateral or bilateral. If it is combined with a horizontal deviation, it is usually esotropia and rarely exotropia. It is associated with a V-pattern (Fig. 8.1). In some cases the adducted eye deviates downward (strabismus deorsoadductorius) (overaction of the superior oblique) and is associated with an A-pattern (Fig. 8.2).
The *V-syndrome* (Fig. 8.1) is defined as significant increase (15Δ) in convergence or decrease in divergence when looking down. The *A-syndrome* (Fig. 8.2) consists of a significant increase (20Δ) in convergence or decrease in divergence when looking up. The V-syndrome implies an overacting inferior oblique, the A-syndrome an overacting superior oblique muscle (Holland 1968; Burian, v. Noorden 1974). A partial V-pattern seen only in superior gaze can be called a *Y-syndrome*. A partial A-syndrome with the deviation only occurring in down gaze can be considered an *inverted Y-syndrome;* it occurs primarily with exodeviation. An X-pattern exists when divergence increases when looking up and looking down.
Strabismus fixus (Fig. 8.3) results when, because of fibrosis or contracture of extraocular muscles or tissues, the eyes are locked in a position of extreme adduction or abduction.

Dissociated Vertical Deviation

This may be monocular or more frequently binocular. When fusion is disrupted, the nonfixing eye deviates upward and extorts; when the cover is removed, the eye returns to its normal position (alternating hypertropia, phoria, or alternating sursumduction). In this case a phenomenon first described by Bielschowsky

(1931) can be elicited. When a filter is placed in front of the fixing eye, the elevated nonfixing eye rotates downward, sometimes even below the horizontal, and incyclotorts. Another kind of dissociated vertical strabismus is the continuously varying vertical deviation of a severely amblyopic eye when the healthy eye is focused straight ahead.

Pseudostrabismus

In pseudostrabismus both visual axes intersect at the fixation point. The cover-uncover test fails to elicit movement from either eye. The strabismic appearance in small children is frequently due to epicanthus. Variations in the kappa angle (failure of the optical axis and visual axis of the eye to coincide) may erroneously lead to the diagnosis of strabismus. A positive kappa angle simulates exotropia; a negative kappa angle, esotropia. The kappa angle is measured monocularly. The eye fixates a light in the center of the Maddox scale at a distance of one meter; the position of the corneal reflex is observed. If the corneal reflex is centered, the angle is 0 degrees. If the reflex is eccentric, fixation is shifted along the Maddox tangent scale until the reflex centers on the cornea. The kappa angle can then be read from the markings on the Maddox scale. Hamburger (1960), Aust (1966) and Burian; v. Noorden (1974) have investigated the relationship of angles gamma, kappa, alpha and lambda.

Strabismus is often simulated during the first few months of life as a result of the *strong convergence tendency of the infant.* This usually disappears before the infant reaches the age of one year.

Sensory Aspects

Fixation (central-eccentric) — Objective angle of squint — Subjective angle — Normal correspondence — Anomalous correspondence — Testing for correspondence — Dominance — Fusion — Binocularity — Testing binocularity — Depth perception.

Sensory and motor behavior of the two eyes is as if they were one single organ (the imaginary cyclopian eye).

Fixation

In order to make a proper diagnosis with regard to size of deviation, correspondence, amblyopia, etc., it is important to know whether the fovea is being used for fixation *(central fixation).* Central fixation may exist despite deep amblyopia.

In *eccentric fixation* the fovea is no longer the carrier of the principal visual direction. The eccentric retinal point used for fixing has acquired the sensation of "straight ahead." In spite of the ocular deviation, the patient has the sensation that he is looking straight at the object. In *eccentric viewing* the target is imaged upon the edge of a central scotoma, but the fovea still carries the principal visual direction and the patient, therefore, has the impression that he is looking past the object.

Determination of Fixation

Fixation is easily determined with the visuscope. The patient is asked to look directly at the visuscope star. If the star is passively projected onto the foveola and the patient has the sensation of looking straight at it, the principal visual direction is with the fovea. Sometimes the patient may perceive the star projected onto the fovea as being straight ahead; but, when asked to actively fixate the star, he does so eccentrically. Fovea and eccentric fixing position then have two spatial orientations. In this situation the star may be seen double.

Objective Angle of Deviation

The objective angle of deviation is that amount of strabismus found with the alternating cover test. Increasing strength prisms (1 degree = about two prism diopters) are held before one eye until all motion (redress movement) on covering the fixing eye stops (angle of deviation is neutralized). This test is not valid in the presence of deep amblyopia or ec-

centric fixation. The cover test is one of the most important means of assessing the ocular motor and sensory status. This is particularly true in children. Alternate cover and cover-uncover is done. The uncovered eye is observed.
In addition to convergent, divergent, and vertical deviations, cyclodeviations are demonstrable with the cover test.
In heterophoria the covered eye deviates under the cover to return to its original position when uncovered. The fixing eye does not move during this time. With muscle paresis, the secondary deviation is larger than the primary deviation (see page 47).
Redress movements of the uncovered eye are frequently larger with alternate cover than cover-uncover testing. If deep amblyopia (poor fixation) is present, the objective angle of squint cannot be determined accurately with the cover test.

Subjective Angle of Deviation

The subjective angle of squint is the angle where the two arms of the synoptophore are positioned so that the patient sees the images of the two eyes as superimposed. In normal correspondence the subjective and objective angle of deviation are the same (see Fig. 8.5 a). In anomalous correspondence the subjective angle is smaller than the objective angle. If the subjective angle is zero, harmonious and anomalous correspondence exists (see Fig. 8.5 b). If the angle is between zero and the objective angle, unharmonious and anomalous correspondence exists (see Fig. 8.5 c).

Normal Correspondence

If the posterior halves of each eye are placed like hollow bowls one into the other, all retinal points which lie on top of each other are *corresponding retinal elements*. Corresponding retinal elements have a common visual direction. This means that, if corresponding retinal elements are stimulated, the stimulus is seen in the same direction in space and binocular single vision results. If an object is imaged upon disparate retinal elements (Fig. 8.5 a), diplopia results and correcting eye movements

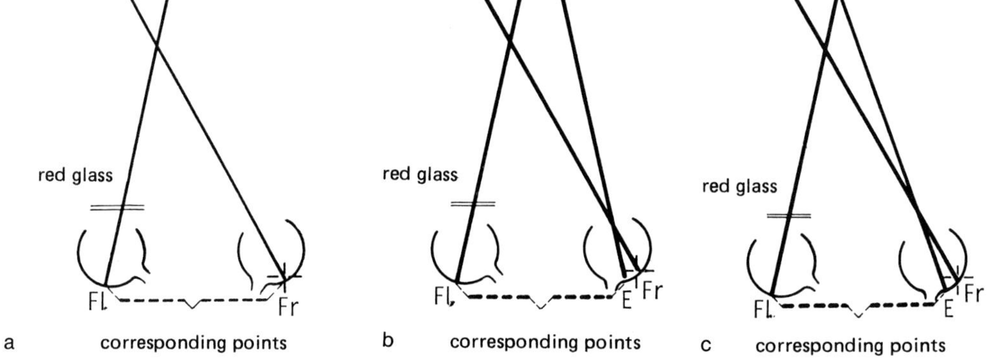

Fig. 8.5 Testing retinal correspondence on the Maddox scale using a dark red glass and after image cross (as per Cüppers). a) Normal correspondence; b) Harmonious anomalous correspondence; c) Unharmonious anomalous correspondence

Fl = fovea of the fixing eye
Fr = fovea of the deviating eye
E = retinal point corresponding to the foveola of the fixing eye

(fusional movements) are triggered. The amplitude of fusion is determined with prisms, and measures two degrees vertical vergence, six degrees divergence and 14 to 45 degrees convergence.

Anomalous and Variable Correspondence

Harmonious *anomalous correspondence* exists if the subjective angle of deviation is zero (Fig. 8.5 b). With unharmonious correspondence the subjective angle is smaller than the objective angle (Fig. 8.5 c).
Retinal correspondence can be *variable* and adapt itself to the situation of the moment. In intermittent exotropia normal correspondence may be present while the eyes are straight, but anomalous correspondence may be found in the deviated position.

Testing Correspondence

The Hering afterimage test is a quick and practical method for determining retinal correspondence. A vertical afterimage is created in one eye and a horizontal afterimage in the other. With normal retinal correspondence the two afterimages are seen as a perfect cross; with abnormal correspondence, the vertical afterimage appears displaced to the left or to the right of the horizontal one (see Figs. 8.5 a, b, c; 8.6).
This can also be accomplished by producing an afterimage in only one eye and then having the patient fix the center light of the Maddox scale with the other eye. The afterimage produced in the first eye will be projected onto the Maddox scale at the angle of anomaly. The synoptophore, the congruence test of Tschermak (1899) and the phase-difference haploscope (Aulhorn 1966) are other methods of testing for retinal correspondence. The foveo-foveal test by Cüppers and other modifications of this test are cited by Aust (1966) (see Fig. 8.5). This test is done on the Maddox tangent scale using a red glass and afterimage.

Esotropia

The red glass is placed before the fixing, afterimage cross on the deviating, eye.

Normal correspondence (Fig. 8.5 a): Objective and subjective angles are the same. Afterimage cross and red light are superimposed; their distance from the white light equals the objective and subjective angles of squint.
Harmonious anomalous correspondence (Fig. 8.5 b): red and white light are superimposed.
Subjective angle = 0.
Objective angle = distance between afterimage cross and (red and white) light.
Objective angle = angle of anomaly.
Unharmonious anomalous correspondence (Fig. 8.5 c):
Subjective angle of squint = distance between red and white light on the Maddox scale.
Objective angle = distance between the afterimage cross and the white light on the Maddox scale.
Angle of anomaly = distance between the red light and afterimage cross = objective minus subjective angle.

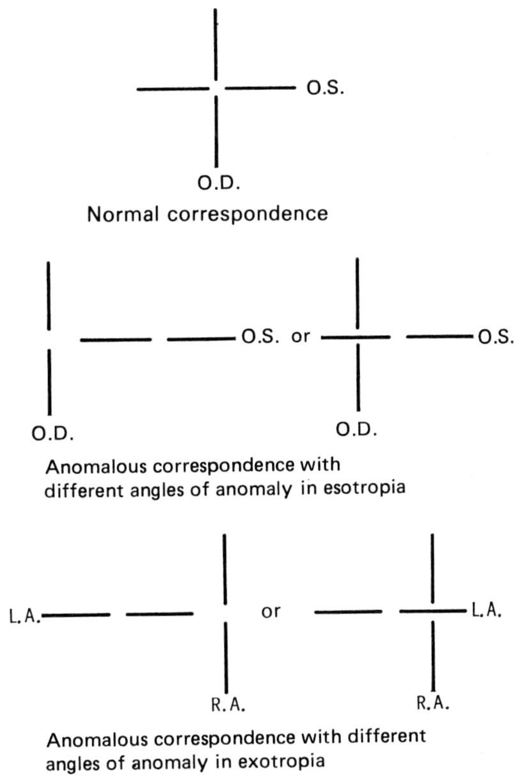

Fig. 8.6 Hering afterimages with normal and anomalous correspondence

The red glass must be dark enough to shut out everything but the fixation light or the deviating eye will be suppressed. This is not a natural way of viewing and raises real objections regarding the validity of such test methods.

Dominance

Even though amblyopia may not be present, one of the two eyes is usually leading. The two eyes are normally in a state of rivalry concerning binocularity. There may be summation of the images of the right and left eye or one eye can dominate over the other. The dominance may be so pronounced that a form of monocular vision results. Some retinal areas in one or both eyes dominate; they may shift dominance continuously so that the binocular visual field appears to have a mosaic-like construction.

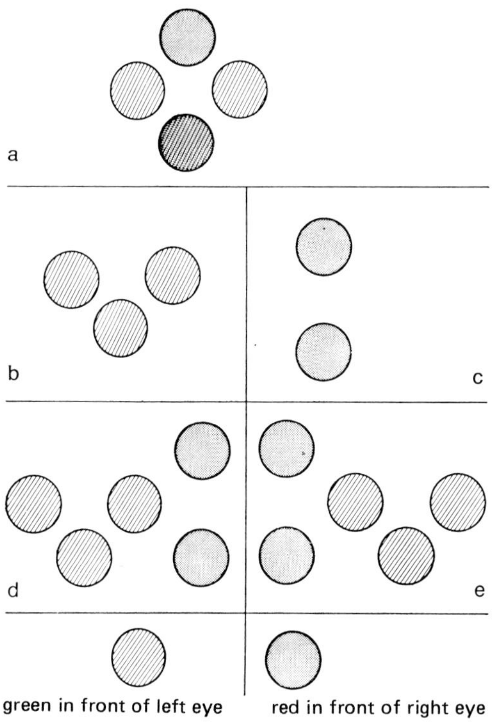

Fig. 8.7 a-e a) Worth four-dot test with binocular vision (orthophoria, or with harmonious anomalous correspondence); b) and c) Worth four-dot test with monocular suppression; d) Worth four-dot test in (latent or manifest) esodeviation with normal or unharmonious anomalous correspondence without suppression; e) Worth four-dot test in (latent or manifest) exodeviation and normal or unharmonious anomalous correspondence without suppression

Fusion

Fusion is the involuntary drive to see a single image. This drive is of greatest importance for binocular vision. Fusion may be tested with prisms or a haploscope. Fusional capacity lies between −5 degrees (divergence) and +30 degrees (14 to 45 degrees) (convergence). The fusional vertical range is only 1 to 3 degrees.

Binocularity

The question of binocularity involves testing for simultaneous binocular perception, fusion, and stereopsis (see page 47).

The following is possible (Worth 1929):

a) Superimposition: The image presented to the left eye is superimposed onto the one presented to the right eye, e.g., the lion is seen inside the cage; the ball, in the box (synoptophore).

b) Superimpositioning with fusion: On the synoptophore two nearly identical pictures are presented to the two eyes, e.g., a cat has no tail in one picture and no whiskers in the other. If fusion is present, the cat is seen as a whole (with tail and whiskers).

c) Superimpositioning + fusion + stereopsis: Identical pictures are presented, but pictures are displaced and imaged, therefore, on disparate retinal points. The sensation of stereopsis is present, e.g., three circles where one has been slightly displaced.

Testing Binocularity

Binocular vision can be tested in the following ways:

1. If a vertical prism is introduced in front of one eye and vertical diplopia is appreciated, binocularity exists.

2. A base-out prism produces crossed diplopia. If fusion and binocularity are present, the base-out prism induces convergence; the two images will be fused and single vision results.

3. Most persons are slightly heterophoric. When fusion is interrupted by covering one eye, this eye deviates slightly. The movement the eye makes to pick up fixation when uncovered is objective evidence of binocularity.

4. With a stereoscope one can present almost

similar pictures to each eye. If the discrepancies visible on only one of the two pictures are incorporated in the single image, fusion and binocularity exist.

5. Stereopsis is present when the horizontally displaced parts of the stereoscopic picture evoke a sensation of depth.

6. A wide variety of devices are available for testing stereopsis. Those devices employing polarized light probably allow the most quantitative measurement of depth perception.

To test binocularity the Worth four-dot test is used. The patient wears a pair of red-green glasses and looks at two green, one red and one white dots of light (see Fig. 8.7 a). One eye sees three green (two green, one white), the other, two red (one red, one white) lights (see Figs. 8.7 b, 8.7 c). When fusion exists, four lights are seen. If one eye is suppressed, only three green or two red lights are seen. When there is no suppression and an angle of deviation exists, five lights (three green, two red) are seen. The distance between them is the subjective angle of squint. The images are uncrossed with esodeviations and crossed with exodeviations (see Figs. 8.7 d, 8.7 e). In harmonious ARC without suppression, the Worth dots are seen as in orthophoria (see Fig. 8.7 a). Unharmonious ARC in a previously untreated strabismus will give a separation between the Worth dots which is smaller than the objective angle of squint.

Crossed diplopia in esotropia is paradoxical anomalous correspondence; it indicates a previous effort to treat the deviation.

7. The impression of three dimensions is best obtained with similar pictures where parts of the picture are slightly displaced obliquely.

In the Titmus test or AO vectorgraph, polarized material and polarized spectacles are used for stereo testing.

8. The best method to explore stereo vision is the haploscope.

Depth of Field

(see Binocularity, page 46)

All object points stimulating corresponding retinal elements lie on the horopter. Every point on the horopter is perceived binocularly as single. The greater the degree of convergence, the smaller the horopter radius. Object points lying outside of the horopter, but within Panum's fusional area, are still not seen double; instead there is a sensation of depth. Points outside of Panum's area evoke diplopia (physiologic diplopia). Uncrossed diplopia gives a feeling of distance, crossed diplopia of nearness. Vertically displaced images do not produce a sensation of depth.

Muscular Gaze Paralysis

Paralysis of the Extraocular Muscles (Paralytic Strabismus)

Signs of ocular muscle paralysis — Double vision — Monocular diplopia — Special forms of eye muscle paralysis, ophthalmoplegia, Marcus-Gunn phenomenon, myopathies: chronic progressive external ophthalmoplegia, ocular myositis — Endocrine myopathy — Ocular myotonia — Pseudomyopathies — Myasthenia gravis — Neurogenic causes — Etiology of extraocular muscle paralysis — Etiology of paralysis of the third nerve — Etiology of paralysis of the sixth nerve.

Signs of Extraocular Muscle Paresis

When an extraocular muscle is paretic, the direct antagonist overacts and the eye assumes its characteristic position of deviation. The *primary angle of deviation* (fixing with the nonparetic eye) is smaller than the *secondary angle* (fixing with the paretic eye). This is because the amount of innervational input required is greater for fixing with the paretic than with the normal eye.

The angle of deviation increases with gaze in the direction of the action of the paretic muscle. *Diplopia* occurs. The double image (from the paretic eye) appears displaced in the direction of action of the paretic muscle. Since the deviation and distance between the double images increase when gazing in the direction of action of the paretic muscle, the patient attempts to minimize symptoms by constantly looking in the opposite direction. This is possible only by turning the head. The *head is turned* in the *direction* of action of the *paretic muscle*. If the patient fixes with the paretic eye and is asked to point at an object with his finger, he will *point past* it in the direction of action of the paretic muscle (Graefe pointing test).

Anomalous head posture may indicate the presence of paralytic strabismus (possibly congenital). Nystagmus, less pronounced in one direction of gaze, may lead to a compensatory head position. Only after these causes of an anomalous head posture are ruled out should torticollis of other etiology (orthopedic, sternocleidomastoid) be considered.

Methods of investigation of paretic extraocular muscles (Hamburger 1960; Burian and v. Noorden 1974).

1. On cover-uncover testing, the primary angle of deviation (fixing with the normal eye) is smaller than the secondary angle (fixing with the paretic eye). With increasing duration of the paresis, the difference between primary and secondary angles declines, and concomitance is approached.

2. Ductions. The range of excursion is normally about 10 mm in the horizontal, 4.5 mm on depression and 7 mm on elevation.

3. Double image testing:
a) Red glass,
b) Lancaster or Hess screen,
c) Zeiss coordimeter,
d) Prisms,
e) "Beißbrettchen" (Hofmann-Bielschowsky),
f) Harms tangent scale.

The paretic deviation goes through several stages (Hamburger 1960). Weakness of the paretic muscle is immediately followed by overaction of the ipsilateral antagonist. Contracture of this antagonist occurs in longstanding paralysis. When the patient fixates with the paretic eye, the contralateral antagonist of the paretic muscle underacts (inhibitional palsy of the contralateral antagonist).

In longstanding paresis, secondary contracture of the ipsilateral antagonist and contralateral synergist occurs. With time what is at first a purely functional change evolves into an anatomic one. The head position, however, changes little in contrast to the demonstrable diplopia. On occasion paresis of one of the horizontal muscles leads to an esotropia which becomes progressively more concomitant.

Diplopia (Binocular, Monocular)

The primary symptom of *paresis* (see page 47) or mechanical restriction (see page 57) of *extraocular muscles* is diplopia. This may be present even with poor visual acuity in one eye. A small residual visual field such as with retinal detachment may still lead to aggravating double vision.

The *blurred images* of uncorrected refractive errors or *unequal images* in anisometropia are often erroneously interpreted by the patient as diplopia.

Improper centering or positioning of *spectacles* can cause diplopia.

Monocular diplopia occurs with subluxated lenses; for example, ectopia lentis in Marfan's syndrome. The eye then has two focal points. The patient may see past the lens with +11.0 diopters or through the lens with −6 or −8 diopters. Due to a lack of zonular tone, the lens is more spherical in these cases and myopia results. *Nuclear cataract* can also cause monocular diplopia; the lens then has two or more focal points. When anterior or posterior lenticonus have been present since birth, diplopia is not appreciated (Gramberg-Danielsen 1957).

Peripheral iris colobomata such as from iridodialysis, traumatic iris perforations, or polycoria can lead to monocular diplopia. On rare occasions monocular diplopia is caused by *high irregular astigmatism, poorly fitting contact lenses, tear film, air bubbles in the anterior chamber, or transparent foreign bodies or cysts.* Monocular dipolopia seen with *uncorrected astigmatism* is actually a double contour.

Monocular diplopia may also occur with *retinal detachment*. When *anomalous* and *normal correspondence* exist *simultaneously*, monocular diplopia may be appreciated (for instance, during orthoptic treatment).

Paresis of Specific Extraocular Muscles

Only the angle of deviation and the double images will be considered. The head turn is always in the direction of the paretic muscle action.

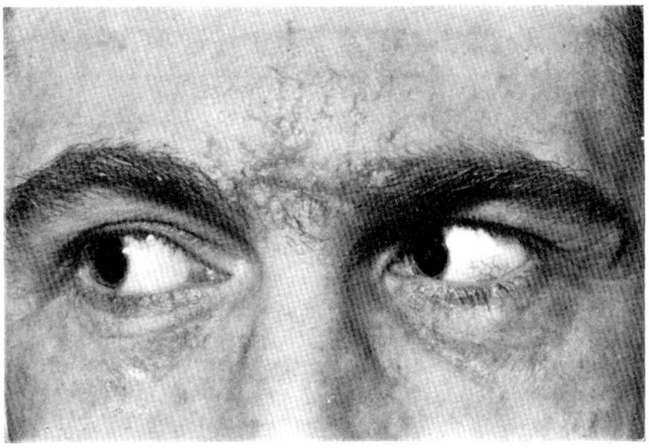

Fig. 8.8 a Left lateral rectus paresis: gaze right

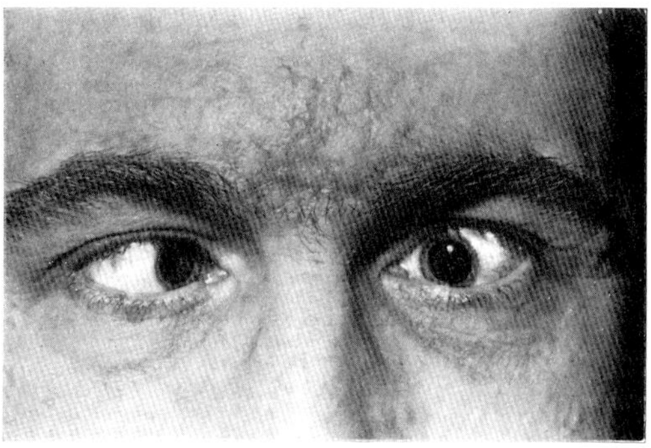

Fig. 8.8 b Left lateral rectus paresis: gaze left

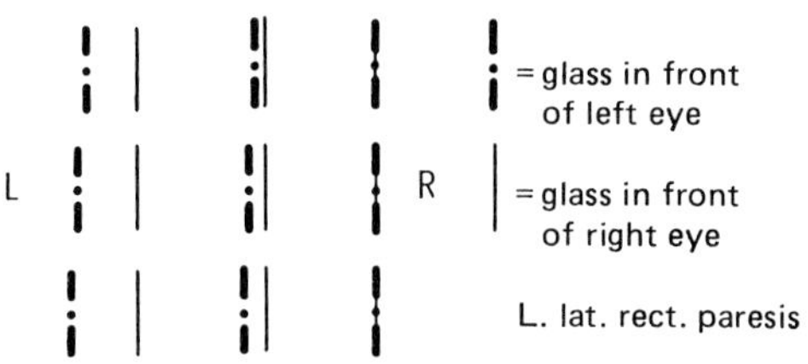

Fig. 8.8 c Diplopic images with left lateral rectus paresis

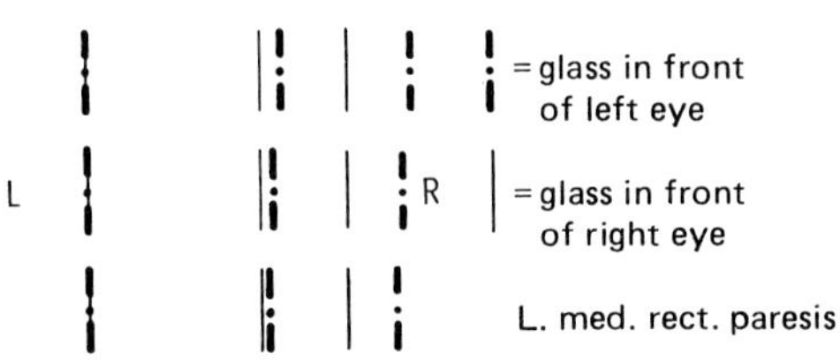

Fig. 8.9 Diplopic images with left medial rectus paresis

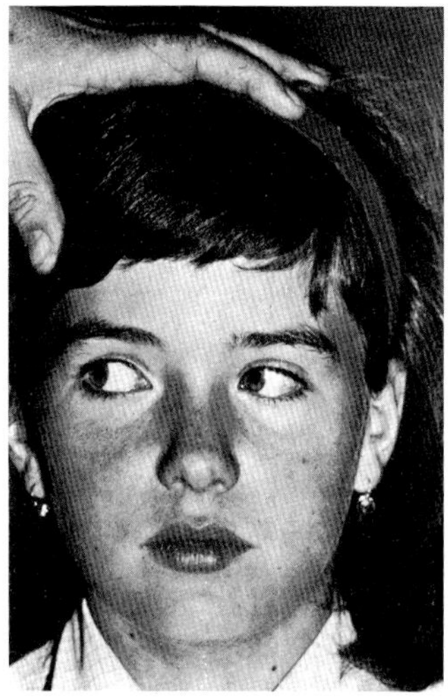

Fig. 8.10 a
Left superior rectus paresis: gaze right and up (♀ 10 yrs.)

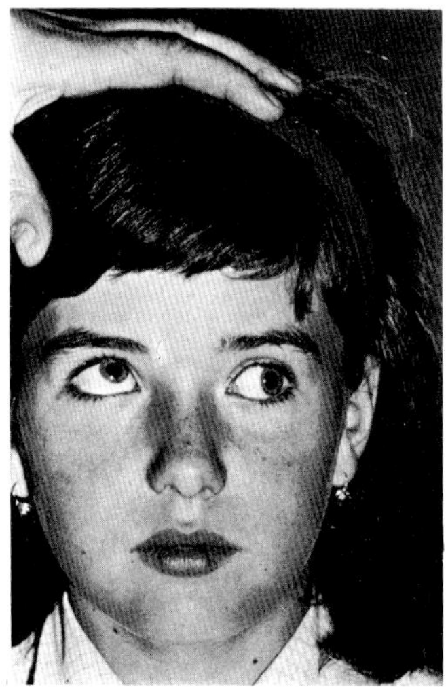

Fig. 8.10 b
Left superior rectus paresis: gaze left and up (♀ 10 yrs.)

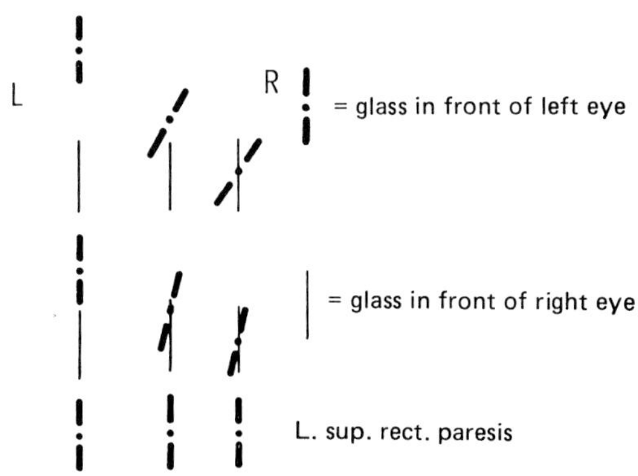

Fig. 8.10 c Diplopic images with left superior rectus paresis

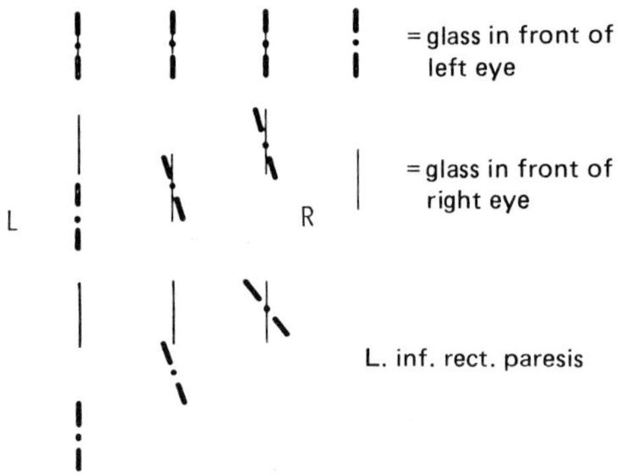

Fig. 8.11 Double images with left inferior rectus paresis

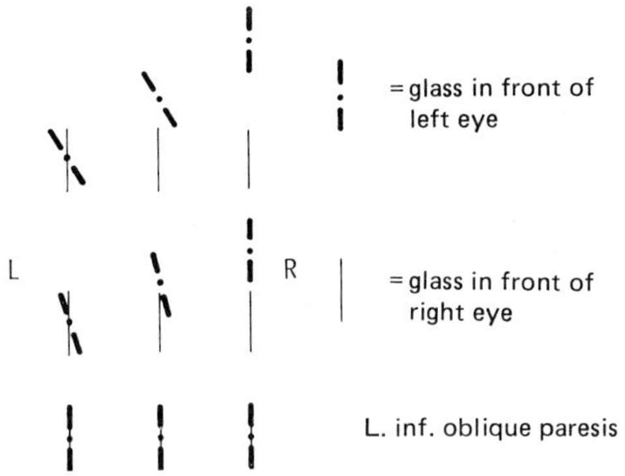

Fig. 8.12 c Double images in inferior oblique paresis, left eye

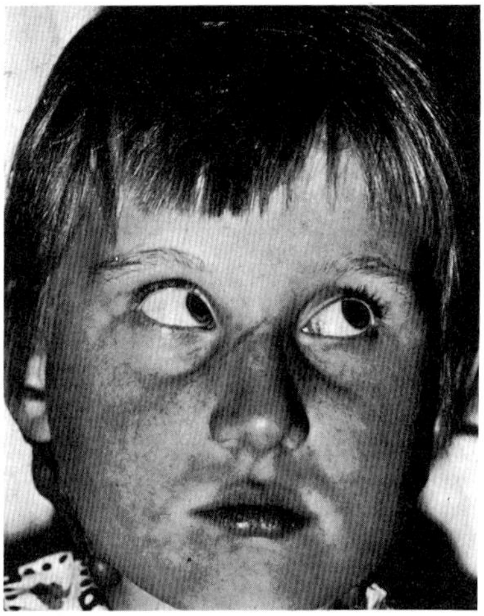

Fig. 8.12 a Left inferior oblique paresis: gaze up and to the left (♀ 6 yrs.)

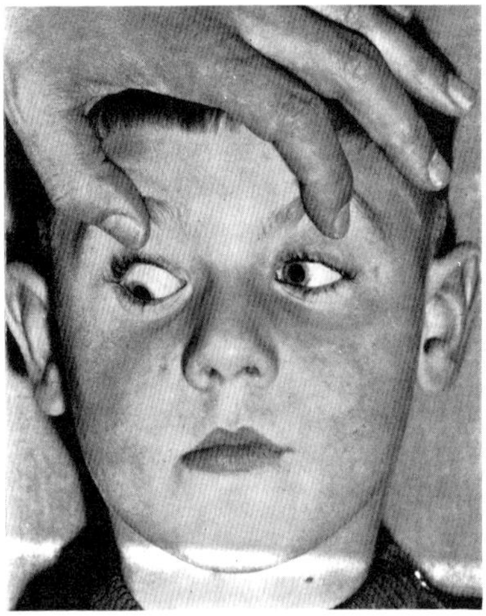

Fig. 8.13 a Left superior oblique paresis: gaze down and right (♂ 8 yrs.)

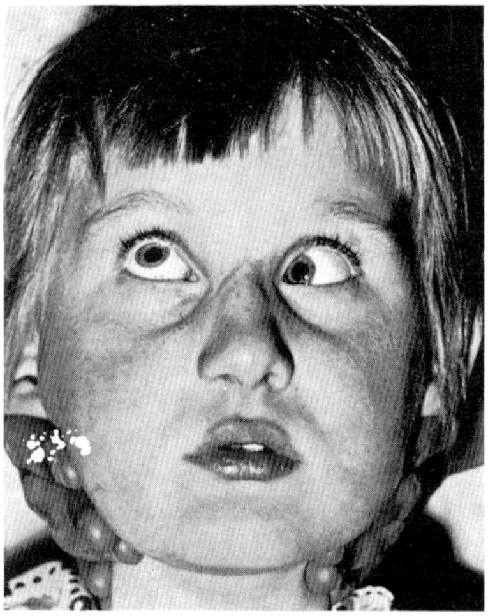

Fig. 8.12 b Left inferior oblique paresis: gaze up and right (♀ 6 yrs.)

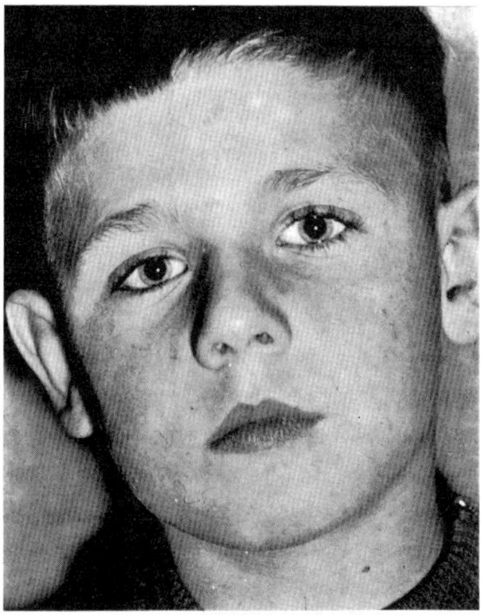

Fig. 8.13 b Left superior oblique paresis: head is turned and tilted to the right, the chin is depressed

1. **Paresis of the lateral rectus** (abducens): The paretic eye lags when gazing to the respective side (Figs. 8.8 a, 8.8 b). The separation of uncrossed double images increases on gaze to the paretic side (Fig. 8.8 c). Head turn is to the left when the left external rectus muscle is paretic.

2. **Paresis of the medial rectus:** The paretic eye lags to the respective side on inward gaze while crossed diplopic separation of images increases on gaze to the paretic side (Fig. 8.9). With paresis of the left internal rectus muscle, head turn is to the right.

3. **Superior rectus paresis:** The paretic eye lags on gaze up and out (Figs. 8.10 a, 8.10 b). There is a failure of the normal cyclorotation when gazing upward and inward; the double image of the paretic eye is tilted (Fig. 8.10 c). In paresis of the left superior rectus muscle, the head turn is to the left and the chin is elevated.

4. **Inferior rectus muscle paresis:** The paretic eye lags on gaze down and out. The normal cyclorotation on gaze down and inward is absent and the double image of the paretic eye is tilted (12 o'clock meridian out) (Fig. 8.11). With paresis of the left inferior rectus muscle, the head is turned to the left and the chin is depressed.

5. **Paresis of the inferior oblique:** The paretic eye lags on gaze up and in (Figs. 8.12 a, 8.12 b). The normal cyclorotation on gaze up and out is absent. The image of the paretic eye tilts out (12 o'clock meridian). Diplopia is greatest on gaze up and in (Fig. 8.12 c). With paresis of left inferior oblique the face turns to the right, the head tilts to the left, and the chin is elevated.

6. **Paresis of the superior oblique** (M. trochlearis): The paretic eye lags on downward and inward gaze (Figs. 8.13 a, 8.13 b). The normal incyclotorsion on gaze down and out is absent, while the double image of the paretic eye is tilted inward (12 o'clock meridian). The distance between the double images is greatest on gaze down and in (Fig. 8.13 d). With paresis of the left superior oblique, the head is turned right and tilted toward the right shoulder, the chin is depressed. On forced head tilt to the side of the superior oblique paresis, the paretic eye elevates (Bielschowsky test) (Fig. 8.13 c). A secondary overaction of the inferior oblique occurs when a paresis of the superior oblique is present.

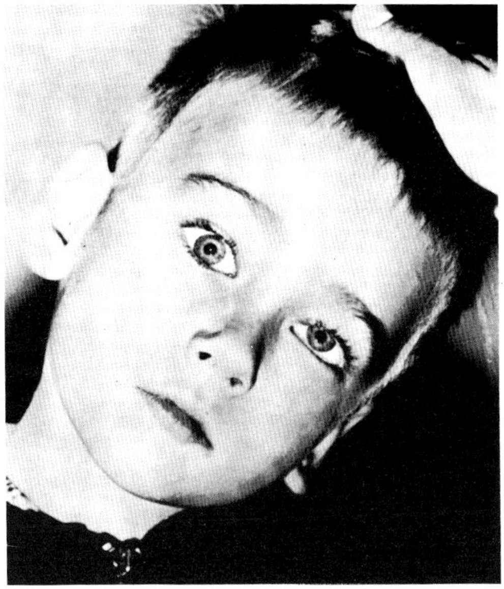

Fig. 8.13 c Left superior oblique paresis: Bielschowsky test = when the head is tilted to the paretic side, the paretic eye deviates up

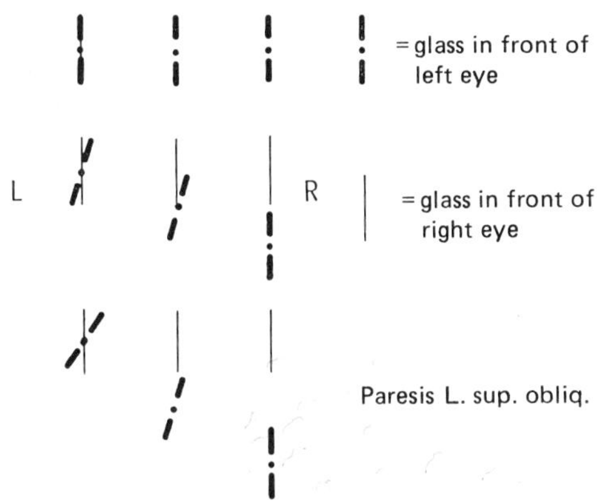

Fig. 8.13 d Double images in left superior oblique paresis

The most common ocular cause of torticollis is a congenital paresis of the fourth nerve with overaction of the inferior oblique.

7. **Paralysis of the oculomotor nerve:** Behind a ptotic upper lid, the eye is turned down (intact superior oblique) and out (intact lateral rectus). If the pupil is nonreactive and accommodation is lost, the internal eye muscles are also involved and total (complete) palsy of the third nerve exists.

Ophthalmoplegia

Ophthalmoplegia externa is a paresis of extraocular muscles. Primary etiologies of acute ophthalmoplegia include (Abrahamson and Horwitz 1954):

1. Vascular diseases (aneurysms of the internal carotid artery or circle of Willis; diabetic vasculopathy);
2. Trauma with orbital fractures or hematomas in the orbit;
3. Intracranial neoplasm;
4. Orbital cellulitis secondary to sinusitis;
5. Ophthalmoplegic migraine;
6. Myasthenia gravis.

Marcus-Gunn Phenomenon

The Marcus-Gunn phenomenon consists of slight ptosis and, at times, paresis of the superior rectus muscle. On opening the mouth or deviating the lower jaw to the unaffected side, the ptotic lid will elevate **(jaw winking)** (Fig. 10.6). The lid, therefore, alternately opens and closes when the individual chews, yells, laughs, etc. An oculomotor-facial-trigeminal synkinesis is present; the origin is unknown. It may be nuclear, supranuclear, or a congenital misdirection of nerve fibers (for review of the literature, see Kanter 1955).

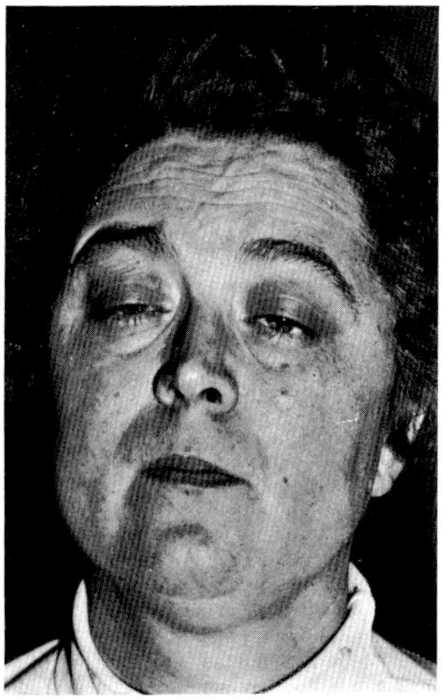

Fig. 8.14 Chronic progressive external ophthalmoplegia, facies myopathica

Myopathies

The following myopathies of the extraocular muscles can be differentiated (Papst 1969; Davidson 1970):

Chronic Progressive External Ophthalmoplegia with Degeneration of Muscle Fibers

Ocular Myositis

1. Acute (exophthalmic ocular myositis)
2. Chronic (oligosymptomatic ocular myositis)
3. Neuromyositis

Endocrine Myopathy (dysthyroid, diencephalo-hypophyseal)

Ocular Myotonia associated with changes in the skeletal muscles

1. Myotonia congenita
2. Myotonic dystrophy

Diseases of the extraocular muscles simulating myopathy (pseudomyopathies)

Ocular Myasthenia

Electromyography and biopsy are the best ways to differentiate the various external ocular myopathies (Papst 1969). Despite little muscular reaction, electromyography shows intense electrical activity. The various myopathies include (Papst 1969; Huber 1971):

Chronic Progressive External Ophthalmoplegia

This was formerly known as ophthalmoplegia externa chronica progressiva nuclearis of von Graefe. The hallmark of this disease is a slowly progressing paralysis of the extraocular muscles with bilateral ptosis and normal pupillary reaction (Figs. 8.14, 10.7). Onset is between the ages of ten and twenty; it progresses slowly for decades. The facial muscles become myopathic, thereby leading to a lack of emotional expression. The head is tilted back; the forehead is wrinkled in an effort to overcome the ptosis. Inheritance is variable (Best 1931; Erdbrink 1957; Esslen and Papst 1961), and can be sex-linked (Beckett and Netsky 1953). The etiology is an increasing dystrophy of the extraocular muscles (Kiloh and Nevin 1951; Schwarz and Lin 1954; Esslen and Papst 1961). Aside from the progressive external ophthalmoplegia and facial myopathy (facies myopathica), no other neurologic signs are present. The purely muscular nature of the disease is seen with electromyography and on biopsy (Papst et al. 1958). On maximum innervational effort, there is a great deal of electromyographic activity without any clinical sign of eye movement. EMG amplitude is diminished. Electromyographic evidence indicates that this is a primary muscle dystrophy.

Ocular Myositis

Acute exophthalmic myositis includes pain, diplopia, unilateral exophthalmos, edema of the lid and conjunctiva as well as paresis of extraocular muscles unrelated to nerve distribution. Many of these cases are probably due to inflammatory pseudotumor. An allergic or immune reaction may be involved. Scleritis, iridocyclitis, inflammatory retinal detachment and neuritis are frequent sequelae. Elevated temperature, increased erythrocyte sedimentation rate and leukocytosis are frequent. The illness tends to recur.
In chronic (oligosymptomatic) ocular myositis, virtually no signs of inflammation are present. Extraocular muscles innervated by various nerves become paretic in both eyes. The paralysis may last for weeks or months and remits spontaneously. Permanent disturbances of movement may remain. The disease resembles ocular myasthenia, but it fails to respond to Prostigmin. There is a discrepancy in myositis between the strong motor input detected electromyographically and the lack of resultant ocular movement. In contrast to dystrophy of the ocular muscles, *no decline in EMG amplitude* is found.

Endocrine Myopathy

Endocrine myopathy is associated with greater or lesser degrees of exophthalmos. Histologically, there is a marked thickening of extraocular muscles with edema and a mononuclear cell infiltration (myositis). Later fibrosis sets in. Diplopia may precede, follow, or be unassociated with, exophthalmos. The most common involvement is the inability to elevate the eye. The medial (and lateral) recti simulating abducens paresis are the next most commonly involved. All extraocular muscles may be involved. Other typical symptoms include: lid lag (Graefe's sign), lid retraction (Dalrymple's sign), stare and infrequent blinking (Stellwag's sign), and convergence paresis (Möbius' sign) (see page 339).

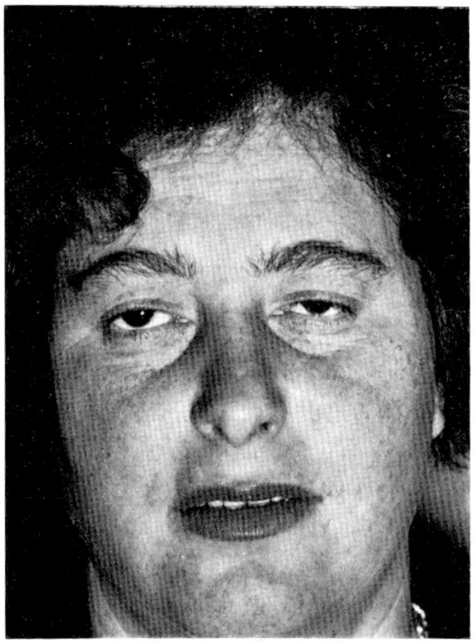

Fig. 8.15 Myasthenia gravis (♀ 32 yrs.)

Ocular Myotonia

Myotonic dystrophy (Steinert) rarely leads to limitation of ocular movement. Ptosis and orbicularis weakness are far more common. In *myotonia congenita* (Thomsen) the myotonic reaction may involve the levator of the lid. On down gaze it is unable to relax rapidly enough.

Myopathy-like Afflictions of the Extraocular Muscles

These may occur with trauma, injury, hematomas, trichinosis, amyloidosis, collagen disorders (dermatomyositis, lupus erythematosus, rheumatoid arthritis).

Myasthenia Gravis (Erb-Goldflam)

In about half the cases, the onset of myasthenia gravis begins with ocular symptoms, specifically ptosis and diplopia (Fig. 8.15). This is followed by paresis of individual muscles, then groups of muscles in either one or both eyes. Myasthenia may appear at any age, including infancy. Symptoms are worse in the evening than in the morning (fatigability). Pupillary reactions and accommodation are normal. Ten percent of all cases begin before puberty (Manz and Schmidt 1970). The Tensilon test is diagnostic, especially when carried out with electromyography. Ten to fifteen seconds after injection of 5 to 10 mg of Tensilon (edrophonium chloride), an increase in the amplitude and frequency of discharges is recorded for several minutes. This is correlated with an improvement in ocular motility and distinguishes myasthenia from similar disorders such as ocular muscle dystrophies, chronic myositis, or neurogenic paresis where the Tensilon test is negative. Eye muscle disorders which clinically resemble myasthenia can be produced by carcinomatosis, intoxications (mustard gas, tobacco, uremia, botulism), and central nervous system disorders (encephalitis epidemica, Wernicke's polyneuritis).

Neurogenic Oculomotor Muscle Disturbances

In these disorders, motor units for innervation cannot be measured electromyographically. Days or weeks after denervation, the denervated ocular muscle will show fibrillation potentials which are independent of any voluntary innervation.

Etiologies of Extraocular Muscle Paresis

The etiology of neurogenic paralysis of the extraocular muscles is primarily nuclear, nerve, or muscle damage after inflammation (infection, starvation, vitamin deficiencies), vascular disorders, expanding intracranial lesions, progressive degenerative disorders (MS) and trauma (Remky 1963). Twelve to eighteen days after infection with ophthalmic *zoster*, neurogenic extraocular muscle paresis may occur. Isolated muscles or groups of muscles may be affected. Total ophthalmoplegia with paresis of the internal ocular muscles may occur (Priggert 1957). A variety of *intoxicants* can produce external and internal ophthalmoplegia: substances poisoning the protoplasm of nerve cells (mercury, manganese, lead, fluoride, and also snake, bee and scorpion venom), hematotoxic agents (carbon monoxide), lipid solvents (halogen and mercury compounds), carbon disulfide, and benzene (Heydenreich 1966).

In chlorine dioxide poisoning, pupillary and abducens paresis are primary symptoms. Bromide poisoning can cause both internal and external ophthalmoplegia. Chronic thallium poisoning leads to optic neuritis as well as ophthalmoplegia. Carbon monoxide poisoning can cause severe central nervous system disturbances with diplopia, neuritis, ophthalmoplegia, paresis of accommodation as well as micropsia or macropsia. Carbon disulfide poisoning may mimic the symptoms of multiple sclerosis. Optic neuritis, muscle paresis, and loss of pupillary afferent reflex can occur. The symptoms of hydrocyanism include: fixed pupils, nystagmus, blindness, dizziness, vomiting, and muscle cramps (see page 121, 316).

A number of toxic agents are recognized as **occupational hazards** (Merté, 1969, 1972):

Arsenic: External and internal ophthalmoplegia, optic nerve and retinal damage.
Lead: Internal and external ophthalmoplegia, optic neuritis.
Mercury: External ophthalmoplegia, nystagmus.
Saltpeter, nitroglycerine: Ophthalmoplegia.
Carbon disulfide: External and internal ophthalmoplegia, nystagmus, optic neuritis.
Manganese: Weakness of convergence.
Caisson disease – "the bends" – (rapid reduction of atmospheric pressure): extraocular muscle paresis, ptosis, nystagmus, fixed pupils, lid and retinal hemorrhages can occur.

Medications of various sorts may lead to dysfunction of ocular muscles, e.g., isoniazid = INH, streptomycin. Furan derivatives (furaltadone, nitrofurantoin) used for urinary tract infections can cause ophthalmoplegia and nystagmus (Dralands and Garin 1972). Vincristine and vinblastine are described as causing paresis of ocular muscles as well as optic neuritis and corneal hypoesthesia (Albert et al. 1967).

Teratogenic agents, especially *thalidomide* (see page 245), produce abducens paresis or occasionally oculomotor nerve paresis. Horizontal gaze paralysis in Duane's syndrome has also been reported.

Etiologies of Oculomotor Nerve Pareses

In *thalidomide teratogenesis* the stage of gestation when the drug was taken is directly related to the type of defect (Papst 1963). Disorders of ocular movements, often with facial nerve paresis (Fig. 8.16 a), aniridia, and malformation of the ears (Fig. 8.16 b) are related to the ingestion of thalidomide 35 to 39 days after the last menstruation. When taken during the fortieth to forty-second day of gestation, microphthalmia and anophthalmos with phocomelia of arms and legs is more common. Colobomata of the iris and choroid are also seen.

Congenital anomalies of ocular movements produced by thalidomide include: facial paresis (Fig. 8.16), specifically Möbius' syndrome; sixth nerve paresis; paresis of the oculomotor nerve; horizontal gaze palsy; and Duane's syndrome.

Elevated intracranial pressure will, at the onset, irritate pupillary fibers and cause miosis. With further increase in damage, mydriasis occurs. The root of the oculomotor nerve may be pressed against the bone as it enters the cavernous sinus (edge of the clivus) or against the posterior cerebral artery (Fischer-Brügge 1951). Supratentorial pressure from a subdural hematoma, temporal lobe tumor or supraclinoid aneurysm can press the oculomotor nerve against the edge of the clivus and, thereby, damage its blood supply. Clinically, this results in what Fischer-Brügge calls the "clivus edge syndrome." First, there is a brief period of miosis after which the pupil is dilated and reacts sluggishly. Various extraocular muscles served by the oculomotor nerve become involved. Painful damage of the trigeminal nerve and loss of consciousness are possible. There appears to be a strong relationship between the "clivus edge syndrome" and ophthalmoplegic migraine (Remky 1954) since localized dilatation and swelling of the *posterior cerebral artery* with compression of the third nerve is considered to be a mechanism for ophthalmoplegic migraine (recurrent third nerve paresis with headaches). Aneurysms of the posterior communicating artery are, however, more likely responsible.

Basilar involvement of the third nerve can also occur with inflammation (lues, tuberculosis, purulent meningitis), tumors, basilar skull fractures.

Traumatic paresis of the oculomotor nerve can be caused by nuclear lesions, damage to the nerve root, or compression of the nerve against the clivus.

Due to the proximity of the oculomotor nerve to the pyramidal tract, lesions in the ventral midbrain will lead to Weber's syndrome: ipsi-

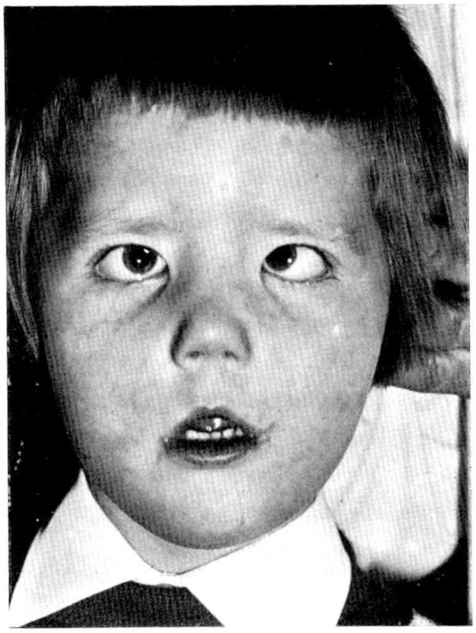

Fig. 8.16 a Thalidomide (Contergan) damage with bilateral facial and abducens nerve paresis (Moebius' syndrome) (♀ 4 yrs.)

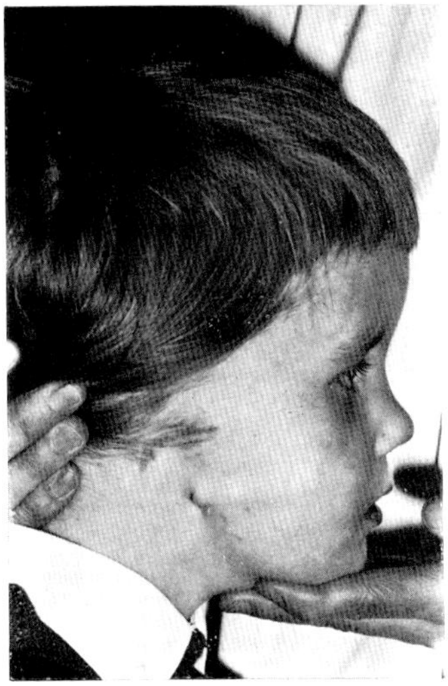

Fig. 8.16 b Thalidomide (Contergan) damage with maldevelopment of the outer ear and Moebius' syndrome) (♀ 4 yrs.)

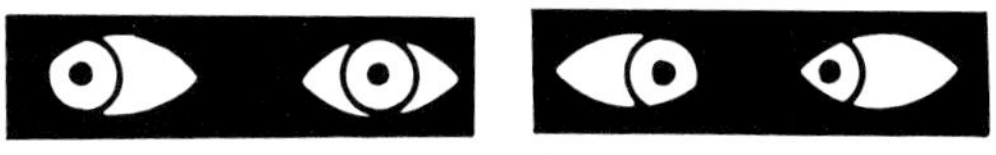

a b

Fig. 8.17 a–b Ophthalmoplegia internuclearis on left side: a) at looking to the right; b) at convergence.

lateral oculomotor nerve palsy with contralateral spastic hemiplegia (face, arm, leg).

Ptosis and *pupillary disturbances* are among the *first signs of progressive damage to the oculomotor nerve. Progressive damage to the oculomotor nucleus*, however, first involves the extraocular muscles and the ptosis occurs last, "the final curtain".

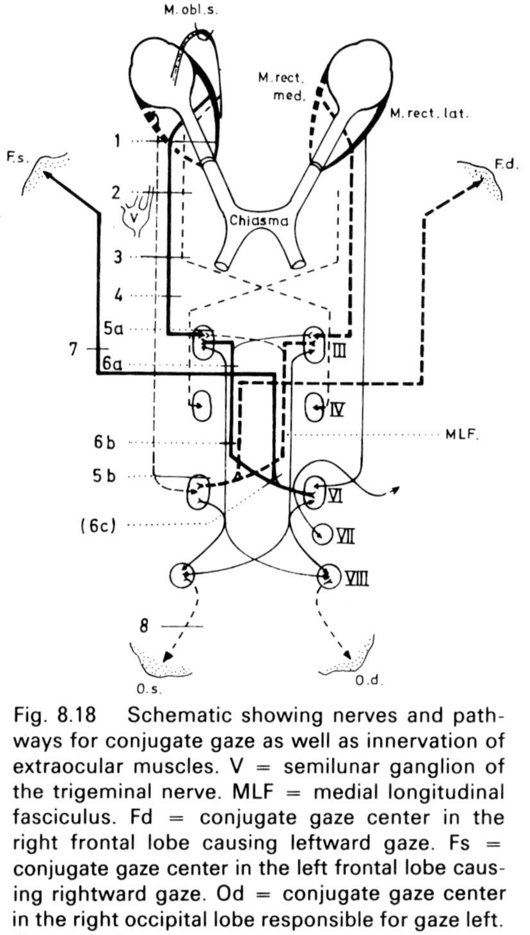

Fig. 8.18 Schematic showing nerves and pathways for conjugate gaze as well as innervation of extraocular muscles. V = semilunar ganglion of the trigeminal nerve. MLF = medial longitudinal fasciculus. Fd = conjugate gaze center in the right frontal lobe causing leftward gaze. Fs = conjugate gaze center in the left frontal lobe causing rightward gaze. Od = conjugate gaze center in the right occipital lobe responsible for gaze left. Os = conjugate gaze center in the left occipital lobe responsible for gaze right. **1**, lesion in the orbit involving one or more muscles or nerves; **2**, lesion involving nerves in or at the superior orbital fissure; **3**, lesion of nerves at the base of the skull; **4**, lesion involving one or both oculomotor nerves in the interpeduncular fossa; **5 a**, lesion of root or nucleus of III; **5 b**, lesions of root or nucleus of VI; **6 a** and **6 b**, lesion in the left MLF: supranuclear paresis, left medial rectus; **6 c**, lesion in the (posterior) left MLF: loss of all rightward movement except on convergence; **7**, lesion in pathway from left frontal lobe center for conjugate gaze: eyes deviated left unable to gaze right; **8**, damage to oculomotor pathways in the optic radiations: loss of following movements and optokinetic nystagmus

Congenital aneurysms occur mainly in the circle of Willis. They frequently act like pituitary tumors. Spontaneous subarachnoidal hemorrhages are usually caused by leaking aneurysms. Overall mortality is 45 percent with the first and 70 percent with the second episode. Four-fifths of all ocular motility disturbances caused by aneurysms involve the *oculomotor nerve*.

Unless *complete remission of total nerve paresis* occurs within the first few weeks after onset, it is not to be expected. *Misdirection of regenerating* third nerve fibers is common if the first signs of remission occur after three or more months. Association movements result. Lid retraction with adduction of the paretic eye (Fuchs' sign) is typical (Figs. 8.19 a, 8.19 b, 8.19 c). The same may occur on down gaze (pseudo-Graefe sign) (inferior rectus fibers go to the levator of the lid). Adduction, or occasionally abduction or pupillary constriction, occurs with vertical gaze. Bulbus retraction on looking upward by simultaneous retraction of superior and inferior recti has been described (Holland 1966). The Marcus-Gunn phenomenon can be explained in the same way (see page 52).

Etiology of Sixth Nerve Paresis

Sixth nerve paresis is the most *common cranial nerve involvement* in *brain tumors* or with *elevated intracranial pressure*. The abducens nerves are particularly vulnerable due to their long course and sharp angle over the petrous ridge through Dorello's canal. Gradenigo's syndrome, consisting of trigeminal pain with abducens and facial nerve paresis is usually caused by an ostitis or periostitis in the petrous bone. This occurs with mastoiditis and middle ear infections. Meningitis, tumors, basilar skull fractures, and elevated intracranial pressure are all causes of sixth nerve palsy.

Cerebellopontine angle tumors (acoustic neuroma, meningioma, glioma) cause abducens palsy with inner ear symptoms, facial paresis, corneal hypoesthesia, nystagmus, cerebellar signs and bilateral papilledema. *Traumatic abducens paresis* occurs with fractures in the petrous pyramid, by compression against the inferior anterior cerebellar artery, hematomas, and edema.

Due to the proximity of the facial nerve and abducens nucleus, damage to the abducens nucleus is usually associated with ipsilateral *facial nerve paralysis*.

Atherosclerosis or *vascular diseases* in *diabetes mellitus* frequently cause nuclear oculomotor and abducens palsy. *Encephalomyelitis, tuberculous meningitis, lues* and *poliomyelitis* are other causes of oculomotor palsies, especially of the abducens nerve.

Orbital Limitations of Eye Movements

From trauma (see blow-out fractures, page 62).

Orbital tumors rarely cause nerve damage, but they do displace and mechanically restrict muscles. The direction of globe displacement is indicative of the tumor location. Exophthalmos need not be present for tumors to restrict motion.

Cysticercus or Echinococcus infestations of the orbit produce pain, exophthalmos, and muscle paresis early in the disease. Papilledema is a later manifestation.

Inflammatory pseudotumor can cause a similar picture but would respond favorably to corticosteroid therapy (see page 350).

Congenital Loss of Motility

Duane's retraction syndrome — Superior oblique tendon sheath syndrome (Brown's syndrome) — Congenital ptosis — Möbius' syndrome (bilateral congenital nuclear palsy) — Ullrich Turner syndrome -- Status dysraphicus — Synkinesis.

Congenital lack of motility of individual muscles or muscle groups may be caused by muscular aplasia, abnormal insertion of muscles, or lesions in nerve nuclei. With congenital lesions, diplopia is not appreciated. There is a compensatory head posture in about one-half the cases. This is particularly true of congenital superior oblique palsies. Head tilt or turn may persist even when binocular vision is lost.

The Stilling-Türk-Duane **retraction syndrome** is particularly common. There is a lack of abduction (Fig. 8.20 a). On adduction the globe retracts and the palpebral fissure narrows (Fig. 8.20 b). The etiology was traditionally thought

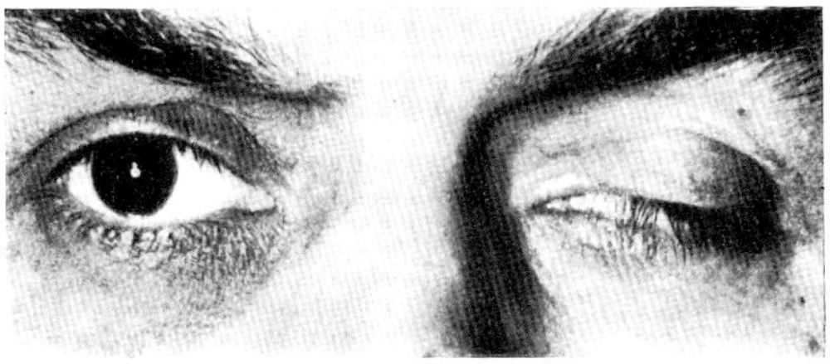

Fig. 8.19 a Long-standing third nerve paresis on the left: gaze straight ahead includes ptosis

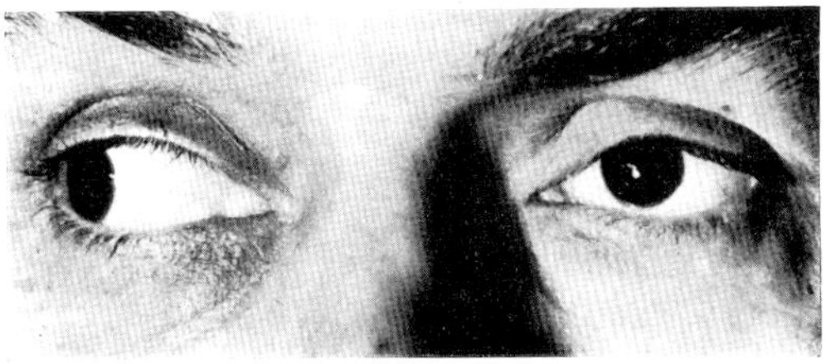

Fig. 8.19 b Long-standing third nerve paresis on the left: on gazing right aberrantly regenerated nerve fibers from the medial rectus cause left lid elevation (synkinesis)

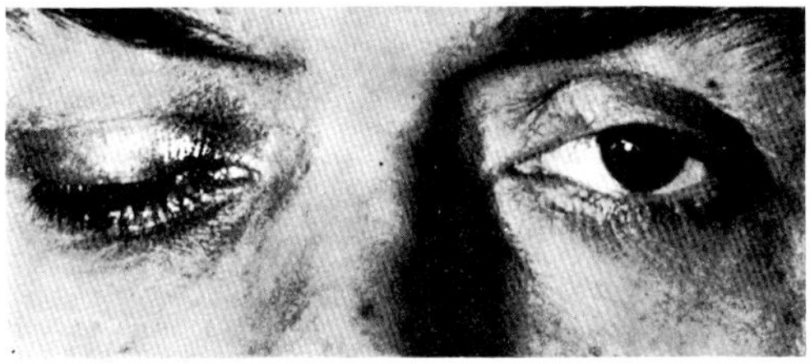

Fig. 8.19 c Long-standing oculomotor paresis on the left: on down gaze the upper lid retracts (pseudo-Graefe sign) owing to a misdirection of inferior rectus nerve fibers to the levator palpebrae (synkinesis)

to be a fibrous anomaly of the muscle (Weekers et al. 1956). Recent research indicates that innervation is paradoxical (Papst 1960; Huber 1969; Burian and v. Noorden 1974). On adduction, both the external and internal rectus muscles are activated. This leads to retraction of the globe and narrowed palpebral fissure. On abduction the lateral rectus muscle fails to fire = Duane's syndrome I. Synergistic = paradoxic innervation usually involving the lateral rectus and any one or a combination of other extraocular muscles on the same side.

Duane's syndrome II (Malbran) consists of a limitation of adduction with retraction of the globe and of the palpebral fissure narrowing. Abduction, on the other hand, is intact. Electromyography shows the lateral rectus fires maximally in both abduction and adduction.

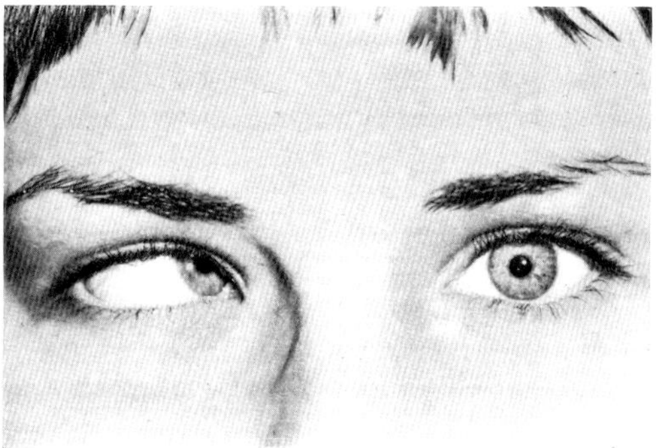

Fig. 8.20 a Retraction syndrome of Stilling-Türk-Duane on the left: gaze left = lack of abduction with large lid fissure (♀ 21 yrs.)

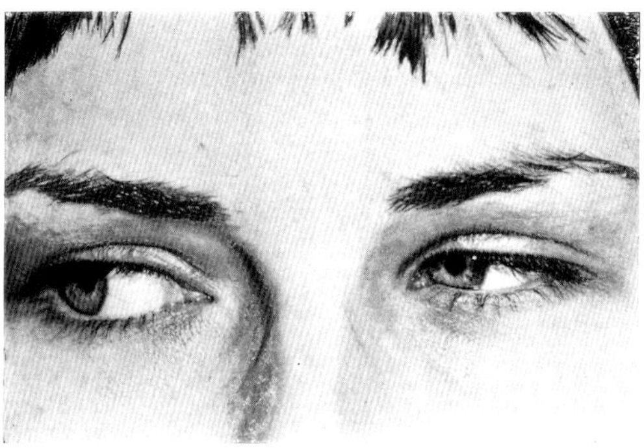

Fig. 8.20 b Stilling-Türk-Duane retraction syndrome on the left: gaze right = limited adduction with retraction and narrowing of the left palpebral fissure (♀ 21 yrs.)

Additional rare paradoxical synergistic innervations (not real palsies) of muscles innervated by different nerves imitate a nerve palsy; for example, simultaneous innervation of the lateral rectus, with the inferior or superior rectus or other muscles innervated by the third nerve (for references, see Papst 1966).

The **superior oblique tendon sheath syndrome** (Brown's syndrome) simulates inferior oblique paresis (limitation of elevation on adduction [Fig. 8.21]). This is caused by anomalies of the superior oblique tendon and its sheath which limit inferior oblique action. Of importance diagnostically is the fact that forced duction is negative with true inferior oblique paresis but positive in Brown's syndrome. Papst and Stein (1969) found a false synergistic innervation (analogous to Duane's syndrome) between the superior and inferior obliques in Brown's syndrome.

Unilateral or bilateral **congenital ptosis** with inability to elevate the ptotic eye (double elevated palsy) is not uncommon.

Möbius' syndrome consists of a bilateral sixth and seventh nerve palsy (Fig. 8.16 a). This can be associated with malformations of the pinna (Fig. 8.16 b), deformities of the skull, mental retardation, and difficulty in chewing.

Turner's syndrome (Ullrich-Turner syndrome) is usually seen in females with 45 chromosomes (one X is missing). It is associated with congenital palsy of cranial nerves and a webbed neck (pterygium colli) (Wollensak et al. 1962).

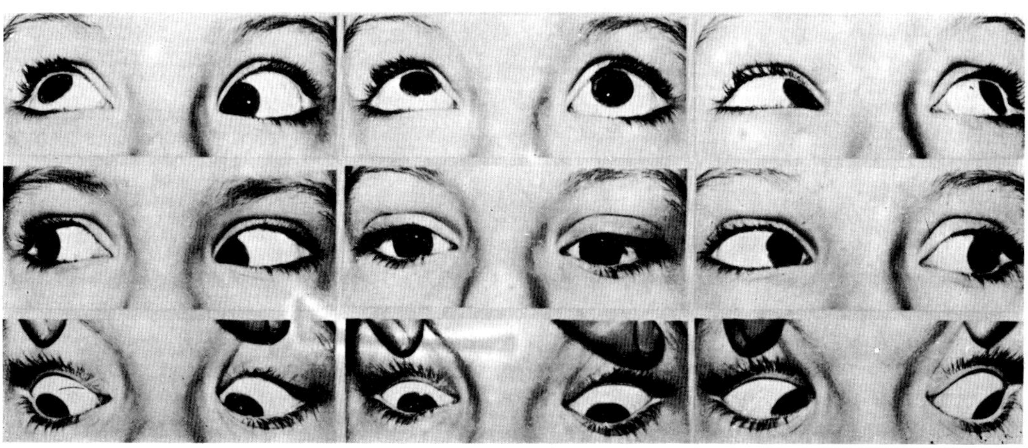

Fig. 8.21 Brown's syndrome on the left (♂ 5 yrs.) = simulating left inferior oblique paresis

Ocular findings with **status dysraphicus** include Horner's syndrome, heterochromia, facial abducens and trigeminal nerve paresis. *Congenital* or *acquired oculomotor nerve palsies* can result in misdirection of nerves leading to **synkinesis** (see page 56 [Fig. 8.18 a, b, c]). Such an aberrant innervation of the levator palpebrae could be one cause of the Marcus-Gunn phenomenon (see page 52) (Fig. 10.6).

Gaze Paresis (Supranuclear Lesion)

Bilateral horizontal gaze palsy — Associated internuclear ophthalmoplegia — Horizontal and vertical gaze palsy — Gaze nystagmus — Skew deviation (Hertwig-Magendie) — Oculogyric crisis — Convergence — Divergence paresis — Conjugate deviation — Etiology of gaze palsies.

With bilateral **paresis of conjugate gaze,** there is inability to look to either side. The most important supranuclear associated palsies are horizontal due to pontine lesions and vertical due to lesions near the superior colliculi (see page 59). **Internuclear ophthalmoplegia** is differentiated into anterior and posterior lesions. Posterior internuclear ophthalmoplegia, as used by Lutz, implies normal adduction but abnormal abduction. This is so rare that its very existence is disputed. Cogan, therefore, uses the term posterior internuclear ophthalmoplegia when convergence is normal, and anterior internuclear ophthalmoplegia when there is associated involvement of convergence with paralysis of the medial rectus on attempted lateral gaze. The lesion is on the side of the involved medial rectus (Fig. 8.17 a, b).
Internuclear ophthalmoplegia may be unilateral or bilateral. The bilateral lesions are predominantly demyelinating in nature. Symptoms typically found in association with internuclear ophthalmoplegia include (Kommerell 1971):
a) Dissociated nystagmus (*nystagmus ataxique* in the French literature). The nystagmus is usually uniocular and occurs only in the abducting eye on lateral gaze.
b) Ocular dysmetria in the adducting eye. This consists of end point oscillatory movements before the object is finally fixated.
c) Slowing of adduction on lateral gaze.
Internuclear lesions may also produce disturbances of disconjugate gaze. *Paralysis of convergence:* While *convergence* is impossible the patient is able to adduct the medial rectus. With *paralysis of divergence,* the external recti work normally on voluntary gaze to either side but fail to relax on distance gaze; the result is convergent strabismus.
Internuclear disconjugate gaze palsies can be produced by encephalitis, multiple sclerosis, tumors, elevated intracranial tension, intoxications, acute effects of alcohol and also by hysteria (Remky 1971). The Kestenbaum distance test is helpful for the differential diagnosis between disconjugate gaze palsies and muscle paresis:
With paretic muscles, diplopia is proportional to the distance of the object. If there is a paresis of convergence, diplopia will not decrease as rapidly as expected when the object is moved closer. The reverse occurs with paresis of divergence (Remky 1971).
Supranuclear **paresis of horizontal gaze** can be pontine (or cortical). **Vertical gaze palsy** implies a lesion in the region of the superior colliculus. Voluntary elevation of the eyes is impossible, but elevation occurs with passive doll's eye movement. *Vertical gaze paresis* (Parinaud's syndrome) caused by lesions in the region of the superior colliculi is frequently associated with impairment of the pupillary reaction and convergence (see page 324). The closer to the nucleus a supranuclear lesion is located, the more asymmetric the resulting defects. Vertical gaze paresis caused by a lesion in the vicinity of the nuclei will show elevation of the other eye when the paretic eye is fixing. With a supranuclear paresis of the medial rectus, normal convergence is retained (see page 55, Fig. 8.17) (Remky 1971).

Gaze-paretic nystagmus occurs with regression of the paralysis. Paresis of gaze could also be considered as incomplete nystagmus: the tonic divergence is not followed by redress movement. Conversely, nystagmus can be considered as incomplete gaze paresis where the tonic deviation is corrected for short periods (Remky 1971). Nystagmus may precede the paresis or remain as a postparetic symptom. Nystagmus can be diminished or even absent when gaze palsy is complete. The *etiology* lies in damage to the brain stem. This occurs with vascular lesions (basilar, posterior cerebral, vertebral, and inferior posterior cerebellar arteries), primary and metastatic tumors, and inflammatory processes.

Skew deviation (Hertwig-Magendie syndrome) is rare. The eye on the side of the lesion deviates downward; the other deviates upward. The etiology is an interruption of communicating pathways from the vestibular nuclei to the medial longitudinal fasciculus and nuclei of the ocular muscles.

Oculogyric crises are conjugate, spastic, vertical movements (visual spasms). They may last from a few seconds to 24 hours. They are caused by irritative lesions in the extrapyramidal system and occur with Jacksonian epilepsy, organic brain damage, encephalitis epidemica, schizophrenia, parkinsonism, ocular dysmetria, cyanide poisoning and ocular flutters (see page 65).

Phenothiazine can also produce oculogyric crises in which the eyes and entire head are spastically contorted.

Pure **divergence** or **convergence paresis** is a *dissociated gaze palsy*. In most instances one is not dealing with true convergence paresis but with exophoria, unilateral amblyopia, or a functional disorder. *Divergence paresis* causes uncrossed diplopia at distance which does not increase on lateral gaze; it decreases as the object moves closer, until crossed diplopia occurs. The onset of the diplopia is frequently sudden and may be associated with headaches. Cortical damage (with coma) may include a period of **déviation conjugée** where the patient "looks at the lesion."

Lesions in the pons may cause a conjugate deviation to the opposite side.

Etiology: Muscle and gaze palsies can be *congenital* (see page 54); the result of *trauma* (with or without bone fractures); hemorrhages; *meningitis* or *encephalitis*, especially encephalitis epidemica; multiple sclerosis; syphilis; and tuberculosis. A variety of infectious etiologies also exist, especially in children: measles, diphtheria (between the third and ninth week after onset), flu, polio (usually fourth to eleventh day), toxoplasmosis, malaria, leptospirosis, zoster ophthalmicus (second to third week), mumps, rheumatoid arthritis (usually sixth nerve), encephalitis epidemica and trichinosis. Vascular etiologies include *cavernous sinus thrombosis*, carotid artery thrombosis, and *intracranial aneurysms* (Rougier et al. 1962) as well as various benign and *malignant tumors*. On occasion it is seen with *myasthenia gravis* or *Graves' disease* as well as *intoxication* from various substances such as sulfonamide, streptomycin, digitalis, tetanus antitoxin (Sachsenweger 1966), botulism, lead and carbon monoxide (Remky 1971). Ophthalmoplegia occurs in pulseless disease (Takayasu's syndrome).

Paresis of Extraocular Muscles with Various Syndromes

Superior oblique fissure syndrome — Orbital apex syndrome — Blow-out fracture — Cavernous sinus syndrome — Pterygopalatine fossa syndrome — Gradenigo's syndrome — Cerebellopontine angle syndrome — Benedikt's syndrome and Weber's syndrome — Nothnagel's syndrome (bilateral partial oculomotor paresis with cerebellar ataxia) — Pontine syndromes — Quadrigeminal plate lesions — Ophthalmoplegic migraine.

The **superior orbital fissure syndrome** (Remky 1971; Huber 1971) (see page 339) is a combination of oculomotor, trochlear, and abducens nerve involvement which eventually leads to complete ophthalmoplegia. Hypoesthesia, (frontal branch of the trigeminal nerves), venous obstruction (superior ophthalmic vein), and miosis complete the picture. Exophthalmos with slight depression of the globe may occur.

In aneurysms, abducens paresis usually occurs early. Venous thrombosis can cause exophthalmos, papilledema, subconjunctival and subcutaneous hemorrhages.

The damage takes place in the area of the superior orbital fissure. The optic nerve may be involved. Etiologies include: tumors (sphenoid sinus meningiomas, metastatic), trauma (orbit, basilar and sphenoid wing fractures), carotid aneurysms of the cavernous sinus as well as inflammations (periostitis, orbital cellulitis resulting from sinusitis).

The orbital apex syndrome is very similar to the superior orbital fissure syndrome except that the optic nerve is primarily more involved; papilledema leading to optic atrophy, central or

Type of Paresis, Combination of Pareses	Probable Location of Responsible Lesion
Loss of voluntary gaze (after Sachsenweger)	
Total loss of voluntary gaze	Bilateral lesions in frontal lobes (foot of second frontal convolution, area 8)
Loss of horizontal gaze with retention of vertical gaze	Bilateral pontine lesion or unilateral lesion which also compresses contralateral centers
Paresis of conjugate gaze in one direction with conjugate deviation in the other direction. Reflex movement of fixation, convergence, and equilibrium are maintained	Lesion in cortex of one cerebral hemisphere (with transient symptoms) or subcortical (with permanent deviation)
Loss of voluntary and reflex gaze to one side with maintained vestibular function	Lesion in medial longitudinal fasciculus
Loss of voluntary as well as reflex gaze	Extensive pontine lesion involving medial longitudinal fasciculus and frequently third and fourth nerve nuclei
Conjugate paresis of upward gaze	Lesion in region of superior colliculi
Conjugate paresis of upward as well as horizontal gaze	Lesion in region of quadrigeminal plate
Loss of reflex gaze (after Sachsenweger)	
Loss of conjugate gaze in both directions	Lesion in area of posterior commissure
Loss of conjugate horizontal gaze with loss of convergence	Large pontine lesion
Loss of cortical reflex gaze with normal convergence	Lesion in pons, cortex (specifically subcortical)
Gaze paresis with loss of vestibular reflex movement	Not an isolated cortical gaze palsy; lesion includes pons

Type of Paresis and Combination of Paresis	Probable Location of Responsible Lesion
Combination of palsies (after Sachsenweger)	
Horizontal gaze paresis combined with abducens nerve palsy, with or without ipsilateral seventh nerve involvement	Lesion in lower pons
Gaze palsy with ipsilateral hemiplegia	Hemisphere disease
Gaze palsy with crossed hemiplegia	Lesion in pons
Gaze palsy, ipsilateral hemiplegia and seventh nerve palsy	Lesion in cortex and subcortex
Ipsilateral gaze palsy and seventh nerve palsy combined with contralateral hemiplegia	Pontine lesion
Gaze paresis and head turn in direction of gaze palsy in comatose patient	Cortical or subcortical lesion
Gaze palsy and head turn toward opposite side of gaze palsy in comatose patient	Lesion in pons, rarely in hemispheres

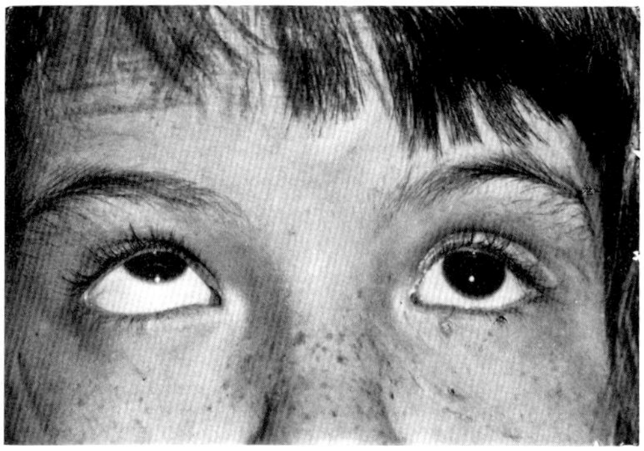

Fig. 8.22 a Left blowout fracture: upward gaze = marked restriction (♂ 11 yrs.)

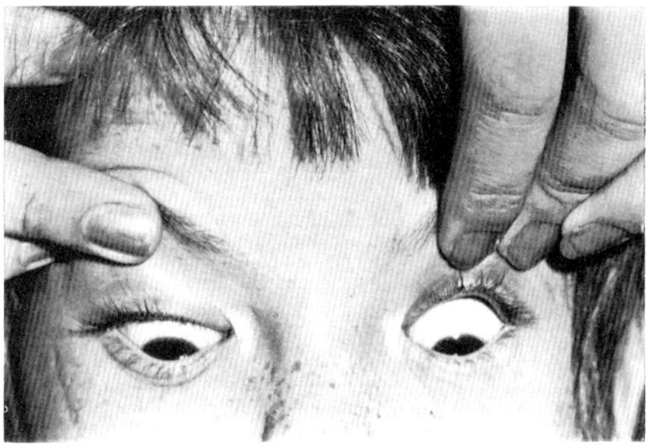

Fig. 8.22 b Left blowout fracture: downward gaze = minimal restriction (♂ 11 yrs.)

peripheral visual field loss. Exophthalmos (anterior displacement) with mechanical restriction of movement is more prominent than in the superior orbital fissure syndrome. Etiologic considerations are similar in the two syndromes.

Blow-out fractures (see page 339): Resulting from trauma (blows with fist, tennis ball, etc.). A sudden rise in intraorbital pressure causes an orbital floor fracture through which orbital tissues herniate and become entrapped. The result is endophthalmos of 3 to 4 mm and limitation of upward gaze (Fig. 8.22 a). Downward gaze is less restricted (Fig. 8.22 b). Forced duction is positive. Cutaneous sensitivity in the area of distribution of the inferior orbital nerve is frequently decreased. The roentgenogram may show a tissue mass in the maxillary antrum. Tomography is particularly helpful for showing the bony defect (Jones 1966). Orbitography using contrast material will also show the defect (Milauskas et al. 1966).

Cavernous sinus syndrome: Frequently caused by aneurysms in the region of the cavernous sinus.

Arteriovenous fistula will produce pulsating exophthalmos (Fig. 15.12), and orbital bruit. The differential diagnosis of pulsating exophthalmos includes *orbital varices* and *encephalocele*.

Ophthalmoplegia (cranial nerves III, V, VI) with trigeminal involvement may complete the picture of cavernous sinus syndrome. If orbital pulsations are absent, one can differentiate between a) anterior cavernous sinus syndrome where only the first branch of the trigeminal nerve is involved (same as the superior orbital fissure syndrome) and b) posterior cavernous sinus syndrome involving the entire motor and sensory branches of the trigeminal nerve. The causes of nonpulsating cavernous sinus syndrome include: metastatic carcinomas, malignant tumors originating at the base of the skull or from the nasopharynx, trigeminal neuromas, or inflammatory cavernous sinus thrombosis (fever, exophthalmos, chemosis).

Pterygopalatine fossa syndrome: Lesions in the pterygopalatine fossa cause anesthesia and neuralgia in the region of the second division of the trigeminal nerve, loss of lacrimation and, possibly, abducens nerve paresis. Etiology: tumors, injury, luetic periostitis.

Gradenigo's syndrome consists of acute otitis media with mastoiditis, ipsilateral *sixth nerve paresis* and *trigeminal neuralgia*. This may be combined with facial nerve paresis on the same side. Later, headaches as well as *oculomotor* and *trochlear nerve* involvement may be seen.

Etiology: acute otitis media, pachymeningitis, mastoiditis involving the apex of the pyramid, tuberculosis, lues.

The earliest signs of the **cerebellopontine angle syndrome** are corneal hypoesthesia and unilateral loss of hearing. Later, nystagmus, papilledema, facial and extraocular muscle palsies are added. It is usually caused by slowly growing tumors such as acoustic neuromas and sometimes by meningiomas.

A dorsal midbrain lesion causes **Benedikt's**

syndrome: ipsilateral oculomotor paresis, contralateral hemitremor (red nucleus). Occasionally contralateral hemianesthesia (lateral lemniscus) is included.

Weber's syndrome consists of oculomotor palsy and contralateral spastic hemiplegia. It is caused by a lesion in the region of the peduncle.

In **Nothnagel's syndrome,** the red nucleus, pyramidal tracts, and medial lemniscus are affected. Expansion of the lesion on the side of the oculomotor palsy can include the medial longitudinal fasciculus, thereby causing a gaze palsy.

Contralaterally, choreoathetosis, spastic hemiparesis and hemianesthesia are found. The cause is midline lesions of the oculomotor nuclei and cerebellar tracts which result in bilateral partial oculomotor nerve paresis with cerebellar ataxia *(Nothnagel's syndrome).*

Due to the proximity of structures, pontine syndromes usually involve the sixth and seventh cranial nerves. In the ventral medial pontine syndrome, the pyramidal tracts are involved at the level of the pons (Millard and Gubler). *Millard-Gubler* syndrome consists of ipsilateral abducens and facial paresis with contralateral hemiplegia.

The inferior lateral pontine syndrome consists of crossed hemianesthesia as well as ipsilateral abducens and facial (peripheral) nerve involvement.

In *Foville's syndrome,* nuclear abducens paresis is combined with a lesion of the medial longitudinal fasciculus. The clinical signs are ipsilateral: abducens paresis, peripheral facial nerve paresis, and gaze paresis to the same side. When deafness is also present (involvement of the root of the eighth cranial nerve), it is the dorsolateral-caudal pontine syndrome (Gasperini).

Damage to the area of the quadrigeminal plates may cause vertical gaze paresis. At times disturbance of the pupillary light reflex may be present. *Recurrent ophthalmoplegic migraine* (Möbius) (see page 80) usually begins in childhood. The patient may have unilateral headaches, diplopia and vomiting for hours to weeks. The intervals between attacks become progressively shorter. After the age of fifty, the attacks decrease. The third nerve is almost always involved; the sixth or fourth cranial nerves are seldom affected. Remky (1954) assumes a biphasic course similar to migraine: spasm with miosis and scintillating scotoma followed by a hypotonic phase with mydriasis and oculomotor paresis. The clinoid edge syndrome may be related (Fischer-Brügge 1951). Other causes which have been thought to produce this clinical picture are vascular spasm; vasculitis caused by allergic, toxic and endocrine factors; syphilis; meningitis; polyneuritis; aneurysms; subarachnoid hemorrhages; and tumors (Sachsenweger 1966).

Involuntary Ocular Movements

Nystagmus

Congenital nystagmus or nystagmus acquired in early childhood is not appreciated as such. In contrast, acquired nystagmus results in apparent movement of the environment which, after years, may only be perceived as blurred vision on gaze in the direction of maximal activity of the nystagmus.

Physiologic nystagmus — Pathologic nystagmus (pendular nystagmus, jerk nystagmus, localization of lesions causing nystagmus, hysterical [voluntary] nystagmus).

Nystagmus is an *involuntary rhythmic movement of the eyes.* The movement can be fast or slow; the excursions large (gross) or small (fine); they can be horizontal, vertical or rotary (Goddé-Jolly and Larmande 1973; Burian and von Noorden 1974). *Hysteric nystagmus* is caused by accommodation and convergence (small pupils) and, therefore, is not a true nystagmus. The random eye movements of blind individuals are also not true nystagmus.

Jerk nystagmus is generally differentiated from *pendular nystagmus.* In jerk nystagmus there is a fast and a slow component. The nystagmus is always named after the direction of the fast component (nystagmus to the right, left, up or down). Pendular nystagmus becomes a jerk nystagmus when the position of gaze is away from the midline. It is, therefore, necessary to specify whether the nystagmus is present on straight ahead gaze or at some degree of deviation.

Physiologic Nystagmus

1. Moving objects evoke optokinetic nystagmus (slow phase is on fixing the object and, therefore, in the direction of movement of the object; fast phase is on refixation).

2. Vestibular nystagmus is produced by acceleration or deceleration of body movement.

3. Cervical reflex nystagmus arises on active movement of the head.

Pathologic Nystagmus

The following should be differentiated:

Pendular nystagmus

1. Nystagmus with amblyopia, albinism, aniridia, achromatopsia;
Hereditary fixation nystagmus;
Latent nystagmus produced by covering one eye or seen only on gaze in certain directions;
2. Miners' nystagmus;
3. Acquired pendular nystagmus in multiple sclerosis;
4. Seesaw nystagmus.

Jerk nystagmus

1. Vestibular and cerebellar nystagmus;
2. Central, pathologic nystagmus;
3. Retraction nystagmus (nystagmus retractorius);
4. Nystagmus in muscle paresis;
5. Nystagmus in poisonings.

Localization of lesions leading to nystagmus
Hysterical (voluntary) nystagmus

Any nystagmus may be enhanced or inhibited by extravestibular, ocular, and cortical influences.

Pendular Nystagmus

Pendular nystagmus is usually ocular in origin. It can, however, be *congenital* or appear in early childhood together with *bilaterally decreased vision* (cataracts, corneal scars, albinism, achromatopsia, aplasia of the macula lutea, aniridia or without known cause = amblyopia). Visual acuity is usually in the range of 20/60 to 20/200.

Latent nystagmus occurs when one eye is covered. The fast phase is toward the uncovered eye.

In a manifest "ocular" nystagmus, optokinetic stimulation will reverse the direction of the nystagmus.

A manifest ocular nystagmus worsens, both in frequency and amplitude, when one eye is covered. This explains why binocular acuity is better than monocular acuity.

The nystagmus tends to be less severe in one direction of gaze (position of rest). This leads to the compensatory head position that these patients usually demonstrate.

Hereditary fixation nystagmus is a familial pendular nystagmus. The patients have a position of gaze where the nystagmus is least and, therefore, also a head turn. Amblyopia is usually not present. Congenital hereditary nystagmus may be latent and not manifest until one eye (usually the better eye) is covered.

In *spasmus nutans* nystagmus-like eye movements occur.

Miners' nystagmus is a pendular nystagmus of varying speed which occurs in persons who work in dark subterranean installations. Improved illumination, alcohol, sedatives, and accommodation reduce miners' nystagmus. The role of darkness, noise, explosions, or methane gas in producing miners' nystagmus has not been clarified.

Acquired pendular nystagmus: Acquired jerk or pendular nystagmus can occur in multiple sclerosis.

Seesaw nystagmus: In this vertical pendular nystagmus, the direction of movement of the two eyes is opposite; one eye goes up, the other down. The elevating eye shows incyclotorsion; the depressing eye extorts (Arnott 1965; Slatt and Nykriel 1964; Arnott and Miller 1970). Amplitude and frequency of the nystagmus vary with the direction of gaze. The vertical excursion is more prominent in the abducted eye, the rotary component in the adducted eye. Exotropia is frequently seen in association with seesaw nystagmus.

The etiology of seesaw nystagmus includes: cerebral trauma, inflammation, vascular or congenital cerebral processes, and brain tumors. Since seesaw nystagmus is particularly associated with sella tumors, Schmidt and Kommerell (1969) postulated a diencephalic lesion. The lesion could be in the superior region of the medial longitudinal bundle or near the posterior commissure (Jensen 1959, see page 65).

Jerk Nystagmus

A jerk nystagmus has a slow (irritation) and a

fast (fixation) phase. The nystagmus is incorrectly categorized as being to the right or left, depending on the fast phase.
When the nystagmus is congenital or was acquired early in life, there is no sensation of oscillopsia. When the nystagmus is acquired later in life, the object fixated gives the sensation of moving. Amplitude and frequency of movement of the environment are a function of the degree of nystagmus.
A physiologic end-point nystagmus occurs in half the population on extreme lateral gaze (slow phase to midline = fatigue, fast phase laterally = fixation).
Optokinetic or *railroad nystagmus* is obtained when a person moves while fixing a stationary object (slow phase). Refixation on the next object is the fast phase.

Labyrinthian or *vestibular nystagmus* can be evoked by rotation, caloric, mechanical, or galvanic stimulation of the inner ear. A nystagmus occurs with unilateral pathology of the labyrinth.
Central pathologic nystagmus is seen in a variety of cerebral processes (most marked with cerebellar lesions). This is particularly true of encephalitis, multiple sclerosis, severe cranial trauma, tumors and intoxications (such as alcohol, nitro-binding and amido-binding aromatic compounds [see page 122]).
In cyanide poisoning, spasm of upward gaze and nystagmus occur. Gaze pareses (pons, quadrigeminal plate regions) may begin as gaze nystagmus (see page 59). The Marinesco-Sjögren syndrome has a particularly striking nystagmus associated with it. There is spinocerebellar ataxia, oligophrenia, microphthalmos, bilateral cataracts, and nystagmus.
Retraction nystagmus is rare (nystagmus retractorius) and usually results from a lesion in the brain stem near the cerebral aqueduct and nucleus of the oculomotor nerve (Thiébaut et al. 1957).

The usual causes are tumors, inflammation, or vascular lesions in the region of the cerebral aqueduct involving the oculomotor and trochlear nerve nuclei as well as their supranuclear pathways and medial longitudinal bundle. With retraction nystagmus there is a loss of the pupillary light reaction, convergence paresis, and an irregular nystagmus; the ocular movements are uncoordinated (Lyle and Mayfield 1954).
Paretic muscle nystagmus becomes manifest on gaze in the direction of action of the paretic muscle.
Nystagmus occurs as an *occupational hazard* or from **toxic effects** (Merté 1969, 1972), for example with:

Nitronaphthalene: nystagmus, pupillary disturbances, optic neuritis, severe keratitis and conjunctivitis.
Mercury: nystagmus, extraocular muscle palsies.
Carbon disulfide: nystagmus, internal and external ophthalmoplegia, optic neuritis.

Drugs such as streptomycin and INH may also produce nystagmus. Piperazine (used against nematodes) can produce nystagmus, ataxia, hallucinations and disturbed accommodation.

Localization

The higher up in the brain stem a lesion is located, the greater the tendency for the gaze paresis or nystagmus to be vertical. Bulbar nystagmus is rotary. Seesaw nystagmus is primarily rotary. Since bitemporal field loss is frequently present, parachiasmatic lesions (trauma, tumors, demyelinating diseases, vascular involvement, infections, and malformations) should be considered (Remky 1971).
Hysteric nystagmus is a very rapid vibratory movement of the eyes associated with pupillary constriction and convergence.
It is seen with maximal accommodation on a functional (neurotic) basis.
Superior oblique muscle myokymia is a monocular tremor with vertical and rotary components which lasts for 3 to 10 seconds and occurs at irregular intervals (sometimes several times per minute). The patients complain of oscillopsia during these attacks. The oscillopsia disappears when the superior oblique muscle is severed from the globe. It is unclear if the pathologic stimulus is to be found in the fourth nerve nucleus or the superior oblique muscle fibers (Hoyt and Keane 1970).

"Dancing Eyes" Syndrome

In the "dancing eyes" syndrome (oscillopsia with myoclonic ataxia) (Brune et al. 1971), rapid intermittent conjugate oscillation of the eyes is present which is enhanced by voluntary

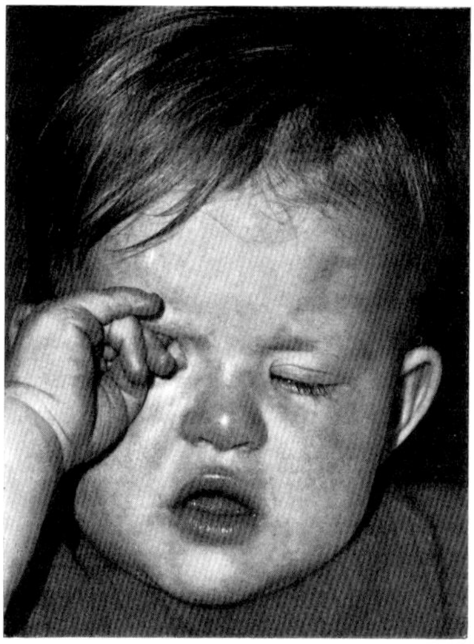

Fig. 8.23 Oculodigital phenomenon (♀ 1 yr.)

gaze in any direction. Myoclonic jerks of the trunk and extremities also occur. When lying down, the abnormal movements may cease entirely. When standing or attempting to walk, they may make any coordinated muscular effort impossible. Severe emotional irritability is present. The etiology is thought to be infectious damage in the area of the brain stem and cerebellar vermis. **Opsoclonus** is chaotic myoclonic movement at the beginning of fixation. *Etiology:* encephalitis, poliomyelitis (Sachsenweger 1966).

Myotonic Rigidity in Parkinsonism

In parkinsonism there is a myotonic rigidity of the muscles leading to cogwheel or interrupted movements. Lid stare with infrequent blinking, *weakness of extreme lateral gaze* and *convergence* are present. The face is rigid and mask-like.
Causes: Lesions in the striate body after epidemic encephalitis, with paralysis agitans (parkinsonism), or arteriosclerosis.

Gaze spasms or fits = oculogyric crises (see page 60) occur with paralysis agitans as tonic-spastic vertical deviations or as up and out deviations. Rarely do they occur in convergence.

Psychomotor Disturbances in Blind Children

Three groups of psychomotor disturbances are seen in blind children (Mackensen 1956):

1. General motor anomalies (hyperkinesia, rhythmic movements, stereotyped movements).

2. Mimicry (mask faces, grimacing, facial contortions).

3. Behavior specifically involving the eyes includes movement to evoke changing patterns of light and shade as well as pressing or rubbing the eyes (oculodigital phenomenon [see Fig. 8.23]).

The *oculodigital phenomenon* begins in the first year of life. It usually disappears by the time the child is five or six years of age, but it may persist until the early teens.

Ataxia and Spasticity in Ocular Syndromes

Ataxia is seen in ataxia-telangiectasia (Louis-Bar's syndrome); in congenital spinocerebellar ataxia with dwarfism, retardation and congenital cataracts (Marinesco-Sjögren syndrome); in retinitis pigmentosa with vestibulocerebellar ataxia, mental retardation and congenital deafness (Hallgren's syndrome). Refsum's disease and the Bassen-Kornzweig syndrome are also associated with ataxia.
Spasticity is found in the Sjögren-Larsson syndrome with oligophrenia, congenital ichthyosis and macula changes consisting of retinal aplasia. Cockayne's syndrome may have an associated spasticity.

References

Abrahamson, I. A., I. D. Horwitz: Acute ophthalmoplegia. Amer. J. Ophthal. 38 (1954) 781–787

Adelstein, F., C. Cüppers: Augenmuskellähmungen. In: Bücherei des Augenarztes, 46: 246–278, ed. by F. A. Hamburger, F. Hollwich. Enke, Stuttgart 1966

Albert, D. M., V. G. Wong, F. S. Henderson: Ocular complications of vincristine therapy. Am. Arch. Ophthalm. 78 (1967) 709–713.

Arnott, E. J.: Vertical see-saw nystagmus. Trans. ophthal. Soc. U. K. 84 (1965) 251–257

Arnott, E. J., S. J. H. Miller: See-saw nystagmus. Trans. ophthal. Soc. U.K. 90 (1970) 491–498

Aulhorn, E.: Phasendifferenz-Haploskopie, eine neue Methode zur Trennung der optischen Eindrücke beider Augen. Klin. Mbl. Augenheilk. 148 (1966) 540–544

Aust, W.: Pleoptik und Orthoptik. Karger, Basel 1966

Beckett, R. S., M. G. Netsky: Familial ocular myopathy and external ophthalmoplegia. Arch. Neurol. Psychiat. (Chicago) 69 (1953) 64–72; ref. in Zbl. ges. Ophthal. 60 (1953) 314

Best, F.: Die chronische progressive Ophthalmoplegie. In: Kurzes Handbuch der Ophthalmologie, Vol. VI, ed. by F. Schieck, A. Brückner. Springer, Berlin 1931 (pp. 504 to 505)

Bielschowsky, A.: Die Motilitätsstörungen der Augen nach dem Stande der neuesten Forschungen. In: Handbuch der gesamten Augenheilkunde, 2nd Ed. Vol. VIII, Part I, Chapter XI, Supplement I, ed. by A. Graefe, Th. Saemisch. Springer, Berlin 1932

Brückner, R.: Exakte Strabismusdiagnostik bei $^1/_2$- bis 3jährigen Kindern mit einem einfachen Verfahren, dem Durchleuchtungstest. Ophthalmologica (Basel) 144 (1962) 184–198

Brune, G., G. Hertel, W. Grüninger: Syndrom der tanzenden Augen mit myokloner Ataxie. Klin. Mbl. Augenheilk. 158 (1971) 41–48

Burian, H. M., G. K. von Noorden: Binocular vision and ocular motility. Mosby, St. Louis 1974

Chajutin, S. M.: Die Grenznormen des latenten Schielens bei Aufnahme in die Sommerschulen. Vestn. Oftal. 16 (1940) 148–155; in: Zbl. ges. Ophthal. 46 (1941) 420

Clausen, W., J. Brauer: Beiträge und Gedanken zur Lehre von der Vererbung des Strabismus concomitans. Z. Augenheilk. 50 (1923) 313–334

Cogan, D. G.: Internuclear ophthalmoplegia, typical and atypical. Am. Arch. Ophthal. 84 (1970) 583–589

Davidson, S. I.: Ocular myopathy. Trans. ophthal. Soc. U.K. 90 (1970) 139–159

Duke-Elder, S.: Neuroophthalmology. System of ophthalmology XII, Kimpton, London 1971

Duke-Elder, S.: Ocular motility and strabismus. System of ophthalmology VI. Kimpton, London 1973

Cords, R.: Die Physiologie der Augenbewegungen. Die Pathologie der Augenbewegungen. In: Kurzes Handbuch der Ophthalmologie, Vol. III, ed. by F. Schieck, A. Brückner. Springer, Berlin 1930 (pp. 440–651)

Dralands, L., P. H. Garin: Médicaments anti-infectieux. Soc. Bull. d'Ophtalm. 160 (1972) 326–389.

Erdbrink, W. L.: Ocular myopathy associated with retinitis pigmentosa. Arch. Ophthal. 57 (1957) 335–338

Esslen, E., W. Pabst: Die Bedeutung der Elektromyographie für die Analyse von Motilitätsstörungen der Augen. Karger, Basel 1961

Fischer-Brügge, E.: Anatomische Ursachen funktionaler Kreislaufstörungen des Gehirns und am N. oculomotorius. Bruns' Beitr. klin. Chir. 181 (1951) 323–336

Goddé-Jolly, D., A. Larmande: Les Nystagmus. Masson, Paris 1973

Gramberg-Danielsen, B.: Monokulare Doppelbilder. Klin. Mbl. Augenheilk. 130 (1957) 610–617

Haase, W.: Zur Diagnose und Therapie des Nystagmusblockierungssyndroms (elektroangiographische Untersuchungen). Klin. Mbl. Augenheilk. 157 (1970) 500–514

Hamburger, F. A.: Stellungsanomalien. In: Der Augenarzt, Vol. III, ed. by K. Velhagen. Thieme, Stuttgart 1960 (pp. 817–1109)

Hamburger, F. A., F. Hollwich: Augenmuskellähmungen. Bücherei des Augenarztes, 46. Enke, Stuttgart 1966

Harms, H.: Erbleiden des Auges. In: Handbuch der Erbkrankheiten, Vol. V, ed. by A. Gütt. Thieme, Leipzig 1938

Heydenreich, A.: Chemisch-toxische Schäden der Augen (Vergiftungen, Berufskrankheiten). Klin. Mbl. Augenheilk. 149 (1966) 145–165

Holland, G.: Über Beginn und Ursache des frühkindlichen Schielens. Sitzungsbericht 111. Versammlg. Rhein.-Westf. Augenärzte 1965

Holland, G.: Prognose und Verlauf der Oculomotoriusparese. Ber. dtsch. ophthal. Ges. 67 (1966) 69–73

Holland, G.: Bedeutung des A- und V-Syndroms beim frühkindlichen Schielen. Klin. Mbl. Augenheilk. 152 (1968) 739–751

Hollwich, F., H. Gernet, E. Damaske: Zum Euryblepharon. Ber. Ver. Rhein.-Westf. Augenärzte 119 (1969) 9–11

Hoyt, W. F., J. R. Keane: Superior oblique myokymia. Arch. ophthal. (Chicago) 84 (1970) 461–467

Huber, A.: Duane's retraction syndrome, Strabismus 1969. Kimpton, London 1970

Huber, A.: Eye symptoms in brain tumors. Mosby, St. Louis 1971

Jaensch, P. A.: Zur Klinik der supranuclearen Medialisparese und internuclearen Ophthalmoplegie. Albrecht v. Graefes Arch. klin. exp. Ophthal. 125 (1931 a) 592–613

Jaensch, P. A.: Zur Klinik der internuclearen Ophthalmoplegie (34. Tagung d. Vereinig. Mitteld. Augenärzte) Klin. Mbl. Augenheilk. 86 (1931b) 392

Jaensch, P. A.: Verletzungen, physikalische Schädigungen und Giftwirkungen. In: Der Augenarzt, Vol. V, ed. by K. Velhagen. Thieme, Leipzig 1963 (pp. 837–946)

Jensen, O. A.: See saw nystagmus. Brit. J. Ophthal. 43 (1959) 225–229

Jones, D. E. P.: Blow-out fracture of the orbita. Trans. ophthal. Soc. U. K. 86 (1966) 271–280

Kanter, D.: Zum Marcus Gunnschen Phänomen. Klin. Mbl. Augenheilk. 126 (1955) 50–59

Kestenbaum, A.: Nystagmus. Review of the literature. Fortschr. Augenheilk. 7 (1946–1954) 221–286

Kestenbaum, A.: Clinical methods of neuro-ophthalmological examination, 2nd Ed. Grune & Stratton, New York 1961

Kiloh, L. G., S. Nevin: Progressive dystrophy of the external ocular muscles. Brain 74 (1951) 115–143

Kommerell, G.: Die internukleäre Ophthalmoplegie. Nystagmographische Analyse. Klin. Mbl. Augenheilk. 158 (1971) 349–358

Krümmel, H.: Differentielle Phorometrie. Klin. Mbl. Augenheilk. 120 (1952) 134–143

Lang, J.: Einfache Differentialdiagnostik und gezielte Behandlung des Strabismus convergens. Klin. Mbl. Augenheilk. 155 (1969) 457–475

Lang, J.: Mikrostrabismus. Bücherei des Augenarztes, 62. Enke, Stuttgart 1973

Lyle, D. J., F. H. Mayfield: Retraction nystagmus: A case report. Amer. J. Ophthal. 37 (1954) 177–182

Mackensen, G.: Die Psychomotorik blinder Kinder. Bücherei des Augenarztes, 26. Enke, Stuttgart 1956

Manz, F., D. Schmidt: Diagnostik der okulären Myasthenie im Kindesalter. Klin. Mbl. Augenheilk. 157 (1970) 173–182

Merté, H. J.: Arbeitsmedizinische Fragen in der Ophthalmologie. Karger, Basel 1969

Merté, H. J.: Arbeits- u. Sozialmedizin. In: Lehrbuch der Augenheilkunde, ed. by T. Axenfeld, H. Pau. Fischer, Stuttgart 1973

Milauskas, A. T., G. F. Fueger, R. R. Schulze: Clinical experiences with orbitography for the diagnosis of blowout fractures of the orbital floor. Trans. Amer. Acad. Ophthal. Otolaryng. 70 (1966) 25–39

Ogle, K. N.: Researches in binocular vision. Saunders, Philadelphia 1950

Papst, W.: Thalidomid und kongenitale Anomalien der Augen. Ber. dtsch. ophthal. Ges. 65 (1963) 209–215

Papst, W.: Paralytischer Strabismus infolge paradoxer Innervation. Ber. dtsch. ophthal. Ges. 67 (1966) 84–101

Papst, W.: Okuläre Myopathien, Klinik, Pathologie, Elektromyographie und Therapie. Almanach für die Augenheilkunde. Lehmann, München 1969 (pp. 25–39)

Papst, W., E. Esslen: Zur Ätiologie der angeborenen Abducenslähmung. Kln. Mbl. Augenheilk. 137 (1960) 306–327

Papst, W., H. J. Stein: Zur Ätiologie des Musculus obliquus superior-Scheidensyndroms. Klin. Mbl. Augenheilk. 154 (1969) 506–518

Papst, W., E. Esslen, H. G. Mertens: Die oculäre Muskeldystrophie sog. Ophthalmoplegia externa chronica progressiva. Klin. Mbl. Augenheilk. 132 (1958) 691–707

Papst, W., H. G. Mertens, E. Esslen: Die chron. okuläre Myositis. Klin. Mbl. Augenheilk. 134 (1959) 374–396

Parks, M. M.: Ocular motility and strabismus. Harper and Row. Hagerstown, Maryland, New York, London 1975

Passow, A.: Über den Einfluß des Sympathicus auf Wachstum und Pigmentbildung, zugleich ein Beitrag zur Kenntnis des Status dysraphicus und seiner okularen Symptome, insbesondere der Heterochromie. Klin. Mbl. Augenheilk. 116 (1950) 561–578

Priggert, W.: Augenmuskellähmungen beim Herpes zoster ophthalmicus. Klin. Mbl. Augenheilk. 131 (1957) 72–77

Remky, H.: Zur Pathogenese der ophthalmoplegischen Migräne. Albrecht v. Graefes Arch. klin. exp. Ophthal. 155 (1954) 518–524

Remky, H.: Grundlagen der neuroophthalmologischen Diagnostik. In: Der Augenarzt, Vol. V, ed. by K. Velhagen. Thieme, Leipzig 1963 (pp. 129–255)

Remky, H.: Blicklähmungen und Nystagmen. Klin. Mbl. Augenheilk. 158 (1971) 313–325

Rougier, J., G. Allègre, G. Lapras, Ph. Léopold: Les anévrysmes carotidiens intracraniens bilatéreux: valeur séméiologique des signes oculaires. Ann. Oculist. (Paris) 195 (1962) 13–30

Sachsenweger, R.: Augenmuskellähmungen. Ein Handbuch für Ophthalmologen, Neurologen und Internisten. VEB Thieme, Leipzig 1966

Schapero, M.: Amblyopia. Chilton Book Co., Philadelphia 1971

Schmidt, D., G. Kommerell: Schaukel-Nystagmus (Seesaw Nystagmus) mit bitemporaler Hemianopsie als Folge von Schädelhirntraumen. Albrecht v. Graefes Arch. klin. exp. Ophthal. 178 (1969) 349–366

Schober, H., K. F. Leisinger: Einäugige Doppelbilder und Reafferenzprinzip und ihre Bedeutung für die Theorien des binocularen Sehraums und der Schielwinkelbestimmung. Klin. Mbl. Augenheilk. 130 (1957) 824–837

Schwarz, G. A., C. N. Liu: Chronic progressive external ophthalmoplegia. Arch. Neurol. Psychiat. (Chicago) 71 (1954) 31–53

Slatt, B., F. Nykiel: See-saw nystagmus. Amer. J. Ophthal. 58 (1964) 1016–1021

Thiébaut, M. F., N. Matavulj, M. O. Metzger: Trois cas de nystagmus retractorius. Bull. Soc. franç. Ophtal. 70 (1957) 50–62

Tschermak, A.: Über anomale Sehrichtungsgemeinschaft der Netzhäute bei einem Schielenden. Albrecht v. Graefes Arch. kln. exp. Ophthal. 47 (1899) 508–550

Weekers, R., P. Moureau, J. Hacourt, A. André: Contribution a l'etiologie du syndrome de retraction oculaire. Acta ophthal. (Kbh) 34 (1956) 343–346

Weigelin, E.: Beurteilung des intracraniellen Kreislaufs mit Hilfe der Netzhautarteriendruckmessung. Docum. ophthal. 8 (1954) 183–245

Wollensak, J., A. Fleischer-Peters, O. Hövels: Über die angeborenen okulo-fazialen Lähmungen (Möbius-Syndrom). Klin. Mbl. Augenheilk. 140 (1962) 383–396

Worth, C.: Squint-its causes, pathology and treatment, Vol. I. Tindall, London 1929

9 Pain and Symptoms Arising from or Localized in the Eye

In *eye-related headaches*, a differentiation must be made between those which occur without any external or ophthalmoscopically *visible* changes (asthenopic) and those with *visible changes in the eyes* or their adnexa which are usually inflammatory. Conversely, *headaches* can *radiate to the eyes*.

Asthenopia

Accommodative asthenopia (hyperopia, myopia, astigmatism, anisometropia, presbyopia, accommodative paresis) — Muscular asthenopia (heterophoria, paresis of ocular muscles, convergence insufficiency, hysterical nystagmus) — Asthenopia from dazzling (dazzling in the normal eye, photophobia with opacities of the refractive media, with mydriasis, asthenopia with artificial light) — Neurotic asthenopia.

Asthenopia must be considered if the appearance of the eye is normal but complaints increase during the course of the day or with extended close work.

Asthenopia actually means "weak vision." The term does not mean "weak sight" in the sense of myopia or decreased acuity. Rather, asthenopia is a comprehensive term for the disturbances and complaints discussed below. Asthenopic symptoms include: blurring of objects with a melting or fading of the environment; lack of stamina for close work; easy fatigability; lack of patience for close work; pulling or pressure behind the eyes; dull pains in, around, or behind the eyes and forehead; supraorbital headaches; dull aches deep within the skull; and vertigo to the point of vomiting. All of these symptoms are intensified during the course of the day as the demands of close work or concentrated effort increase.

Accommodative asthenopia occurs with presbyopia, hyperopia, overcorrected myopia, accommodative paresis, astigmatism, and any blurring of objects which in turn requires that the object be held closer to the eyes, thereby demanding increased accommodation. *Accommodative asthenopia* is to be differentiated from *muscular asthenopia* such as seen with heterophorias, ocular muscle paresis, and convergence insufficiency. Asthenopia occurs with *dazzling* and the use of *artificial light*. *Neurotic asthenopia* is associated with emotional strain, fatigue, hysteria, etc. In addition to the above-mentioned causes, asthenopia can also be caused by a *combination of factors*. Inflammation of the lids or conjunctiva aggravates asthenopic symptoms.

Refractive errors and ocular deviations may combine and reinforce each other. In many cases, therefore, it is impossible to separate accommodative and muscular etiologies. Moreover, the psychologic condition of the moment plays a major role in asthenopia. There is a huge variation in the subjective susceptibility of individuals to all of these symptoms. As a result, only a small percentage of patients with refractive errors or heterophorias ever suffer from asthenopic symptoms. Of 2316 such patients, Lanchner (1953) found asthenopic complaints in 5.7 percent. Cause and effect are often interchanged since the headache may be blamed for difficulty with close work.

Frequently, asthenopia is artificially produced by improper glasses (excess minus sphere = hyperopia), incorrect cylinder lenses (astigmatism) and heterophoria (prismatic effect of decentered glasses).

Accommodative Asthenopia

Hyperopia (see page 24)

Since, in the hyperopic individual, the globe is too short for his refractive power, he must accommodate at distance in order to see clearly. Any nearer points of interest require additional accommodative effort. Depending on age (decreasing range of accommodation) and degree of hyperopia, hyperopic asthenopia occurs. For varying periods of time, everything is seen clearly and then everything blurs. After a period of "rest" or with increased effort, things are clear again. Fatigue, a dull headache, and a feeling of pressure behind the eyes which radiates to the brow occurs with prolonged periods of reading or near work. Symptoms are absent early in the day but increase during the course of the day. Frequently, the patient is heterophoric (see page 37). Moderately hyperopic individuals (below 3 diopters) are rarely bothered during the first two decades of life. If then, they are bothered it is only by very fine close work, or with emotional or generalized fatigue. In this regard, the proper working distance for close work (usually 30 to 35 cm) is important. Asthenopic symptoms in young, even emmetropic, patients occur when the habitual working distance is much less than this and greater effort of accommodation and convergence is therefore required.

Young amblyopic and hyperopic patients often move objects close to the eyes in order to get a larger, albeit blurred, retinal image. In this way they clinically simulate myopia (see page 25).

In "nervous," "overworked," emotionally unstable persons with functional overlay, the dull eyebrow headaches may occur with minimal hyperopia. The degree of subjective discomfort is also greater with pain over the entire head (brow, temples, occiput) and neck. Actual migraine episodes including nausea and vomiting are simulated. Symptoms are aggravated by physical exertion, illness, or emotional strain such as studying for examinations.

Myopia (see page 25)

Myopia with (real or relative) elongation of the globe normally does not cause eye ache or headache. Rarely, an individual with uncorrected myopia will complain of pressure around the eyes. This is probably the result of the patient converging at close distances without appropriately accommodating (accommodation and convergence are related). Symptoms are usually absent in myopia, even when intermittent exotropia is present.

Myopic individuals involved with close work (seamstresses, students, etc.) get so close to the object that their head is held forward in an uncomfortable position. This constant stretching of neck muscles produces pain in the shoulders and neck as well as *headaches*. The situation is different when the myopic individual is *overcorrected;* he then has an artificial hyperopia and needs to accommodate to see clearly at distance. The myopic individual with proper correction, who previously needed less accommodation than the emmetropic individual (and, therefore, has an underdeveloped ciliary muscle), may now develop the dull *eyebrow headaches* of accommodative asthenopia such as seen with hyperopia.

Astigmatism (see page 24)

The primary complaint of an astigmatic individual is poor, blurred vision. With hyperopic astigmatism this is particularly true at close distances; in myopic astigmatism, at far distances. Asthenopic symptoms may occur. Clear distance or near vision requires effort, especially over a long period of time. *Asthenopic symptoms* such as *pressure* and *pulling* of the eyes, *vertigo,* or even *migraine headaches* with *vomiting* can be related to astigmatism. These symptoms are probably the result of a constant shifting of accommodation between the two axes and circle of least confusion. High astigmatism, like any congenitally acquired cause of poor vision, usually causes no other complaints. There may be exceptions where asthenopic symptoms have been present very early. In the vast majority of cases, asthenopic complaints (easy fatigability, dull *pressure* in the eyes or head) only develop when increased demands are made on vision such as with fine work, or with a decline in general well-being (overexertion, debilitating diseases, etc.).

The prismatic correction should be accurate to the nearest one-quarter diopter. Correction to one-eighth diopter is superfluous. The cylindrical axis, on the other hand, needs to be as precise as possible. This becomes more important as the power of the correcting cylinder increases. The prevalence of astigmatism varies between 5 percent and 50 percent depending on which level (one-half, two-thirds, one diopter) is considered physiologic.

Artificial astigmatism is frequently created by improper cylindrical corrections.

Since irregular astigmatism causes blurred vision but not headaches, it need not be considered here. It is usually the result of corneal scarring or damage.

Anisometropia (see page 24)

On rare occasions a significant difference in the refractive error of the two eyes will lead to *asthenopic complaints* (dull *eyebrow pain* and *headaches)* of an *accommodative nature.* The more hyperopic eye is usually amblyopic. A difference greater than three to four diopters in the corrective lenses of the two eyes is usually not tolerated by the patient. Children are an exception.

Presbyopia (see page 28)

If the elderly patient fails to wear the appropriate presbyopic prescription regularly, he is forced to exert a correspondingly greater accommodative effort in order to see clearly at near distances. This leads to *asthenopic complaints,* such as fatigability, *dull eye pain* radiating to the forehead, *headaches,* and occasionally nausea.

Paresis of Accommodation (see page 28)

With isolated pupillary and accommodative paresis (internal ophthalmoplegia), the young patient is forced to make an increased, perhaps futile, effort of accommodation; this leads to *asthenopic complaints* (rapid tiring, *dull eyebrow pain,* etc.). Increased *light sensitivity* from the dilated pupil is an added factor.
Objects appear minified with both accommodative and convergence paresis (accommodative micropsia, convergence micropsia).

Muscular Asthenopia

Heterophoria (see page 37)

In *orthophoria* the eyes have the same visual direction, even after one eye is covered. If the covered eye deviates, *heterophoria* (latent strabismus) exists. Some degree, however minimal, of heterophoria is present in 75 percent of the population. *Esophoria* (latent in-turning) differs from *exophoria* (latent out-turning) and from *hyperphoria-hypophoria* (latent vertical deviation). *Cyclophoria* (latent rotation around the visual axis) is also seen.

Improperly fitting glasses that produce a prismatic effect may create an *artificial heterophoria* leading to significant asthenopic complaints: fatigability, dull headaches, etc.
If normal fusion is present, the heterophoria is compensated by the increased tone of selected muscles. The asthenopic symptoms, therefore, are *muscular asthenopia.*
The usual complaints include a feeling of pressure or pain about the eyes that leads to dull headaches; the headache increases during the course of the day or with close work. Concentrated distance vision (driving, watching movies) creates similar symptoms. These may be *diffuse headaches* leading to *vertigo, nausea,* or even *vomiting.* The complaints are rarely of decreased vision, diplopia that arises with fatigue, or burning of the eyes. The constant headaches associated with these asthenopic symptoms often do not permit prolonged work; depression may therefore result. In the absence of organic disease, such patients are then labeled as neurotic, with functional overlay, as "neurasthenic," etc. Conversely, asthenopic symptoms will appear in emotionally unstable, psychologically exhausted, "overworked," neurotic individuals with minimal heterophoria. The psychogenic component of asthenopic complaints also explains why one patient will have them with minimal heterophoria, but they may be absent in other patients with marked heterophoria.
The fact that 75 percent of the population are heterophoric indicates that usually even high heterophoria is asymptomatic. Hyperphoria tends more often to be symptomatic since the vertical range of fusion is limited (about two prism diopters). Esophoria is least symptomatic because near work convergence takes place normally.

It is incorrect to think that asthenopic complaints may be absent in high heterophoria because the drive to keep the eyes straight, which is present in small phorias, is unsuccessful and therefore absent in high phorias. Once the deviation is no longer latent (phoria) it is manifest (tropia).
To measure a phoria, the patient must be wearing his appropriate correction. Furthermore, since the phoria is suppressed through the fusional mechanisms, fusion must be interrupted. This is done by covering one eye or by using the Maddox rod. The Maddox rod is placed in front of one eye while the patient fixes upon a light. The rod changes the light

to a line. The patient, therefore, sees a point light source with one eye and a line with the other. These are such dissimilar images that no fusional impulse arises and, if a phoria is present, the point and line images separate. Various other methods of investigating phorias (prisms, Maddox phorometer) are not dealt with here.

Extraocular Muscle Paresis (see page 47)

Diplopia, especially of recent onset, may be so disturbing that the patient becomes dizzy or even falls. The forced head deviation and the need to concentrate may lead to eye aches and headaches in addition to the symptoms of the underlying disease (orbital or nerve) (see Ophthalmoplegic Migraine [page 80]).

Convergence Insufficiency (see page 60)

In convergence insufficiency as with heterophoria, there is a feeling of *forced effort, fatigue, pressure, ocular tension,* and *headaches* (sometimes migraine-like). These patients frequently have the feeling of underachieving and tend to be hypochondriacal. Diplopia can occur. Convergence insufficiency is most prevalent in weak, anemic or emotionally exhausted persons with a decrease in fusional capacity. Exophoria is frequently present. Since accommodation and convergence are related, the patient must be tested with his proper correction. The individual with uncorrected myopia frequently has difficulty with convergence.

Hysteric (Voluntary) Nystagmus

The most marked muscular asthenopia is seen with *hysterical nystagmus* (see page 65). The patient converges forcibly, the pupils constrict and there is a very fine, rapid ocular oscillation (500 to 1200 cycles per minute). If maintained for any length of time, this maximal accommodative and convergence effort produces symptoms of *pressure* and *pain.* The patient may ascribe the symptoms to some previous trauma (combat neurosis).

Asthenopia from Dazzling

(see page 30)

Dazzling in the Normal Eye

When certain light intensities are exceeded, the patient is no longer able to discriminate between various luminance levels and is dazzled. Dazzling is both a psychological and a physiological phenomenon. It may involve the whole retina *(Ganzfeld)* or only a small part of the visual field (contrast). Dazzling is *absolute* when the total light level is simply too high. It is relative, for example, when the dark-adapted driver is blinded by oncoming headlights.

The eye is protected from dazzling by retinal adaptation, pupillary constriction, and narrowing of the palpebral fissures.

Sparsely pigmented (iris, pigment epithelium, choroid) eyes are generally more sensitive to dazzling than dark, heavily pigmented eyes. Sudden dazzling such as occurs with spotlights or going from a dark room into the bright outdoors can cause sharp ocular pain. Constant dazzlement produces *dull headaches* which radiate from the brows and temples to the occiput. The constant squinting that goes along with dazzling contributes to this pain. The necessary contraction of the frontalis muscle may lead to occipital neuralgia (Griffith 1934, 1935). Dazzling caused by oncoming headlights is a particular problem. The *headaches* experienced by some night drivers are only partly due to dazzling. The constant *squinting,* emotional strain, and increased alertness required contribute significantly to the driver's discomfort.

Dazzling by Opacities of the Refractive Media

Opacities in the refractive media (cornea, aqueous humor, lens, vitreous body) scatter light and dazzle the patient at what would otherwise be acceptable levels of illumination. The patient may be incapacitated by sunlight or automobile headlights. Again, diffuse dull headaches occur. Any ocular inflammatory disease will increase the patient's normal level of photophobia and susceptibility to dazzling.

Dazzling Through Pupillary Dilatation

If the pupil fails to constrict with increasing levels of light, too much light will fall into the eye. If the light level is high enough, the patient will be dazzled and may eventually develop the *diffuse headaches* described. For the differential diagnosis of a dilated pupil (paresis) see page 323. Pupillary dilation with pain, fright, etc., is a sympathetic response.

Fluorescent Lights and Asthenopic Symptoms

Fluorescent lights seem particularly to evoke asthenopic complaints. The patients are *easily tired, listless,* complain of *pressure* or *pulling* behind the eyes as well as *dull brow headaches.* In his definitive work on illumination, Schober (1953) points out that shadows are as important to vision as light. The flat diffuse light of indirect illumination creates an unfamiliar shadowless environment. To avoid this, fluorescent lights should be mounted above windows or perpendicular to the working surface. Schober attributes the asthenopic symptoms to the lack of shadows which causes a constant, futile change of accommodation. It is important to check that all such patients have the proper refraction.

Fluorescent lighting in the daylight spectrum, when insufficiently intense, gives the impression of poor vision. People do not look "well" in such light. Psychologically, this creates a feeling of being ill, lethargic, headaches, etc. Such problems are alleviated by changing the spectrum or intensity of illumination.

Headaches and Other Symptoms Produced by Diseases of the Eye and Its Surroundings

Ciliary neuralgias — Conjunctivitis — Diseases of the lids — Diseases of the cornea — Episcleritis — Scleritis — Ocular injuries — Iridocyclitis — Choroiditis, retinitis, cataracts — Optic nerve involvement (neuritis and retrobulbar neuritis) — Glaucoma — Diseases of the orbit — Lacrimal diseases and diseases of the bony orbit — Oculonasal reflex neuralgia (Sluder-Charlin syndrome).

Ciliary Neuralgias

Ciliary or *iris* pain is caused by pressure irritation of trigeminal nerve endings. This occurs with trauma, inflammation (iritis, iridocyclitis) or glaucoma and is a *stabbing* or *pulling* pain. Ocular pains occur which are either unrelated to visible disease or are out of proportion to the degree of involvement. When there is a persistent iritis, iridocyclitis or secondary glaucoma, severe pains may persist in spite of *hypo-anesthesia of the globe* (Pau 1950) or blockage *of the gasserian ganglion.* Such pains, described as dull headaches or also as tearing or boring behind the eyes, seem to have a sympathetic causality. In exceptional situations *secondary meningeal irritation* may cause such headaches. The trigeminal nerve carries the acute pain of injury to the iris or ciliary body as well as the *stabbing pain* of accommodation seen with iritis. The pain conducted by the trigeminal nerve could be labeled *ciliary pain.* In contrast the duller, pressure-like headaches of the autonomic nervous system are best labeled *ciliary neuralgias.* This occurs with longstanding iritis, iridocyclitis, scleritis, etc., and appears to require a summation of subthreshold irritants before coming to consciousness. The severe, at times unbearable, pain associated with glaucoma seems to belong more to the ciliary neuralgias of the autonomic system than to trigeminal ciliary pain. Since it is usually impossible to separate *ciliary pains* and *ciliary neuralgias,* such headaches should not be classified according to their origin (cerebrospinal or autonomic).

Headaches and Other Symptoms Produced by Diseases of the Eye and Its Surroundings

If the main symptoms are *burning* and *itching,* diseases of the lid and conjunctiva are the primary consideration. When edema is present, allergic processes such as eczema and urticaria must be considered. Chalazion, lid abscess or other localized inflammatory processes are at fault when redness, edema and *pain are localized.* Herpes zoster produces particularly severe unilateral ocular and trigeminal neuralgia. The diagnostic vesicular lesions in the area of the distribution of the trigeminal nerve may be fleeting, sparse, or even absent.

Corneal erosion (ulcer, foreign body, chemical burn, etc.) produces burning, sensation of a foreign body or sand, or severe pain in the eye.

Sharp corneal pain in spite of hypo-anesthesia implies the diagnostic choices of herpes simplex, herpes zoster, or vaccinia, in that order. Dull, pressing pain radiating to the head occurs in interstitial keratitis, scleritis (may be unbearable radiating ciliary neuralgia), iritis, and iridocyclitis. In acute iritis, sharp stabbing pain occurs with accommodation. In episcleritis the pain is circumscribed and elicited by pressure. There is a continuum of pain types and physical findings from phlyctenulosis to episcleritis and scleritis. Optic nerve neuritis or retrobulbar neuritis causes pain, especially during movement of an eye which is otherwise free of irritation. The visual acuity is markedly decreased. In older persons temporal arteritis must be considered, especially when facial pains, pain on chewing, or tender, thickened temporal arteries are present. Episodes of pain and blurred vision suggest glaucoma (acute angle closure, chronic congestive glaucoma, secondary glaucoma).

With inflammation of Tenon's capsule, exophthalmos and chemosis accompany marked pain on moving the globe. With orbital cellulitis there is generalized malaise. Noninflammatory exophthalmos only when bending over is no more a diagnostic problem than headaches associated with pulsatile exophthalmos or orbital hemorrhage.

Localized swelling and pain in the orbit aids in the diagnosis. Lacrimal gland processes involve the upper temporal orbital region; lacrimal sac inflammation, the lower nasal orbital region; sinusitis, the upper nasal orbital region.

Oculonasal reflex neurosis (see page 78) produces unilateral eye-nose-head pain, lacrimation and rhinorrhea.

Diseases of the Lids and Conjunctiva

Conjunctivitis, blepharitis and blepharoconjunctivitis cause *burning*, itching, and a *foreign body sensation* when blinking.

Conjunctivitis

In addition to the various forms of acute *conjunctivitis* (see page 121), a "physiologic" conjunctivitis *(conjunctivitis chronica simplex)* results from chronic irritation by wind, dust, etc. The patients complain of *heavy lids, burning, itching eyes* and *foreign body sensation*. It appears that the majority of such patients are female, neurotic, and emotionally unstable. On waking, many patients find their eyes "glued shut" because of "sleep," "matter," or secretions. Symptoms are aggravated by hot, dry weather and wind.

Conjunctivitis complaints appear in *ectropion* (spastic, senile, paralytic, cicatricial) with conjunctival catarrh and heavy lacrimation.

Inflammations of the Lids

(see page 91)

Diseases of the Lid Margins

Most chronic inflammations of the lid margins are constitutional (see page 106) and relatively asymptomatic until irritated by excessive smoke, wind, or dust. *Foreign body sensation*, dry eyes, and a feeling of *heaviness* are present. Dry weather aggravates the symptoms. Symptoms are particularly pronounced with *ulcerative blepharitis*.

Diseases of the Lid

Eczema of the lids and face produces varying degrees of *burning* and *itching* depending on the degree of edema, redness, scaling, weeping, pustule or blister formation. If skin maceration at the lateral canthi causes rhagades, *localized pain* occurs. This in turn causes reflex lid spasm.

Depending on the severity, diseases of the lids (herpes simplex, vaccinia, erysipelas, lid abscess, syphilitic chancres, tuberculosis, molluscum contagiosum, mycotic infections, etc.) produce varying degrees of *pain, heaviness*, or *foreign body* sensation.

Inflammation of the Glands of the Lid Margin

(see page 91)

Acute pain differentiates *inflammation of the lid* or more particularly of the lid margin (hordeolum, hordeolosis, lid abscess) from chronic chalazion where there is a localized feeling of *tension and pressure*. Occasionally, the *preauricular* lymph nodes are swollen. The entire lid is edematous, occasionally the cheek or brow is involved. The pain is relieved only when the inflammatory cyst ruptures and the pus drains.

Ophthalmic Zoster

Zoster ophthalmicus produces *unilateral neuralgia* of the eye and face. Vesicles form on the conjunctiva and cornea; iritis and secondary glaucoma may occur.

Tearing, photophobia, and neuralgia may be present several days before vesicle formation. The patients complain of *unilateral pain* in the eye and face. The neuralgia usually persists even after the vesicles have healed and the characteristic scars have formed. With corneal involvement or secondary glaucoma, the respective symptoms are added.

Diseases of the Lids with Corneal Involvement

Entropion (spastic, senile, cicatricial) produces strong *localized stabbing pain*, a *foreign body sensation, rubbing, photophobia, tears and the feeling of "sand" in the eyes.* The lid margin turns inward and the lashes rub on the cornea. Lid spasm, corneal erosions and ulcers result. A similar foreign body sensation is caused by *misdirected lashes (trichiasis, distichiasis), foreign bodies under the lid, meibomian lithiasis* (after infarction of the meibomian gland), *scars* and *chalazions under the upper lid.*

Diseases of the Cornea (see page 142)

Corneal Erosions (see page 148)

Any corneal erosion causes sharp stabbing pain, foreign body sensation, tearing and photophobia. With *recurrent erosions* the history alone gives the diagnosis. An undetermined period after minor corneal injury the patient awakens with sharp eye pain and tearing. The decrease in tear secretion at night allows adhesions to form between the lid and corneal epithelium. When the eye is opened, the epithelium is torn loose.

The *familial corneal dystrophies* (granular, macular, lattice) develop epithelial irregularities and erosions causing episodic inflammation, pain, and tearing.

Superficial punctate keratitis, potentially leading to filamentous keratitis with burning and dryness, is brought about by a number of causes. These include actual dry eyes such as in Sjögren's syndrome *(keratitis sicca)*, irritation from smoke, hydrogen sulfide, ultraviolet light (welding arc burns) and herpes keratitis. *Dry eyes* and foreign body sensation occur with inadequate blinking (*lagophthalmic keratitis* = exposure keratitis) from facial nerve paresis, exophthalmos, and lid contractures. If the lids remain partially open at night, the eye dries out and exposure keratitis develops on the lower third of the cornea. This eventually leads to ulceration.

Corneal Ulcers (see page 159)

Every corneal ulcer causes foreign body sensation and pain. The pain may be extremely severe and radiate from the eye to the brow and head *(ciliary neuralgia)*. Symptoms are least with marginal ulcers, ulcers caused by *diplobacilli* (Hemophilus duplex), fungi (keratomycosis), and *keratomalacia* (vitamin A deficiency). Pain is greatest with *serpiginous ulcers* and may be neuralgic in *rodent ulcer* (Mooren's ulcer).

A *neuroparalytic* keratitis may appear soon or years after alcohol injection or electrocautery of the trigeminal ganglion (gasserian). In spite of the sharply demarcated central ulcer, the eye is normally pain-free unless iritis or secondary glaucoma are also present. In this case a *ciliary neuralgia* occurs (see page 73).

Severe *acid* and especially *alkali burns* (lime, artificial fertilizers, aniline dyes, etc.) cause long, protracted, *painful* inflammation and ulceration with a strong tendency for corneal vascularization and conjunctival shrinkage.

Hypoesthesia and Symptomatology

A hallmark of *corneal herpes* (see page 152) is localized ocular *pain* in the face of decreased corneal sensitivity *(anesthesia dolorosa)*. The *pain* frequently radiates to the head in a *neuralgiform* fashion. The keratitis may be superficial, usually dendritic, but also filiform or punctate. It may be deep, as in metaherpetic or disciform keratitis. Characteristically, a dull pressing pain radiates from the globe to the area of distribution of the first or all three branches of the trigeminal nerve (neurotropic virus). The patient may feel systemically ill. These pains are particularly marked with ophthalmic zoster involving cornea and conjunctiva (see page 155). Involvement of the nasociliary nerve (blisters at the tip of the nose) is a sign of involvement of the first trigeminal nerve branch and the eye. The cornea, conjunctiva, or even the iris may be affected. Pain in the area of distribution of the first branch of the trigeminal nerve may precede blister formation by hours or even weeks and may persist long after the vesicles have resolved. The pain is then usually *neuralgic* in nature. The patient may be febrile before and during the vesicular eruption. The relationship between *herpetic keratitis* and *topical steroid use* should be stressed.

Vaccination (inadvertent) of the cornea and conjunctiva produces similar symptoms.

Parenchymatous (Interstitial) Keratitis

Luetic interstitial keratitis is usually manifest between the ages of five and twenty. Initially, the lesion is asymmetric with an unpredictable interval between the two eyes. There is marked photophobia and ciliary pain radiating to the orbit and brow. Other forms of *interstitial keratitis* have similar symptoms.

Episcleritis – Scleritis (see page 181)

Usually *episcleritis* is fairly pain-free, except on *direct pressure* to the involved area. The pain on pressure in *scleritis* varies with the degree of involvement. Some cases are accompanied by a virtually intolerable *ciliary neuralgia* which radiates to the head (see page 73).

Ocular Injury

Pain on *ocular injury* varies with location (conjunctiva, cornea, sclera, iris), severity, duration, accompanying inflammation, and secondary complications (glaucoma, iridocyclitis, enophthalmos, etc.).

Diseases of the Inner Eye

Iridocyclitis (see page 195)

Subjective complaints of pain in iridocyclitis depend on the severity and duration of inflammation. They are most pronounced with acute, severe, fresh invölvement and least pronounced in chronic uveitis, in spite of marked protein flare in the anterior chamber. *Photophobia* and *tearing*, presumably from irritation of trigeminal nerve endings, may be the principal symptoms.

Acute iridocyclitis is accompanied by a *painful pressure* in the eye which may radiate in *neuralgiform* fashion to the brow, temples, or entire head. A minimal meningeal irritation may play a role in producing this pain. *Iris movement* (pupillary constriction), accommodation or light produces sharp, stabbing pain in the eye. Conversely, pupillary dilation (such as with l-epinephrine) may cause severe, virtually unbearable pain that radiates from the eye to the head. The patients frequently complain of *neuralgias* in the area of distribution of the trigeminal nerve. Pupillary dilation (mydriasis) brings dramatic relief from the pain. If the cyclitis is particularly strong or localized, the area of the ciliary body may be *pressure sensitive.*

Choroiditis, Retinitis, Lenticular Damage

Diseases of the choroid may produce photopsias (scintillations, sparks), decreased vision and scotomata (diffuse) but do not cause *eye* or *head pain*. Such pain occurs only if the *ciliary* body or *iris* are involved. An accompanying mild meningitis such as in acute tuberculous or luetic chorioretinitis also produces pain.

Diseases of the retina, unless accompanied by secondary glaucoma (hemorrhagic retinitis, central vein thrombosis, retinal glioma, etc.), do not cause pain. Headaches are part of diseases also affecting the retina (atherosclerosis, hypertensive retinopathy, etc.). Involvement of the lens produces pain only if it leads to secondary glaucoma. This may occur with (sub) luxation of the lens or injury to the capsule which results in the release of lens protein. Lens protein may escape through an intact, but metabolically damaged, capsule (hypermature cataract, Fuchs' heterochromia complicata iridocyclitis) and cause glaucoma.

Diseases of the Optic Nerve

Neuritis and Retrobulbar Neuritis (see page 307)

Optic neuritis, in contrast to retrobulbar neuritis, rarely causes pain. The underlying disease may, however, be responsible for headaches. Inflammation of the optic nerve may be endogenous and *primary,* or *secondary to meningitis, opticochiasmatic arachnoiditis, orbital cellulitis, chorioretinitis, iridocyclitis* or *endophthalmitis.* Poisoning with neurotoxic agents should be mentioned (see page 310). Severe systemic involvement (diarrhea, vomiting, confusion, coma), headaches and visual loss occur with *methyl alcohol intoxication.*

Retrobulbar neuritis: In contrast to optic neuritis, in addition to subjective visual loss, *pain is present with eye movement. Orbital pain* may be evoked by passive mechanical pressure which pushes the globe backward. Dull orbital pain and *headaches around the temples* also occur.

The most impressive symptom in this illness is a rapid onset of what can be profound visual loss and possibly total blindness. Often some, even complete, recovery of vision occurs. The vision loss appears primarily as a central scotoma.

Temporal Arteritis (see page 311)

Temporal arteritis (Horton) almost exclusively affects older patients (60 to 80 years). The patients may have rheumatoid symptoms, a low grade fever, and a pathognomonic elevated sedimentation rate (rule of thumb: sedimentation rate equals or exceeds the patient's age). *Headaches* occur often, especially in the temples over the temporal artery and also in the occiput. *Pain* often occurs with mastication, or is more severe in the evening. The temporal artery itself may be *pressure sensitive.* The disease usually presents unilaterally with blurring of the optic disk, anemia ("acute ischemia," Siegert). The severe, usually total visual loss presents acutely. Unless steroid therapy is begun, the other eye almost invariably becomes involved.

Glaucoma (see page 223)

Open angle glaucoma (glaucoma simplex) usually does not produce *ocular pain* or *headaches.* The acute glaucoma attack causes pain (decompensating glaucoma, acute angle closure, congestive or acute inflammatory glaucoma). The subjective symptoms are alarming. A tearing, boring pain radiating to the entire orbit, brow, and skull begins suddenly in the eye. The area of distribution of the *trigeminal nerve* is preferentially involved. The pain may become so unbearable that the patient begs to have his eye removed. *Nausea* and *vomiting* (trigeminal = vagal connection) is an important clinical sign. Migraine, trigeminal neuralgia, and even stomach ulcers are common false diagnoses. The differentiation from acute iritis (= iridocyclitis) is crucial; the intraocular tension makes the diagnosis. With iritis, however, the pupil is constricted; with acute glaucoma it is middilated.

Prodromal attacks of headaches and milder ocular pain occur with chronic (= congestive) glaucoma. The attacks may last minutes or hours. With chronic congestive glaucoma, the signs and symptoms depend on the severity of the pressure rise (see page 223). *Headaches* and epithelial edema often occur in the morning (peak diurnal pressure).

The pain may be a simple dull eye ache.

Secondary glaucoma such as with interstitial keratitis, serpiginous ulcers, iritis, iridocyclitis, subluxated lens, injured lens capsule, choroiditis, central vein thrombosis, retinitis pigmentosa, retinal detachment, intraocular tumors, angle recession, etc., may be asymptomatic (glaucoma simplex) or symptomatic. *Ocular pain* and *headache* may be constant, episodic, or even resemble the worst acute glaucoma attack (with the danger of permanent blindness).

Diseases of the Orbit

Tenonitis (see page 349)

Tenonitis causes exophthalmos which is usually less pronounced than with orbital cellulitis. Lid edema and conjunctival chemosis are present. There is a restriction of motion and *marked pain* when an attempt is made to move the eye. Due to the pain, the patient turns his head in order to avoid all eye movements. *Neuralgias* radiating into the orbit and to the forehead may be prodromal or accompany the acute inflammation.

Orbital Cellulitis (see page 348)

With orbital cellulitis there is marked lid and conjunctival edema, exophthalmos and a frozen immobile globe. *Dull pressing pain* in the orbit and forehead is reported. If there is deep involvement, the *pain* may be *pulsatile*. Usually the patient is systemically ill. Orbital cellulitis differs from tenonitis in that the latter has less exophthalmos and lid or conjunctival edema, greater pain when the eye is moved, and no systemic symptoms.

Inflammation of the Bony Orbital Wall and Orbit (see page 349)

It is important to realize that most cases of *osteitis* and *periosteitis* result from the penetration or perforation of *sinusitis* into the orbit. The sinuses must be examined. Most common locations are the frontal and ethmoidal sinuses. The inner upper nasal quadrant is *edema tous* and *tender.*

Intermittent Exophthalmos (see page 341)

Orbital varices are painless. Bending over or a Valsalva maneuver causes a *proptosis* of a few millimeters to 2 or 3 cm. The protrusion may take a minute or longer to become visible as the veins fill. The direction of displacement of the globe depends on the location of varices in the orbit. In the erect position, exophthalmos disappears. A *dull pain* or heavy feeling of the globe may be present with the intermittent exophthalmos. Nausea, vomiting, and vertigo when bending over can tip off the diagnosis. Vision usually remains normal. Optic atrophy with decreased acuity can occur.

Pulsating Exophthalmos (see page 340)

Rupture of the carotid artery within the cavernous sinus (usually traumatic, rarely idiopathic) leads to sudden severe stabbing and boring *ocular pain* and *headache*. Nausea, vomiting, vertigo, and even coma occur. The patient hears a bruit synchronous with the pulse. The physician hears the bruit when auscultating the orbit. After a few days or a few weeks, a marked exophthalmos of up to 20 mm develops. Orbital as well as conjunctival, episcleral, and retinal vessels become congested because of the arteriovenous shunt. The globe and entire orbit pulsate. There may be a palpable thrill.

Hemorrhages and Tumors of the Orbit

Orbital *hemorrhage* following *blunt injury* to the orbit and ophthalmic artery results in a marked *feeling of pressure,* deep orbital and head pain. There is exophthalmos, the globe is immobile, the conjunctiva and lids are a dark red-blue.

Until inflammation or orbital tissue displacement is present, rare *parasitic infestations* (Echinococcus, Cysticercus, filariasis, trichinosis, etc.) as well as *orbital tumors* and *pseudotumors* remain asymptomatic.

Diseases of the Bony Orbit and Lacrimal System (see page 111)

Inflammation of the Lacrimal Gland

Acute dacryoadenitis involves an inflammation of both the orbital and palpebral portions of the lacrimal gland, which becomes tender. When the upper lid is raised, the swollen gland is visible in the superior temporal quadrant. The skin and even the entire side of the face may be edematous.

Inflammation of the Lacrimal Drainage System

Except for constant tearing and some conjunctivitis, a chronic dacryocystitis may be relatively asymptomatic. An acute cellulitis can flare up around the lacrimal sac with *swelling, tenderness,* and *pain*. The patient then becomes febrile.

Oculonasal Reflex Neurosis (see Velhagen, Tosch)

Sluder, the rhinologist, (1908) described a syndrome of inflammation of the mucous membranes lining the sphenoid sinus and irritation of the pterygopalatine ganglion. *Retro-orbital* and *maxillary pain* radiating to the *neck* and *shoulder* as well as rhinorrhea, swelling of nasal mucosa and conjunctiva, conjunctivitis, photophobia and tearing result. Symptoms disappear when a pledget soaked in cocaine and adrenalin is placed beneath the posterior end of the middle turbinate near the pterygopalatine ganglion.

Maggiori separates the *Sluder syndrome* of the *pterygopalatine* or *sphenopalatine* ganglion into

1. *Neuralgiform* where the *pain* radiates to the *root of the nose, orbits, jaws, teeth, eye,* and *ear.*

2. *Sympathetic form* with *exophthalmos, mydriasis, photophobia* and *tearing.*

The posterior nasal structures are primarily involved.

In addition to these, there is the *nasociliary* or *anterior ethmoidal nerve syndrome* described by Charlin (1936). These limited episodes of *orbital* and *supraorbital pain* are more severe than the ocular findings would indicate. The pain, unilateral around the eye and nose and radiating to the jaw and forehead, is very similar to a trigeminal neuralgia. Episodes of tic-like *pain* uncontrolled by medication occur, especially at night. Valleix's trigger points are found at the inner superior orbital rim and base of the nose. The eye is involved in a variety of ways. Tearing, lid edema, conjunctival hyperemia, corneal changes (ulcers, infiltration, punctate keratitis), iritis, cyclitis, and even hypopyon occur. Profuse rhinorrhea and anatomic changes in the nose develop, especially at the inferior turbinate (hypertrophy, ulcers, malformation of the turbinate).

Insufflation of the nasal mucosa with a cocaine-adrenalin mixture leads to rapid relief. As with any reflex neurosis, the psychological value of cocainization in affecting a cure is unknown.

Headaches Arising Independently of the Eyes but with Ocular Involvement

Vasomotor Headaches

Migraine — Ophthalmoplegic migraine — Vasomotor headaches and central retinal artery pressure.

Migraine

In addition to symptomatic headaches (refractive errors, oculomotor disturbances, disease, intoxication, etc.), *idiopathic headaches* which are not a symptom of other processes play an important role. Of the vascular headaches, migraine is the most significant. Ocular prodromes are the most frequent aura preceding a migrainous attack. If the eye findings (*scintillating scotomata* or other *visual disturbances*) dominate the attack, one speaks of ocular migraine *(Migraine ophthalmique associée ou accompagnée [Charcot]).*

Most migrainous scotomata begin at a point near the center of the visual field and expand toward the periphery. The reverse also occurs. The visual field defect clears in the same way as it appeared. The visual field which first became involved is also the first to clear.

Homonymous hemianopia and the majority of scintillating scotomata presumably result from vasoconstriction (cortical) in the area of distribution of the posterior or middle cerebral arteries. The rare altitudinal hemianopias may be caused by interruption of retinal circulation. There are isolated reports in the literature of bilateral spasm of the superior or inferior branch of the central retinal artery (Koenig 1953).

Most "scintillating" scotomata appear in only one half of the visual field as bright flimmering spots or dark areas of shadow. Dark, foggy patches surrounded by a bright zigzag (picket fence) border may last no more than twenty minutes. The scotoma is often very mobile and micropsia exists. The entire phenomenon may last for seconds or minutes, rarely for hours. The headaches, usually hemicranial, above the eye, brow, temples and occiput, begin immediately after the prodrome. Although they can cause unbearable throbbing with nausea and vomiting, they may be minimal or entirely absent. The patient may be *photophobic* and insist on staying in a dark room.

Migraine can probably be initiated by a variety of stimuli. Trigeminal irritation from refractive errors, heterophoria, optical irritation, and blinding light have been implicated (Matzdorff 1939).

Ophthalmoplegic Migraine (see page 63)

In ophthalmoplegic migraine as described by Charcot (1936), neurologic deficits lasting from 12 to 24 hours or longer follow hemicrania. Transient ophthalmoplegia (periodic oculomotor nerve paresis [Möbius 1936]) with *headaches* is differentiated from migraine. Nonetheless, it is undoubtedly true that a picture similar to ophthalmoplegic migraine may be produced by disease processes such as aneurysms, basilar tumors, arteriosclerosis, myasthenia gravis, etc. Remky (1954) believes that vascular migraine without oculomotor symptoms may evolve into a classic ophthalmoplegic form. Ophthalmoplegic migraine is primarily a pediatric disease. The interval between attacks is usually long and irregular. A strong, one-sided headache with *eye pain* ends several days later with complete or partial oculomotor nerve palsy. The trochlear or abducens nerves are seldom involved. Trigeminal paresthesias and *supraorbital* pain as well as facial nerve paresis occur. The pains resolve as the paresis sets in. The painful episode of the illness may last for days or even weeks. Resolution of the oculomotor paresis takes much longer.

Since the *nerve palsy* begins hours after onset of the headaches, the vasodilatory phase of migraine is probably responsible. There may be a direct compression of oculomotor nerves by dilated cerebral vessels. Another possibility is that edema or a disturbance of permeability, which has been shown to be present in migraine, is responsible. Carotid artery and posterior communicating artery *aneurysms* must be ruled out in ophthalmoplegic migraine. *Recurrent aneurysmal hemorrhage* may cause transient oculomotor nerve paresis and hemicephalgia. In this case, meningism and a bloody spinal fluid are usually present.

Vasomotor Headache and Central Retinal Artery Pressure

The ophthalmologist may aid in the differential diagnosis of *vasomotor headaches*. Weigelin (1954 b) recommends measuring the central retinal artery pressure via the method of Baillart. This pressure is then compared with the patient's blood pressure. With normal intracranial circulation, there is a close relationship. Elevated central retinal artery pressure is seen with dilatation of large vessels leading to the head or with constriction of peripheral intracranial vessels. A low central retinal artery pressure is found with constriction of the large arteries to the brain or dilatation of peripheral intracranial vessels.

Weigelin (1954 b) gives the following formula:

CRAPm = 0.475 (SBPm − IOP) + IOP

(CRAPm = mean central retinal artery pressure;

SBPm = mean systemic blood pressure;

IOP = intraocular pressure.)

Mean systemic and central retinal artery pressure is defined by Weigelin (1954 b) as the diastolic pressure plus 42 percent of the difference between the systolic and diastolic pressures. Among 602 *headache patients*, three groups could be differentiated:

a) 33.5 percent had dilatation of peripheral intracranial vessels,

b) 11.5 percent had constriction of peripheral intracranial vessels,

c) 10.5 percent had a tendency for spasm of intracranial vessels.

The last group was diagnosed by the vasoconstriction stimulation test of Hines and Brown whereby an inordinate amount of intracranial vascular constriction occurred.

Intracranial circulatory disturbance was not present in 44.5 percent of the patients. Clinically, the three groups cannot be differentiated from each other. In all cases there were episodic or permanent *headaches* which were variously described as *pressure*, throbbing or stabbing pain in the forehead, temples, or occasionally in the occiput or over the entire cranium. Generally the patients were under forty years of age. A diagnosis of vasomotor headaches was made when no other etiology could be found for the pains and when other signs of mild autonomic circulation disturbances were present (hyperemia, tremors, cold feet, etc.).

After commotio cerebri about 30 percent of the patients have intracranial circulatory findings. Remky (1953) feels that elevation of the mean central retinal artery pressure when moving from a sitting to a lying position indicates retinal capillary pooling and, therefore, arteriolar hypotony. Conversely, decline of the mean central retinal artery pressure in this situation indicates blockage of outflow with poor retinal perfusion and arteriolar hypertonia. During the *headache* (103 patients with migraine and some with migraine-like headaches were examined), there is either a *hypertonic* or *hypotonic* disturbance. These would correspond to the *vasoconstrictive* and *vasodilatory* forms of migraine. The vasodilatory form was three times as prevalent as the vasoconstrictive. The vasodilatory form without oculomotor nerve palsies can decompensate to the vasoconstrictive type. Scintillating scotomata and hemianopia were seen only in the angiospastic form.

Elevation of retinal artery pressure in the face of constant systemic blood pressure was described as a separate clinical entity by Espildora (1931 a, b, c). The *retinal artery pressure* (measured via Baillard) was elevated as high as 130/60. This was interpreted as indicative of a disturbance of the carotid artery. The patients complained of hypoesthesia of the limbs and menstrual irregularity. *Headaches* and *vertigo* occurred, especially at night.

Giraud (1949) found a similar elevation of intracranial vascular and retinal arterial pressure (as measured with ophthalmodynamometry) to exist in headache patients who had otherwise normal systemic blood pressure and circulation. Functional or organic disturbances of vascular tone were the presumed etiology and occasionally represented a prodrome of generalized intracranial disease (arteriosclerosis, generalized hypertension, space-occupying lesions).

Sinusitis

Sinusitis can cause pain localized in the eyes.

Giant Cell Temporal Arteritis

Often there is pain irradiating from the temporal region towards the head and sometimes towards the shoulder. About the possibility of opticomalacia see page 312.

Trigeminal Neuralgia

The pain of trigeminal neuralgia may be localized in the eye.

Diseases of the Brain and Intracranial Pressure

Pain with *brain tumors, elevated intracranial pressure, central nervous system syphilis, meningitis, cardiac and circulatory decompensation* is frequently localized "behind" the eyes.

Headache is a symptom of elevated intracranial tension, as is vomiting and *papilledema*. Every patient with unexplained headaches needs a fundus examination.

A further sign of elevated intracranial pressure is the onset of *bilateral sixth nerve paresis*. The long intracranial course makes the abducens nerve particularly vulnerable. Oculomotor nerve signs such as unilateral mydriasis and fixed pupil can be a sign of elevated intracranial pressure. Pupillary signs are common in *post-traumatic epidural* and *subdural hematomas*, especially in chronic subdural hematomas. The patient is confused for days or weeks after the injury. Downward displacement of the brain by any mass lesion may press the oculomotor nerve against the edge of the clivus, thereby producing pupillary dilatation and ptosis.

Acute subarachnoid hemorrhage has a sudden onset with severe, diffuse, often occipital headaches. The mortality rate is 25 percent. There may be a palsy of extraocular muscles along with the associated meningism and bloody cerebral spinal fluid. An oculomotor nerve paresis is common if the etiology was a posterior communicating artery aneurysm. Aneurysm of the anterior cerebral artery can cause bilateral optic atrophy and bitemporal hemianopia, even before any bleeding occurs. Subarachnoid hemorrhages may produce papilledema and massive pre-retinal hemorrhages (Rintelen 1969).

References

Charcot: Cited by A. Bielschowsky. In: Handbuch der Neurologie Vol. IV, ed. by O. Bumke, B. Foerster. Springer, Berlin 1936 (p. 209)

Charlin, C.: Syndrome du nerf nasal par toxémie bacillaire. Ann. Oculist. (Paris) 173 (1936) 25–31

Espildora, C.: Die Hypertension der Retinaarterien bei allgemeiner Hypertension. Arch. Oftal. hisp.-amer. 31 (1931a) 456–469

Espildora, C.: Retinaler Überdruck vasculärer Genese ohne allgemeine Hypertension. Arch. Oftal. hisp.-amer. 31 (1931b) 487–504

Espildora, C.: L'hypertendu artériel céphalique. Ann. Oculist. (Paris) 168 (1931c) 923–931

Giraud, M. G.: Les céphalées de l'hypertension cérébro-rétienne solitaire. Schweiz. med. Wschr. 1949, 884

Griffith, A.: The eyes as a cause of headache Brit. med. J. 1934, MMMDCCCXLI, 296–297, Zbl. ges. Ophthal. 32 (1935) 523

Koenig, F.: Über die Ophthalmoneurologie der Migräne. Ophthalmologica 125 (1953) 363–366

Lanchner, A. J.: Headache in ophthalmic practice. Zbl. ges. Ophthal. 60 (1953) 289

Matzdorff, P.: Reflektorisch bedingte und reflektorisch ausgelöste Migräneanfälle. Nervenarzt 12 (1939) 225

Möbius: Cited by A. Bielschowsky. In: Handbuch der Neurologie Vol. IV, ed. by O. Bumke, B. Foerster. Springer, Berlin 1936 (p. 211)

Pau, H.: Die Ciliarneuralgie als vegetativer Schmerz. Klin. Mbl. Augenheilk. 116 (1950) 578–583

Pau, H.: Der Kopfschmerz aus augenärztlicher Sicht. In: Kopfschmerzen, ed. by J. Krischek, Karder, Basel 1958

Remky, H.: Netzhautkreislaufbefunde bei Migräne und verwandten Formen des Anfallkopfschmerzes. Albrecht v. Graefes Arch. klin. exp. Ophthal. 154 (1953) 58–64

Remky, H.: Zur Pathogenese der ophthalmologischen Migräne. Albrecht v. Graefes Arch. klin. exp. Ophthal. 155 (1954) 518–524

Rintelen, F.: Kopfschmerz und Auge. Klin. Mbl. Augenheilk. 154 (1969) 304–315

Schober, H.: Die Ursachen asthenopischer Beschwerden bei Beleuchtung durch Leuchtstofflampen. Klin. Mbl. Augenheilk. 123 (1953) 462–474

Sluder, G.: The role of ganglion spheno-palatinum in nasal headaches. Med. J. N. Y. 1908

Velhagen, K.: Klinisches und Theoretisches zur Neuralpathologie und -therapie des Auges. Albrecht v. Graefes Arch. klin. exp. Ophthal. 150 (1950) 459–489

Weigelin, E.: Diagnose und Behandlung vasomotorischer Kopfschmerzen. Medizinische 1954a, 75–79

Weigelin, E.: Beurteilung des intracraniellen Kreislaufes mit Hilfe der Arteriendruckmessung. Docum. ophthal. 1954b, 183–245

10 Lids

Abnormal Movement of the Lid

Increased blinking — Decreased blinking — Squinting — Myoclonic tic — Blepharospasm — Retraction of the upper lid (Dalrymple's sign) — Lid lag (Graefe's sign) — Lid stare (Stellwag's sign) (see page 339) — Difficulty in everting the lid (Gifford's sign) — Synkinesis of lid and globe — Bell's phenomenon.

The normal rate of blinking is three to seven times per minute.

Increased blinking occurs with any inflammation, fatigue, or strenuous close work. A psychopathic tic or blepharospasm also increases the frequency of blinking.

Decreased blinking occurs with endocrine ophthalmopathy (Stellwag's sign), parkinsonism and hysteria. It is also seen in contact lens wearers and with ingestion of alcohol.

Squinting is a sign of refractive error, especially of myopia or astigmatism. The patient creates a stenopeic slit. Patients may squint to decrease light entering the eye.

Myoclonic tic involves clonic contractures of isolated orbicularis fibers. It occurs with emotional strain and fatigue but may represent some localized disease process.

Reflex **blepharospasm** occurs with any lid, corneal or conjunctival irritation. It may be seen in parkinsonism, brain tumors (acoustic neuromas), brain abscess, aneurysms, cerebrovascular accidents, tertiary lues, or as irritation during recovery from seventh nerve paresis. Functional blepharospasm occurs in hysteria, after dazzling, or with diplopia.

With **lid retraction** (Dalrymple's sign), there is a widened lid fissure and exposure of a sickle-shaped area of sclera above the cornea. The most common cause is endocrine exophthalmos (thyrotoxicosis). Parkinsonism is a rare cause. Drops of 3 to 10 percent cocaine will lead to lid retraction. Lid retraction may be physiologic in the small child (Fig. 10.1).

Graefe's sign is a lag of the upper lid on down gaze (Fig. 10.3). It is seen in thyrotoxicosis and hysteria.

Stellwag's sign or lid stare is infrequent blinking. This is symptomatic of thyrotoxicosis hysteria and postencephalitic parkinsonism.

Gifford's sign is a difficulty in everting the upper lid. It is typical of thyrotoxicosis.

Synkinesis of lid and globe (see paresis of extraocular muscles, page 56). Bell's phenomenon is a physiologic synergistic up and out deviation of the globes on lid closure. The phenomenon may be reversed with facial nerve paresis or absence of both upper lids.

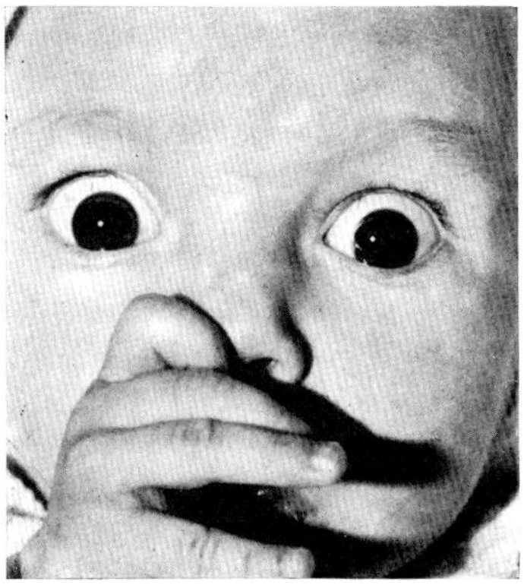

Fig. 10.1 Retraction of the upper lid in an infant (♂ 3 months)

Widening of the Lid Fissure

Facial nerve paresis — Exophthalmos — Vertical gaze palsy — Buphthalmos, high myopia — Post medial rectus tenotomy — Lid contracture — Paradoxical innervation.

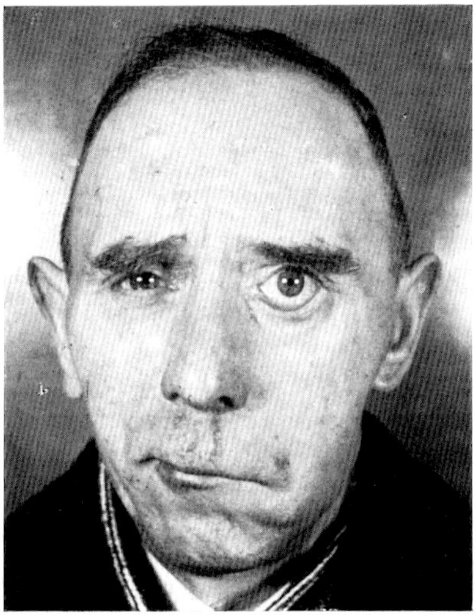

Fig. 10.2 Left facial paresis with lagophthalmos. Note paretic ectropion (♂ 53 yrs.)

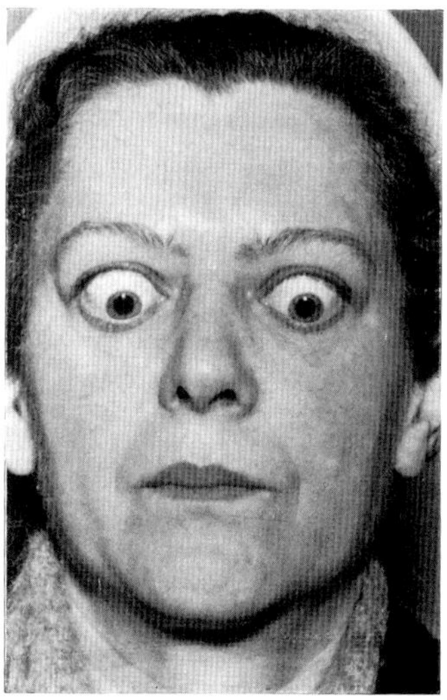

Fig. 10.3 Endocrine exophthalmos: Graefe and Dalrymple's sign

Facial nerve paresis, *orbicularis oculi muscle paresis* with *lagophthalmos (Fig. 10.2):* Normally the cornea is wetted throughout the day. Decreased tear secretion and drying occur at night. The cornea is protected by Bell's phenomenon. In lagophthalmos the lower third of the cornea is exposed. Erosions, ulcers, and even perforation may occur. One usually finds a piling up of gray, vascularized connective tissue *(lagophthalmic keratitis)* (Fig. 13.32). Paralytic ectropion is common. Facial nerve paresis is caused by trauma, tumors, and inflammatory processes. Isolated muscles may be affected by *vaccinia* (see page 95). Leprosy (see page 94) can also cause facial and trigeminal nerve paresis with corneal anesthesia.

A widened lid fissure occurs with **exophthalmos** from any cause, especially endocrine (Fig. 10.3); but it may also be secondary to edema, hematoma, orbital tumors, and sympathetic irritation. Fear or fright has the same effect.

Vertical gaze paresis (Parinaud) (see page 59) is seen with lesions near the superior colliculi. There is an associated lid retraction with widening of the interpalpebral fissure.

A widened lid fissure can be caused by an enlarged globe as is seen in **buphthalmos** in congenital or infantile glaucoma. It can be idiopathic due to **high myopia** or a **scleral staphyloma.**

Slipped muscle after medial rectus tenotomy causes a widened lid fissure.

Cicatricial lids: congenital or acquired (chemical or thermal burns, scleroderma) scarring shortens the lids and widens the interpalpebral fissure.

The lid fissure widens intermittently with **paradoxical innervation** following oculomotor nerve palsy (see page 56) as in the Marcus-Gunn phenomenon.

Narrowing of the Interpalpebral Fissure

Ptosis with oculomotor nerve paresis — Congenital ptosis — Ptosis and limitation of lid movement — Ptosis with progressive external ophthalmoplegia — Ptosis in myasthenia gravis — Ptosis with dermatomyositis — Horner's syndrome — Ptosis with poisoning — Causes limited to the lid — Blepharospasm — Microphthalmia — Tumors — Narrow lid fissure with meningocele — Mucocele.

Ptosis occurs with **oculomotor nerve paresis** (see page 51) which includes the levator palpebrae superioris. The upper lid can no longer be elevated and complete ptosis exists (Fig. 10.4).

Congenital ptosis (Fig. 10.5) of the upper lid is usually bilateral and genetically dominant. With secondary ptosis the superior rectus muscle is usually paretic. Epicanthus, blepharophimosis, and other hereditary malformations are present. In congenital aplasia of the levator of the lid, the superior lid fold is missing.

The patients attempt to elevate the lids with the frontalis muscle and tilt their head backward to look out from under the lid.

The Ullrich-Turner syndrome (see page 89) includes webbed neck (pterygium colli), lymphangiectasia, lax skin around the eye, ptosis, cataract, atypical retinitis pigmentosa, paralytic strabismus, abducens and facial nerve paresis.

There is an abnormal karyotype (XO, chromatin-Barr body negative). Ptosis may be seen with other chromosomal aberrations: Grouchy's syndrome, trisomy D (13) and E (18) and the Hirschhorn-Cooper syndrome (see page 329).

Ptosis and lid synkinesis: A peculiar picture of ptosis occurs in the Marcus-Gunn phenomenon (Fig. 10.6 [see page 52]). The lid elevates when the patient chews, opens his mouth or the jaw is deviated to the ptotic side (jaw winking). Traditionally the etiology is thought to be misdirected cross innervation between the oculomotor nerve and the pterygoid nerve (motor branch of the trigeminal nerve).

An abnormality of supranuclear innervation may also be the cause (Kanter 1955).

Synkinesis of lid and eye occurs with aberrant regeneration of a variety of extraocular nerves, especially the oculomotor nerve (see page 56). The lid may elevate on adduction, abduction, or depression (Fig. 8.19 c) and may depress with adduction.

Progressive external ophthalmoplegia (v. Graefe) (Fig. 10.7) includes bilateral ptosis and an increasing extraocular muscle palsy (Fig. 8.14). This is a muscular dystrophy (myopathy) (Kiloh and Nevin 1951; Beckett and Nettsky 1953; Papst et al. 1958).

Ptosis with myasthenia gravis (see page 53). During the course of the day eye movements worsen (Fig. 8.15). The condition is reversed within minutes by parenteral administration

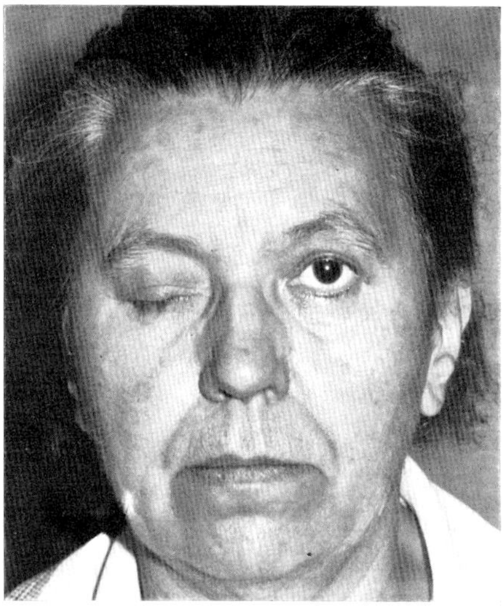

Fig. 10.4 Ptosis-oculomotor nerve palsy (♀ 68 yrs.)

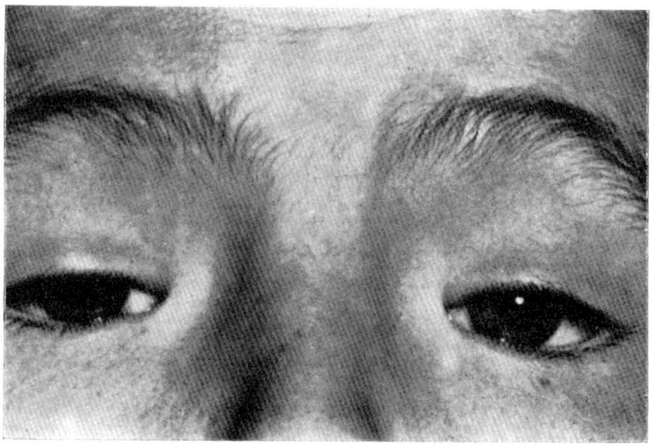

Fig. 10.5 Congenital ptosis (with epicanthus)

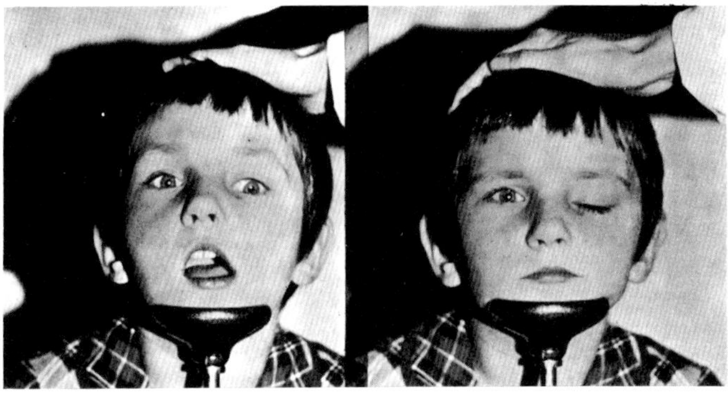

Fig. 10.6 Marcus-Gunn phenomenon (♀ 9 yrs.)

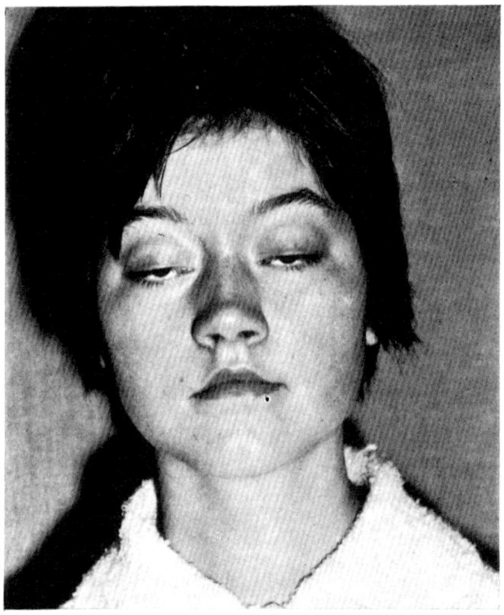

Fig. 10.7 Ophthalmoplegia progressiva (♀ 16 yrs.) = chronic progressive ocular muscle dystrophy

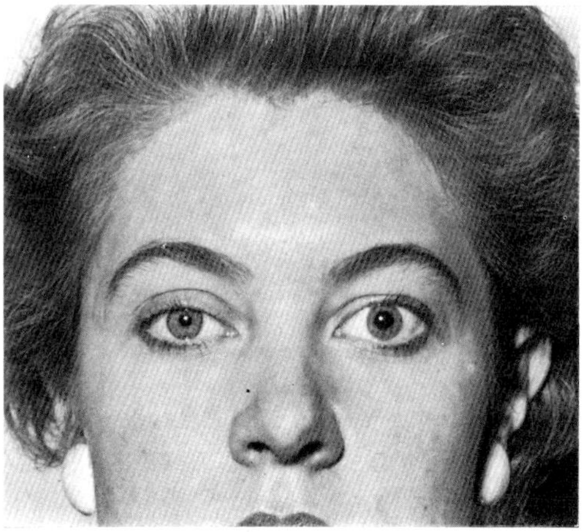

Fig. 10.8 Horner syndrome, right eye (miosis, ptosis, enophthalmos)

of cholinesterase inhibitors (physostigmine, Prostigmin, Tensilon, etc.).

Ptosis in dermatomyositis: Symptoms include extraocular muscle myositis, episcleritis and poikiloderma.

Horner's syndrome (sympathetic dysfunction) is usually unilateral but can be bilateral. Unilateral sympathetic damage can be caused in the neck (stellate ganglion) by a cervical rib; disorders may be present at the apex of the lung; Klumpke's paralysis or syringomyelia may also be found. Horner's syndrome (Fig. 10.8) includes miosis, ptosis, and enophthalmos. Motion of the lid is normal with sympathetic ptosis. If present from infancy, the iris on the involved side remains less pigmented (heterochromia) than on the uninvolved side.

Ptosis can result from poisoning from lead, arsenicals, dichlorodiethyl-sulfide, carbon monoxide, and botulism.

Ptosis due to processes localized on the lid occurs with inflammation, conjunctival scarring, pemphigus, chemical burns, diphtheria, etc. Tumor, amyloidosis, trachoma, lid edema, hordeolum, chalazion, pachydermoperiostosis, etc., weigh down the lid and thereby cause ptosis.

Blepharospasm narrows the lid fissure. It is seen with trigeminal neuralgia as well as with inflammation of the anterior segment of the eye and lids, especially scrofula (Fig. 10.3). It may also occur with facial nerve involvement, postencephalitic tetany, parkinsonism, tabetic crises, dazzling, functional (hysteric) blepharospasm, and tic.

Microphthalmos: A narrowed lid fissure occurs with congenital microphthalmos, high hyperopia (small eye), and phthisis bulbi.
Tumors as a cause of narrowed lid fissure: Orbital and lid tumors such as hemangioma (Fig. 25.17), dermoid, basal cell carcinoma, plexiform neuroma (Fig. 10.45), lacrimal gland tumors, osteoma, sarcoma, and facial hemihypertrophy in von Recklinghausen's disease can all produce narrowed lid fissures.
Meningoencephalocele (Fig. 25.8) or **mucocele** (Fig. 25.16) can cause narrowed palpebral fissures.

Malformation and Maldevelopment of the Lid

Ablepharia, microblepharia – Blepharophimosis – Ankyloblepharon – Cryptophthalmia – Obliquity of the lid fissure (mongoloid, antimongoloid) – Broad eyelids (euryblepharon) – Blepharochalasis and senile epiblepharon – Symblepharon – Lid colobomas – Epicanthus.

Ablepharia is lack of lids; microblepharia is underdeveloped lids.
Blepharophimosis: Marked narrowing of the lid fissure in the horizontal and vertical directions (Fig. 10.9). This may be congenital, associated with ptosis and epicanthus, or acquired from scarring or lid shrinkage (trachoma, pemphigus, burns).

Waardenburg's syndrome is an autosomal dominant disorder which includes (Aasved 1962): lateral displacement of the inner canthi (telecanthus) and lacrimal puncta, blepharophimosis (99 percent), hyperplasia of the root of the nose (78 percent), hyperplasia of the medial portion of the eyebrow (45 percent), partial or complete heterochromia of the iris (25 percent), congenital deafness (20 percent), white forelock (17 percent) and vitiligo.

Ankyloblepharon: Fusion of the upper and lower lids is called ankyloblepharon. It may be congenital (Fig. 10.10) or acquired. It is frequently associated with anophthalmos or microphthalmos.
Cryptophthalmos: The lids are also not developed in congenital cryptophthalmos where the globe is rudimentary or severely deformed (Badtke 1961).
Oblique lid fissures: The lid fissure may be slanted. In a mongoloid slant, the lateral canthus is higher than the medial. In an antimongoloid slant, the situation is reversed.
The differential diagnosis of mongoloid slant includes: Asians; Down's syndrome; Laurence-Moon-Biedl-Bardet syndrome (see page 286); Klinefelter's syndrome (see page 330); congenital chondrodystrophic calcification syndrome of Conradi with cataract, optic atrophy, flat root of the nose, large head; and anhidrotic ectodermal dysplasia.
Antimongoloid slant may occur as a congenital anomaly, combined with separation of the lateral canthus from the globe.
(Franceschetti and Avanca 1960 [see page 331]).
Antimongoloid slant is more frequent in the oculoauriculovertebral syndrome (Goldenhar) (see page 331), oculomandibulodyscephaly (Hallermann-Streiff) (see page 332), mesodermal dystrophy (Marchesani) (see page 252), in craniofacial dysostosis (Crouzon), acrocephalosyndactyly (Apert), Turner's syndrome, trisomy 18 (E-trisomy) (see page 329). Scarring can cause antimongoloid slants.
Wide eyelids: Congenital broad eyelids (over 30 mm) are called *euryblepharon* (Fig. 10.11). The lid fissure is lengthened; the lateral canthi may fall away from the globe and "pockets" may form at the lid angles. Conjunctivitis and

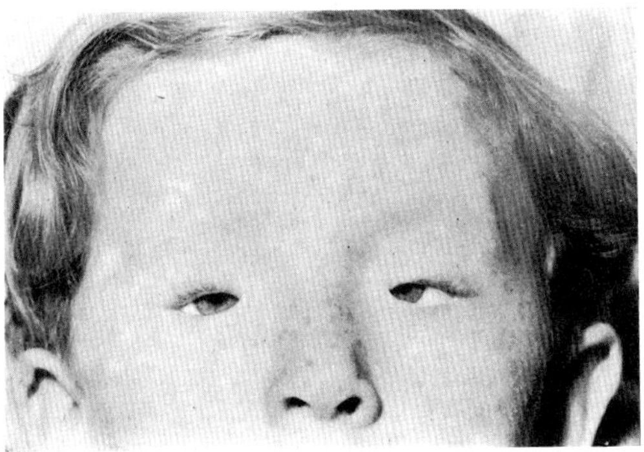

Fig. 10.9 Blepharophimosis (with ptosis and epicanthus)

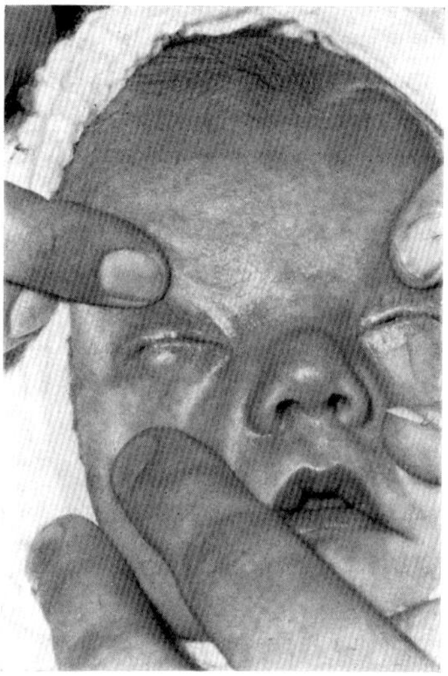

Fig. 10.10 Congenital ankyloblepharon (♂ 14 days)

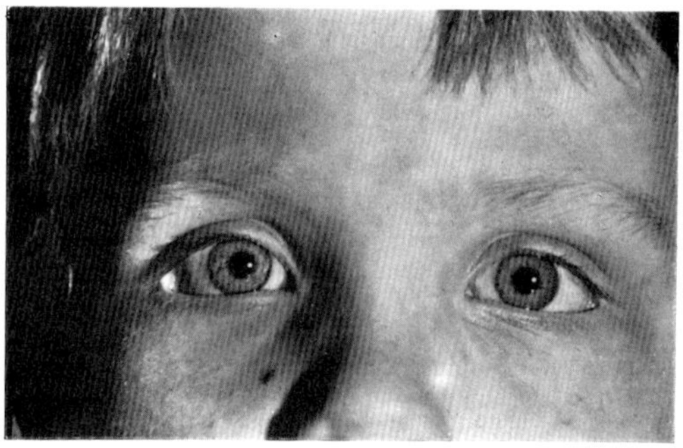

Fig. 10.11 Euryblepharon (♂ 6 yrs.)

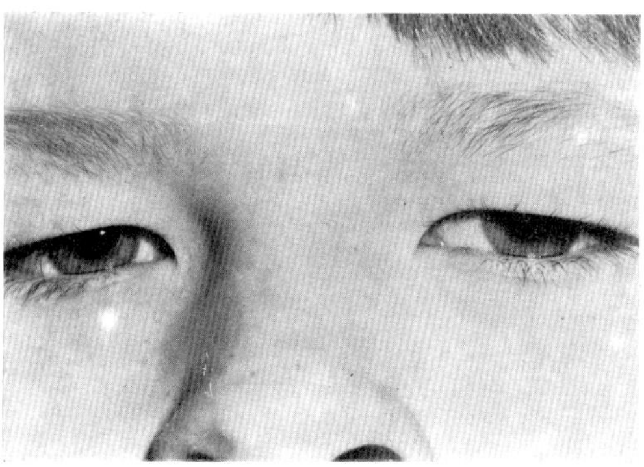

Fig. 10.12 Blepharochalasis (♂ 8 yrs.)

lacrimation result. The eyebrows are frequently fused (Hollwich et al. 1969).

Elschnig's syndrome is elongation of the lid fissure with downward displacement of the lateral angle. Ectropion of the lower lid as well as cleft lip and palate may occur.

The lid fissure of the adult European is normally 27 to 30 mm long and 10 to 14 mm wide. The ratio of length to width is about 3:1 in the adult and 2:1 in infants.

Blepharochalasis; dermatochalasis (senile epiblepharon): Blepharochalasis occurs when excess skin of the upper lid hangs over the lid fissure. This is a congenital defect first appearing at puberty or in early childhood (Hadley 1939; Löhr 1949) (Fig. 10.12). There is atrophy of all skin layers as well as loss of fascia and ectasia of subcutaneous vessels. Orbital fat and lacrimal gland may herniate. The excess, wrinkled skin of the lid hangs over the cilia and may block vision.

Blepharochalasis of the lower lid is reported (Stein 1930).

Asher's syndrome consists of blepharochalasis, duplication of the mucous membrane of the upper lip, and intermittent swelling of the upper lid. Spina bifida and pectus excavatum may be present (Klemens 1939; Eisenstodt 1949).

The laxity of the upper lid that causes skin to hang over the lid fissure is called *dermatochalasis, senile epiblepharon,* or *cutis laxa senilis* (Fig. 10.13). Dermatochalasis of the upper and lower lid (skin fold) presses the cilia against the cornea. It occurs in infants and tends to disappear with age. It is caused by an excess of subcutaneous fat (Fig. 10.18).

Symblepharon is fusion of the bulbar and palpebral conjunctiva. This leads to scarring and foreshortening of the fornix (Fig. 10.14). The etiology includes acid, alkali, or thermal burns; trauma; diphtheria; trachoma; pemphigoid; etc.

Coloboma of the lid is a triangular congenital defect, usually between the inner and middle third of the upper lid (Fig. 10.15). In the lower lid, it is between the middle and outer thirds (Badtke 1961). Lid colobomata are frequently traumatic in origin (Fig. 10.16). Congenital lid colobomata are usually associated with other ocular (microphthalmos, uveal colobomata, dermoids, etc.) or facial malformations (clefts, mandibulofacial dysostosis, etc.).

Typical facial clefts may be oblique or hemifacial (mouth-eye-face). Usually there is a lower lid coloboma near the inner canthus. The lower lid is rarely missing entirely. Atypical facial clefts are less common. The cleft extends from the mouth laterally and is associated with a lateral coloboma of the lower lid.

Lid colobomata are part of the oculoauricular syndrome (Goldenhar, see page 331) and oculomandibulofacial dysostosis (Franceschetti, see page 331).

Epicanthus: Mongoloid fold or epicanthus (Figs. 10.5, 10.9) is a common anomaly. A crescent-shaped fold of skin extends from the upper lid (rarely the lower lid [epicanthus inversus]) across the inner canthus. Inverse epicanthus almost always has an associated congenital ptosis. Mongoloids virtually always have an epicanthus. Inheritance is dominant and may be associated with other congenital defects such as esotropia, ptosis, shortened lid fissure, hypertelorism, etc. Children frequently have a small degree of epicanthus which disappears in the second decade of life as the base of the nose develops. Epicanthus is found with chromosomal anomalies: Down's syndrome (trisomy 21), Lejeune's syndrome (cri du chat) (deletion of chromosome 18), Klinefelter's syndrome (multiple X plus Y) (see page 330), and Turner's syndrome (XO).

The Ullrich-Turner syndrome (see page 330) is sometimes classified as a phacomatosis (see page 296). Epicanthus and hypertelorism are common. Zunin and Mariotti (1953) found fundus anomalies in nine of their patients. Hypoplasia of the optic disk was found in one-third of the cases and hyperplasia in the remaining two-thirds. Numerous tortuous ciliary retinal arteries were described. Situs inversus of the retinal vasculature was found in one patient. Common anomalies in Turner's syndrome include absence of the caruncle, lacrimal gland hypoplasia, anomalies of the eye lashes, abducens and facial nerve palsy. Fülling and Pünder (1965) describe equatorial chorioretinal pigmentary changes, hyperopic astigmatism, and esotropia.

Epicanthus, cataract, and elastic skin occur in the Ehlers-Danlos syndrome. Hyperextensibility of the joints (india-rubber man) is also found.

Renofacial dysplasia (Potter's disease) is associated with epicanthus, hypertelorism, spina bifida, club foot, renal and genital malformations.

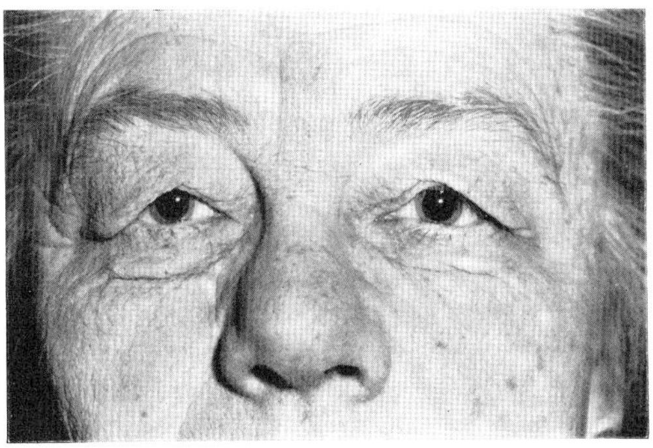

Fig. 10.13 Dermatochalasis (♀ 67 yrs.)

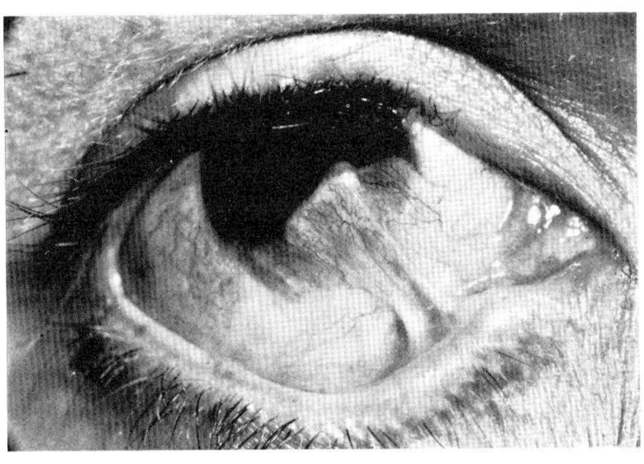

Fig. 10.14 Symblepharon following a burn, secondary pterygium (♂ 21 yrs.)

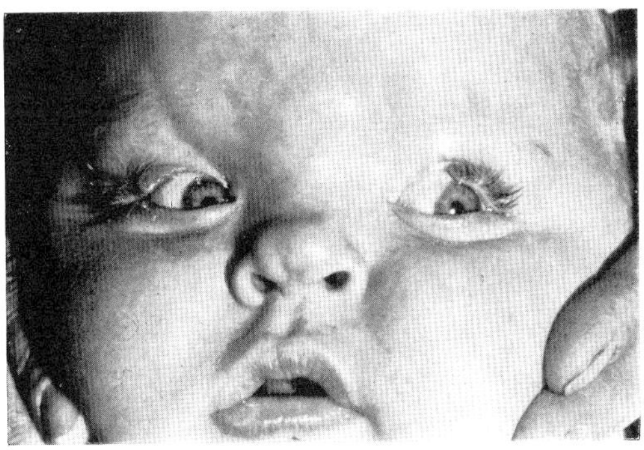

Fig. 10.15 Congenital lid coloboma (♂ 6 months)

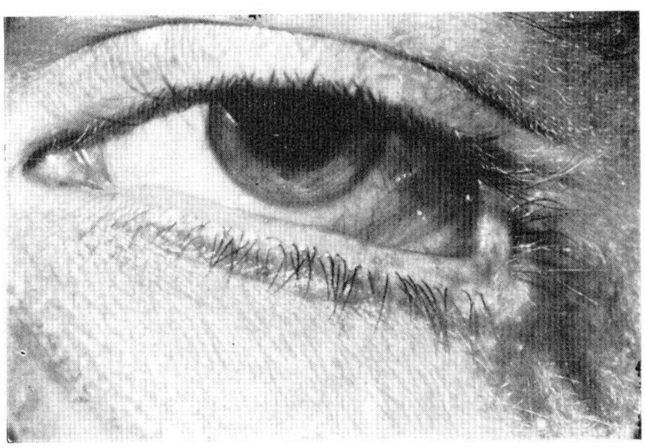

Fig. 10.16 Acquired, traumatic lid coloboma (♂ 20 yrs.)

Displacement of the Lids

Ectropion — Entropion.

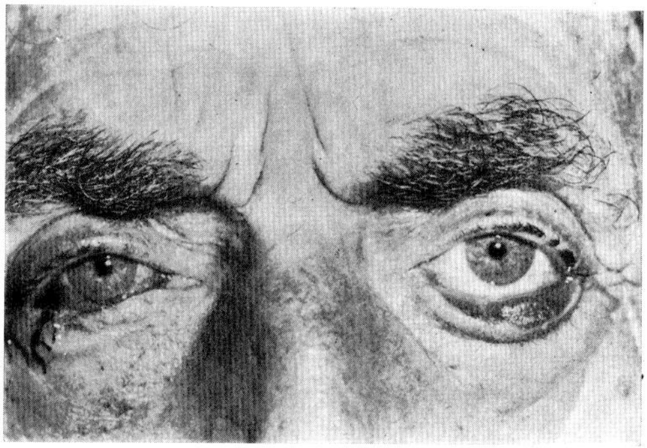

Fig. 10.17 Senile ectropion on the left; postsurgical correction on the right (♂ 72 yrs.)

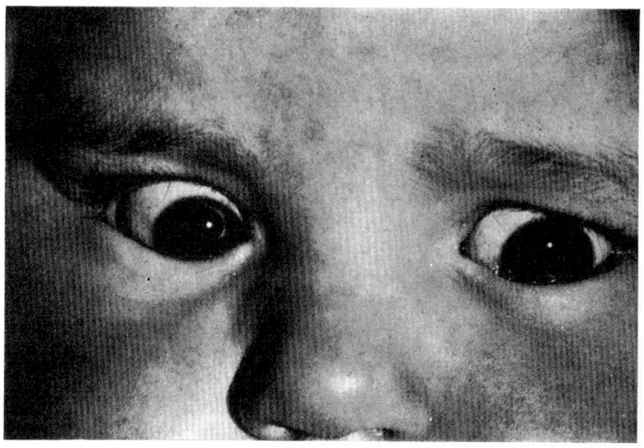

Fig. 10.18 Entropion in an infant (♂ ½ yrs.)

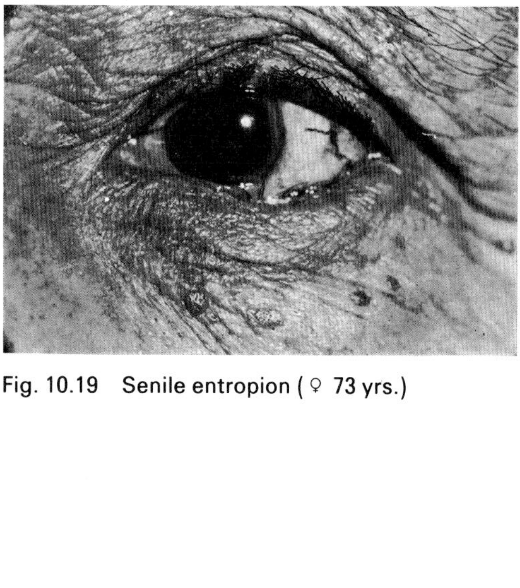

Fig. 10.19 Senile entropion (♀ 73 yrs.)

Ectropion or eversion of the lids occurs when the lower lid falls away from the globe. Tears tend to pool because the punctum is no longer in contact with the lacrimal lake. Epiphora, chronic conjunctivitis and chemosis result. The ectropion is made worse by constant rubbing.

Senile ectropion is caused by an age-dependent loss of tone of the orbicularis oculi muscle (Fig. 10.17). *Cicatricial ectropion* occurs secondary to scarring, of the skin (Plate I, Fig. 2, page 128 a) after chemical or thermal burns.

Ectropion is caused by any significant traumatic or inflammatory shrinkage or loss of lid substance. Causes include lupus vulgaris, tuberculosis, luetic periostitis, osteomyelitis with contracting fistulas, ichthyosis, scleroderma, xeroderma pigmentosa, yaws, etc.

Facial nerve palsy affecting the orbicularis oculi muscle produces a *paralytic ectropion* (Fig. 10.3) with lagophthalmos (this word is derived from the old myth that hares sleep with their eyes open). *Spastic ectropion*, as with scrofula, is caused by spasm of the outer fibers of the orbicularis oculi muscle.

The conjunctiva in the area of the ectropion is thickened, dry, and hyperemic. Epiphora or weeping results because the lacrimal punctum cannot drain tears.

Entropion: When the lids turn inward, the lashes rub on the globe (trichiasis). This produces corneal erosion and ulcers. Congenital entropion (Fig. 10.18) is a rare occurrence and usually disappears within a few months. Entropion is usually a *senile* phenomenon (Fig. 10.19) or *cicatricial*. The latter is caused by scarring of the conjunctiva such as with burns, symblepharon, ocular pemphigoid, trachoma, gonorrhea, or diphtheria.

Spastic entropion is caused by contracture of the inner fibers of the orbicularis oculi muscle. This is seen with severe corneal inflammations such as scrofulous keratoconjunctivitis (blepharospasm), interstitial keratitis, and corneal ulcers. Any blepharospasm, even hysterical blepharospasm, is caused and reinforced by lashes rubbing on the cornea.

Inflammatory Lid Edema

Hordeolum and lid abscess — Chalazion — Urticaria — Eczema — Scrofula — Impetigo — Anthrax — Glanders — Lupus erythematosus — Erysipelas, lid necrosis — Gangrene — With corneal-conjunctival diseases and injuries — Diseases of the orbit — Photodermatitis — Acute viral inflammations — Mycoses — Parasites — Gumma — Primary and secondary lues — Tuberculosis — Sarcoidosis — Leprosy — Chancroid — Acne rosacea, psoriasis.

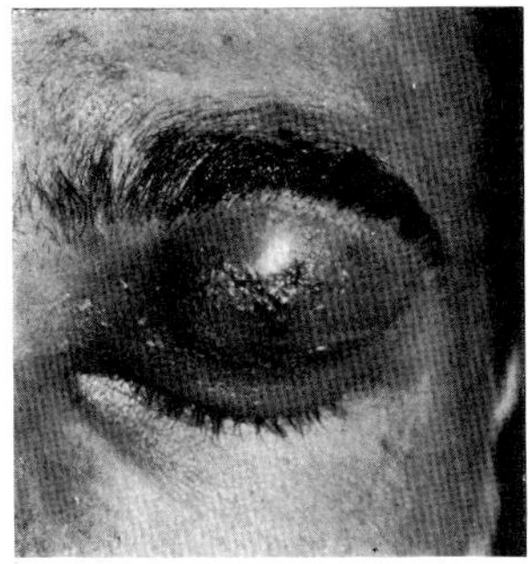

Fig. 10.20 Lid abscess (♂ 18 yrs.)

Due to thin skin and loose subcutaneous connective tissue, the lids swell easily and become edematous. *Hordeolum and lid abscess:* Hordeolum (Plate I, Fig. 3, page 128 a) is a localized, painful, red, edematous inflammatory process with rapid abscess formation. Healing is quick once the abscess drains.

The glands of Zeiss (sebaceous) and Moll's glands (sweat) empty into the ciliary follicles. The meibomian glands (modified sebaceous glands) lie in the tarsal plate.

External hordeolum is an *acute inflammation* of the sebaceous glands at the lid margin. *Internal hordeolum* is an *acute inflammation* of the meibomian gland. The causal agent is usually staphylococcus. In some cases multiple foci of inflammations exist *(hordeolosis)*. These may abscess, fuse with one another, and cause a true lid abscess (Fig. 10.20). A *lid abscess* may be secondary to orbital cellulitis (exophthalmos, chemosis, systemic signs), periostitis (localized edema, marked pressing pain of the thickened orbital rim), infected laceration, dacryoadenitis (painful edema, redness under the upper outer lid), sinusitis (X-ray), etc. See inflammations of the orbit (page 348).

Chalazion is a *chronic inflammation* of the meibomian gland (Fig. 10.21; Plate II, Fig. 1, page 128 b). This may be secondary to an unhealed internal hordeolum or the result of a primary retention of secretions. These round, red to yellow, immobile, nontender nodules in the tarsal plate may cause localized lid edema. Histologically, lymphocytes, epithelioid cells, and giant cells are seen. Pedunculated granulomas have been observed (granuloma pyogenicum).

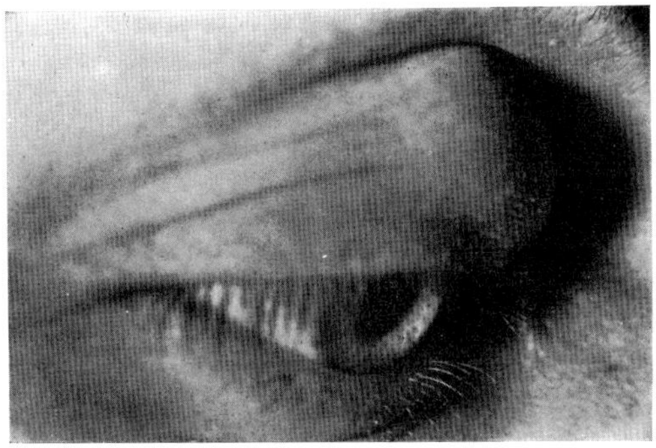

Fig. 10.21 Chalazion of the upper lid (♀ 13 yrs.)

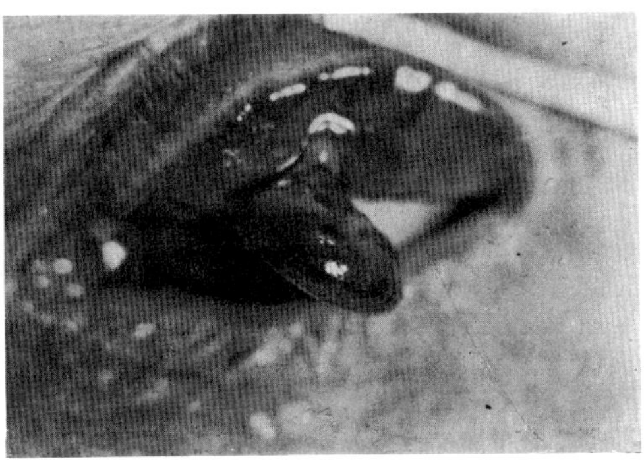

Fig. 10.22 Granuloma pyogenicum (♂ 68 yrs.)

Chalazions are frequently transient and recurrent but may remain unchanged for weeks to months. They may disappear spontaneously, break through to the conjunctiva, or result in a granuloma pyogenicum (Fig. 10.22) or a giant chalazion. Chalaziosis (e. g., multiple chalazions) may occur. Chalazion has been observed in infants (Minamik 1939).

A histologic search for basal cell carcinoma must be made if a chalazion has an irregular surface, ulcerates, or is slowly expansive. Meibomian gland adenocarcinoma frequently simulates recurrent chalazion.

Urticaria (hives); eczema: *Urticaria* causes conjunctival itching, burning, redness, edema, even blister formation. Corneal edema, erosions and iritis have been observed. Causes include nettles, cowslip, insect bites, jellyfish stings, poison ivy, poison oak, etc. Some foods (strawberries, fish, etc.) are particularly allergenic and cause hives in susceptible patients. *Eczema of the lids* (see page 122) produces burning, itching, edema, and a feeling of tension. In the acute stage eczema is usually wet. When chronic, however, it is dry with scaling and crust formation (Plate II, Fig. 2, see page 128 b).

Topical medications (antibiotics, atropine, sulfonamides, anesthetics, mercurials, iodine and chamomile) are notorious for causing lid eczema. Eczema may be seen with local or parenteral use of gold (toxic), arsenicals, iodides, bromides, antihypertensives, hyponotics or sedatives. Cosmetics are a major cause of contact dermatitis (eczema) around the eyes. Other agents include plastics (eyeglass frames), animal hair, feathers, grasses, flowers, soaps, tar, caoutchouc, poison oak, poison ivy, etc.

Streptomycin causes chronic, particularly recalcitrant blepharoconjunctivitis (Charamis 1949; Mejer 1949, 1950). Due to the high incidence of penicillin allergy, penicillin should not be used topically (Plate II, Fig. 3, page 128 b) (Schubert 1967).

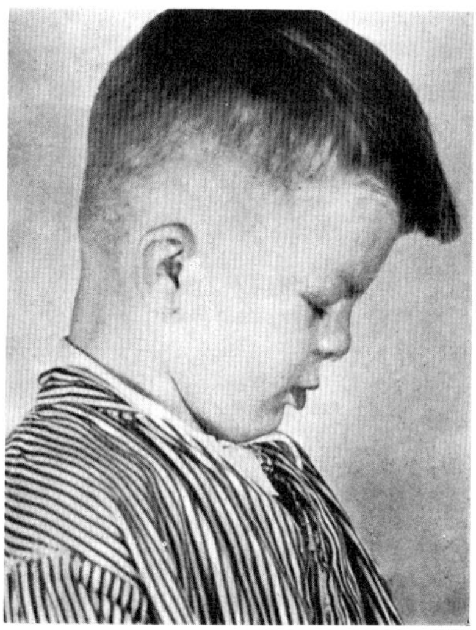

Fig. 10.23 Blepharospasms in scrofulosis (♂ 6 yrs.)

Oral medications can also cause eczema of the face or lids. Notorious agents include barbiturates, bromides, iodides, and quinine. Allergenic foods include milk, cheese, eggs, fish, strawberries, mushrooms, and legumes.

Eczema of the lids may spread to the face, hands, and rest of the body. Cornea and conjunctiva (see page 122) can become involved.

Scrofula: *Scrofulosis* is a specific entity (tuberculosis) which, when it involves the eyes, includes *lid eczema* and phlyctenular keratoconjunctivitis. The angles of the lids, mouth, nares, and ears may all be eczematous. Diet, sanitation, physical wellbeing, and a history of allergies play a role in this disease. Like keratitis, poorly healing lid rhagades cause *blepharospasm* (Fig. 10.23). At first this is a purely symptomatic reflex blepharospasm, but it may persist as a functional blepharospasm after the underlying process (scrofulous keratitis) has healed.

Impetigo: The red blisters and yellow scabs of *impetigo contagiosa* are the result of a localized streptococcal skin infection. It is primarily seen in children with poor hygiene. The lesions are spread by scratching and may ultimately cover the entire face.

Anthrax (Bacillus anthracis) of the lids is rare. After an incubation period of two to three days, a malignant pustule or edema develops. Regional lymph nodes are tender and swollen. The first sign is an itchy red spot that evolves into a blue-red pustule. The pustule characteristically develops a black scab. At first the lid is pale white but it then becomes blue-red. Anthrax is acquired by handling animal products.

Glanders (Pseudomonas mallei) in its chronic form occasionally affects the lid. These are poorly healing nodules. Farcy is the same disease in horses and is the usual source of infection for man.

Lupus erythematosus: Since lupus erythematosus primarily affects exposed parts of the body, the lids are also involved. The first sign is lid edema, then hyperkeratosis, seborrhea, and finally atrophy of the skin (Cordes and Aken 1947; Rohrschneider and Ehring 1953). Conjunctival (see page 268) (Lutz 1932; Vilanova et al. 1956) and corneal hyperkeratosis occur (Pillat 1935; Doesschate 1956) (Fig. 10.24).

Of the 48 patients with lupus erythematosus examined by Pillat (1935), 16 (33 percent) had chorioretinal lesions; 14 were old and two were active. The lesions were usually uniocular, peripheral, and varied from one to five per eye. Cotton-wool spots, dilated retinal veins (Hotz 1957; Kato and Omoto 1957), retinal hemorrhages, and circumscribed chorioretinal lesions occur (for review of the literature, see Schreck 1960). The disseminated disease affects heart, kidneys, spleen, bone marrow, stomach, and intestinal tract.

Erysipelas; lid necrosis: *Erysipelas* (St Anthony's fire) causes a rock-hard, erythematous, and eventually gangrenous lid. It is a streptococcal infection with high fever. Lid involvement is usually secondary to facial erysipelas and is seldom caused by a lid laceration or primary infection. After an incubation period of one to two days, a sharply delimited area of skin edema occurs. High fever is present. Complications include lid gangrene, keratitis, iritis, and neuritis (from orbital thrombophlebitis) accompanied by optic atrophy.
Quincke's edema is differentiated by its lack of systemic illness and fever; herpes zoster, by its segmental distribution.
Limited necrosis and even *lid gangrene* are an exception (Plate II, Fig. 4, page 128 b). The etiology is infectious (diphtheria, staphylococci, streptococci, lues, fungi, etc.). Diabetes, marasmus, and lues are frequent underlying factors.

Keratoconjunctival injury and disease: Inflammatory lid edema may be caused by corneal ulcer, *gonoblennorrhea* (Fig. 12.4), acute *trachoma, conjunctival diphtheria,* etc. *Insect bites* are a primary consideration. *Trichiasis* seldom leads to lid edema. *Lacerations,* especially if infected, cause pronounced lid edema.

Photodermatitis of the lid (see page 135): *Solar eczema* (sun burn) is physiologic.
Photoallergic dermatitis (see page 135) is pathologic and caused by exposure of hands, face, etc., to ultraviolet light. Erythematous, wet, papular eczema results. If *exogenous,* the usual cause is drug absorption, *aniline dyes,*

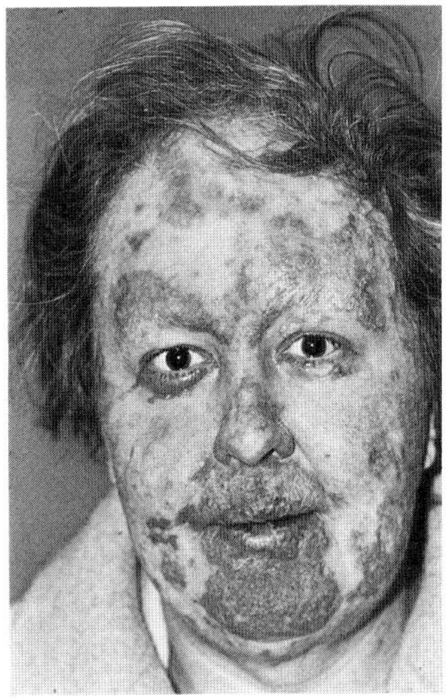

Fig. 10.24 Erythema of the face and lids (♀ 48 yrs.)

hydroquinone, hydrocarbons, sulfonamides. Endogenous causes include *hematoporphyrinuria* (see page 366) and *xeroderma pigmentosum.* The latter begins in the second or third decade with erythema, inflammation, and pigmentation. Finally, atrophy, leukoplakia, and scarring of the skin may occur. Ulcerated skin lesions develop into tumors (spindle cell melanoma [Plate II, Fig. 5, page 128 b]). Death from a metastatic lesion frequently occurs before the patient reaches the age of twenty. The eyes are involved through ulceration of the lids which extends to the conjunctiva and globe.

Acute viral inflammations: Vesicle formation is more prominent in acute viral exanthema than is lid edema (herpes simplex, zoster, vaccinia, variola) (see page 95).

Mycoses: Fungal skin infections also involve the lids (Hofmann 1965, François 1968). In the case of *actinomycosis* (gram-positive bacterium), it is usually an extension from infection of the jaw. Subcutaneous infiltration, nodules, and fistulizing abscesses develop. The nodules in *sporotrichosis* are smaller, grow more slowly, and fuse into each other. The lids become edematous and indurated ulcers develop. The draining lymph node can become flocculent. Ultimately, the infection spreads to the lacrimal sac and orbit. The differential diagnosis

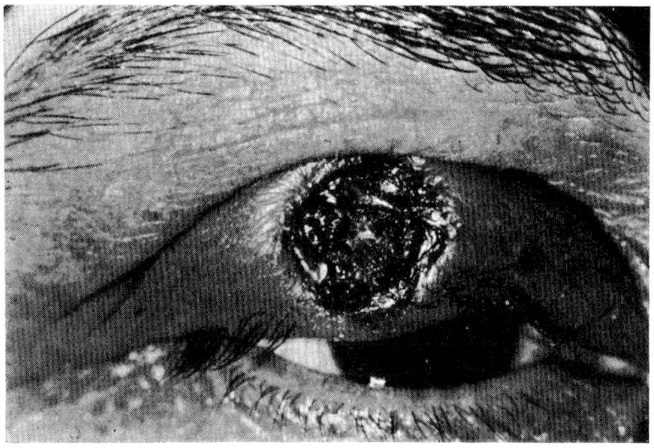

Fig. 10.25 Round, firm, chronic mycotic ulcer (blastomycosis) of the upper lid (♂ 34 yrs.)

includes syphilitic gumma and tuberculous granuloma. In children, *Trichophyton* (tinea, ringworm) can involve the lids or eyebrows. These are scaly round lesions healing at the center.

Candidiasis of the lids may be primary or secondary. Lid edema and erythema with small pustules or an eczema-like reaction results.

Thrush and *leptothrix* can cause lid erythema and pustule formation.

Blastomycosis of the lid causes ulcerating papules. More commonly a well circumscribed ulceration occurs (Fig. 10.25). This may cause scarring with contracture and distortion of the lid. The *differential diagnosis* includes gumma, lupus vulgaris, basal cell carcinoma, and sporotrichosis (with preauricular lymphadenopathy).

Rhinosporidosis causes polyp-like growths which bleed easily.

Animal parasites (see page 198): Lid edema secondary to parasites is primarily seen in the tropics. *Ophthalmomyiasis* (fly larvae) (see page 199) is a markedly painful lid edema with chalazion-like granulomas from which the larvae can be expressed. *Trichinosis* frequently begins with lid edema.

Filariasis (elephantiasis) causes recurrent lid edema.

Leishmaniasis (oriental boil, dumdum fever) causes pseudochalazion, edema, and lid abscesses. The cornea, tear ducts, and conjunctiva may be secondarily involved. Corneal abscess formation and even perforation can occur.

Sleeping sickness (trypanosomiasis) may cause edema of the lids and orbit as well as interstitial keratitis, iridocyclitis, neuritis, and extraocular muscle paresis (rare).

Primary luetic lid involvement is rare (Pôstić 1940). It was seen in Russia and the Balkans because of the custom of licking wounds. Of 100 extragenital primary lesions, four to five were in the region of the eyes (Löhlein 1931). After three weeks, a hard chancre develops with edema of the preauricular or submaxillary lymph nodes.

The rash of secondary lues (maculas, papules, or pustules) may also involve the lids (Löhlein 1931; Pôstić 1940). Gummatous lid involvement may occur years after a primary infection or in congenital lues.

Tuberculosis: In contrast to lupus vulgaris, primary tuberculosis of the lid is rare. Lid tuberculomas are also rare in this day and age (Plate III, Fig. 1, page 128 c).

Lupus vulgaris usually involves the lids secondarily and may cause marked ectropion formation.

Skin nodules of varying size are a major finding in *sarcoidosis*.

Tuberculoid leprosy frequently involves the lids. Lepromata infiltrate and cause hypertrophy (pseudochalazion), especially in the upper lids. Eyebrows and lashes may turn white and fall out. The classic leonine facies develops. Paresis of the facial nerve with lagophthalmic keratitis and of the trigeminal nerve with corneal hypoesthesia or anesthesia is described. Conjunctival, episcleral, or scleral nodular infiltrates may extend to the cornea as interstitial keratitis. In most cases, as much as three-fourths of the cornea is involved. At first the corneal infiltrates follow the course of corneal nerves. Later, there is pannus and even staphyloma formation. There may be nodules in the iris and chronic iridocyclitis may be present. Complications include synechiae, secondary glaucoma, and cataracts. The eye is affected in 72 percent of patients with leprosy (Schields and Waring 1974). Löwe (1955) found 50 percent of the patients in Kashmir with ocular leprosy to be blind. Chorioretinitis and extraocular muscle palsies also occur.

The age at which the risk is greatest for contracting leprosy (Mycobacterium leprae) is between five and fifteen years of age. In some 90 percent of cases, the eyes will be involved (Elliot 1951; Bouzas 1956).

Chancroid (ulcus molle, Hemophilus ducreyi) rarely involves the lids. When it does, there may be multiple soft superficial ulcers with undermined edges.

Acne rosacea and psoriasis may appear on the lids.

Vesicular Inflammations of the Lids

Acute viral inflammations (herpes simplex, zoster, vaccinia, variola) — Erythema multiforme (Stevens-Johnson syndrome, mucocutaneous ocular syndrome, [Fuchs]) — Pemphigus vulgaris — Benign mucosal pemphigoid — Epidermolysis bullosa — Drug-induced bullae — Polymorphic light eruptions (hydroa vacciniforme).

Acute viral infections can cause lid edema and vesicle formation.

Herpes simplex: After a fever, herpes simplex lesions may appear on the lid (Fig. 10.26) as small clear vesicles with an erythematous base. They usually heal without sequelae.

Ophthalmic zoster: Zoster in the distribution of the ophthalmic division of the trigeminal nerve (Fig. 10.27 [see page 34, 155]) forms grouped vesicles which leave scars after healing. Photophobia, lacrimation, neuralgias, and a generalized malaise may appear prior to vesicle formation. The accompanying ciliary neuralgias can last for months or even years.

In ophthalmic zoster (nasociliary nerve), the possibility of corneal infiltrates, erosions, iritis, therapeutically recalcitrant secondary glaucoma and paresis of ocular muscles (especially the oculomotor nerve) should be considered (see page 155). An associated internal ophthalmoplegia with a fixed dilated pupil may be present; retrobulbar neuritis is rare.

Vaccinia: Following vaccinations the eye may become involved. The patient scratches the inoculation site and transfers infectious material to the lids and eyes. More rarely there is hematogenous dissemination. Spread from the vaccination site is particularly likely in children who already have blepharitis (Fig. 10.28). There is a firm lid edema. Vesicles which evolve into wet, smeary, white, pus-coated ulcers arise. The ulcers are often confluent with "kissing lesions." There is a preauricular lymphadenopathy. With autoinfection the lesions appear after four to eleven days and with heteroinfection after one to two weeks. If the globes are not involved, the lesions heal after two to three weeks. The cornea is involved in about one-third of cases.

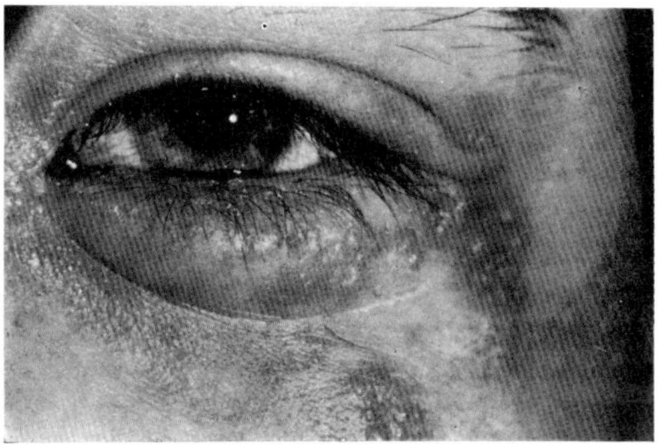

Fig. 10.26 Herpes simplex (♀ 19 yrs.)

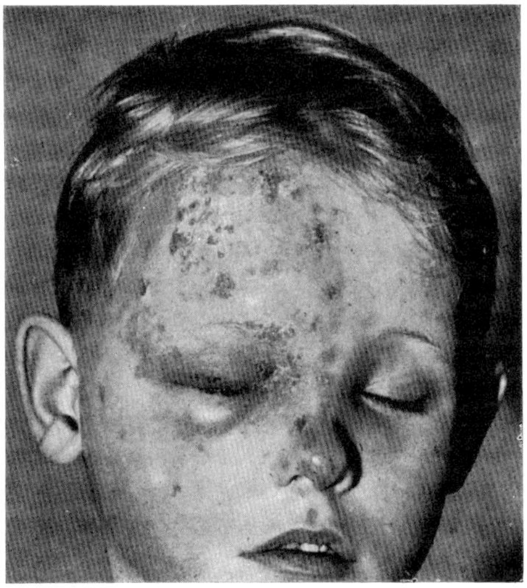

Fig. 10.27 Ophthalmic zoster with involvements of the nasociliary ramus (♂ 5 yrs.)

Corneal infiltrates appear six to eight days after vaccination (Sédan et al. 1953). The lesions are small, white, limbal infiltrates and are rarely disciform. They appear just as the lid margins begin to improve (Bruens 1944). With generalized hematogenous spread, isolated muscle palsies, chorioretinitis, central serous retinopathy, central vein thrombosis, optic neuritis, vitreal haze, and panophthalmitis can occur (Rosen 1948).

Diphtheria is a primary consideration in the *differential diagnosis*. Usually the pharynx is also involved and hemorrhagic pseudomembrane formation is present. Diphtheroid ulcers and kissing lesions are less discrete. Luetic chancres are firm with painful lymph nodes.

With smallpox and chickenpox, the systemic illness is striking. Local isolated lid involvement is almost never found.

Smallpox (variola vera): In smallpox there is a spotty involvement of skin and mucous membranes by nodular pustules. The eyes can be affected. Prior to vaccination, smallpox was one of the most common causes of blindness. In India 20 percent of all blindness is caused by smallpox (Strehl 1962). Lid pustules cause marked lid edema. The conjunctiva is rarely affected. Corneal involvement is in the form of ulcers and rarely interstitial keratitis (Zade 1932).

Erythema multiforme: A number of vesicular inflammations are brought together under the heading of *mucocutaneous ocular syndrome* (Plate III, Fig. 2, page 128 c) or *erythema multiforme*. Proppe (1948) reviewed the diversity of signs, symptoms, and disease entities included in this classification.

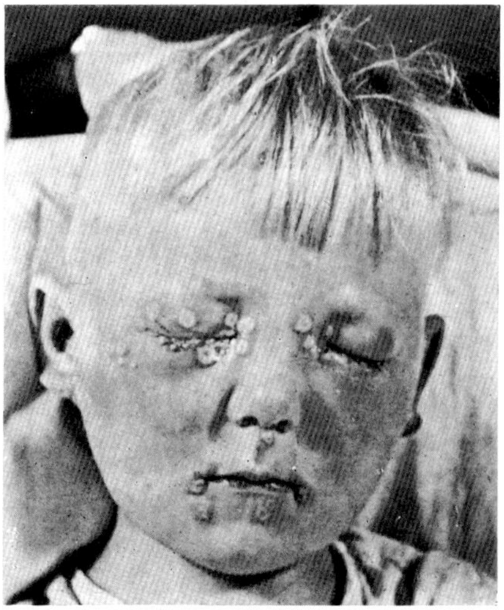

Fig. 10.28 Vaccinnia (♀ 3 yrs.)

Fuchs (1876) was the first to describe a pseudomembranous conjunctivitis in association with erythema multiforme. He called the entity "herpes iris conjunctivae."

The ectodermal layers of the eye (lids, cornea, conjunctiva) are primarily involved. There is a mild, bilateral, acute conjunctival inflammation with minor lid edema. In addition to the conjunctival inflammation and blister formation, thick (2 to 3 mm) pseudomembranes form. They are smooth-surfaced and peel off easily, but recur within hours.

After two to three weeks, the membranes become thinner and slowly disappear. The conjunctiva may return to normal or, depending on the severity of involvement, scarring, entropion, ectropion (Mattson and Carlberg 1953), and symblepharon may remain (Wolff 1949; Rougier et al. 1958).

Corneal involvement ranges from noninvolvement to punctate keratitis, bullae, ulcers, and severe stromal thinning (François 1954; Mattson and Carlberg 1953). Corneal scars and even staphyloma result. The skin lesions also appear on the lids. The conjunctival process may involve the lacrimal puncta and canaliculi causing membranous scars (Mamelock and Laval 1955). It may go deeper to produce a scleritis (Contino 1952; Godtfredsen 1954; Naróg 1956). Keratitis or scleritis may involve the iris, ciliary body, or choroid secondarily (Schreck 1960).

Proppe includes Baader's dermatostomatitis, ectodermosis erosiva pluriorificialis (Fiessinger-Rendu), Stevens-Johnson syndrome, pseudomembranous conjunctivitis, and stomatitis in the entity of acute mucocutaneous ocular syndrome (Fuchs) (= erythema multiforme). For causal agents, see page 127.

The *differential diagnosis* of pseudomembranous conjunctivitis includes diphtheria, pemphigus, and hoof-and-mouth disease (Carleton 1949; Raffin 1922; Thies 1950; Krataka 1955; Schreck 1960). In erythema multiforme the lid edema is soft. With diphtheria it is firm and there is a painful preauricular lymphadenopathy. According to Proppe, the nail beds remain uninvolved in erythema multiforme but are involved in foot-and-mouth disease. Pemphigus vulgaris has typical skin involvement. The late cicatricial changes of benign mucous pemphigoid cannot be differentiated from late scarring of erythema multiforme.

Scarring in benign mucous pemphigoid is severe. The process almost inexorably progresses to total shrinkage, scarification, and drying out of the conjunctival sac.

In **pemphigus vulgaris** (see page 128), there is vesicle formation over the entire body including lids and conjunctiva (Plate VI, Fig. 2, page 128 f). At first the vesicles are clear. Later they become opaque, rupture, and dry out. Symblepharon, trichiasis, xerophthalmia and corneal opacities result. Pemphigus vulgaris is an adult disease. It develops over a period of many years and is eventually fatal.

Benign mucosal pemphigoid is primarily limited to the conjunctiva (Fig. 12.10), but other mucous membranes may be involved (nose, mouth, pharynx, genitalia). The disease is bilateral and also known as essential shrinkage of the conjunctiva (see page 128).

Hereditary dystrophic epidermolysis bullosa (see page 128 [Fig. 10.29]): Recessive dystrophic epidermolysis bullosa has ocular involvement. The dominantly inherited epidermolysis bullosa simplex does not (Lutz 1932; Riecke 1931; Siemens 1937). Dystrophic epidermolysis bullosa is manifest within the first years of life.

Mechanical trauma (rubbing) causes bulla formation. The bullae break readily and heal by scarring. Conjunctival shrinkage and trichiasis result (Linser 1907; Katayama 1933). Corneal bullae with erosion and scarring are reported (Bogrow 1911; Cohen and Sulzberger 1935, Bäfverstedt and Granström 1940; Machionini 1938; Lemmingson 1953).

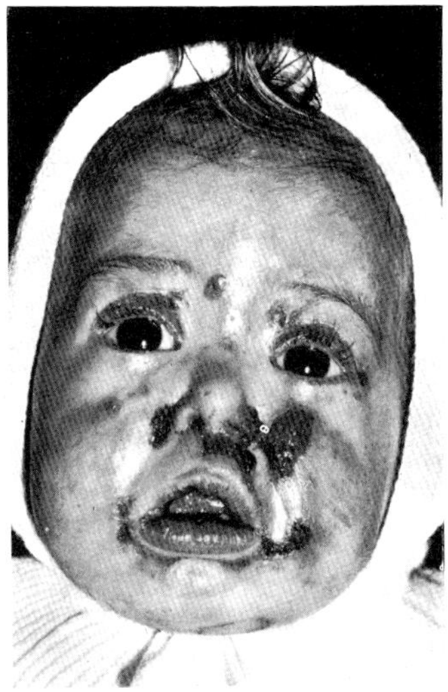

Fig.10.29 Epidermolysis bullosa hereditaria (♀ 7 months)

Drug-induced (allergic) bullae (see page 128 [Plate III, Fig. 3, page 128 c]). Allergic drug reactions cause the clinical picture of erythema multiforme or pemphigus (barbiturates, aminopyrine, antipyrine, arsphenamine, penicillin, streptomycin, sulfonamides and anesthetic agents (see page 128).

Behçet's syndrome, which consists of recurrent iritis with hypopyon formation, low-grade fever, and oral, genital and cutaneous ulcers, belongs to the mucocutaneous uveal syndrome (see page 203).

Polymorphic light eruptions (hydroa vacciniforme) (see page 93): There is a solar dermatitis with bulla formation. Ocular involvement includes photophobia, tearing, conjunctivitis, keratitis, blepharospasm, and inflammation of the lids. The male:female ratio is 10:1. Porphyria (see page 366), drug reactions and xeroderma pigmentosum are underlying causes. Skin malignancies are common in xeroderma pigmentosum.

Noninflammatory Lid Edema

Angioneurotic and allergic edema — Melkersson-Rosenthal syndrome — Vasociliary (Charlin) syndrome — Various causes of lid edema (renal, cardiac, collaterals) — Subcutaneous emphysema — Myxedema — Tumors and pseudotumor — Elephantiasis — Amyloidosis — Progressive scleroderma.

Angioneurotic edema, Quincke's edema (giant urticaria), *allergic edema* (Fig. 10.30): These are a transition to inflammatory edema. In children etiologic agents include antigenic, foreign proteins such as parasites (ascaria, pinworms) (see page 198, Conrads and Heinmüller 1959). In ascariasis recurrent lid edema is equivalent to the transient eosinophilic lung infiltrates.

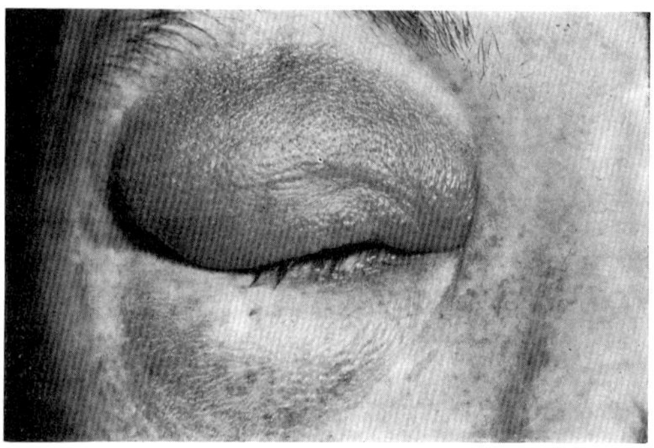

Fig. 10.30 Allergic edema (♀ 37 yrs.)

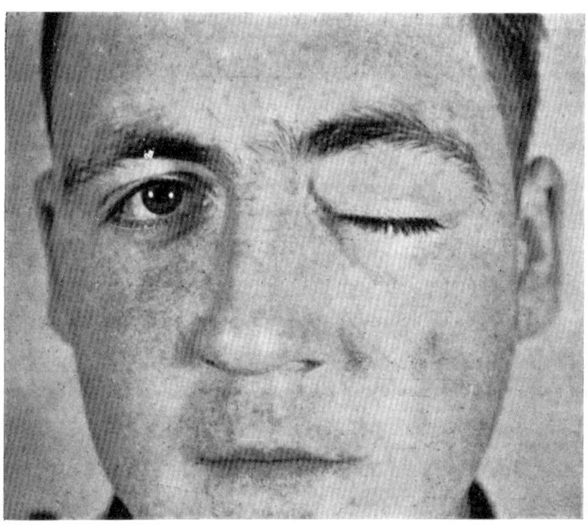

Fig. 10.31 Air emphysema after fracture of the lamina papyracea (♂ 21 yrs.)

Trichinous lid edema is particularly severe.

Melkersson-Rosenthal syndrome includes recurrent facial and lid edema, furrowed tongue, and facial nerve paresis.

Vasociliary (Charlin) syndrome is unilateral. There is lid edema, conjunctivitis, rhinorrhea, and possibly keratitis (see page 78).

Various causes for lid edema: *Renal or cardiac edema, infectious mononucleosis, diphtheria, scarlet fever, trypanosomiasis, malaria, malnutrition, cachexia, or local trauma with circulatory disturbances* around the eye. On rare occasions, frontobasilar skull fracture with dural laceration allows cerebrospinal fluid to seep beneath the lids.

Subcutaneous emphysema (Fig. 10.31): This occurs primarily with fracture of the lamina papyracea. Caisson disease (decompression syndrome) and gas gangrene are other causes. There is a characteristic crepitus on palpation. The edema (air) shifts on pressure.

Myxedema: Hypothyroidism produces a firm dry edema. The skin has a yellowish cast (Fig. 25.11).

Tumors and pseudotumors (see page 103) (eosinophilic or basophilic granulomas, chalazia) also cause lid edema (see page 103).

Meningoceles or encephaloceles occur in infants and produce edema over the medial canthi and root of the nose.

Elephantiasis is a marked permanent thickening and hypertrophy of the lids. Tumors such as neurofibromatosis, hemangiomas, or lymphangiomas can be responsible.

True elephantiasis (elephantiasis nostras) results from blockage of the lymph drainage system. This occurs with trauma, surgery, infection (recurrent erysipelas, leprosy, lues, tuberculosis) and chronic eczema (Melkersson-Rosenthal syndrome) (see page 33).

Pachydermoperiostosis (Touraine-Solente-Golé) is a rare hereditary disorder. Elephantiasis of the lids caused by meibomian gland cysts and connective tissue hypertrophy is one manifestation.

Amyloidosis causes thickened lids and a gray discoloration of the conjunctiva. The conjunctiva bleeds easily (Plate VII, Fig. 5). The most common causes are local paramyloidosis, plasmacytosis or secondary to chronic inflammation, particularly trachoma.

Progressive scleroderma: This is a collagen disease (autoimmune connective tissue disorder). Ocular findings include mild chronic lid edema, decreased tearing, keratitis sicca, and hypertensive retinopathy.

Congestive Hyperemia

Congestive hyperemia occurs with cavernous sinus thrombosis, pulsating exophthalmos (Plate XXXI, Fig. 6), orbital vein thrombosis, malignant (endocrine) exophthalmos (Plate XXXI, Fig. 5), and severe blepharospasm.

Subcutaneous Hematoma and Hemangiomas

The loose subcutaneous connective tissue around the eyes allows rapid diffusion of blood (Fig. 10.32). Periorbital hematoma with skull fracture is a classic example. Other causes include whooping cough, blood dyscrasia, hemorrhagic disorders, vitamin C (scurvy, Möller-Barlow disease in children), vitamin K deficiency, and caisson disease. Most periorbital subcutaneous hemorrhages will reabsorb within two to three weeks.

In any perforating injury causing a lid hematoma one must consider the possibility of orbital wall fractures and even cerebral damage. All too often injury to the bony orbit (usually orbital roof) with laceration of the dura remains unrecognized until the patient develops a meningitis.

Hemangiomas are common. Lid hemangiomas almost always regress before the age of one or two (rarely, five or six) (Proppe and Hauss 1963; Holland 1968). Nevus flammeus (Sturge-Weber) is associated with glaucoma (see page 226), especially when the upper lid is involved.

Discoloration of the Lids

Infectious exanthems, telangiectasias — Hypopigmentation (albinism, vitiligo) — Hyperpigmentation (melanosis, nevus of Ota, acanthosis nigricans, Peutz-Jegher's syndrome) — Exogenous hyperpigmentation.

Infectious exanthems: measles, scarlet fever, varicella, etc.

Telangiectasias

Ataxia telangiectasia (Louis-Bar's syndrome) combines cerebellar ataxia as well as skin and conjunctival telangiectasias. The syndrome is one of the phakomatoses (see page 296). Patients suffering from angiokeratoma corporis diffusum (Fabry) (see page 257, Fig. 22.2) have skin telangiectasias.

Hypopigmentation: This is congenital in *albinism* (Plate XIII, Fig. 3, page 192 e) and ac-

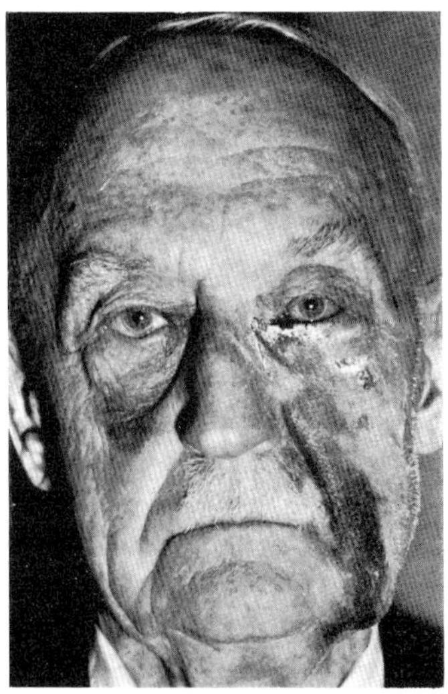

Fig. 10.32 Left periorbital hemorrhage spreading to the right side and down the face (♂ 86 yrs.)

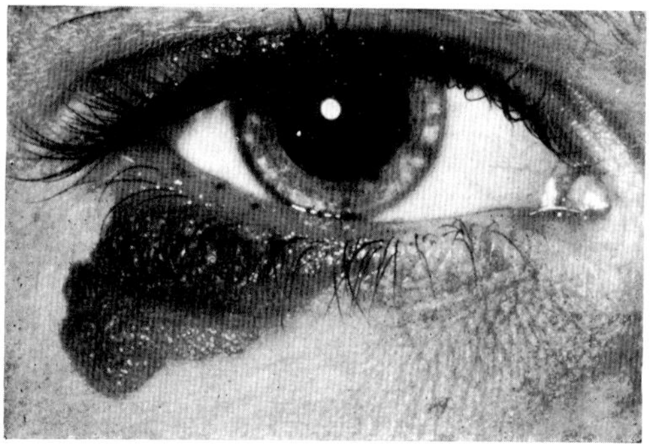

Fig. 10.33 Nevus of the lower lid (♀ 18 yrs.)

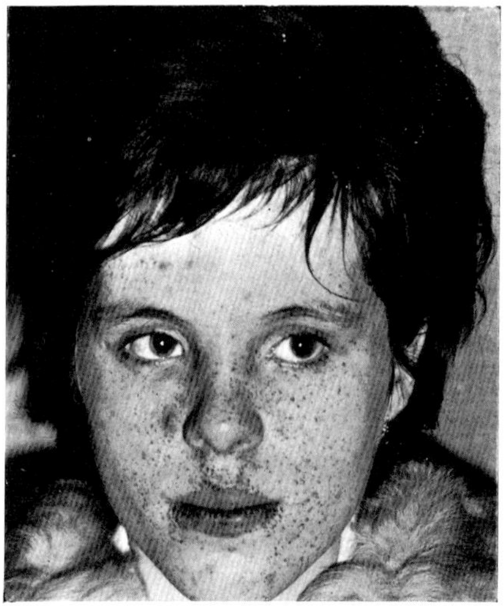

Fig. 10.34 Peutz-Jeghers syndrome: numerous freckles on the face and lids (♀ 21 yrs.)

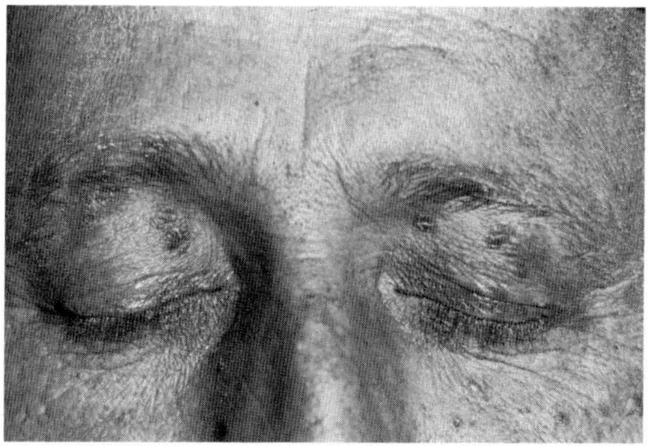

Fig. 10.35 Psoriasis of the lids (♂ 45 yrs.)

quired with *vitiligo*. Vitiligous patches consist of white depigmented areas with a slightly hyperpigmented border. Eyelashes and eyebrows may also be depigmented (poliosis). The iris may become depigmented in certain uveitides (Vogt-Koyanagi-Harada) (Hoff 1954).

Vitiligo is also seen in Waardenburg's syndrome (see page 87), kwashiorkor, leprosy and pinta (spirochete: Treponema carateum).

Hyperpigmentation occurs in four forms:

a) Congenital or endogenous *melanosis*. Addison's disease (Plate III, Fig. 4, page 128 c), hyperthyroidism, hemochromatosis (iron-storage disease), ochronosis (see page 119), incontinentia pigmenti (Bloch-Sulzberger syndrome). In pregnancy irregular, poorly delineated brown patches may appear on the face (chloasma gravidarum). Nevi of different size and color are common on the lids (see page 104).

b) *Nevus of Ota* (Fig. 10.33) is a blue-gray melanosis in the area of the first and second trigeminal nerve branches. Skin, sclera, iris, uvea, conjunctiva, and even the optic disk are discolored (Kraus and Jung 1968). Sometimes the cornea is involved. It is more common in pigmented races and in women (4:1). It is usually inherited as an autosomal dominant. Peak incidence is during the first three years of life or between the ages of 12 and 20 (Hidano et al. 1967).

c) In *acanthosis nigricans* a gray-black discoloration and hyperkeratosis occur, especially along skin folds and the neck. Lids and eyebrows may be involved. The usual etiology is an endocrine disorder.

d) In *Peutz-Jegher's syndrome* freckles abound on the face, lids, extremities, and around the mouth. There is an associated intestinal polyposis caused by the mutation of a single gene (Fig. 10.34).

e) Psoriasis can cause slightly elevated brown scales or spots on the lids (Fig. 10.35).

Exogenous hyperpigmentation: Prolonged use of silver *(argyrosis), mercury*, or compounds containing *arsenic* can cause exogenous hyperpigmentation and deposition of these materials in connective tissue. *Chrysiasis* (auriosis) is a gray discoloration of the skin by deposition of gold particles. The discoloration is most noticeable on the lids. The conjunctival discoloration is more green. Gold, like arsenic, can cause severe dermatitis.

Melanodermatitis (Plate III, Fig. 5, page 128 c) may be caused by light-sensitive substances (see page 135). The most severe photodermatitis, *xeroderma pigmentosum* (see page 93), has its onset by age two or three. Exposed areas of skin become hyperemic, inflamed, and develop pigmented spots, atrophy and scarring. There is a high incidence of verrucous ulcerations and tumors (carcinomas, melanomas).

Sarcoidosis (see page 201) may have brown to brown-red lid nodules accessible for biopsy.

Atrophy of the Skin of the Lid

Atrophy of the skin occurs after radiation, with blepharochalasis (see page 86), scleroderma, secondary to scarring, burns, and chronic irritation (lupus vulgaris, fungi).

Cysts and Pseudotumors of the Lids

Retention cysts — Comedo — Milia — Sebaceous cysts — Molluscum contagiosum — Sarcoidosis — Hyperkeratosis — Xanthelasma — Lipidosis.

Retention cysts of the glands of Zeiss are white, and may be the size of a pinhead or a pea. Retention cysts of the sudoriferous glands

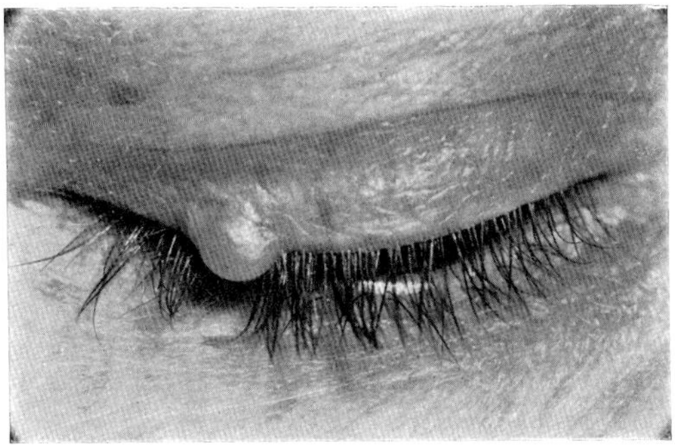

Fig. 10.36 Moll gland retention cyst (♀ 70 yrs.)

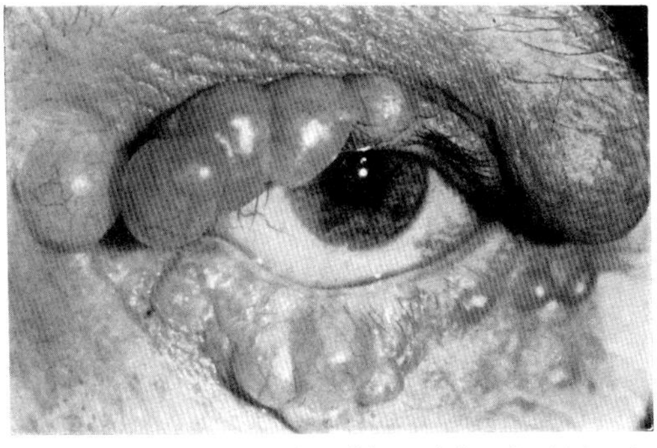

Fig. 10.37 Cysts and solid nodules in Urbach-Wiethe's disease (lipoid proteinosis) (♂ 55 yrs.)

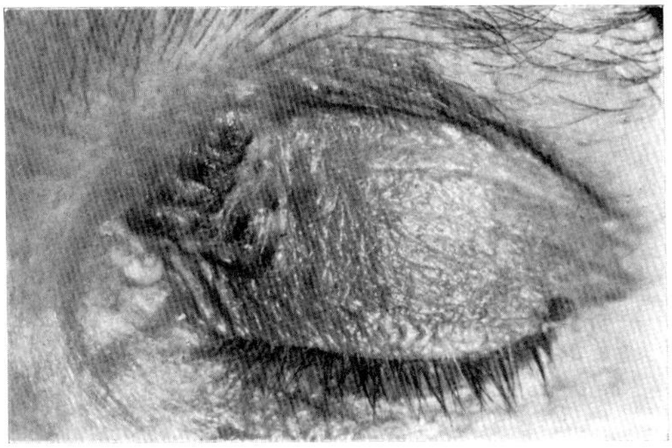

Fig. 10.38 Comedo (♀ 59 yrs.)

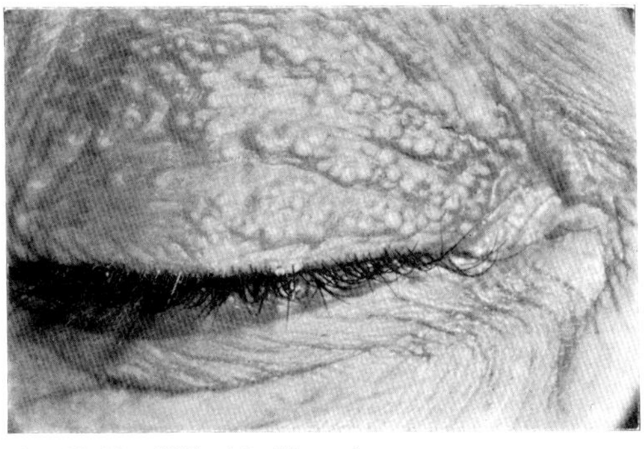

Fig. 10.39 Milia (♀ 44 yrs.)

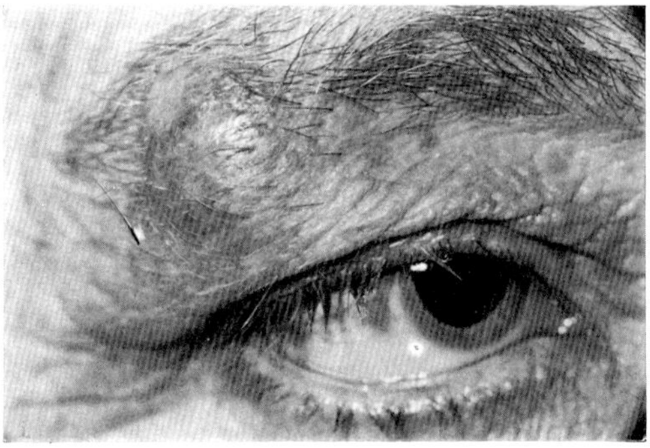

Fig. 10.40 Sebaceous cyst of the upper lid (♀ 57 yrs.)

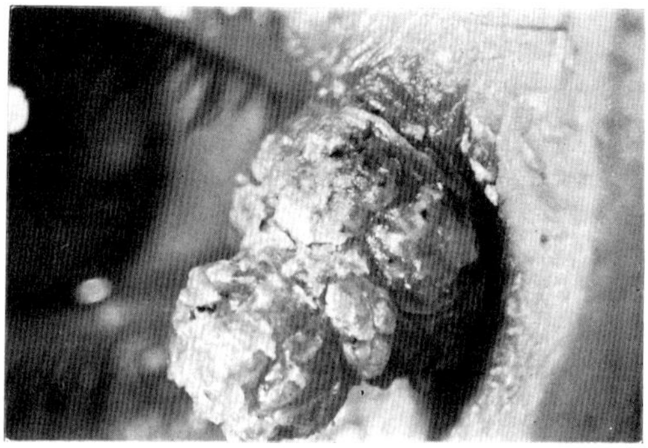

Fig. 10.41 Cutaneous horn (♂ 75 yrs.)

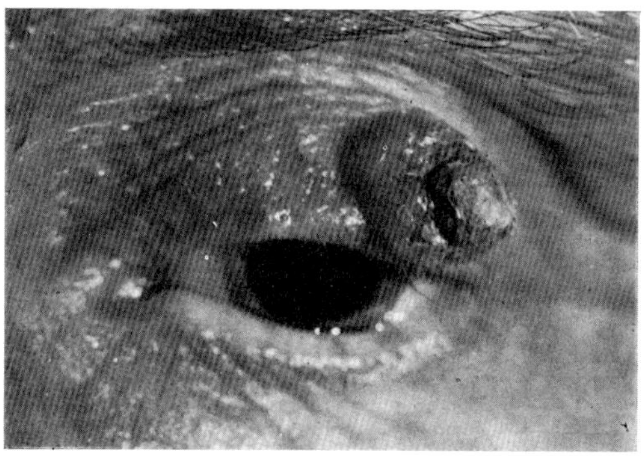

Fig. 10.42 Hyperkeratosis (♂ 58 yrs.)

of Moll are more glass-like (Fig. 10.36). These are noninflammatory cysts at the lid margin which grow slowly over a long period and may dry out spontaneously.

Retained secretions of the meibomian gland produce a yellow-gray discoloration which, when it turns white, is called a *calcified infarct* of the meibomian gland. This usually occurs in older patients. The hard, inspissated matter may rub on the cornea causing corneal abrasions and foreign body sensation.

Lipoid proteinosis (Urbach-Wiethe disease) (Fig. 10.37) is a hereditary disproteinemia with deposition of homogenous hyaline material in skin and mucous membranes. The lids characteristically develop glassy, gray-blue cysts at the lid margins (François et al. 1968; Bacskulin and Bacskulin 1965).

Comedo (blackheads) (Fig. 10.38) are common retention cysts of dermal sebaceous glands.

Milia (Fig. 10.39) are yellow-white hard, round, pinhead-sized keratin aggregates.

Sebaceous cysts also occur on the lid (Fig. 10.40).

Molluscum contagiosum: These are small, 1 to 5 mm, virus-induced, umbilicated, pearly nodules (acanthoma) which may afflict the lids. The incubation time is unknown. The lesions desquamate material into the cul-de-sac producing chronic conjunctivitis and keratitis. The differential diagnosis includes syringoma (sweat gland adenomas of the skin).

Sarcoidosis: Boeck's disease may appear as red-brown nodules of the lids (see page 201).

Cutaneous horn; hyperkeratosis: Cutaneous horns (Fig. 10.41) and other senile hyperkeratotic lesions such as senile keratosis (10.42) or seborrheic keratosis (often pigmented), are common and should be biopsied if malignancy is suspected.

Xanthelasma (Plate III, Fig. 5, page 128 c) are yellow, bilateral, cholesterol-laden plaques appearing medially on the lids of older persons.

Lipoidoses affect the lids (Franceschetti and Avanza 1958) as tuberous xanthoma, disseminated xanthoma, or pearly nodules in Urbach-Wiethe's disease (see above).

Disseminated xanthomatosis, Hand-Schüller-Christian disease and Gaucher's disease may all show conjunctival deposits. Lipid deposition in the cornea occurs with disseminated xanthomatosis, dermoid cornea, lipid keratopathy, secondary fatty degeneration and arcus senilis. Arcus lipoides is seen in aging individuals or in association with primary and secondary lipoidoses, hypercholesterinemia, or hyperlipidemia. Within the eye juvenile xanthogranulomatosis involves uveal tissues. Lipemia retinalis occurs with elevated serum triglycerides.

Tumors of the Lids

Hemangioma — Neurofibroma — Benign epithelial lesions — Malignant epithelial tumors — Pigmented tumors — Lymphomas, myelosis.

Tumors of the lid may be differentiated as inflammatory or degenerative, epithelial, mesenchymal, neuroectodermal or melanocytic (Lund 1969).

Hemangioma: Hemangiomas of the lid (Fig. 10.43) are common. They frequently appear as *telangiectasias* in the newborn and almost invariably regress by the age of two or three. This is in contrast to the persistent *cavernous hemangiomas* (Fig. 10.44) which may be hereditary (see phacomatoses: Sturge-Weber [see page 296], Plate III, Fig. 6, page 128 c). Hemangiomas can usually be emptied by compression. They are easily recognized when superficial but may simulate pigmented tumors or blastomas when deep.

Neurofibromatosis involves the lids or other parts of the body (Hager 1958). Elephantiasis, neurofibroma, plexiform neuroma (Fig. 10.45), café-au-lait spots, proptosis (may be pulsatile), and ectropion formation are some of the pleomorphic lid manifestations in von Recklinghausen's disease (Meyer 1939; Shapland 1950; Magni 1956). In the cornea thickened corneal nerves, Descemet's membrane, and stromal opacities can be observed.

Gray-yellow iris nodules (neurofibromas) are common (Unger 1947; Pietruschka 1952). Choroidal nodules (Stemmermann 1953) as well as ciliary body and choroidal neuromas occur (Kreibig 1940). Optic nerve gliomas (and neuromas) are frequent manifestations of von Recklinghausen's disease (Schmincke 1956). Optic atrophy is common (especially in children) (Dresner and Montgomery 1949). Glaucoma occurring early enough in life causes buphthalmos (Böck 1948).

Von Recklinghausen's disease is a dominantly inherited phacomatosis of variable penetrance.

Benign epithelial tumors: *Papilloma.* Keratoacanthoma may appear as a crater with a central keratin plug. Since it resembles molluscum contagiosum, it is also called *molluscum sebaceum.* Growth is rapid for six to eight weeks; the lesion then resolves.

Dermoids presumably arise from congenitally retained ectoderm. They are most common su-

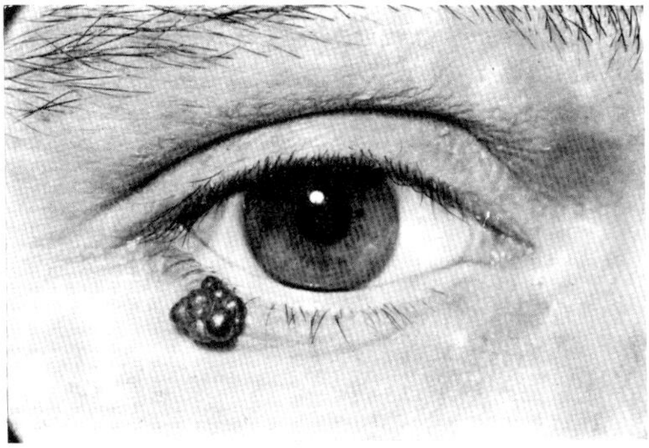

Fig. 10.43 Botryoid hemangioma (♀ 6 yrs.)

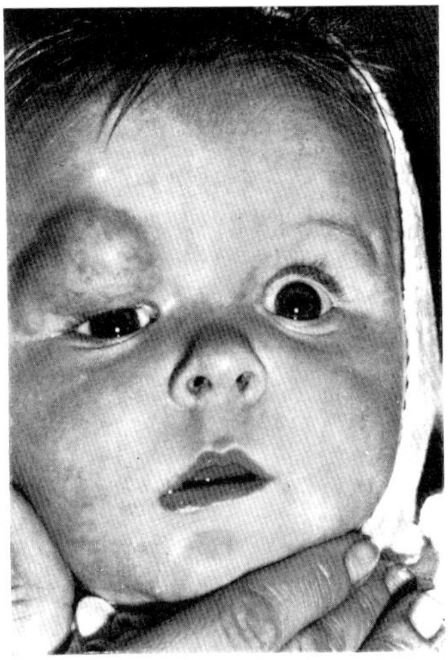

Fig. 10.44 Cavernous hemangioma (♀ 6 months)

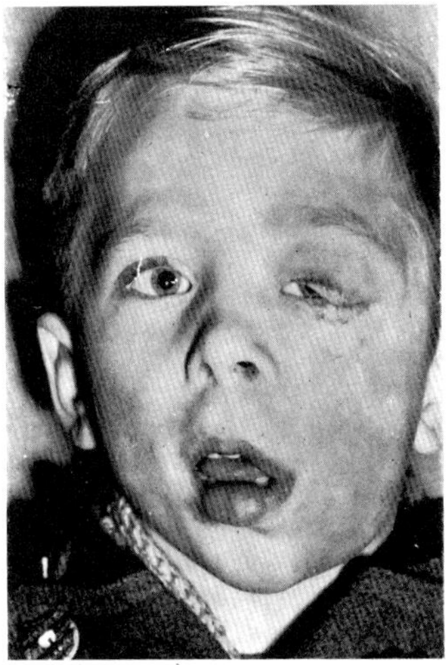

Fig. 10.45 Von Recklinghausen's neurofibromatosis; plexiform neuroma with elephantiasis (♂ 11 yrs.)

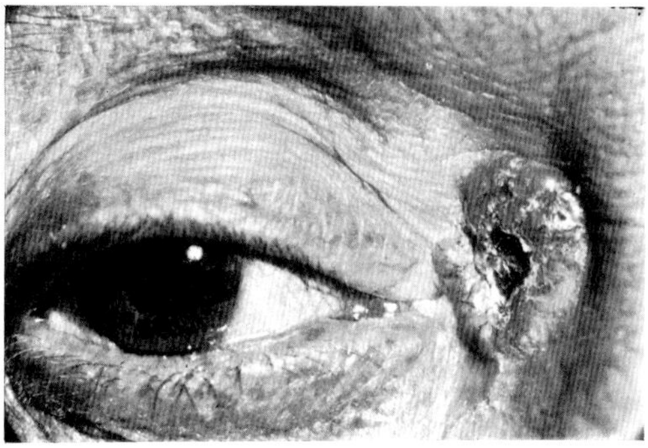

Fig. 10.46 Basal cell carcinoma (♂ 57 yrs.)

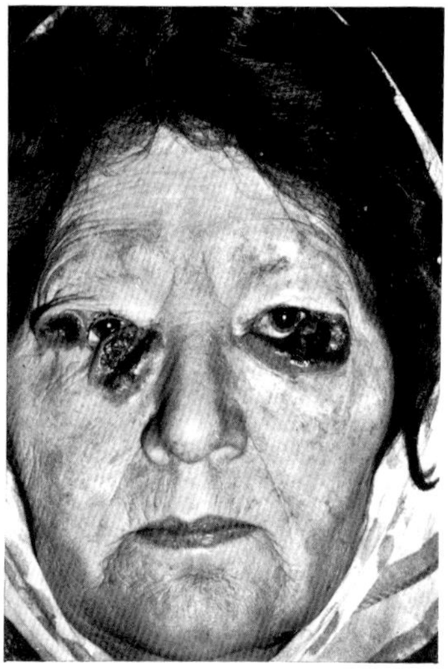

Fig. 10.47 Squamous cell carcinoma at three different locations on the lids (♀ 69 yrs.)

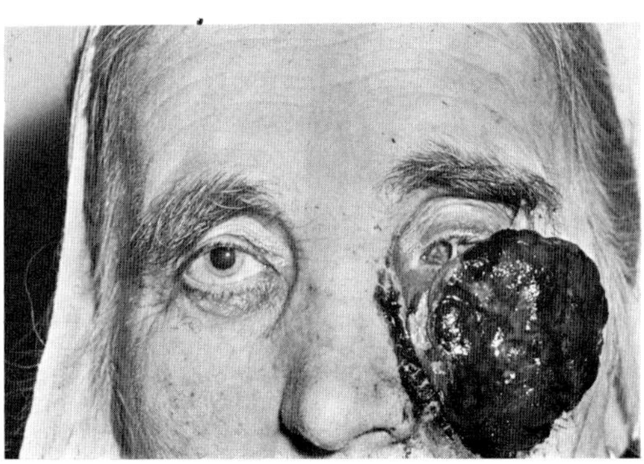

Fig. 10.48 Large keratoacanthoma of the lids (♀ 70 yrs.)

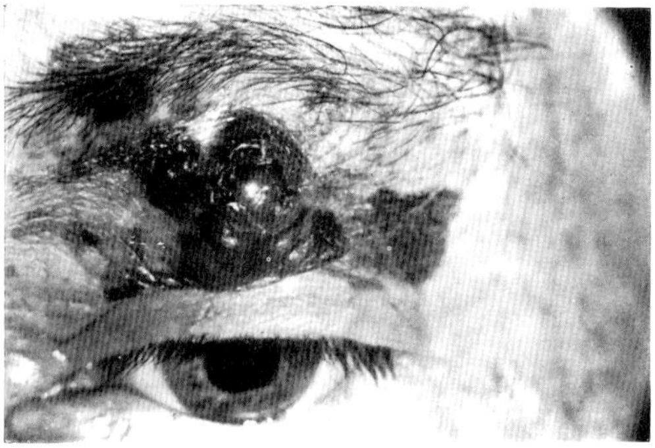

Fig. 10.49 Malignant melanoma arising from a pigmented nevus present since childhood (♀ 69 yrs.)

perior and temporal near the lacrimal gland. A superior nasal mass implies mucocele. Lipomas and *lipodermoids* are another consideration. Sebaceous cysts commonly occur on the lids.

Benign calcified epithelioma of Malherbe is a rare, hereditary tumor of childhood occurring mainly in females; it simulates dermoid or sebaceous cysts. This cellular, pleomorphic tumor grows slowly. Diagnosis is made on biopsy (Lohse and Tost 1967).

Benign *adenomas* arise from meibomian glands and as narrow plaques from sweat glands.

Malignant epithelial tumors: The most common malignant lid tumor is basal cell carcinoma (rodent ulcer) (Fig. 10.46). Basal cell carcinoma is seven times more common than squamous cell carcinoma (Reeh 1963). The tumor grows slowly and does not metastasize. It is a nodular, pearly-edged lesion with central ulceration and bleeds easily. Metastasizing squamous cell carcinoma (Fig. 10.47) and adenocarcinoma are found less often. Adenocarcinomas of the meibomian gland or, less frequently, of the Zeiss or Moll glands simulate chalazia. Clinically, lid cancers may be difficult to differentiate from *benign papillomas, warts, precancerous lesions* (senile keratoma) and keratoacanthoma (molluscum sebaceum) (Fig. 10.48) (Rodenhäuser 1957).

Pigmented tumors: The differential diagnosis of pigmented lid lesions includes pigmented nevi and *diffuse melanosis*. *Blue nevi* (Plate IV, Fig. 1, page 128 d) are dysontogenetic dermal lesions not involving the epidermis (see page 117).

Precancerous melanosis is a transitional form between the benign and malignant stage. The conjunctiva is preferentially involved with shifting patches of pigmentation. Melanomas of the lid are extremely malignant. Pigmentation is variable. The surface can be glassy and it bleeds easily. The differential diagnosis includes hemangioma and pigmented basal cell carcinoma. Urinary melanin is usually not elevated until metastases are present in the liver. Growing *nevi* should be suspected of *malignant melanoma* (Fig. 10.49). *Juvenile xanthogranulomas* occur everywhere, including lids and iris. They are yellow, elevated nodules which can undergo spontaneous remission (Fig. 10.50). Lymphoid and reticulum cell sarcomas afflict the lids.

Lymphomas and myelosis (Fig. 10.52): Lymphosarcoma, especially giant follicular lymphoma (Brill-Symmer's disease) causes unilateral or bilateral lid swelling, orbital masses with exophthalmos and lacrimal gland infiltration. Lymphomas produce nodules (Fig. 10.52). All types of lymphomas and leukemia can cause tumor-like infiltrates (Fig. 10.51).

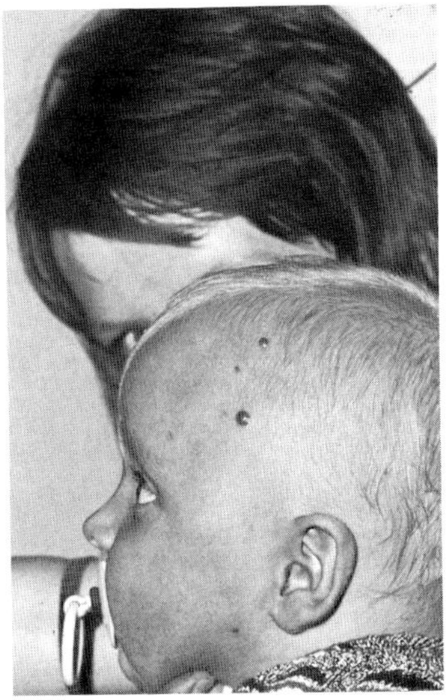

Fig. 10.50

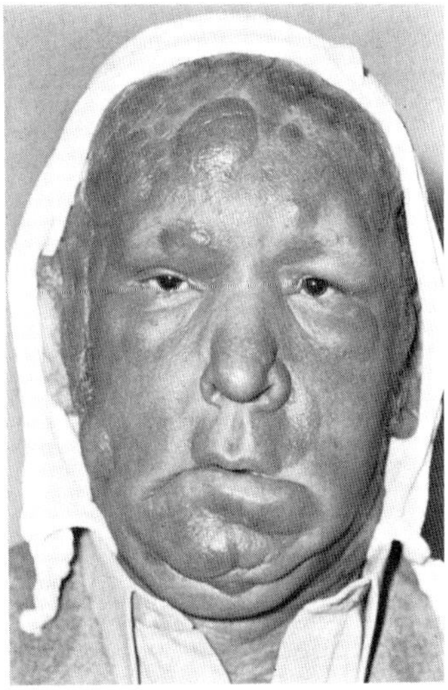

Fig. 10.51

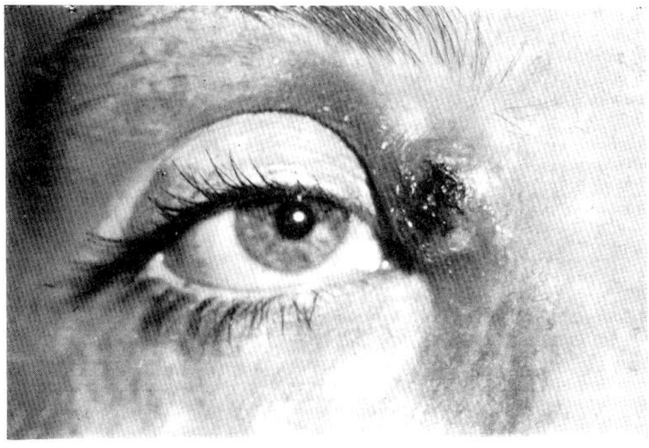

Fig. 10.50 Several large pea to bean sized xanthomatous nevi on the head (♂ ½ yr.)

Fig. 10.51 Lymphocytic leukemia with infiltrates in the face and lids (♀ 56 yrs.)

Fig. 10.52 Poorly healing ulcer at the inner canthus; histology: lymphogranuloma (♀ 23 yrs.) ▶

Trauma, Chemical or Thermal Burns, Occupational Diseases

Trauma and burns are not usually a diagnostic problem (see page 356).

Occupational diseases: Merté (1969, 1972) lists the following occupational diseases of the lids:

Arsenicals: Lid edema, blepharitis, keratitis, conjunctivitis, optic neuritis. Arsenic trichloride, hydrogenated arsenic and atoxyl all cause irritation and inflammation.

Nitrobenzene and aminobenzene *(methemoglobin formers):* Aniline (aminobenzene), chloraniline and nitroaniline, toluene, xylene, toluidine, phenyldiamine, paraphenyldiamine and benzidine may all cause blepharitis, conjunctivitis, keratitis, lid discoloration, and inflammation.

Halogenated hydrocarbons: Chlorinated naphthalin (perna) causes inflammation of the sebaceous glands.

Vanadium and beryllium; Blepharitis and conjunctivitis.

Tar, pitch, resin: Precancerosis and skin cancers.

Inflammations of the Lid Margin (Blepharitides)

Squamous blepharitis – Ulcerating blepharitis – Pubic lice – Angular blepharoconjunctivitis.

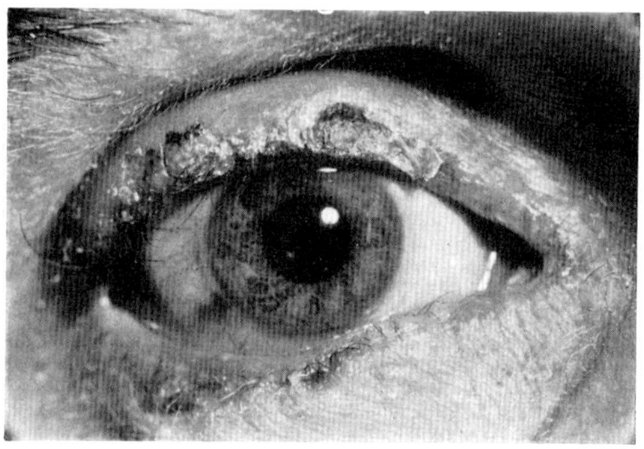

Fig. 10.53 Ulcerating blepharitis (♂ 30 yrs.)

Squamous blepharitis (seborrheic blepharitis): The equivalent of seborrheic dermatitis of the lid margins is common. The lid margins are hyperemic; yellow scales and conjunctivitis develop. Brow and scalp hair is invariably involved. Treatment must include all areas of scalp and face. Light skin, avitaminosis, endocrine disorders, generalized debility, irritants (dust, smoke, refractive errors, close work) all seem to constitute a predilection for this disease.

Ulcerating blepharitis: Bloody ulcers and scale formation occur on the lid margin. There is loss of lashes (madarosis) (Fig. 10.54). This is a staphylococcal infection (Fig. 10.53).

Blepharitis is associated with chalazion and hordeolum formation. In older persons meibo-

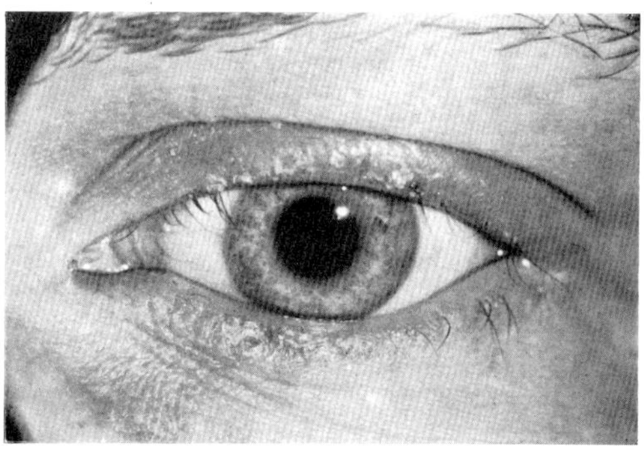

Fig. 10.54 Ulcerating blepharitis with madarosis (♀ 26 yrs.)

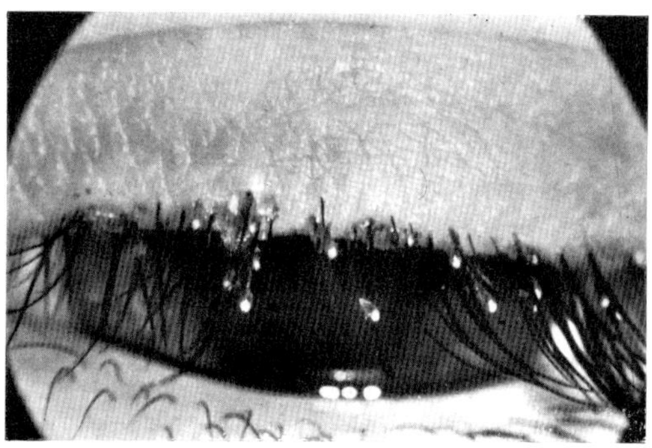

Fig. 10.55 Pubic lice and nits (♀ 7 yrs.)

mian gland infarcts are common. The regenerating lashes may be misdirected and scrape the cornea, thus causing trichiasis. Squamous hyperplasia of conjunctival epithelium causes dryness and irritation of the eye.
Pubic lice: Phthirus pubis (Fig. 10.55) produces blepharitis and conjunctivitis. The protruding end of the parasite and the nits reveal its presence.
Angular blepharoconjunctivitis: Conjunctivitis associated with dermolysis at the lateral canthus is characteristic of staphyloccus or Morax-Axenfeld diplobacillus infection (Plate IV, Fig. 2, page 128 d).

Cilia

Trichiasis — Distichiasis — Loss of lashes — Poliosis.

Trichiasis: Misdirection of lashes with corneal irritation may be caused by scarring or may be secondary to burns, injury or inflammation.
Distichiasis: A hereditary disorder where a second row of lashes arises from the orifices of the meibomian glands. These lashes rub the cornea (Fox 1962). The disease is manifest at puberty. Pigmented nevi at the lid margin may be associated with extra or misdirected rows of eyelashes (nevus pigmentosus pilosus, (Fig. 10.56). *Loss of the eyelashes:* The upper (150) and lower (75) lashes are replaced every five months. Loss of lashes (Fig. 10.57) occurs with a variety of disorders: ulcerating blepharitis, vaccinia, eczema, mycoses, lues, burns, fever, poisonings (thallium, arsenic). Hypervitaminosis A causes a reversible loss of lashes. Generalized alopecia is another cause.
Poliosis is congenital in albinism and Waardenburg's syndrome (see page 87). It is acquired with blepharitis, trachoma, inflammatory scarring, uveitis (sympathetic ophthalmia, Vogt-Koyanagi-Harada's disease). Other causes of poliosis include: trigeminal neuralgia, trauma, encephalitis, fright (?), vitiligo, and progressive hemifacial atrophy.

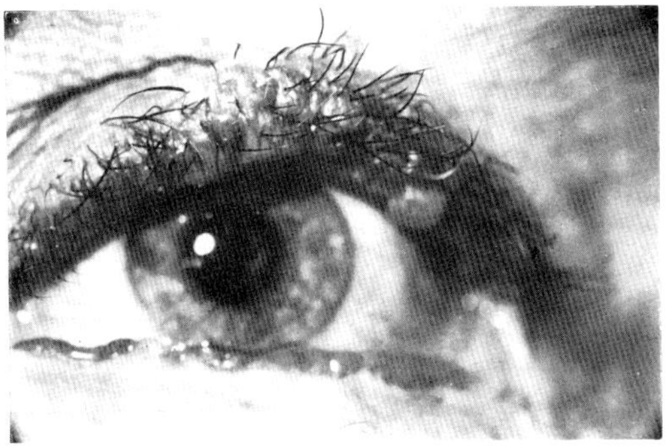

Fig. 10.56 Hairy pigmented nevus (♀ 35 yrs.)

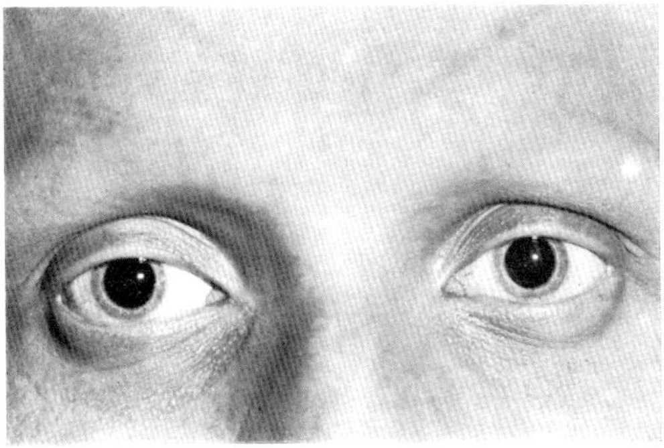

Fig. 10.57 Total alopecia (♀ 24 yrs.)

Eyebrows

Loss of the outer third of the brows — Hypertrophy of the inner third — Duplication of eyebrows.

Hertogh's sign (Fig. 10.58) is described as *lack of the outer third of the eyebrows.* Causes include autonomic nervous system dysfunction, endocrinopathies, diphtheria, neurodermatitis, scleroderma, hypothyroidism, and hypogona-

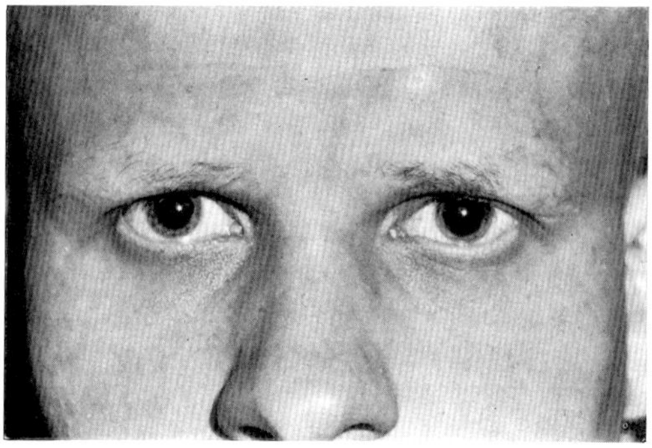

dism (Schönfeld 1947). It is an integral part of keratosis follicularis spinulosa decalvans (Siemens 1937).

Waardenburg's syndrome (see page 87) includes telecanthus, *hyperplasia* of the root of the nose and inner third of the eyebrows. A double row of eyebrows is occasionally found (Cascio 1965).

◀ Fig. 10.58 Hertogh's sign (♂ 28 yrs.)

References

Aasved, H.: Waardenburg's syndrome. Acta ophthal. 40 (1962) 622–628

Ascher, K. W.: Blepharochalasis mit Struma und Doppellippe. Klin. Mbl. Augenheilk. 65 (1920) 86–97

Bacskulin, J. V., E. Bacskulin: Beitrag zur Klinik der Hyalinosis cutis et mucosae, Lipoid-Gluko-Proteinose Urbach-Wiethe. Acta ophthal. 43 (1965) 610–628

Badtke, G.: Die Mißbildungen des menschlichen Auges. In: Der Augenarzt, Vol. IV, ed. by K. Velhagen. Thieme, Stuttgart 1961

Bäfverstedt, B., K. O. Granström: Fall von Epidermolysis bullosa hereditaria dystrophica mit Augensymptomen (Erosio corneae recidivans). Zbl. Haut- u. Geschl. Kr. 65 (1940) 517

Beckett, R. S., M. G. Netzky: Familial ocular myopathy and external ophthalmoplegia. Arch. Neur. (Chicago) 69 (1953) 64–72; ref. in: Zbl. Ges. ophthal. 60 (1953) 314

Böck, J.: Über eigenartige Gefäßveränderungen im Auge bei v. Recklinghausenscher Neurofibromatose. Dtsch. ophthal. Ges. 53 (1948) 275–282

Bogrow, S.: Zur Kenntnis der atypischen bullösen Hautaffektionen. Arch. Derm. Syph. (Berlin) 110 (1911) 75–84

Bouzas, A.: Ponction camérulaire et étude de l'humeur aqueuse prélévée dans des maladies des yeux d'origine lépreuse. Bull. Soc. franç. ophtal. 69 (1956) 488–497

Bruens, E.: Über Keratitis vaccinulosa. Gleichzeitig ein Beitrag zur Behandlung der Vaccineerkrankung des Auges. Albrecht v. Graefes Arch. klin. exp. Ophthal. 147 (1944) 83–104

Carleton, Alice: Vesico-bullous diseases affecting the eye. Brit. med. J. 1949, MMMMDCXXXII, 835–837

Cascio, G.: Sur la duplicatio supercilii. Ophthalmologica 130 (1955) 231–243

Charamis, J.: Ocular allergy in handlers of streptomycin. Brit. J. Ophthal. 33 (1949) 714–715

Cohen, M., M. B. Sulzberger: Essential shrinkage of conjunctiva in a case of probable epidermolysis bullosa dystrophica. Arch. ophthal. 13 (1935) 374–390

Conrads, H., G. Heinmüller: Beitrag zur Genese des rezidivierenden Lidödems bei Kindern. Klin. Mbl. Augenheilk. 135 (1959) 496–501

Contino, F.: Manifestazione oculare nel corso die malattia di Stevens-Johnson. Probabile genesi virale della forma morbosa. Riv. ital. Tracoma 4 (1952) 5–18

Cordes, F. C., S. D. Aken: Ocular changes in acute disseminated lupus erythematosus. Amer. J. Ophthal. 30 (1947) 1541–1555

Doesschate, J. ten: Corneal complications in lupus erythematosus discoides. Ophthalmologica (Basel) 132 (1956) 153–156

Dresner, E., D. A. D. Montgomery: Primary optic atrophy in v. Recklinghausen's disease (multiple neurofibromatosis). Quart. J. Med. 18 (1949) 93–103

Duke-Elder, S.: The ocular adnexa. System of ophthalmology XIII: 1. diseases of the eyelids, 2. lacrimal, orbital and para-orbital diseases. Kimpton, London 1974

Eisenstodt, L. W.: Blepharochalasis with double upper lip. Amer. J. Ophthal. 32 (1949) 128–130

Elliot, D. C.: An interpretation of the ocular manifestations of leprosy. Ann. N. Y. Acad. Sci. 54 (1951) 84–100

Fanta, H.: Lider und Tränenorgane. Fortschr. Augenheilk. 9 (1959)

Fox, S. A.: Distichiasis. Amer. J. Ophthal. 53 (1962) 14–18

Franceschetti, A., C. Avanza: Sulla manifestazione familiare dell' iperaminoaciduria associata a cataratta congenita. Atti 43 Congr. Soc. oftal. ital. 17 (1958) 530–536; ref. in: Zbl. Ges. ophthal. 79 (1960) 212

François, J.: Les ectodermoses erosives pluriorificielles. Acta ophthal. (Kbh.) 32 (1954) 5–35

François, J.: Les Mycoses oculaires. Masson, Paris 1968

François, J., J. Bacskulin, P. Pollmann: Manifestations oculaires du syndrome d'Urbach-Wiethe; hyalinosis cutis et mucosae. Ophthalmologica 155 (1968) 433–448

Friede, R.: Zur Klinik und Ätiologie des Epicanthus. Klin. Mbl. Augenheilk. 115 (1949) 12–27

Friede, R.: Zur Operation des Epicanthus. Klin. Mbl. Augenheilk. 117 (1950) 178–186

Fuchs, E.: Herpes iris conjunctivae. Klin. Mbl. Augenheilk. 14 (1876) 333–351

Fülling, G., G. Pünder: Augenhintergrundsveränderungen beim Status Bonnevie-Ullrich. Klin. Mbl. Augenheilk. 128 (1956) 724–727

Godtfredsen, E.: Ophthalmological signs and symptoms in mesenchymal diseases. Acta ophthal. (Kbh.) 32 (1954) 717–728

Hadley, H. G.: Blepharochalasis. Acta ophthal. (Kbh.) 17 (1939) 310–313

Hager, G.: Augenärztliche Beobachtungen und Probleme bei der v. Recklinghausenschen Erkrankung. Klin. Mbl. Augenheilk. 132 (1958) 350–363

Heydenreich, A.: Krankheiten der Augenlider. In: Der Augenarzt, Vol. III, ed. by K. Velhagen. Thieme, Stuttgart 1960 (pp. 1–195)

Hidano, A., H. Kajima, S. Ikeda, Mizutanti, H. Miyasato, M. Nitmura: Natural history of nevus of ota. Arch. Derm. Syph. (Chicago) 95 (1967) 187–195

Hoff, F.: Akuter totaler Pigmentverlust. Dtsch. med. Wschr. 79 (1954) 284–287

Hoffmann, D. H.: Pilzinfektionen des Auges. Fortschr. Augenheilk. 16 (1965) 63–217

Holland, G.: Hämangiome der Lider. Klin. Mbl. Augenheilk. 152 (1968) 365–373

Hollwich, F., H. Gernet, E. Damaske: Zum Euryblepharon. Ber. Verein Rhein.-Westf. Augenärzte. 119 (1969) 9–11

Hotz, G.: Augenhintergrundsveränderungen bei Kollagenkrankheit. Ophthalmologica (Basel) 133 (1957) 354–356

Kanter, D.: Zum Marcus Gunnschen Phänomen. Klin. Mbl. Augenheilk. 126 (1955) 50–59

Katayama, R.: Experimental study of tuberculosis in guinea-pigs (I). Results obtained from inoculation in the skin of the abdomen. Acta derm. (Kyoto) 22 (1933) 49–50

Kato, T., S. Omoto: A case of disseminated erythematodes with intensive change in eye. J. clin. Ophthal. (Tokyo) 11 (1957) 390–394

Kiloh, L. G., S. Nevin: Progressive dystrophy of the external ocular muscles (ocular myopathy). Brain 74 (1951) 115–143

Klemens, F.: Blepharochalasis und Doppellippe. Klin. Mbl. Augenheilk. 102 (1939) 588–589

Kratka, W. H.: The bullous dermatosis. Amer. J. Ophthal. 39 (1955) 233–236

Kraus, E., E. Jung: Pigmentierungen der Hornhautrückfläche bei Naevus fusco-coeruleus ophthalmo-maxillaris. OTA. Ber. dtsch. ophthal. Ges. 68 (1968) 442–444

Kreibig, W.: Aderhautveränderungen bei Neurofibromatose (Recklinghausen). Klin. Mbl. Augenheilk. 105 (1940) 369–370

Kümmel, R.: Lider. In: Handbuch der speziellen pathologischen Anatomie und Histologie, Vol. XI/2, ed. by O. Henke, B. Lubarsch. Springer, Berlin 1931 (pp. 139–262)

Lemmingson, W.: Augenbeteiligung bei Epidermolysis bullosa. Klin. Mbl. Augenheilk. 122 (1953) 350–353

Linser, P.: Über die Epidermolysis bullosa hereditaria und ihren Zusammenhang mit der Raynaudschen Krankheit. Arch. Derm. Syph. (Berlin) 84 (1907) 369–386

Löhlein, W.: Erkrankungen der Lider. In: Kurzes Handbuch der Ophthalmologie, Vol. III, ed. by F. Schieck, A. Brückner. Springer, Berlin 1930 (pp. 243–366)

Löhlein, W.: Die entzündlichen Erkrankungen der Lidhaut. Syphilis. In: Kurzes Handbuch der Ophthalmologie, Vol. III, ed. by F. Schieck, A. Brückner. Springer, Berlin 1931 (pp. 289–291)

Löhr, K. Ein Fall von Blepharochalasis im Kindesalter. Klin. Mbl. Augenheilk. 115 (1949) 28–31

Lohse, K., M. Tost: Zur Frage des Epithelioma calcificans Malherbe. Acta ophthal. 45 (1967) 876–882

Lowe, J.: Leprous affection of the eyes. Proc. roy. Soc. Med. 48 (1955) 107–108

Lund, O. E.: Tumoren der Lider. Almanach für die Augenheilkunde. Lehmann, München 1969 (pp. 1–10)

Lutz, W.: Epidermolysis bullosa traumatica hereditaria. Handbuch der Ophthalmologie, Vol. VII, ed. by F. Schieck, A. Brückner. Springer, Berlin 1932 a (p. 304)

Lutz, W.: Lupus erythematodes. In: Kurzes Handbuch der Ophthalmologie, Vol. VII, ed. by F. Schieck, A. Brückner. Springer, Berlin 1932 b (p. 330)

Magni, S.: Rilievi clinici ed istopatologici in alcuni casi di neurofibromi e di neuromi plesiformi a localizzazione orbitaria. Atti 41. Congr. Soc. Oftal. ital. 15 (1956) 281–284

Mamelok, A. E., J. Laval: Stenosis of the lacrimal canals and puncta caused by the Stevens-Johnson syndrome. Amer. J. Ophthal. 40 (1955) 83–86

Marchionini, A.: Über Epidermolysis bullosa dystrophica vegetans. Arch. Derm. Syph. (Berlin) 176 (1938) 347–371

Mattson, R., O. Carlberg: Eye lesions and their treatment in the so-called Stevens-Johnson's syndrome or ectodermosis erosiva pluriorificialis. Acta ophthal. (KbH) 31 (1953) 469–483

Mejer, F.: Durch Streptomycin bedingtes allergisches Lidekzem als Berufskrankheit. Wien. klin. Wschr. 61 (1949) 702–703

Mejer, F.: Durch Streptomycin bedingte allergische Lidekzeme als Berufskrankheiten. Sitzung der Wiener Ophthalm. Ges. vom 13. 6. 1949. Wien. klin. Wschr. 62 (1950) 55

Merté, H. J.: Arbeitsmedizinische Fragen in der Ophthalmologie. Karger, Basel 1969

Merté, H. J.: Arbeits- und Sozialmedizin. In: Lehrbuch der Augenheilkunde, ed. by T. Axenfeld, H. Pau. Fischer, Stuttgart 1973

Meyer, F. E.: Recklinghausensche Neurofibromatose und Auge. Klin. Mbl. Augenheilk. 103 (1939) 44–57

Minamik, K.: Über einen Fall von Chalazion bei einem 4 Monate und 22 Tage alten Säugling. Acta Soc. ophthal. Jap. 43 (1939) 216; ref. in: Zbl. ges. Ophthal. 43 (1939) 493

Naróg, F.: Membranaceous conjunctivitis in Erythema exsudativum multiforme. Klin. oczna 26 (1956) 395–400

Nikolowski, W., R. Seitz: Epithelioma Malherbe im augapfelnahen Hautgewebe. Klin. Mbl. Augenheilk. 136 (1960) 825–836

Ota, M.: Nevus fusco-coeruleus ophthalmo-maxillaris. Jap. J. Derm. 46 (1939) 369

Papst, W., E. Esslen, H. G. Mertens: Die oculäre Muskeldystrophie sog. Ophthalmoplegia externa chronica progressiva. Klin. Mbl. Augenheilk. 132 (1958) 691–707

Passow, A.: Über den Einfluß des Sympathicus auf Wachstum und Pigmentbildung. Zugleich ein Beitrag zur Kenntnis des Status dysraphicus und seiner okularen Symptome, insbesondere der Heterochromie. Klin. Mbl. Augenheilk. 116 (1950) 561–578

Patz, A.: Ocular involvement in erythema multiforme. Arch. Ophthal. 43 (1950) 244–256

Pietruschka, G.: Zur Frage der Irisveränderungen bei der Recklinghausenschen Krankheit. Klin. Mbl. Augenheilk. 121 (1952) 663–672

Pillat, A.: Über das Vorkommen von Chorioiditis bei Lupus erythematodes. Albrecht v. Graefes Arch. klin. exp. Ophthal. 133 (1935) 566–577

Poštić, S.: Ein primäres Abklatschulcus vortäuschende Kontaktgummibildung an den Lidrändern. Klin. Mbl. Augenheilk. 104 (1940) 319–323

Proppe, A.: Die Baadersche Dermatostomatitis, die Ektodermosis erosiva pluriorificialis Fissinger, Rendu, das Stevens-Johnsonsche Syndrom und die Conjunctivitis et Stromatitis pseudomembranaca als Syndroma muco cutaneo-oculare acutum Fuchs. Arch. Derm. Syph. (Berlin) 187 (1948) 392–408

Proppe, A., E. Hauss: Zur Frage der Blutschwammbehandlung. Derm. Wschr. 148 (1963) 330

Raffin, A.: Conjunctivitis, Rhinitis und Stomatitis aphthosa mit Erythema multiforme. Klin. Mbl. Augenheilk. 68 (1922) 216–220

Reeh, M. J.: Treatment of lid and epibulbar tumors. Thomas, Springfield Ill. 1963

Riecke, F.: Epidermolysis bullosa. In: Handbuch der Haut- und Geschlechtskrankheiten, Vol. VII/2, ed. by J. Jadassohn. Fischer, Jena 1931 (p. 222)

Rodenhäuser, J. H.: Zur Klinik und Histologie des Molluscum pseudocarcinomatosum (Molluscum sebaceum, Kerato-Akanthoma). Albrecht v. Graefes Arch. klin. exp. Ophthal. 158 (1957) 468–484

Rohrschneider, W., F. J. Ehring: Die Bewertung der Augenbefunde für die Erkennung der Ätiologie beim Erythematodes. Hautarzt 4 (1953) 451–455

Rosen, E.: Some new concepts concerning ocular complications following vaccination. Ophthalmologica (Basel) 115 (1948) 321–332

Rougier, J., D. Colomb, J. Royer: Syndrome de Stevens-Johnson associé à un syndrome de Gougerot-Sjögren frustre. Bull. Soc. Ophtal. Fr. 1958, 233–237

Schmincke, A.: Recklinghausensche Krankheit. In: Handbuch der speziellen pathologischen Anatomie und Histologie, Part IV, ed. by O. Lubarsch, F. Henke, R. Rössle. Springer, Berlin 1956 (pp. 664–695)

Schönfeld, W.: Dermatologie für Augenärzte. Thieme, Stuttgart 1947

Schreck, E.: Erythema exsudativum multiforme. Dermatologie und Venerologie, Vol. IV, ed. by H. A. Gottron, W. Schönfeld. Thieme, Stuttgart 1960 (pp. 832–835)

Schubert, H.: Kontaktekzeme in Augenumgebung. Klin. Mbl. Augenheilk. 151 (1967) 457–465

Sédan, J., A. G. Ourgaud, P. Guillot: Les accidents oculaires d'origine vaccinale observés dans le département des Bouches-du-Rhône au cours de l'épidémie variolique de l'hiver 1952. Ann. Oculist. (Paris) 186 (1953) 34–61

Shapland, C. D.: A case of neurofibromatosis with extensive involvement of the right upper lid. Trans. ophthal. Soc. U. K. 69 (1950) 319–322

Shields, J. A., G. O. Waring, L. G. Monte: Ocular findings in leprosy. Amer. J. Ophthal. 77 (1974) 880–890

Siemens, H. W.: Dichtung und Wahrheit über die Ichthyosis bullosa mit Bemerkungen zur Systematik der Epidermolysen. Arch. Derm. Syph. (Berlin) 175 (1937) 590–608

Stein, R.: Blepharochalasis des Unterlides. Klin. Mbl. Augenheilk. 84 (1930) 846–851

Stemmermann, W.: Neurofibromatose von Recklinghausen und Sehorgan. Ber. dtsch. ophthal. Ges. 1953, 348

Strehl, C.: Blindheitsverhütung. Klin. Mbl. Augenheilk. 140 (1962) 425–427

Thies, O.: Das Auge bei Erythema exsudativum multiforme. Klin. Mbl. Augenheilk. 116 (1950) 44–53

Thies, O.: Das Syndroma muco-cutaneo-oculare Fuchs. Klin. Mbl. Augenheilk. 119 (1951) 486–494

Unger, K.: Neurofibromatosis iridis (Recklinghausen's disease). Arch. Ophthal. 38 (1947) 754–759

Vilanova, X., C. Cardenal, J. M. Capdevilla: Chronischer Lupus erythematodes der conjunctiva. Dermatologica (Basel) 113 (1956) 226–231

Waardenburg, P. J.: Hyperplasia interocularis cum dystopia lateroversa canthi medialis, blepharophimosis, dyschromia iridocutanea et dysplasia auditiva. Acta ophthal. 35 (1957) 311–324

Wolff, J. E.: Ocular complications in erythema exsudativum multiforme with mucous membrane lesions. Brit. J. Ophthal. 33 (1949) 110–120

Zade, M.: Erkrankungen des Sehorgans in ihren Beziehungen zu den Infektionskrankheiten. Pocken. In: Kurzes Handbuch der Ophthalmologie, Vol. VII, ed. by F. Schieck, A. Brückner. Springer, Berlin 1932 (pp. 182–184)

Zunin, C., J. Mariotti: Le anomalie oculari nello status Bonnevie-Ullrich. Ann. Ophthal. 79 (1953) 359–376

11 Lacrimal System

Lacrimal gland

Hyposecretion (Dry Eyes)

Physiologic decrease in tearing — Pathologic hyposecretion — Pharmacologic causes of hyposecretion — Consequences of hyposecretion — Methods of investigation.

Physiologic Decrease in Tearing

Innervation of the lacrimal gland is not complete during the first months of life. As a result there is no tearing on "crying." There is physiologic decreased tearing in sleep and in deep stages of anesthesia.

Pathologic Hyposecretion (see pages 130–150)

Decreased tearing is seen with lacrimal gland hypoplasia and disruption of nervous pathways controlling tearing.

Facial nerve paresis superior to the geniculate ganglion causes loss of tearing. Once the superior petrosal nerve has branched off below the ganglion, tearing is uninfluenced by a lesion of the facial nerve. Senile involution, atrophy of the lacrimal gland following inflammation, or partial surgical removal of the lacrimal gland are other causes of hyposecretion.

Sjögren's syndrome (see pages 130–150) occurs primarily in middle-aged females (40 to 60 years old). There is a loss of tear as well as salivary and nasal mucous membrane secretions. Polyarthritis and achlorhydria are common associated findings. Sjögren's syndrome is usually classified as a collagen disorder. Other causes for decreased tear secretion include avitaminoses, hepatic disease, hormonal imbalance, and pituitary dysfunction. Avitaminosis A, xerophthalmia, Mikulicz's syndrome, conjunctival scarring (chemical and thermal burns, trachoma, diphtheria, pemphigus vulgaris [Plate VI], pemphigoid [Fig. 12.9], erythema multiforme, and epidermolysis bullosa) should also be considered.

Familial autonomic dysfunction (dysautonomia, Riley-Day syndrome) has congenital lack of tearing. Neuroparalytic keratitis occurs secondary to the corneal anesthesia. Affected children show retarded development, dysphagia, susceptibility to pneumonia, or hyperhidrosis with dehydration. It is genetically recessive (Sorsby 1970).

Congenital anhidrotic ectodermal dysplasia includes aplasia of the lacrimal gland and, therefore, lack of tearing. Prominent curved eyebrows, saddle nose and thick lips are characteristic. Rhinitis, or even ozena, and microphthalmos occur. It is inherited as a sex-linked recessive or dominant (Sorsby 1970).

Hyposecretion Caused by Drugs

Parasympatholytic agents (belladonna, atropine, scopolamine) and botulism cause decreased tearing.

Consequences of Hyposecretion

There is a drying out of the cornea and conjunctiva (xerosis conjunctivae et corneae), filamentary keratitis, superficial punctate keratitis (see page 150), and keratoconjunctivitis sicca (Plate VI, Fig. 6, see page 228 f). Subjective symptoms: burning, itching, photophobia, eyes feel dry and sandy.

Methods of Investigation

For Schirmer's test topical anesthetic drops are given and the end of a standardized (5 mm wide) strip of filter paper is placed in the cul-de-sac. After three minutes the amount of wetting should be 10 mm. Less than 5 mm indicates decreased tear production.

In the fluorescein dilution test (Nover-Jaeger), a drop of 2 percent fluorescein is dropped in the cul-de-sac. Two minutes later, the tears are soaked up with a piece of filter paper and its color compared with standardized fluorescein concentrations.

Hypersecretion

Psychic hypersecretion — Inflammation and irritation — Inadequate drainage — Hypersecretion from various causes — Crocodile tears — Hypersecretion with drugs, bloody tears.

Hypersecretion with epiphora (wet eyes): Tearing results from hypersecretion or inadequate drainage. Tear production over a sixteen-hour waking period is about 0.6 to 1.0 ml. It decreases in sleep.

Emotional factors and reflex mechanisms increase tearing. Pain, sadness, or joy are emotional causes of tearing. Any irritation of the eyes causes reflex tearing.

Inflammation and Irritation

Tearing occurs with *any inflammation* of the anterior portion of the eyes (keratitis, conjunctivitis, blepharitis, episcleritis, scleritis, iridocyclitis). Any injury, foreign body (corneal, conjunctival, lid, scratching lashes), or burn causes tearing. Chemical irritants, onion, formaldehyde, tear gas, etc., may also cause tearing.

Irritation of nasal mucosa by odors, acrid gases, or mechanical methods will evoke a tear response. Irritation of gustatory nerves and even chewing may produce tearing. Other factors include cold, dazzling, yawning, vomiting, migraine, trigeminal neuralgias, and sour foods. Allergic irritation of mucous membranes such as occurs with hay fever is a particularly powerful stimulus for tearing.

Inadequate Tear Drainage

When drainage is inadequate, tearing occurs without irritation. Lacrimal puncta or canaliculi can be absent or stenosed, fail to communicate, or be fistulous. Lacrimal puncta, canaliculi, or the tear sac may be stenosed congenitally, secondary to chronic inflammation or injury, and may be blocked by foreign bodies, lashes, concretions, fungi, actinomycosis, tumors, polyps, etc. Diverticuli and reduplication of the drainage system are further causes for poor drainage. Attempts at irrigation of the drainage apparatus are unsuccessful. Malpositioning of the lids (ectropion, eversion of the lacrimal punctum, entropion with trichiasis, symblepharon) will cause tearing. Irrigation is successful in these instances.

Hypersecretion from Various Causes

Lacrimal gland tumors in their early stages may cause hypersecretion. It is also seen with parkinsonism, hyperthyroidism, and myxedema. Charlin's syndrome (see page 78) involves unilateral tearing, pain, and changes of the anterior segment of the globe. Placing a cocaine-soaked pledget in the nose is diagnostic therapy. The nose must be examined for tumors or other irritants in any case of excessive tearing.

Crocodile Tears

A facial nerve lesion located superior to the geniculate ganglion (prior to separation of the superficial petrosal nerve) causes loss of tearing. If the lesion is below the geniculate ganglion tear production remains normal. Lagophthalmos from the facial paresis allows inadequate drainage. Aberrant innervation of the lacrimal gland by salivary gland nerves produces "crocodile tears." This is seen after facial nerve damage in the region of the geniculate ganglion. Eating, chewing, or any gustatory stimulus causes tearing. They are called *crocodile tears* not because they are large or profuse, but because of the legend that crocodiles cry while eating their victims. Severing the superficial petrosal nerve remedies the problem.

Crocodile tears may occur in Duane's syndrome (Papst 1966; Trieschmann 1973).

Hypersecretion Due to Drugs; Bloody Tears

Parasympathomimetic agents (Mecholyl, doryl, pilocarpine, Prostigmin) cause tearing.

Bloody tears occur with conjunctival papillomas, granulomas, fibromas, hemorrhagic telangiectasia (Rendu-Osler-Weber), and vicarious menstruation or severe muscarine or alkyl-phosphate (E 605) poisoning.

Swelling in the Lacrimal Gland Region

Dacryoadenitis — Acute dacryoadenitis — Chronic dacryoadenitis — Periostitis — Tumors — Cysts — Ectopic lacrimal gland; herniated lobe.

The lacrimal gland has an orbital and a palpebral lobe. Accessory lacrimal glands (glands of Krause) are scattered throughout the conjunctiva, especially in the superior cul-de-sac.

Dacryoadenitis causes a characteristic S-shaped curve of the upper lid (Plate IV, Fig. 3, page 128 d). The swollen tender gland is visible on lid eversion (Fig. 11.1). Chemosis, pre-auricular lymphadenopathy and displacement of the globe inferiorly and nasally may occur.

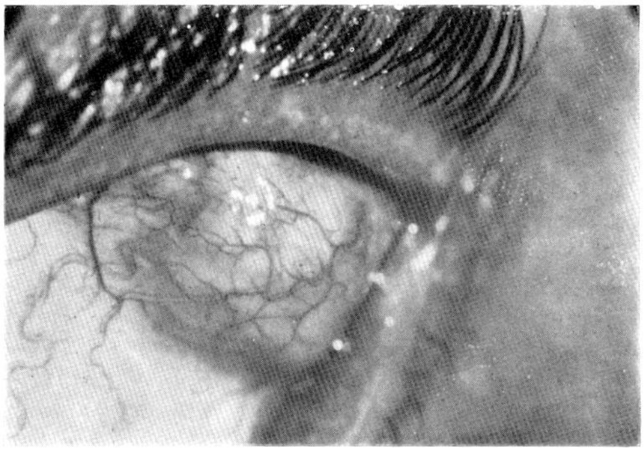

Fig. 11.1 Dacryoadenitis: red swollen lacrimal gland (♂ 46 yrs.)

Acute dacryoadenitis is usually part of a generalized infection (measles, influenza, scarlet fever, diphtheria, infectious mononucleosis, gonorrhea). Mumps may affect both lacrimal glands. Staphylococcal infection and bacterial emboli are rare causes of acute dacryoadenitis. There may be abscess formation.

Differential diagnostic considerations include the following. Chalazion is tender over the tarsus, and lid abscesses may form. Sinusitis, potentially with orbital cellulitis, is usually more nasal; there is a greater degree of systemic illness. Osteomyelitis of the superior temporal orbital rim is rare. There is marked skin edema and pressure on the bone elicits pain. The patient is systemically ill. Radiological otolaryngological consultations are part of the regular workup.

Chronic dacryoadenitis is usually pain-free. There is ptosis and a characteristic S-shaped deformity of the upper lid. Bilateral parotid and lacrimal gland involvement occurs in Mikulicz's syndrome.

Causes of chronic dacryoadenitis include: luetic gumma, tuberculosis, sarcoidosis (see page 201; includes uveoparotid fever = Heerfordt's syndrome), lymphosarcoma, and lymphogranuloma (Hodgkin's disease).

Periostitis: Periostitis of the upper lateral orbital rim may simulate dacryoadenitis with edema and S-shaped deformity of the lid.

Tumors (see page 344): benign *lipodermoids* are the most common tumor in this region. The most common true lacrimal gland neoplasm is the more or less malignant tumor of epithelial and connective tissue origin (Fig. 11.2).

Although the peak incidence is in the third and fourth decades, the tumor has been described in children (McPherson 1966). *Mixed tumors* have also been called myxochondroepitheliomas, fibroepitheliomas, or pleomorphic adenomas. The firm tumor grows slowly (sometimes for years). There is a slow onset of exophthalmos, displacement of the globe and diplopia.

Lymphoma, reticulum cell sarcoma, adenoma, adenocarcinoma, cylindroma, plasmocytoma, angioma, and fibroma are rare. About 5 percent of lacrimal gland tumors develop from lymphoid hyperplasia. When such a tumor grows slowly, it remains isolated and noninfiltrating. It can be called lymphoma. Lymphangiomas, adenolymphoma, plasmocytoma, histiocytoma and oncocytoma may appear as slowly growing noninfiltrating tumors.

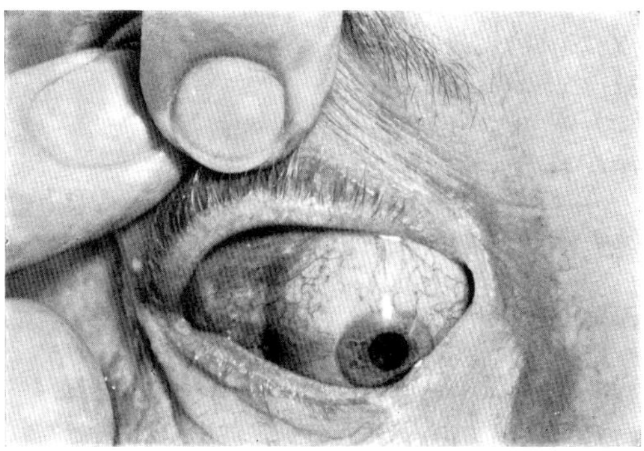

Fig. 11.2 Mixed lacrimal gland tumor (♂ 59 yrs.)

Leukemia and Hodgkin's disease produce a similar clinical picture. Salivary glands, lymph nodes, liver, and spleen are also involved.
Lymphosarcomas are rapidly growing, firm, non-displaceable tumors which frequently arise from the periosteum.
Cysts and displacement of the lacrimal gland. Harmless retention cysts (dacryops), dermoids, and parasitic cysts may all cause swelling and the S-shaped deformity of the upper lid. Displacement (ectopia) of the lacrimal gland can do the same thing. It may be congenital, traumatic, or due to displacement of the gland by progressive exophthalmos.

Lacrimal Passages

Patency of lacrimal passages — Diseases of puncta and canaliculi — Dacryocystitis — Congenital lacrimal sac obstruction — Tumors.

Tears are slightly alkaline and contain 1 percent NaCl. They pass through the lacrimal puncta, canaliculi and lacrimal sac into the nose where they enter below the inferior turbinate. Two percent fluorescein dye instilled in the conjunctival sac will pass into the nose by this route. Staining of a handkerchief or cotton pledget demonstrates the patency of the lacrimal passages. Irrigation of lacrimal passages is performed with the head forward. Liquid runs into the nose and, when the head is tipped backward, the fluid runs into the pharynx causing the patient to swallow.
Injection of radiopaque dyes allows roentgenographic diagnoses (dacryocystogram).
In about 5 percent of patients, reflux from the nose into the conjunctival sac is possible. Air bubbles may be seen at the puncta when these patients blow their nose.

Diseases of the Lacrimal Passages

Diseases of the Lacrimal Puncta and Canaliculi

Double, triple, or even quadruple lacrimal puncta and canaliculi occur congenitally (Bacskulin 1964). Congenital atresia of the punctum or canaliculus is found less frequently.
As a rule, obstruction of the lacrimal passages occurs after burns (chemical, thermal), or by foreign bodies (concretions, cilia, hairs, fungi), trauma or tumors.
Signs of canaliculitis and obstruction caused by fungi (Plate IV, Fig. 4, page 128 d) include tearing, hyperemia, and edema in the punctum and canalicular area. Actinomycotic (gram-positive bacteria) dacryocanaliculitis (Hofmann 1965, François 1968), causes chronic, therapy-resistant inflammation at the inner canthus. Tearing and stringy conjunctival secretions accompany indolent edema of varying degrees in the region of the canaliculus. Dry, gray-yellow, crumbly material or pus can be expressed from the canal. Culture and microscopic examination of this material reveals the causal agent. In mycotic canaliculitis the expressed plug is virtually a pure culture (colony) of the organism. In addition to *Actinomyces* (gram-positive bacteria), less common pathogens are *Aspergillus, Candida, Sporotrichum,* and *Cephalosporium*. Fungi will also infect meibomian glands, conjunctiva, skin of the lids and cornea.

Inflammation of the Lacrimal Sac

Dilated lacrimal sac — Dacryocystitis, cellulitis — Fungal dacryocystitis — Tuberculous dacryocystitis — Syphilis, yaws — Dacryocystitis in trachoma — Differential diagnosis — Complications of acute dacryocystitis.

Stenosis of the lacrimal gland near its entrance into the nose allows accumulation of mucoid, pussy material and dilatation of the lacrimal sac (Fig. 11.3). Diverticula are rare, but cause similar symptoms. Injury to the sac such as fractures of the lacrimal fossa is another anatomic cause of obstruction. Rhinitis, sinusitis, polyps, hypertrophied nasal turbinate and traumatic probing may all obstruct the lacrimal canal.
Superinfection frequently occurs with chronic lacrimal sac obstruction. This leads to acute dacryoadenitis and cellulitis. The primary pathogen is pneumococcus and, on occasion, staphylococci or streptococci (Plate IV, Fig. 5, page 128 d). The acute inflammation will be accompanied by fever, headache, and general

malaise. A fistula between the skin and the lacrimal sac often results. If the borders of the inflammation are sharp, erysipelas is a possibility.
Women are three times more often affected than men. Dacryocystitis can result in a mucocele or pyocele of the lacrimal sac.
Mycotic infections of the lacrimal sac *(actinomyces* [gram-positive bacteria], *candida, aspergillus, sporotrichum, cephalosporium, rhinosporidium)* are rare (Hoffmann 1965). These will cause a low-grade indolent cellulitis with fistula formation, accumulation of brittle concretions or mucopurulent material. Tuberculosis can cause chronic and acute canaliculitis and dacryocystitis in children. Bacterial superinfection is frequent. The lacrimal system may still irrigate freely since the granulomas tend to be pushed aside by the pressure. In most cases the infection fistulizes to the skin. Lacrimal sac fistulas (Fig. 11.4) may be congenital or result from dacryocystitis-cellulitis.
Congenital syphilis, which is less common now than in the past, was formerly an important cause of acute dacryocystitis in children (ages 2 to 12 years). Igersheimer (1928) found *syphilis* to be the cause in 50 percent of acute dacryocystitis in this age group. The cases were frequently bilateral and caused by blockage in the nose from luetic involvement of bone and mucosa (gumma, periostitis, saddle nose, and bony atresia of the nasal passages). Yaws *(Spirochaeta pertenue)* also causes dacryocystitis. The depigmented skin lesions create cicatricial ectropion and tearing. Dacryocystitis is common in trachoma.
Differential diagnostic considerations include hordeolum, furunculosis, and orbital cellulitis; the lacrimal passages irrigate freely in these cases. In dacryocystitis the mass lies below the canthal ligament. Mucoceles or tooth infections are recognized on X-ray films.
Complications of acute dacryocystitis include ulceration, perforation into the nose and through the skin, panophthalmitis, thrombophlebitis, meningitis, and optic atrophy.

Congenital Obstruction of the Lacrimal Passages

At birth there is frequently a persistent unperforated membrane between lacrimal canal and nose (Hasner's fold). This membrane may be present in up to 35 percent of newborns (Schwarz 1949). It normally perforates shortly after birth. Nordlöw and Vennerholm (1953) found nasolacrimal duct stenosis in 6 percent of 1,000 children studied. True atresia of the bony lacrimal canal is rare. Mothers of these patients notice tearing and conjunctival irritation. Pus can be expressed from the swollen lacrimal sac. Frequently the false diagnosis of tumor or conjunctivitis is made.

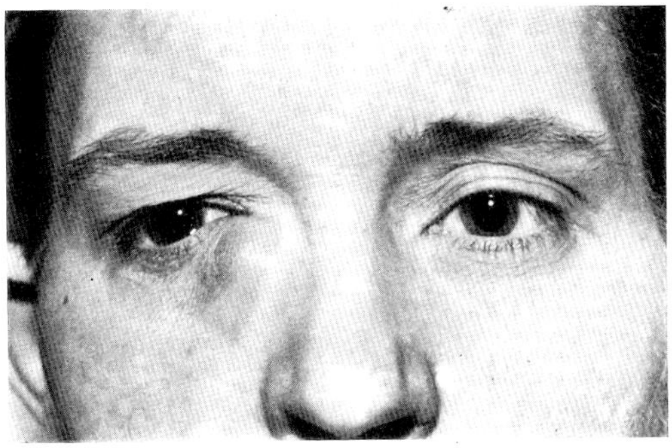

Fig. 11.3 Dacryocystocele (♂ 42 yrs.)

Tumors

Tumors obstructing the lacrimal passages are almost invariably secondary and arise from the skin (basal cell, carcinoma), the nose (polyps, carcinoma), sinuses (carcinoma), periosteum (sarcoma), or are metastatic. Primary tumors are rare (carcinoma, sarcoma, reticulum cell sarcoma, papilloma, granuloma).
Pseudotumors (granulomas) and papillomas are often pedunculated. *Differential diagnostic*

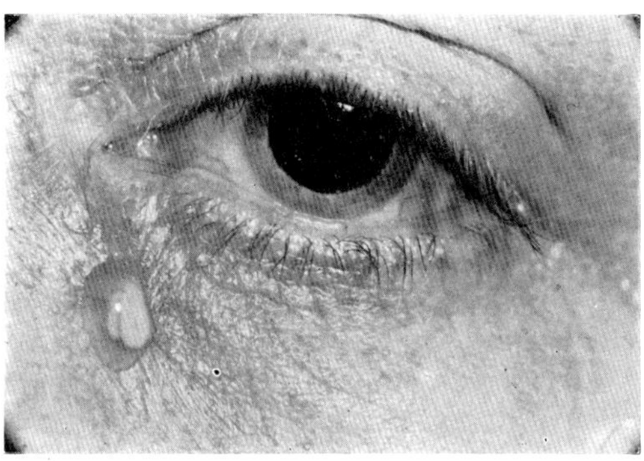

Fig. 11.4 Lacrimal sac fistula (♀ 43 yrs.)

considerations include rare diverticula and cysts of the lacrimal passages. These are either congenital or acquired. The lacrimal passage will irrigate freely, in spite of a diverticulum. The contents, however, can be expressed. A cyst is taut, and may be large. While diverticula visualize with injection of radiopaque dye, cysts do not. They may, however, present as a filling defect.

References

Bacskulin, J.: Punctum lacrimale duplex, triplex und quadruplex. Klin. Mbl. Augenheilk. 144 (1964) 418–428

Badtke, G.: Die Mißbildungen des menschlichen Auges. In: Der Augenarzt. Vol. IV, ed. by K. Velhagen. Thieme, Stuttgart 1961

Duke-Elder, St.: Diseases of the lacrimal apparatus. In: Textbook of Ophthalmology, Vol. V. Kimpton, London 1952 (p. 5201)

Duke-Elder, S.: The ocular adnexa. System of ophthalmology XIII: 1. diseases of the eyelids, 2. lacrimal, orbital and para-orbital diseases. Kimpton, London 1974

Fischer, F.: Die Entwicklung der ableitenden Tränenwege beim Menschen. Karger, Basel 1936

François, J.: Les Mycoses oculires. Masson, Paris 1968

Hoffmann, W. H.: Pilzinfektionen des Auges. Fortschr. Augenheilk. 16 (1965) 63–217

Hogan, M. J., L. E. Zimmerman: Ophthalmic Pathology. Saunders, Philadelphia 2nd Ed., 1962

Igersheimer, J.: Syphilis und Auge. Springer, Berlin 1928

Korting, G. W.: Fehlbildungen der Haut und Hautveränderungen bei Fehlbildungssyndromen. In: Handbuch der Haut- und Geschlechtskrankheiten, Vol. III, ed. by J. Jadassohn. Springer, Berlin 1963 (pp. 375–493)

McPherson, S. D. Jr.: Mixed tumor of the lacrimal gland. Amer. J. Ophthal. 61 (1966) 561–563

Meisner, W.: Die Erkrankungen der Tränenorgane. In: Kurzes Handbuch der Ophthalmologie, Vol. III, ed. by F. Schieck, A. Brückner. Springer, Berlin 1930

Nordlöw, W. J.: Vennerholm: Congenital Atresia of the lacrimal passages: Their occurrence and treatment. Acta ophthal. (Kbh.) 31 (1953) 367–371

Papst, W.: Paralytischer Strabismus infolge paradoxer Innervation. 67. Ber. dtsch. Ophthal. Ges. 1965 (1966) 84–101

Schreck, E.: Veränderungen des Sehorgans bei Haut- und Geschlechtskrankheiten. In: Dermatologie u. Neurologie, Vol. IV, ed. by H. A. Gottron, W. Schönfeld. Thieme, Stuttgart 1960

Schwarz, M.: Die Voraussetzungen einer spontanen Beteiligung von Lidern und Orbita bei den Erkrankungen der Nasennebenhöhlen. Klin. Mbl. Augenheilk. 114 (1949) 535–541

Seidel, E.: Tränenorgane. In: Handbuch der speziellen pathologischen Anatomie und Histologie, Vol. XI/2, ed. by O. Henke, B. Lubarsch. Springer, Berlin 1931

Sorsby, A.: Ophthalmic genetics: Butterworth, London 1970

Stock, W.: Pathologie der Tränenorgane. In: Handbuch der gesamten Augenheilkunde, Vol. IX, ed. by A. Graefe, Th. Saemisch. Springer, Berlin 1925

Trieschmann, W.: Krokodilstränen bei Conterganschäden. Klin. Mbl. Augenheilk. 162 (1973) 546–550

12 Conjunctiva

Discoloration

Subconjunctival hemorrhage — Yellow, gray, blue, brown discoloration.

Conjunctival Hemorrhage

The transparent conjunctiva has no color of its own. Hemorrhage from any cause (ruptured vessels in trauma, arteriosclerosis, coughing [pertussis], sneezing, pressure, anticoagulation therapy), or transmitted (skull fracture) provides color (Plate IV, Fig. 6, page 128 d). Conjunctival bleeding occurs with vicarious menstruation, in caisson disease (decompression syndrome), and in strangulation and compression injuries to the chest. Older patients will have spontaneous subconjunctival hemorrhages for no obvious reasons. Vitamin C deficiency (scurvy, in adults; Möller-Barlow disease, in children) causes hemorrhages around and, on rare occasions, in the eye. Yellow-brown discoloration from hemosiderin may remain for some time after resolution of a subconjunctival hemorrhage.

Yellow Discoloration (see page 100)

The conjunctiva is yellow with bilirubinemia, picric acid, leptospirosis, or brucellosis (Bang's disease or Mediterranean fever). Skin, lung, or oral uptake of aromatic nitro and amino compounds can cause conjunctival icterus. Peripheral neuropathies and retrobulbar neuritis as well as retinal hemorrhages and nystagmus are less common complications. Dinitrobenzene causes cyanosis of the lips and ears as well as a red-yellow discoloration of the hair. Dinitrophenol, formerly used as an appetite suppressant, has been shown to cause cataracts (Jaensch 1963). Conjunctival fat, which is frequent in elderly and Negro patients, causes a yellow discoloration of the conjunctiva (Plate V, Fig. 1, page 128 e).

Gray (Black) Discoloration (see page 100)

Chronic use of compounds containing silver will color the conjunctiva, cornea, and skin (argyrosis) a slate gray. The coloration is most visible in conjunctival folds and at the inner canthus. Oral or parenteral use of compounds containing silver as well as exposure to silver dusts or vapors may discolor the skin and mucous membranes. Atabrine therapy also causes gray discoloration of conjunctiva and caruncle. Acetanilid, nitrochlorbenzine, and phenols (specifically phenylic acid) are other compounds which produce a gray discoloration of the conjunctiva and sclera. The lid fissure area is especially involved. Carbon disulfide produces optic neuritis and motor nerve paresis, as well as conjunctival discoloration (gray). Chrysiasis, gold deposition, has a more gray-green effect. With arsenicals the discoloration is ash-white. Melanosis in chronic arsenic poisoning may be in patches involving the limbus and conjunctiva. Mascara frequently leads to embedding of pigment granules in the tarsal conjunctiva (Jaensch 1963).

Brown Discoloration

Nevus, melanosis, melanoma — Brown discoloration by drugs — Metabolic and vitamin disturbances — Brown discoloration in endogenous ochronosis (alkaptonuria).

Nevus, Melanosis, Melanoma

The conjunctiva may be *pigmented* markedly in Negroes. The same occurs in true melanosis. In *conjunctival melanosis* there are circumscribed, perilimbic, light to dark brown pigmented spots which move with the conjunctiva (Fig. 12.1, Greer 1954; Reese 1955). It is frequently associated with *subepithelial* or *epi-*

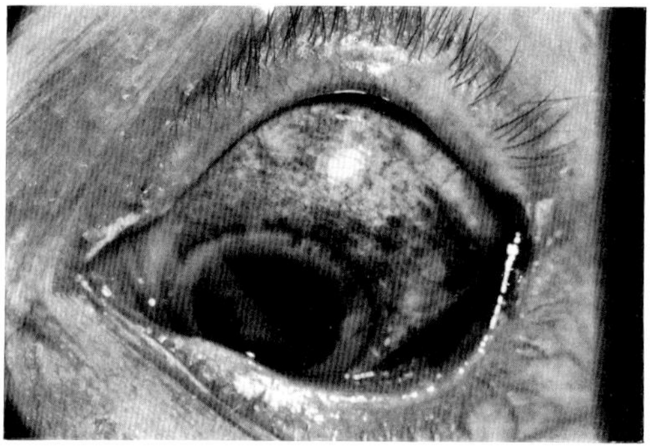

Fig. 12.1 Conjunctival and corneal melanosis (♀ 79 yrs.)

scleral melanosis which does not move with the conjunctiva. These frequently collect like a ring around scleral emissaries (Reese 1955). *Ocular melanocytosis* or *melanosis* is characterized by (Bourquin 1971):

- gray, slate-blue to violet scleral patches of varying size situated around the limbus.
- dark brown or black coloration of the iris. Multiple superficial pigment spots may be present on the iris.
- entire fundus has a darker gray coloration. Melanocytosis is usually unilateral. Conjunctiva, peripheral cornea and even the optic disk may be involved (François 1938). Malignant melanomas develop in 20 percent (Samuels 1953) or 25 percent (Reese 1955).

The *differential diagnosis* includes staphyloma, recurrent scleritis and senile hyaline plaques anterior to muscle insertions (see Fig. 14.2, page 183). These are not true hyperpigmentations but the uvea is visible through thinned sclera. Argyrosis and ochronosis are further considerations.

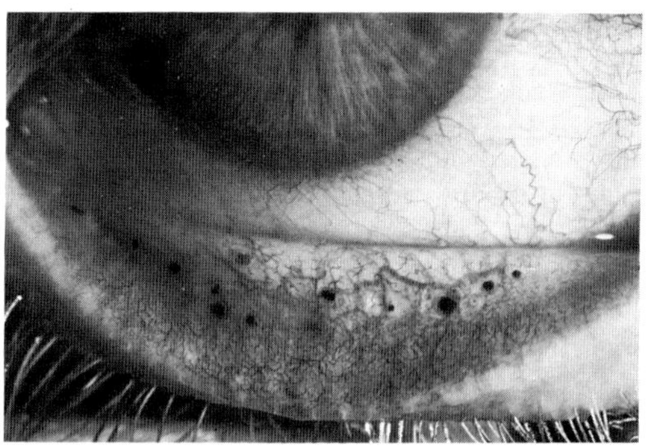

Fig. 12.2 Numerous brown homogeneous conjunctival deposits of variable size following many years of epinephrine use (♀ 66 yrs.)

Ocular melanocytosis (nevus of Ota) is a gray-brown nevoid hyperpigmentation in the distribution of the first trigeminal division. The brow, temple, and eye are affected. It is particularly common in pigmented races (Duke-Elder 1964). There is ocular melanosis and flat, nonelevated, disseminated, blue-gray to violet-brown discoloration of the surrounding skin. Women are more often affected than men. Onset is in the first year of life or at puberty (Hidano et al. 1967).

Pigmented nevi are localized congenital nests of cells (Lund and Kraus 1962). A clear separation between tumor and congenital malformation is impossible. Conjunctival nevi appear before the age of nine in one third and before the age of 30 in two thirds of all cases. About one third of nevi are unpigmented (Reese 1963; Jay 1965).

Pigment deposits (Fig. 12.2) resembling nevi or cysts develop with prolonged use (years) of epinephrine eye drops (Löwenstein, Corwin and Spencer 1963).

Juvenile melanomas (Spitz 1948) of the conjunctiva are rare (Gartmann and Thurm 1960; Thiel 1965). The lesions are red or brown-red, pinhead to pea-sized accumulations of large, bizarre, polymorphic and, at times, multinucleate cells. They are freely moveable over the sclera and may become malignant.

Blue nevi (Plate IV, Fig. 1, see page 128 d) are benign dysontogenic dermal tumors without epidermal involvement (Gartmann 1963 b). Blue nevi rarely occur in the conjunctiva (Greer 1954; Reese 1963; Jay 1965 b).

Precancerous melanosis (Reese 1955, 1963) begins as flat, pigmented spots which expand and develop a granular surface. The disease is usually unilateral and begins between 40 to 50 years of age. The yellow-brown to black lesions may expand onto the cornea (Duke-Elder and Leigh 1965). Conversion to malignant melanoma is a distinct danger. Histologically, there is an increase in pigmentation and in the number of cells in the basal epithelial layer. The cytoplasm is swollen; nuclear degeneration occurs.

Differential diagnosis: Nevi occur in the

younger age group. They are circumscribed, elevated, possibly with small cysts. Melanosis and nevus of Ota also appear (Lund and Krause 1962) early in life. Uvea and skin are also pigmented. Malignant melanoma can originate from normal conjunctiva, nevi, or precancerous melanosis. They are usually situated near the limbus. Color may vary from pale red to deep brown-black. Melanomas bleed easily. A key diagnostic point is their rapid growth (to the size of a pea within one year [Duke-Elder and Leigh 1965]). Histologically, the conjunctival epithelium is replaced by anaplastic pigmented cells of varying size and shape. Mitotic figures are prominent. Melanomas evoke a chronic subepithelial connective tissue inflammation. Often the histologic picture of a melanocarcinoma is found (Allen and Spitz 1953; Reese 1963).

Brown Discoloration Due to Drugs

Phenothiazines, especially in high dosages, can cause photosensitive brown pigmentation of the conjunctiva and sclera (Ayd 1966). Corneal and retinal pigmentation are equally common (Alkemade 1968) (see page 168). Dust, steam, anil-quinoline combinations (benzoquinone, paraquinone, hydroquinone), *phenol derivatives* and *aniline dyes* (occupational hazard) cause brown pigmentation of the conjunctiva and cornea in the region of the lid fissure. *Bromides, chromic acid* and *chromates* also cause brown pigmentation (Jaensch 1963) (see page 122). Sympathomimetics (adrenalin, Eppy, etc.) can result in circumscribed brown areas of conjunctival discoloration after about nine months of therapeutic use. Usually it causes structureless, punctate brown-black deposits (Fig. 12.2) (Mooney 1970).

Brown Coloration Due to Metabolic or Vitamin Disturbances

Bronze diabetes (hemochromatosis, i.e., iron storage disease) and Addison's disease cause yellow-brown discoloration of the conjunctiva. Severe *avitaminosis A* (malabsorption, diarrhea, malnutrition) leads to xerosis (see page 163) and a brown-gray conjunctiva. The brown discoloration of the conjunctiva in chronic liver disease (cirrhosis, carcinoma) may be related to avitaminosis A.

Avitaminosis A is one cause of white, foamy conjunctival plaques (Bitôt's spots) in the interpalpebral fissure.

Gaucher's (storage) (see page 366) disease is associated with thickened conjunctiva in the interpalpebral area. There is a brown pigmentation of the conjunctiva, hepatomegaly and splenomegaly, leukopenia, hypercalcemia, and pigmented spots on the skin. In children the acute disease is lethal.

Various *lipidoses* have yellow-brown conjunctival deposits: xanthomatosis, Hand-Schüller-Christian disease, and Gaucher's disease (see page 366). Yellow-white *crystal deposition* occurs with cystinosis (Plate XI, Fig. 2, page 192 c), and occasionally in gout.

Pinguecula is a common hyaline degeneration of subepithelial connective tissue. It is usually nasal and always situated perilimbically in the interpalpebral fissure area.

Brown Discoloration in Endogenous Ochronosis (Alkaptonuria) (see page 364)

Two thirds of patients with *ochronosis (alkaptonuria)* present with pigmentation in the interpalpebral fissure area (Sallmann 1926) (Fig. 12.3). Comma, punctate and spiraliform conjunctival deposits occur in the same location as pingueculae. The cornea is rarely involved with small, superficial, perilimbic pigment granules. The sclera has round, brown patches (see Fig. 12.3). The pigmentation becomes more noticeable with age. Histologically, there is random distribution of pigment in cornea, conjunctiva and sclera (Seitz 1954; Rodenhäuser 1957).

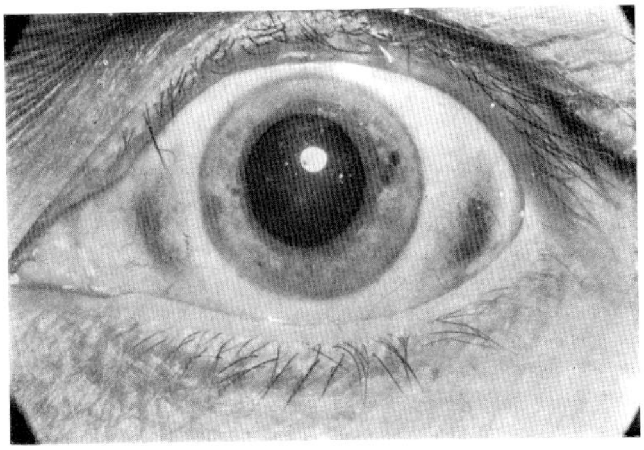

Fig. 12.3 Ochronosis (alkaptonuria) of conjunctiva and sclera in the region of the palpebral fissure (♀ 26 yrs.)

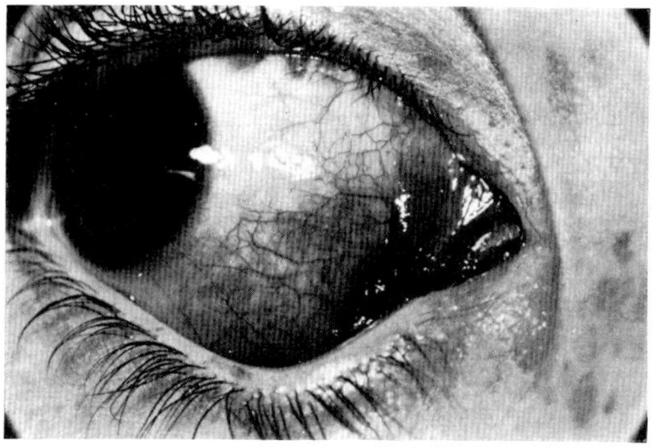

Blue Discoloration of the Conjunctiva

Ink tattoo from pens is dark blue (Fig. 12.4). The history makes the diagnosis obvious. Chronic exposure to *manganese dust* (manganese dioxide mines) causes a blue-red conjunctival and corneal discoloration as well as manganese encephalopathy and retrobulbar neuritis.

◀ Fig. 12.4 Ink pen burn of conjunctiva and caruncula (♂ 34 yrs.)

Conjunctivitis

Signs of conjunctivitis — Acute conjunctivitis — Chronic conjunctivitis — Nodular conjunctivitis — Conjunctivitis with preauricular lymphadenopathy.

Signs of Conjunctivitis

Conjunctival (and ciliary) injection — Conjunctival edema (chemosis) — Secretions — Pseudomembrane formation — Follicles.

Conjunctival (and Ciliary) Injection

Every conjunctival inflammation causes vascular dilatation to a greater or lesser degree. The meibomian glands are normally seen on lid eversion as yellow-white stripes running perpendicular to the lid margin. They are no longer visible in conjunctival inflammation.

Conjunctival injection (Plate V, Fig. 2, page 128 e) increases away from the limbus toward the fornix. Individual dilated vessels are easily recognizable. This differs from *ciliary injection* which is a more diffuse, deeper, blue-red color strongest around the limbus *(perilimbic injection)*. In practice the underlying process causing ciliary injection (scleritis, keratoconjunctivitis, etc.) is associated with tearing, blepharospasm, and rubbing, all of which lead to conjunctival injection. A mixed injection is then the case. Ciliary injection can be diagnosed by topical use of vasoconstrictive drops.

Epinephrine or Neo-Synephrine will constrict conjunctival vessels and expose the deeper ciliary injection.

Conjunctival Edema (Chemosis)

Chemosis occurs when the conjunctival inflammation is sufficiently strong (Plate V, Figs. 5 and 6, page 128 e). It may be so pronounced that the lids no longer close. A purely circulatory disturbance may also cause chemosis. This occurs with advanced exophthalmos and inflammations around the eye (abscess, hordeolum, insect bite, dacryoadenitis, dacryocystitis, posterior scleritis, panophthalmitis, orbital cellulitis, venous sinus thrombosis, and with use of *dionin,* etc.) (see page 34). Chemosis will not include the tarsal conjunctiva since this is immobile and firmly adherent to the tarsal plate. Chemosis only involves the loose, mobile, bulbar, and redundant forniceal conjunctiva. The conjunctiva is closely adherent to underlying tissue for only 1 to 3 mm around the limbus. The semilunar fold at the inner canthus is particularly susceptible to swelling. The plica semilunaris corresponds to the nictating membrane of lower mammals. The caruncle swells slightly. It also lies at the inner canthus, is covered by squamous epithelium, and has fine hairs and sebaceous glands. The lacrimal caruncle may be absent in Turner's syndrome (see page 89). Chemosis is an early sign of trichinosis (see page 198). *Loa loa* (Kreibig 1965) causes unilateral chemosis with burning. The live microfilaria are subconjunctival and move constantly.

Secretions

Every conjunctival inflammation produces secretions. These may be serous, mucoid, fibrinous, purulent, or even bloody, depending on the underlying cause of the inflammation (Plate V, Fig. 3, page 128 e). The lashes become encrusted. After sleeping, the lids may be stuck together with matter, especially in children. There is a generalized increase in tearing.

Pseudomembrane Formation

A fibrinous exudate will form gray-white pseudomembranes (see page 127) (Plate VI, Fig. 1, page 128 f). These strip easily from the conjunctiva, often leaving small hemorrhages. Pseudomembranes form with bacterial (diphtheria, pneumococcal, gonococcal), viral (epidemic keratoconjunctivitis, swimming pool conjunctivitis), allergic and chronic drug-induced conjunctivitis. They are particularly prominent in erythema multiforme (see Fuchs' syndrome, page 127).

Follicle Formation

Certain viruses (epidemic keratoconjunctivitis, swimming pool conjunctivitis) and trachoma typically cause follicle formation (Plate VI, Fig. 4, page 128 f). Most chronic conjunctivitis will cause follicular as well as papillary hypertrophy. Medications such as pilocarpine may cause hypertrophy and aggregation of lymphoid cells (follicles). Children often have conjunctival follicles without signs of inflammation just as they frequently have benign, nonspecific lymphadenopathy. The paving-stone papillae of vernal catarrh are true papillae and not lymphocytic aggregates.

Acute Conjunctivitis

Noninfectious acute conjunctivitis — Bacterial acute conjunctivitis — Viral conjunctivitis — Fungal infections of the conjunctiva — Pseudomembranous conjunctivitis.

Conjunctivitis is either acute or chronic. Subjective symptoms in *acute conjunctivitis* (Plate V, Fig. 2, page 128 e) are burning, foreign body sensation, heaviness of the lids, and pain. Objective signs include hyperemia of even the smallest vessels. The redness increases away from the limbus toward the fornices. The meibomian glands are no longer visible. There is tearing and a watery or serosanguinous discharge. The lids may be stuck together on awakening. The discharge can contain pus or blood and may form pseudomembranes. Follicles are seen with some specific infections and chronic involvement. A conjunctival smear should be made in every case to identify the causal agent.

Noninfectious Acute Conjunctivitis

The patient usually knows the cause in noninfectious, acute conjunctivitis.

Foreign body, burn, occupational disease — Ultraviolet burns — Allergies — Self-induced — Parasites — Protozoa — Conjunctivitis (ophthalmia) nodosa — Worms.

Foreign bodies (smoke, dust, sand, vegetable matter) play a major role, especially in children. **Burns** can result from acids, lye, ink pens, silver nitrate, potassium permanganate, or ether. Inorganic compounds may cause severe *corneal* and *conjunctival burns* or *irritation* (Jaensch 1963): halogenated compounds, hydrochloric acid, chlorine, chromate, chromic acid, hydrogen fluoride, hydrogen sulfide (particularly prone to cause superficial punctate keratitis), sulfur dioxide, sulfuric acid, thioglycolic acid (used in home permanents), ammonia, saltpeter, chlorine gas, tear gas, phosphotrichloride, and pentachloride. The various halogenated aliphatic hydrocarbons are solvents which can cause corneal and conjunctival irritation. Neuropathies and pupillary disruption have been observed. Vaporizing alcohol, formaldehyde, formalin and osmium can cause irritation.

Tar and pitch, either as smoke, dust, or solid particles, cause irritation. Phenol, specifically phenylic acid, can cause chemical burns. Chemical weapons (mustard gas, mace) usually involve the eyes, produce lacrimation, blepharospasm, and possibly chemical burns. Tear gas is in many self-defense pistols, pens, spray cans, etc.

Occupational diseases involving the cornea and conjunctiva include (Merté 1969, 1972):

Arsenicals including arsenic trichloride, arsonium and atoxyl cause arsenic melanosis, conjunctival hyperkeratosis, conjunctival hemorrhage, necrosis and shrinking, corneal ulcer, optic neuritis, and paresis of ocular muscles.

Benzoquinone, aniline derivatives, quinone, paraquinone and hydroquinone induce brown discoloration in the region of the lid fissure, burns, blister formation, and corneal ulcers.
Benzene, toluene, xylol: epithelial damage, neuritis and retinitis.
Nitrobenzene and *aminobenzene* (methemoglobin formers) and nitronaphthalene cause severe corneal and conjunctival inflammation, vesicles, and neuritis. Other agents causing corneal and conjunctival reactions are: nitrobenzene and dinitrobenzene, dinitrophenol, trinitrophenol (picric acid causes the skin to turn yellow), aniline (aminobenzene), chlornitroaniline (band keratopathy), aniline dyes.

Halogenated hydrocarbons: inflammation

Chromium: inflammation and brown coloration

Cadmium: inflammation
Lead: mucous membrane inflammation and optic neuritis
Manganese: blue-red discoloration of the conjunctiva
Carbon monoxide: conjunctival and retinal hemorrhages

Phosphorus, phosphorus trichloride and pentachloride, phosphorus trisulfide and sequisulfide: conjunctivitis and conjunctival icterus

Mercury: conjunctivitis, blepharitis, extraocular muscle paresis

Nitroglycerin: inflammation

Carbon disulfide: burns, sensory disturbances, gray discoloration of the conjunctiva, optic neuritis

Hydrogen sulfide: inflammation

Vanadium and beryllium: conjunctivitis and blepharitis.
Burns cause varying degrees of acute or chronic conjunctivitis.
Ultraviolet radiation (sun, sunlamps, welding arc, lightning, glacier disease or snow blindness, etc.): four to six hours after exposure to ultraviolet radiation, conjunctivitis and punctate keratitis begin. These can be exceedingly severe (ophthalmia photoelectrica) with marked photophobia and blepharospasm (see page 149).

X-ray and radium irradiation can cause a more or less chronic conjunctivitis.

Allergies: Riehm (1957) divides ocular allergies into the idiosyncratic and focal afflictions.
Hypersensitivity reactions (idiosyncratic) (see page 92) may include the eyes in a generalized systemic process. Hay fever, conjunctivitis with urticaria, or drug reaction are examples.
Allergic conjunctivitis is a contact reaction to pollen antigens from flowers, grasses, and plants. These are usually well-known to the patient. Hay fever (Plate V, Fig. 4, page 128 e) is an example. Topical atropine will cause a characteristic skin and conjunctival reaction (Plate II, Fig. 2, page 128 b). Atropine and camomile skin and conjunctival reactions usually require weeks to clear. Topical antigens or haptenes include cocaine, pantocaine (anesthesia keratitis [page 162] [Plate IX, Fig. 3, page 192 a]), iodine, mercury and pilocarpine. Primrose, hair dyes, hair creams, mascara, cosmetics, systemically acting foods such as strawberries, fish, etc., also cause allergic conjunctivitis. In 238 cases of lid eczema, Borrie (1956) found 29 percent to be caused by drugs (two thirds were penicillin [Plate II, Fig. 3, page 128 b] and sulfacetamide). Twenty percent were contact dermatitis (70 percent industrial, 10 percent cosmetic).
Sidi and Mawas (1953) found the majority of iatrogenic conjunctival and lid eczemas to be due to atropine, mercuric oxide, novocaine, sulfonamides, PAS and hair dyes. All cosmetics, creams, lotions, mascara, eye liner, nail polish, hair creams, etc., may be allergenic.
Corneal necrosis and dermatitis have been described after arsphenamine (Ehrlich 606) therapy (Hegner 1917; Meyer 1941). Prolonged use of phenobarbitol may cause an exfoliative dermatitis and conjunctivitis (Stevens-Johnson syndrome, i.e., erythema multiforme and Lyell's syndrome).
Acute topical allergy causes lid eczema (Plate II, Figs. 2, 3, page 128 b), erythema, weeping with blister formation and crusting. There is conjunctival injection, edema, erythema, tearing, burning, and itching.
The key finding in chronic atopic conjunctivitis is follicle formation (Plate VI, Fig. 4, page 128 b).

A self-induced conjunctivitis occurs in psychotics and malingering for secondary gain, etc.

Lime, soap, tobacco, hot cigarette ash, and any variety of drugs or substances may be used. The foreign substance tends to collect in the inferior cul-de-sac and the inflammation is far greater under the lower than the upper lid. A tight nonremovable dressing will establish the diagnosis.

Parasites

Fly larvae (ophthalmomyiasis): Behr (1920) differentiated *ophthalmomyiasis externa*, in which the adnexa (lids, lacrimal gland, conjunctiva, orbits) are affected, from *ophthalmomyiasis interna* where the larva is actually inside the eye (iridocyclitis, vitreal haze, chorioretinitis). *Hypoderma bovis* (Suurküla 1942) and *Wohlfahrtia magnifica* are primary causes of ophthalmomyiasis interna in Northern Europe. The larvae burrow transsclerally into the anterior chamber (Hartmann 1954; Eickemeyer 1957, Krümmel and Brauss 1956).

Common agents in external ophthalmomyiasis are *Oestrus* and *Cephalomyia* (Martini 1946).

Protozoa: In any protozoan infection the conjunctivitis is overshadowed by *systemic symptoms. Amoebic dysentery (Entamoeba histolytica)* causes conjunctivitis with marginal corneal ulcers, iridocyclitis, and chorioretinitis.

Ocular signs of *malaria* are hyperemia of lids and conjunctiva, secondary herpes simplex, and icterus.

Trypanosomiasis (sleeping sickness) causes chemosis and lid edema. Keratitis, iridocyclitis, choroiditis, optic neuritis and extraocular muscle palsies are rare in trypanosomiasis or malaria.

Leishmaniasis is another cause of lid edema and keratoconjunctivitis.

Conjunctivitis (Ophthalmia) Nodosa

The embedding of caterpillar hairs in the conjunctiva evokes a particularly painful, unpleasant, foreign body reaction. The spicules can work their way into the eye *(ophthalmia nodosa)*. Spines of fruits (blackberries) and insects have the same effect.

Infestation by worms: *Ascaris lumbricoides* may cause allergic toxic reactions in the form of keratoconjunctivitis, iridocyclitis, central serous retinopathy, papilledema, and recurrent clouding of the vitreous.

Toxocara causes similar symptoms. The parasite tends to form granulomas either at the posterior pole or peripherally.

Heavy intestinal tract infestation with *Oxyuris vermicularis* may be associated with mild keratoconjunctivitis and lid edema.

Trichina (Trichinella spiralis) specifically afflicts the extraocular muscles causing painful motor disturbances, chemosis, lid edema, and exophthalmos.

In the tropics filariae frequently infect the eyes.

Filaria loa (Loa loa) is endemic to regions of tropical West Africa. The macrofilaria wander through the connective tissues of the lids, conjunctiva, and orbit causing amazingly little reaction.

Onchocerciasis (Onchocerca volvulus) (river blindness) develops with microfilaria-containing skin nodules. From there a general dissemination occurs. A hypersensitivity reaction to dead microfilaria causes conjunctivitis, keratitis, and phlyctenulosis. The microfilaria enter the eye at a late stage and cause iritis, chorioretinitis, and even optic atrophy.

Deposition of the *Schistosoma (Bilharzia)* ova in connective tissue produces a soft, flat granuloma.

Conjunctival cysts due to *Taenia echinococcus* or *Taenia solium (Cysticercus)* are extremely rare.

Acute Bacterial Conjunctivitis

Almost any infectious disease may cause a conjunctivitis, often with keratitis (usually superficial punctate). Bacteria tend to selectively involve the eye. Conjunctivitis can be part of a generalized infection, the primary site of which may be unknown. In contrast viral conjunctivitis is usually part of a systemic infection whose origin is easily determined.

Pneumococcus, Koch-Week's bacillus, Streptococci — Gonococcus — Various agents.

Pneumococcus, Koch-Week's bacillus, streptococci, staphylococci: Acute conjunctivitis is commonly caused by *pneumococcus* and sometimes by the gram-negative *Koch-Week's bacillus*. After a one to two day incubation period, chemosis, pseudomembrane formation, sub-

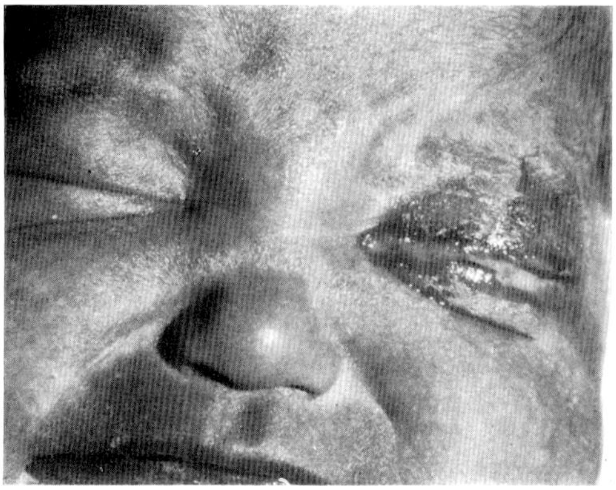

Fig. 12.5 Ophthalmia neonatorum (gonococcal blennorrhea) (♀ 6 days)

conjunctival hemorrhages, lid edema and purulent discharge occur. Koch-Week's bacillus is more common in the Middle East and North Africa.

Staphylococci cause a subacute conjunctivitis, usually with chronic blepharitis. *Streptococci* cause catarrhal inflammation and pseudomembrane formation.

Gonococcal ophthalmia neonatorum may occur despite Credé prophylaxis (1 percent silver nitrate). The incubation period is two to three days. In addition to chemosis and lid edema (lids often swell shut) (Fig. 12.5), there is a profuse purulent exudate. This may literally squirt from the eye when the lids are forced open. At first the exudate is serosanguineous but quickly becomes a thick pus. On conjunctival smear, gonococci are found both intracellularly and extracellularly.

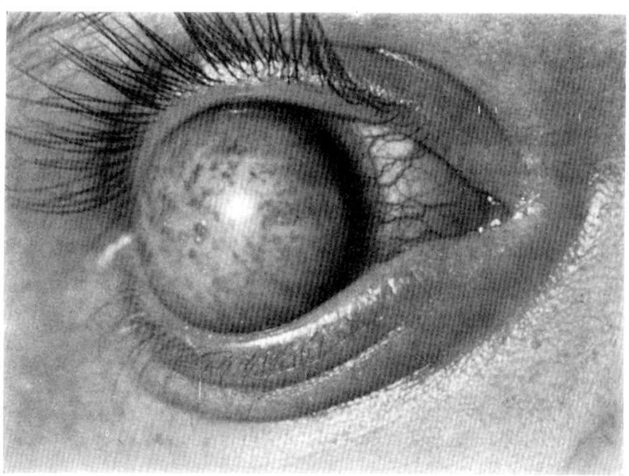

Fig. 12.6 Staphyloma and secondary glaucoma following gonococcal blennorrhea with corneal perforation (♂ 9 months)

The marked chemosis compromises perilimbic vessels and results in necrosis of corneal epithelium. Corneal ulcers with perforation, leukoma adhaerens, secondary glaucoma, and staphyloma result (Fig. 12.6). As the gonococci disappear the discharge turns mucoid. Months after the infection, papillary hypertrophy (postcatarrh) may still be present.

The same clinical picture occurs in adults. In the pre-antibiotic era, corneal perforation was common. In warm climates such as Egypt, flies can spread the gonococcal agent. Of 122 patients for whom this was the form of transmission, "Gonoblennorrhoea epidemica" (Rais 1952) – corneal perforation – occurred in 40. Bilaterality was present in 11. Among children in India, 50 percent of blindness is caused by gonococcal blennorrhea (Wohra 1951). Acute gonococcal conjunctivitis may be metastatic from gonococcal arthritis. Conversely, *hematogenous spread of gonococci* in ophthalmia neonatorum may cause metastatic (mono) arthritis (Di Bella 1923; Prizi 1924; Wahlberg 1925). Rarely do gonococci cause scleritis or episcleritis (Aust 1929).

Intraocular hematogenous spread of gonococci results in severe fibrinous iritis and synechia formation (Siegert 1939).

Differential diagnosis: Silver nitrate irritation (Credé prophylaxis) is far milder and nonprogressive. Inclusion blennorrhea has a longer incubation period (six to ten days), is less symptomatic, and can cause preauricular lymphadenopathy.

Various causal agents: *Haemophilus influenzae* (Pfeiffer), *meningococcus, streptococcus, staphylococcus, diphtheria, and Neisseria* all cause acute conjunctivitis. *Proteinase* formation in *pseudomonas conjunctivitis* creates the danger of corneal ulceration.

Brucellosis (Bang's disease, Malta fever, Mediterranean fever, pig breeder's disease) causes recurrent fever, icterus, conjunctivitis, phlyctenules, punctate keratitis, dacryoadenitis, optic neuritis, chorioretinitis, and extraocular muscle palsies.

Ocular involvement in *plague (Pasteurella pestis)* includes serosanguineous conjunctivitis, keratitis, corneal ulceration, uveitis, and metastatic ophthalmia.

Leptospira (especially *L. icterohaemorrhagiae,*

i.e., Weil's disease; less so in *L. canicola* or *L. grippotyphosa)* may involve the eye: icterus, acute conjunctivitis, episcleritis, fibrinous iridocyclitis with vitreal haze (see page 198), rarely chorioretinitis and neuritis.

Acute Conjunctivitis Due to Viral and Rickettsial Agents

Viral and rickettsial conjunctivitis are often part of a systemic illness, the source of which can be readily determined by the history.

Inclusion conjunctivitis — Swimming pool conjunctivitis — Epidemic keratoconjunctivitis — Herpes simplex and zoster — Rickettsia — Infectious mononucleosis — Varicella — Variola, vaccinia — Mumps — Foot-and-mouth disease, arboviruses — Metastatic conjunctivitis.

In inclusion blennorrhea (paratrachoma) symptoms begin six to ten days after birth and are less severe than with gonorrhea.
Halberstädter-Prowazek inclusion bodies are seen on Giemsa-stained conjunctival smears. There is preauricular lymphadenopathy. The causal agent is the TRIC virus *(Chlamydia oculogenitalis)* (see page 130).
Differential diagnosis: Silver nitrate irritation (Credé prophylaxis) occurs immediately after birth, is nonprogressive, and does not cause lymphadenopathy.
Ophthalmia neonatorum begins two to three days after birth.
Chemosis, lid edema, serous-sanguineous and pus-like exudate are florid. Gonococci are seen in a conjunctival smear.
Swimming pool conjunctivitis (TRIC) is often unilateral and begins eight to twelve days after exposure to the virus in a swimming pool. Conjunctival follicles and preauricular lymph nodes are present. The clinical picture and etiologic agent is that of inclusion body conjunctivitis. The agents of trachoma and inclusion conjunctivitis are exceedingly similar if not the same (Jones et al. 1967). They are, therefore, called TRIC (trachoma inclusion conjunctivitis) virus. Other terms are *Bedsonia, Chlamydia,* or *Chlamydozon.*
Adenoviruses (APC, adenopharyngeal-conjunctival):
Two of the 27 serologic types cause characteristic illnesses.

1. *Pharyngoconjunctival fever*
After a five to six day incubation period, a highly infectious pharyngitis with fever occurs. This is usually caused by adenovirus, type 3. The bilateral conjunctivitis is follicular.

2. *Epidemic keratoconjunctivitis*
Epidemic keratoconjunctivitis sometimes presents with mild fever, malaise, and headaches after an eight day incubation period. Ocular findings include conjunctival erythema, edema of the plica and caruncle (see page 152), chemosis (Plate V, Figs. 5, 6, page 128 e), and ptosis secondary to inflammatory lid edema. Pre-auricular lymph nodes are painful and swollen. The serous discharge dries on the lashes as yellow scales. Pseudomembranes may form (Plate VI, Fig. 1, page 128 f). Five to eight days after the acute conjunctivitis superficial punctate staining occurs. Subepithelial nummular infiltrates develop from this which frequently remain for months, or even years (Fig. 12.7). The causal agent is usually adenovirus, type 8. Spread is by direct contact, usually in ophthalmologists' offices (drops, ointments, fingers, tonometers).
Differential diagnosis: In swimming pool conjunctivitis, the chemosis and pre-auricular lymphadenopathy tend to be less. The cornea remains uninvolved. Due to the difficulty in making a differential diagnosis, the more serious epidemic keratoconjunctivitis should be considered first.
Newcastle (fowlpox) disease is acquired directly by people handling chickens. The acute follicular conjunctivitis is usually unilateral. Both **herpes simplex** and **herpes zoster** may cause

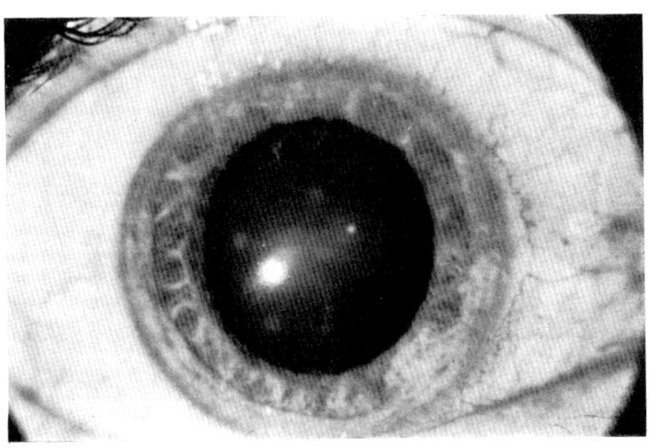

Fig. 12.7 Corneal infiltrates in epidemic keratoconjunctivitis (♂ 58 yrs.)

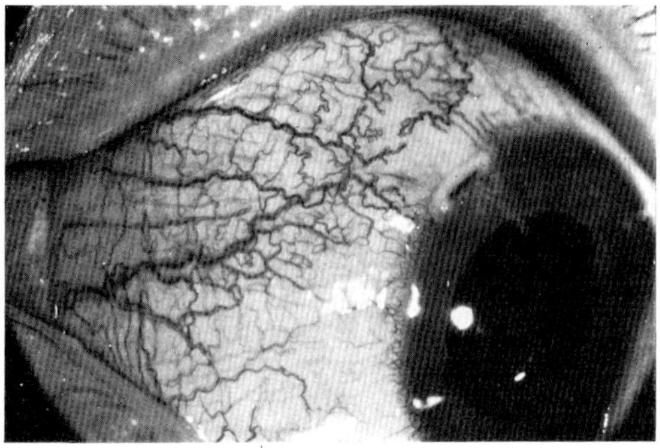

Fig. 12.8 Varicella conjunctivitis with phlyctenules (♂ 7 yrs.)

acute follicular conjunctivitis. Usually, the cornea will be involved with dendritic or disciform keratitis.

Rickettsia: Rickettsial infections (*typhus*, Rocky Mountain spotted fever, Q fever, tsutsugamushi fever) almost always have conjunctival erythema, photophobia and tearing. Exophthalmos, keratitis, iridocyclitis, and extraocular muscle palsies are described. In typhus, retinal hemorrhages and neuritis are more frequent (Sautter 1943).

Infectious mononucleosis (Pfeiffer's glandular fever): Mononucleosis is thought to be a viral illness. It afflicts primarily younger persons. After an incubation period of four to ten days, there is generalized malaise, debility, and lymphadenopathy. Ocular findings include (Tanner 1954):

a) Direct mononuclear cell infiltrates causing follicular conjunctivitis, episcleritis, lid and periorbital edema, dacryoadenitis, sinusitis, rarely uveitis, optic neuritis, retinal edema, and hemorrhages.

b) Neuroophthalmic and central nervous system involvement can cause ocular muscle paresis, ptosis, nystagmus, gaze paresis, hemianopsia, and scotomata.

Varicella lid lesions heal without scarring. Phlyctenules (Fig. 12.8) form when the conjunctiva is involved. Superficial or deep keratitis is rare. The symptoms are similar to those of zoster.

Smallpox (variola vera), like *vaccinia*, may lead to lid (see page 96) and corneal (see page 155) involvement. The incubation period is four to eleven days after which pustules or a smeary, pussy ulcerating conjunctivitis develops. The pre-auricular nodes are painful and swollen.

Mumps (epidemic parotitis) affects salivary and lacrimal glands. Conjunctivitis, episcleritis, scleritis, interstitial keratitis, and optic neuritis are reported.

Hoof-and-mouth disease has an incubation period of three to six days. The mucous membranes (including conjunctiva) develop painful red blisters. This is caused by a virus. Lymph glands are swollen.

Epidemiologically, it is important whether other persons drinking the same raw milk have become infected.

Arbovirus (*ar*thropod-*bo*rne) infections can cause conjunctivitis. These include yellow fever, dengue fever, pappataci fever and Rift Valley fever.

Cat-scratch fever and *Beal's* conjunctivitis are probably viral in origin.

Metastatic conjunctivitis: An *acute conjunctivitis* can be *metastatic*. Measles, rubella, influenza, varicella, scarlet fever, and rarely gonococcus can be the cause. Of importance is that the conjunctivitis follows the exanthem by several days (hematogenous spread). Retinal pigment epithelium dispersion may occur. Metastatic conjunctivitis is always bilateral. Lid and conjunctiva are less inflamed and the erythema is more red-blue and deeper than in other conjunctivitides.

Measles can in addition produce a scrofulous keratitis or even keratomalacia (caused by vitamin A deficiency).

Fungal Conjunctivitis

Mycotic conjunctivitis is rare (Hoffmann 1965) but should be considered in chronic therapy-resistant cases.

Actinomycetes (gram-positive bacteria) form yellow, slightly raised conjunctival nodules. Orbital cellulitis is possible.

Candida conjunctivitis begins as small white punctate lesions that become confluent and form a pseudomembrane. Unlike diphtheria, the pseudomembrane can be stripped from the conjunctiva without bleeding. The cornea may be involved.

Blastomycetes cause a stringy or foamy conjunctival exudate with trachoma-like follicles, pre-auricular lymphadenopathy, conjunctival ulcers, and granulomas.

Sporotrichosis may be one cause of Parinaud's syndrome. Firm yellow-white conjunctival nodules are formed, which later ulcerate.

Rhinosporidium forms dark red vascularized lesions which develop slowly over months. Trichophytosis may cause an allergic conjunctivitis.

Pseudomembranous Conjunctivitis

Diphtheria — Other infections — Oculomucocutaneous syndrome — Pemphigoid — Pemphigus — Dermatitis herpetiformis — Hereditary epidermolysis bullosa — Reiter's syndrome — Wegener's granulomatosis — Ligneous conjunctivitis — Vaccinia — Variola.

Diphtheria is the first choice in any pseudomembranous conjunctivitis. The incubation period is one to two days. Serous, pussy exudate and yellow-gray pseudomembranes form. Removal of the pseudomembranes causes bleeding. The lids are edematous and may be firm with necrotic areas and scarring (entropion and ectropion formation). Corneal ulceration and necrosis may occur. Diphtheria limited to the lid can cause systemic toxicity (nerve paresis, circulatory damage, nephritis, etc.). The infectious agent is *Corynebacterium diphtheriae*.

Other infections: Other agents also cause pseudomembranous conjunctivitis: streptococci, staphylococci, gonococcus, pneumococcus, Koch-Week's bacillus, vaccinia, epidemic conjunctivitis (Plate VI, Fig. 1, page 128 f), herpes simplex, herpes zoster and foot-and-mouth disease.

Oculomucocutaneous syndrome (Fuchs) = erythema multiforme (Fig. 12.9): Pseudomembrane formation is part of this syndrome. The clinical picture is highly varied (see page 96) and, therefore, carries many names (Howard 1963; Schmidt and Lischka 1969).

Synonyms: Fuchs' syndrome, herpes iris conjunctivae (Fuchs), erythema multiforme, dermatostomatitis (Baader), Fiessinger-Renduor Stevens-Johnson syndrome, Lyell syndrome, toxic epidermal necrolysis (Lyell), scalded skin syndrome (Braun-Falco-Geissler), explosive necrotizing epidermolysis (Solterman), acute universal toxic epidermolysis (Korting-Holzman), ectodermosis erosiva pluriorificialis.

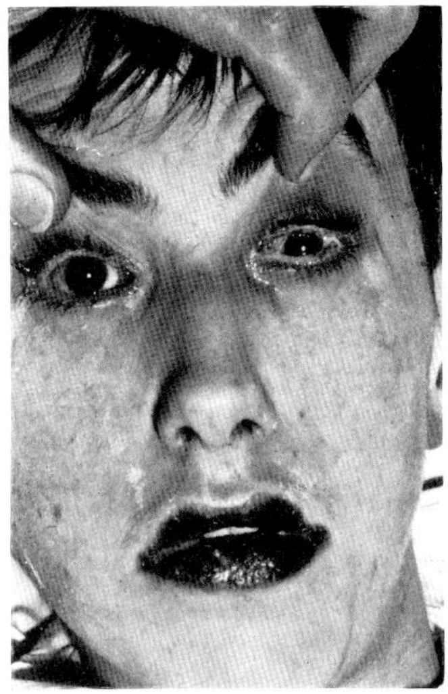

Fig. 12.9 Oculomucocutaneous syndrome (Stevens-Johnson) (♂ 16 yrs.)

The disease starts acutely with fever, rhinitis, pharyngitis, pneumonia, and multiple skin lesions. There are large erythematous areas that develop hemorrhagic blisters. The mucous membranes (nose, pharynx, genitalia, anus) may be involved with yellow-gray pseudomembrane formation (stomatitis, vulvovaginitis, urethritis, etc.). Children and young males are primarily affected. The eye is almost always afflicted.

There is severe bilateral conjunctivitis, chemosis, and lid edema with blistering, ulceration and pseudomembrane formation. Punctate corneal staining, epithelial erosions, and ulcerations occur. Sequelae include scarring, vascularization, symblepharon formation, and total drying out of the conjunctiva.

Both the *oculomucocutaneous syndrome* and *Lyell's syndrome* can be caused by drug toxicity or allergy. In Fuchs' syndrome there is an exudative inflammation of the corium with secondary edema and blister formation in the epidermis. Papules form and develop a central blister. These are frequently distributed symmetrically over the face, arm, and leg. Lyell's syndrome has necrosis of the epidermal cells (Schmidt and Lischka 1969, 1970). Erythematous plaques develop and quickly turn into necrotic bullae. When the skin desquamates, a weeping raw surface remains (scalded skin

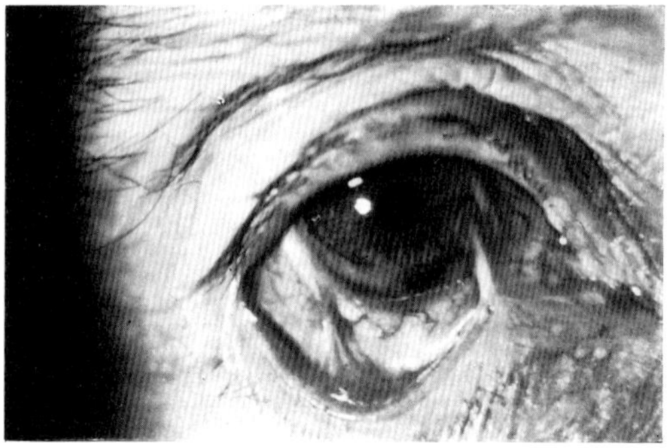

Fig. 12.10 Benign essential conjunctival shrinkage (pemphigoid) (♀ 72 yrs.)

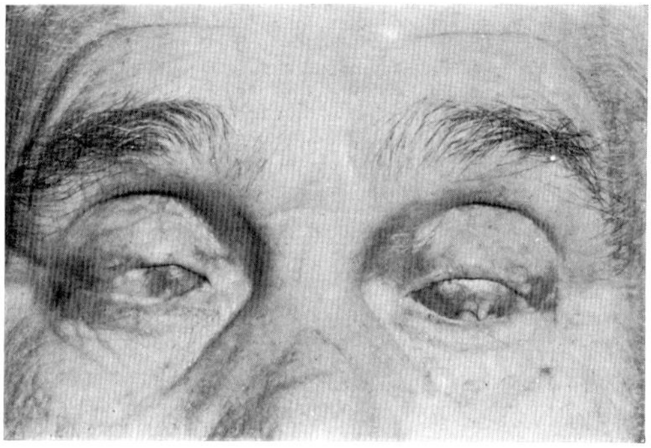

Fig. 12.11 Xerosis in pemphigoid (♀ 82 yrs.)

syndrome). Skin and nails of the extremities may peel off like gloves.

Blisters also form on the conjunctiva. They rupture and become smeary ulcers. Separation of the epidermis when the skin is rubbed (Nikolsky's phenomenon) is a classic sign. Death from metabolic imbalance and cardiovascular collapse occurs in 30 percent of cases. Both Lyell's syndrome and Fuchs' syndrome have photophobia, tearing, blepharospasm, conjunctival bullae, and pseudomembrane formation. The process can last for weeks. Sequelae are cicatricial entropion, symblepharon, trichiasis, loss of tear secretion, xerosis, corneal infiltration, and vascularization.

Bullous eruptions with drug allergies: Any of the entities encompassed in the term oculomucocutaneous syndrome, particularly Stevens-Johnson's and Lyell's syndrome, may result from various medications (Oppel 1964; Pesch and Wessing 1967; Reich and Jünnemann 1970). Pyramidon, antipyrine, phenacetin, barbiturates, arsenicals, sulfonamides, and streptomycin are the most common agents. The Debré-Lamy-Lyell syndrome is often infectious secondary to streptococci, viruses, staphylococcus, mycoplasma, and fungi. An appropriate susceptibility must be present. Fuchs' syndrome may be set off by sunlight, x-rays, vaccination, neoplasms, collagen disorders, vitamin deficiency, contact allergies, pregnancy, and menstruation (Schmidt and Lischka 1969, 1970).

Benign ocular (conjunctival) pemphigoid: *Pseudomembranes* form. The clinical picture is one of essential conjunctival shrinkage (Figs. 12.10, 12.11) (see page 97).

Pemphigus vulgaris produces bullae of the conjunctiva, skin and mucous membranes. The blisters are intraepithelial (acantholysis) and usually do not leave scars. The epithelium desquamates in patches. Corneal and conjunctival vascularization occur (Plate VI, Fig. 2, page 128 f).

Dermatitis herpetiformis (Duhring) produces a similar picture.

Hereditary epidermolysis bullosa (genodermatosis) (see page 97) is a *recessively inherited dystrophy* causing epithelial bullae (Fig. 10.29) of the conjunctiva, cornea, mouth, nose, pharynx, and esophagus. These rupture, causing scarring, shrinkage, and symblepharon formation. Nikolsky's phenomenon is present at various stages of the disorder.

In **Reiter's syndrome** (Fiessinger-Leroy-Reiter) (see page 198), all mucous membranes are inflamed. Males between the ages of 20 and 40 are most affected. Conjunctivitis (subconjunctival metastatic), episcleritis, rarely keratitis, iritis, and neuroretinitis are associated with fever, urethritis, enteritis, and recurrent polyarthritis. Chlamydial infection is thought to be the cause (Jones et al. 1967; Dawson et al. 1970). Mixed forms exist when the uvea is also involved (Bechterew's disease, Behçet's syndrome).

Wegener's granulomatosis is associated with conjunctival necrosis and pseudomembrane formation (see page 182).

In **ligneous conjunctivitis** a true conjunctival membrane several millimeters thick is present. Any effort at removal causes bleeding (Plate VI, Fig. 3, page 128 f.). The membrane reforms quickly after it is removed. The condition is

a) Brick red hyperemia. Individual vessels and their branches are easily identifiable. Vessels move with the conjunctiva.

d) Bright red, tortuous, superficial, arborizing, anastomotic vessels. Originating from the conjunctiva, these vessels pass onto the cornea without interruption.

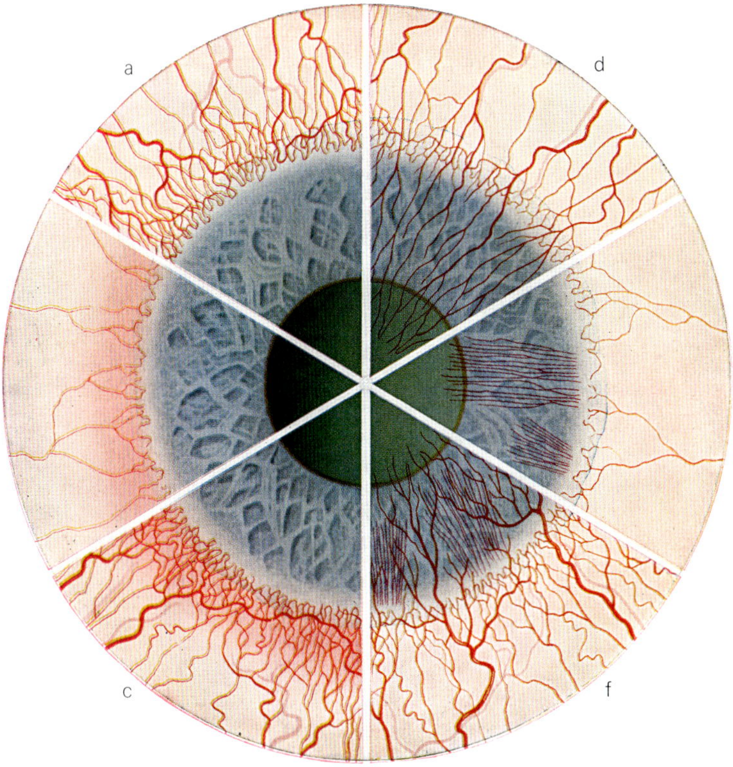

b) Blue-red perilimbal discoloration. Conjunctiva moves over the redness.

e) Dark red, brush-like tufts of vessels in the corneal stroma. Branching is dichotomous. Originating from the limbal arcade, the vessels begin directly the limbus.

Superficial and deep hyperemia of the anterior segment

a) Conjunctival injection
b) Ciliary injection
c) Conjunctival and ciliary (mixed) injection

Superficial and deep neovascularization of the anterior segment

d) Superficial vascularization (pannus)
e) Deep vascularization
f) Deep and superficial (mixed) vascularization

Fig. 1 (from R. Thiel, Atlas of Diseases of the Eye, 6th ed., Thieme, Stuttgart, 1963) (see pages 32, 148)

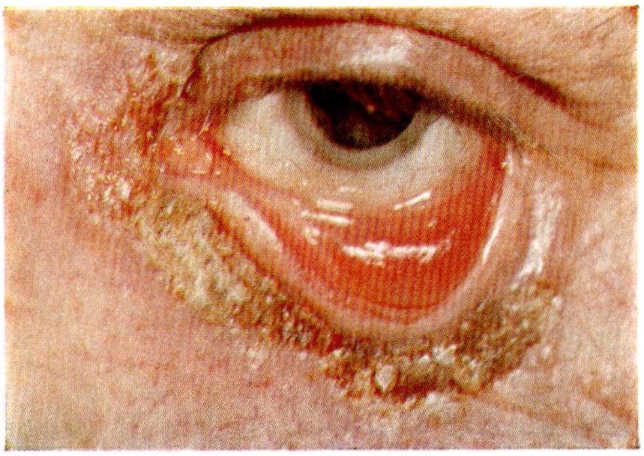

Fig. 2 Cicatricial ectropion following a burn (♂ 64 yrs.) (see page 90)

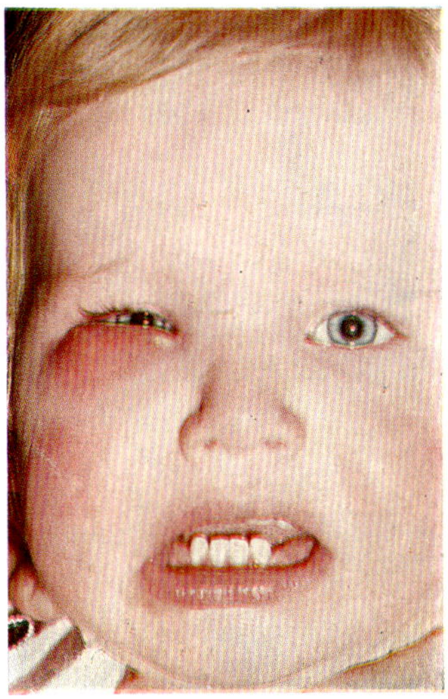

Fig. 3 Hordeolum R. lower lid (♀ 1 yr.) (see page 91)

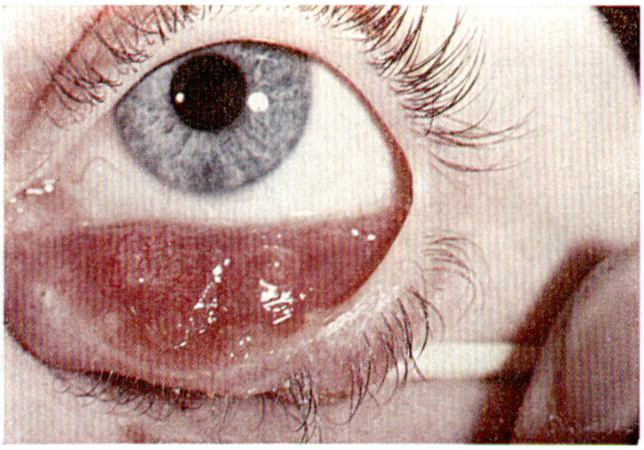

Fig. 1 Chalaziosis, multiple chalazia L. lower lid (♀ 22 yrs.) (see page 91)

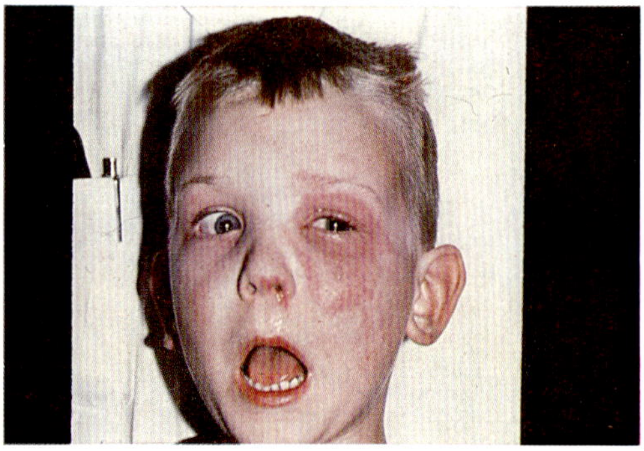

Fig. 2 Atropin dermatitis, L. lids, skin, nostril (♂ 6 yrs.) (see pages 92, 122)

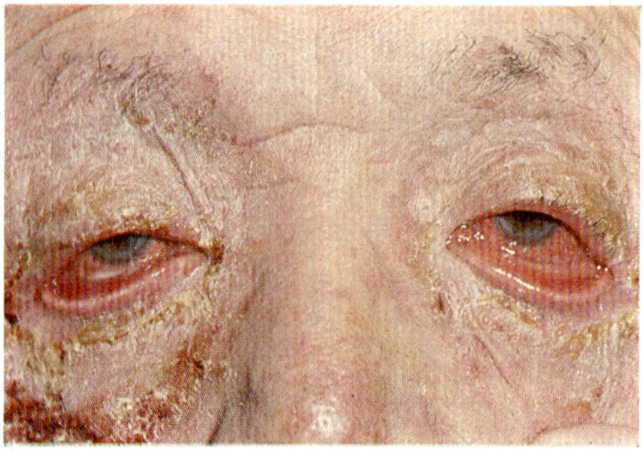

Fig. 3 Penicillin reaction with ectropion (see pages 92, 122)

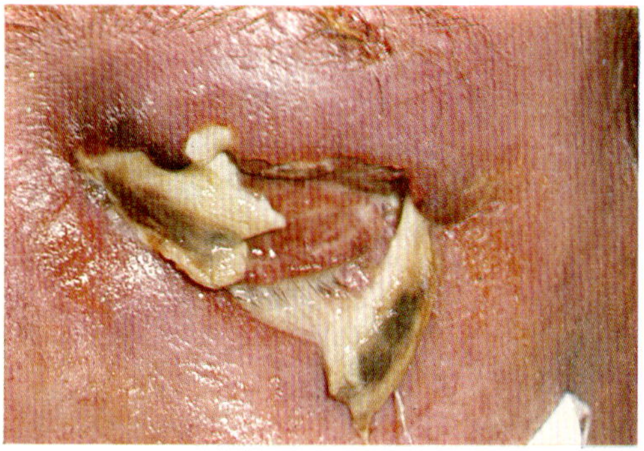

Fig. 4 Gangrene of L. upper lid (staphylococcus aureus) (♂ 46 yrs.) (see page 93)

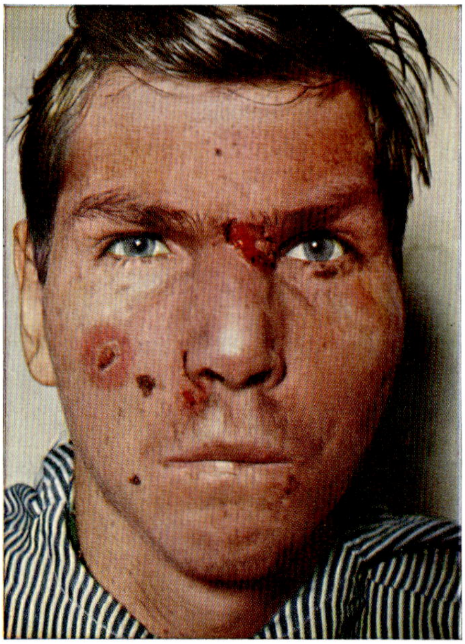

Fig. 5 Xeroderma pigmentosum (from: R. Thiel, Atlas of Diseases of the Eye, 6th ed., Thieme, Stuttgart, 1963) (see page 93)

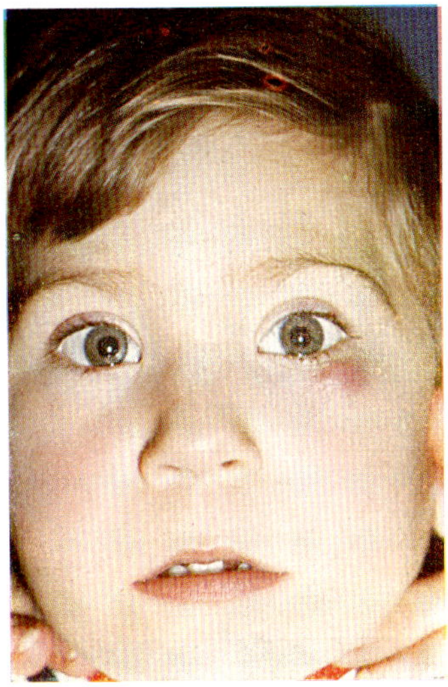

Fig. 1 Tuberculoma of the bony orbit (♂ 11 yrs.) (see page 94)

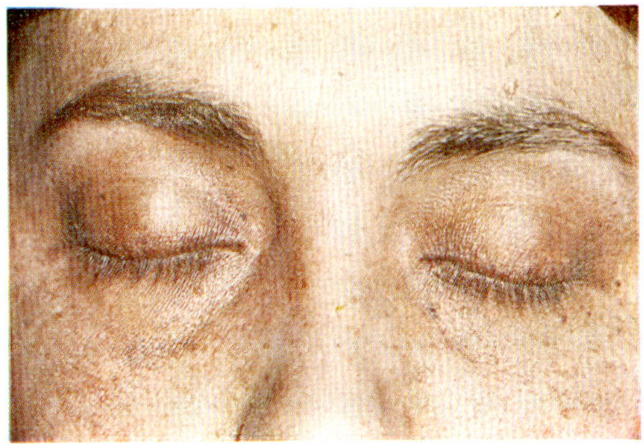

Fig. 4 Pigmentation in Addison's disease (♀ 37 yrs.) (see page 100)

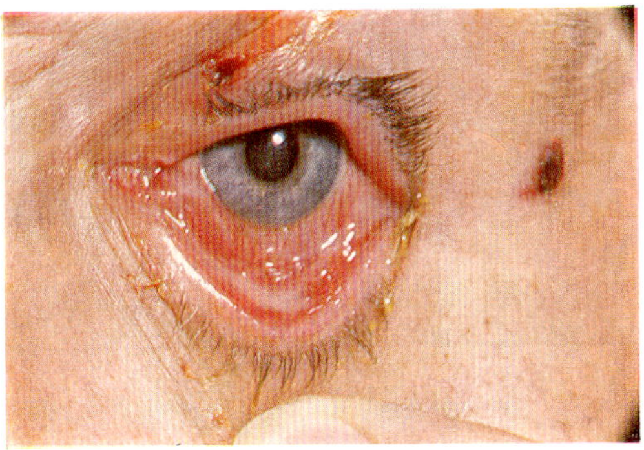

Fig. 2 Mucocutaneous-ocular syndrome (♀ 58 yrs.) (see page 96)

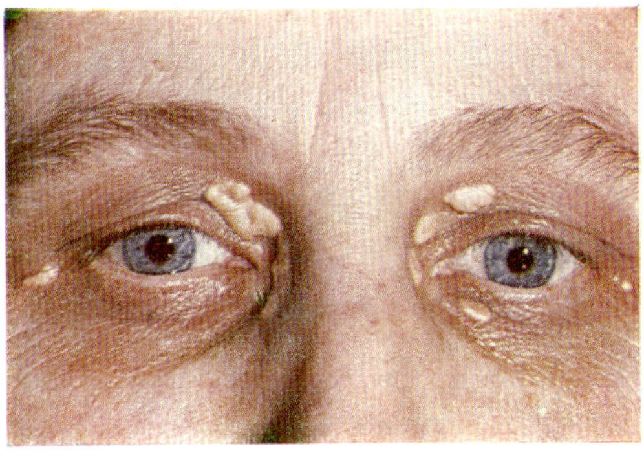

Fig. 5 Hyperpigmentation and xanthelasma in melanodermatitis (♀ 42 yrs.) (see pages 101, 102)

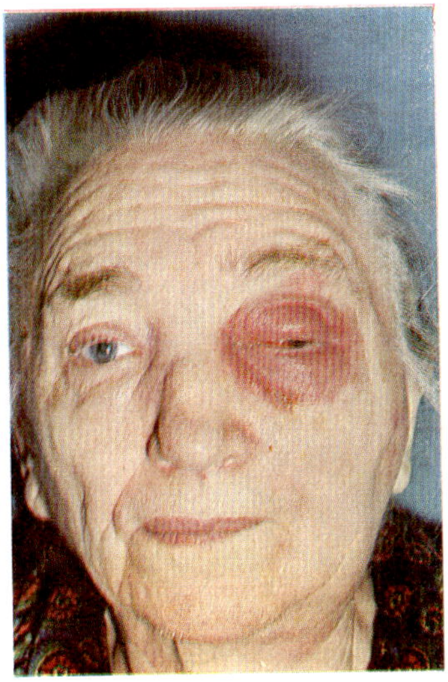

Fig. 3 Allergic reaction to novocaine (♀ 77 yrs.) (see page 97)

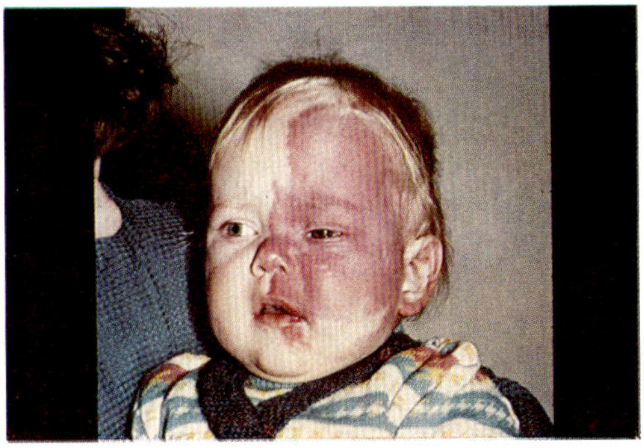

Fig. 6 Sturge-Weber syndrome, i.e., hemangioma in the distribution of the trigeminal nerve (♂ 1¼ yrs.) (see pages 103, 226)

Plate IV (Chapters 10, 11, 12)

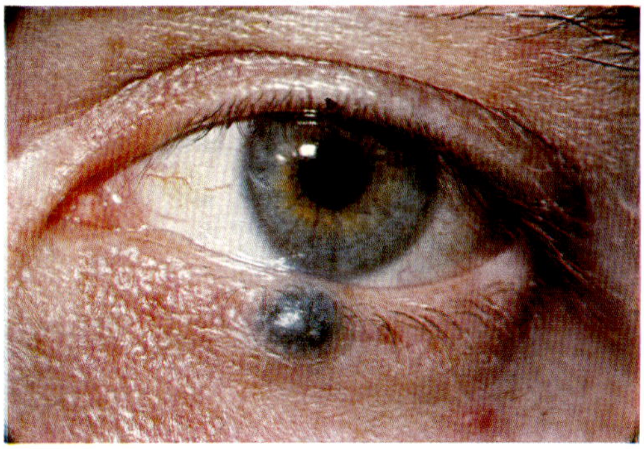

Fig. 1 Blue nevus (♂ 26 yrs.) (see pages 104, 118)

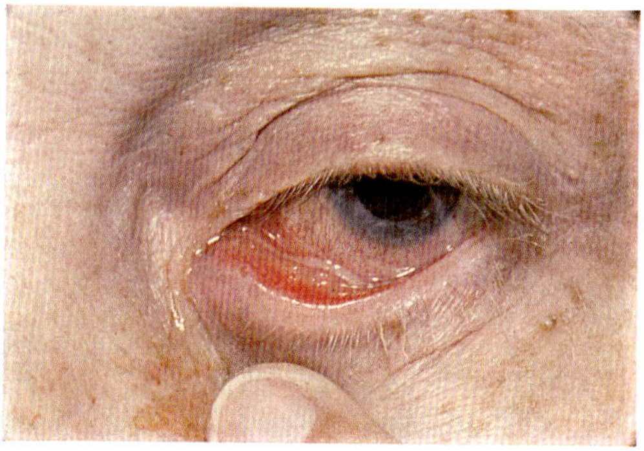

Fig. 4 Imitation of a fungal infection of the lower canaliculus (Actinomycosis; ♂ 53 yrs.) (see page 114)

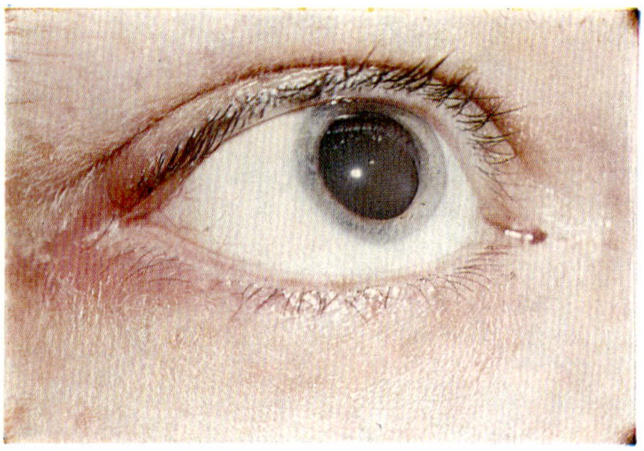

Fig. 2 Angular blepharoconjunctivitis (♂ 30 yrs.) (see pages 107, 130)

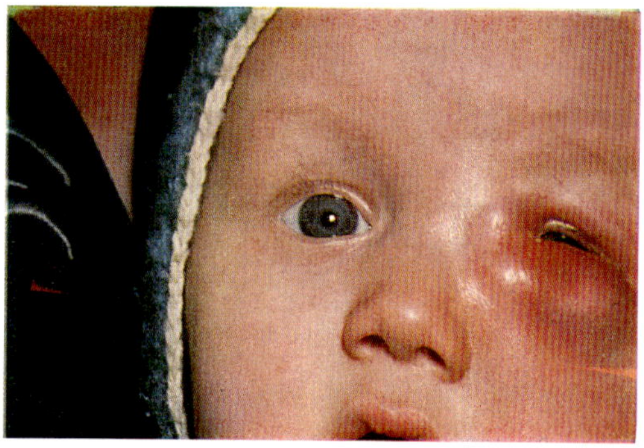

Fig. 5 Dacryocystitis (♂ 1 yr.) (see page 115)

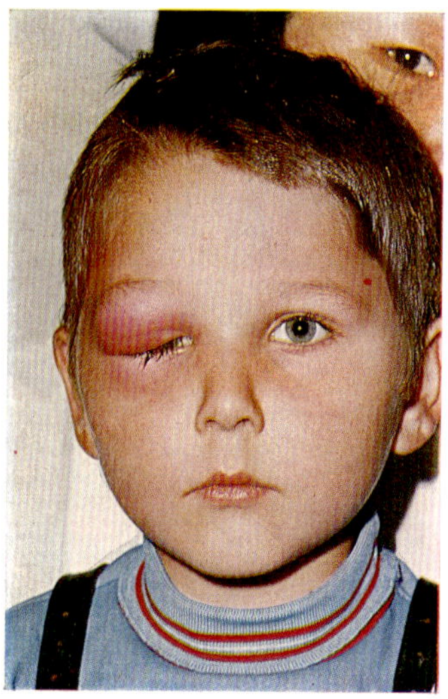

Fig. 3 Acute dacryoadenitis (♂ 4 yrs.) (see page 113)

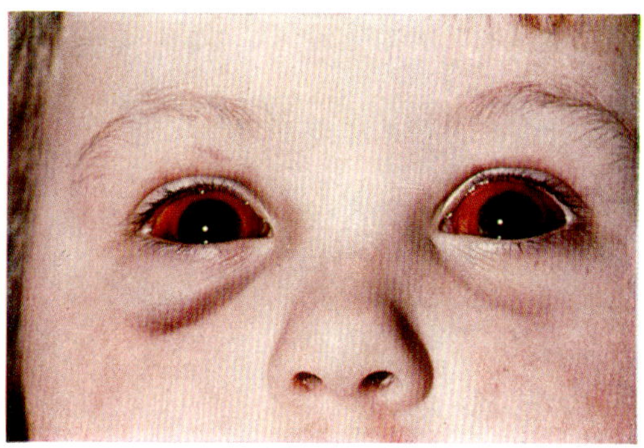

Fig. 6 Conjunctival and lid hemorrhages in whooping-cough (♀ 6 yrs.) (see page 117)

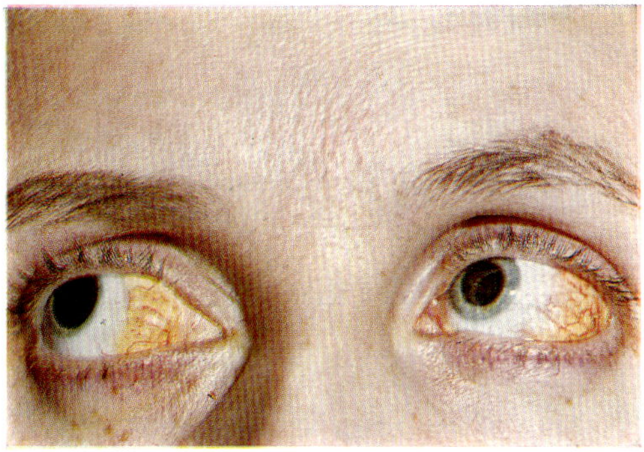

Fig. 1 Lipid deposition in the conjunctiva and episclera (♀ 35 yrs.) (see page 117)

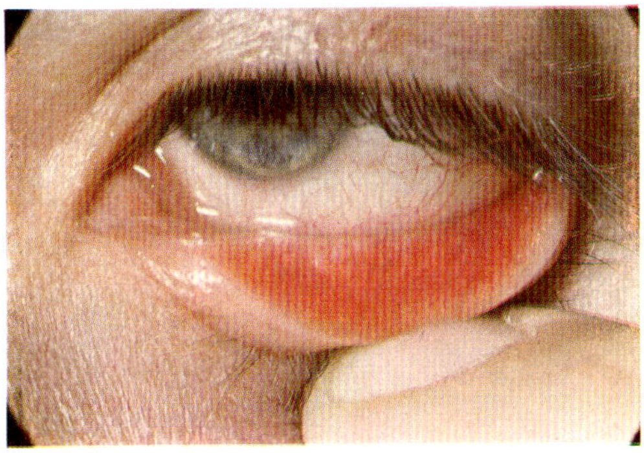

Fig. 4 Allergic conjunctivitis (hay fever) (see page 122)

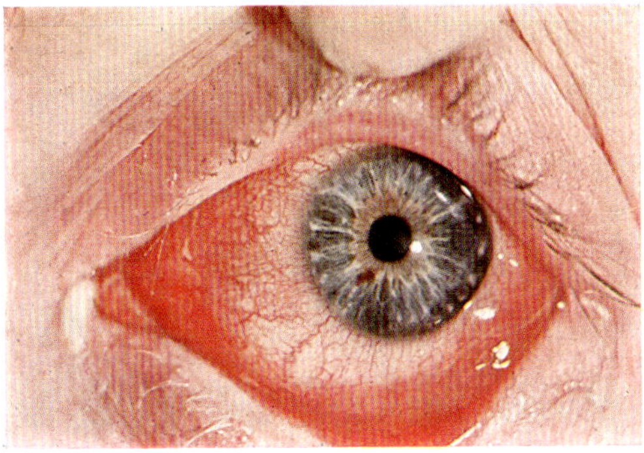

Fig. 2 Acute conjunctivitis (pneumococcus) (♂ 25 yrs.) (see pages 120, 121)

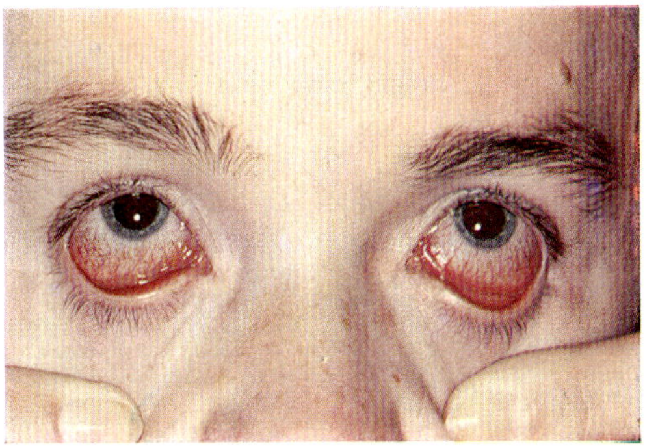

Fig. 5 Epidemic keratoconjunctivitis with chemosis of the caruncle (see page 125)

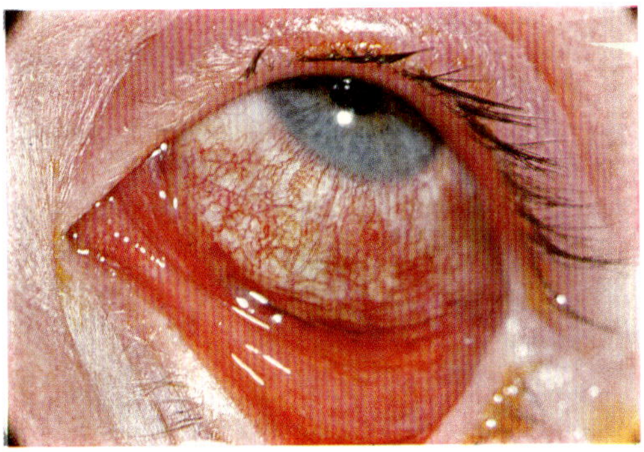

Fig. 3 Hemorrhagic conjunctivitis (♀ 34 yrs.) (see page 121)

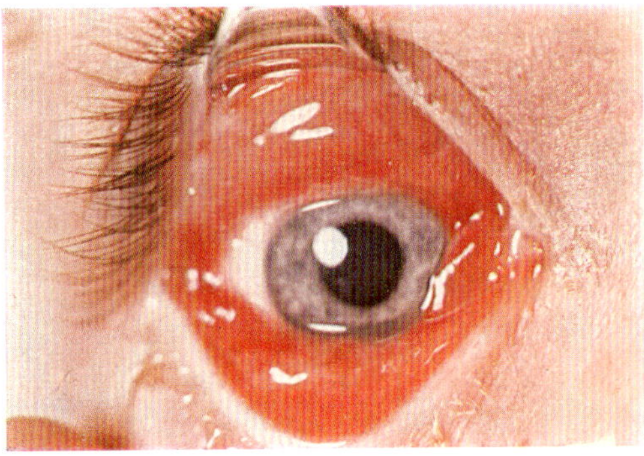

Fig. 6 Conjunctival chemosis in epidemic keratoconjunctivitis (♂ 11 yrs.) (see page 125)

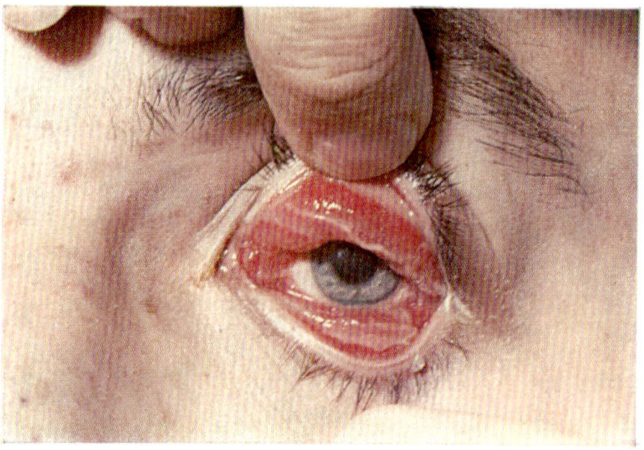

Fig. 1 Pseudomembranous conjunctivitis (epidemic) (see pages 121, 125, 127)

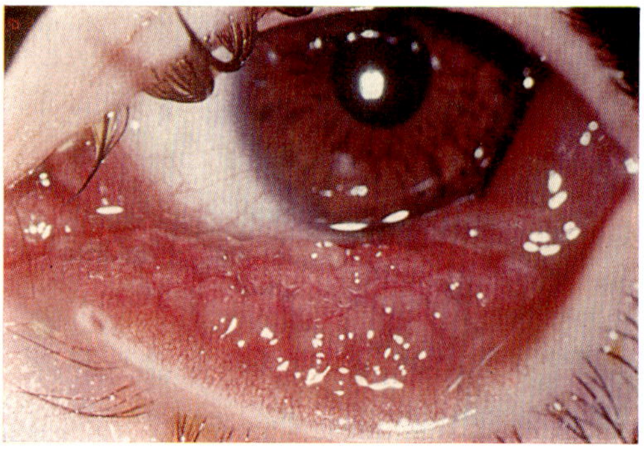

Fig. 4 Follicular conjunctivitis (♀ 3 yrs.) (see page 129)

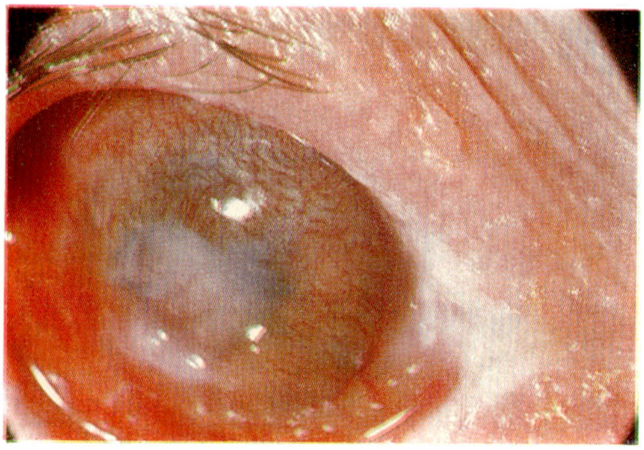

Fig. 2 Pemphigus vulgaris of the conjunctiva and cornea. There is marked conjunctival scarring and superficial vascularization of the conjunctiva (♀ 72 yrs.) (see pages 97, 128)

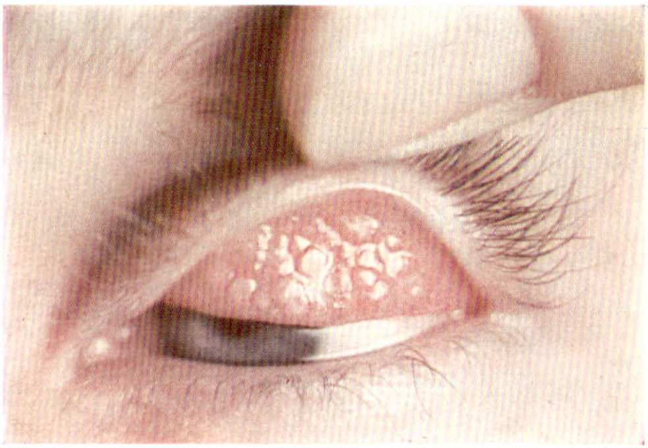

Fig. 5 Vernal conjunctivitis with milky red "cobblestone" papillae (♂ 9 yrs.) (see page 129)

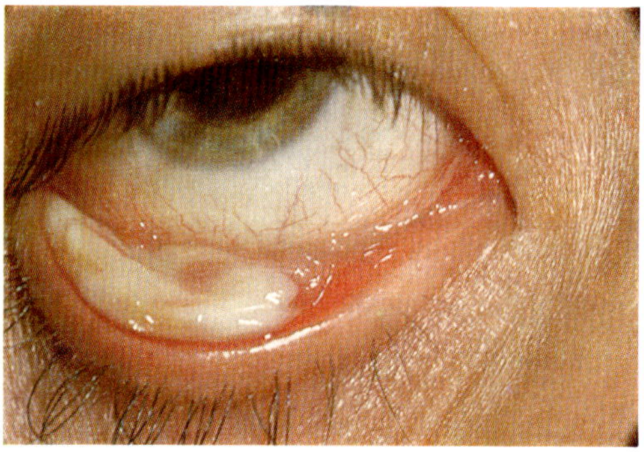

Fig. 3 Ligneous conjunctivitis (♂ 13 yrs.) (see page 128)

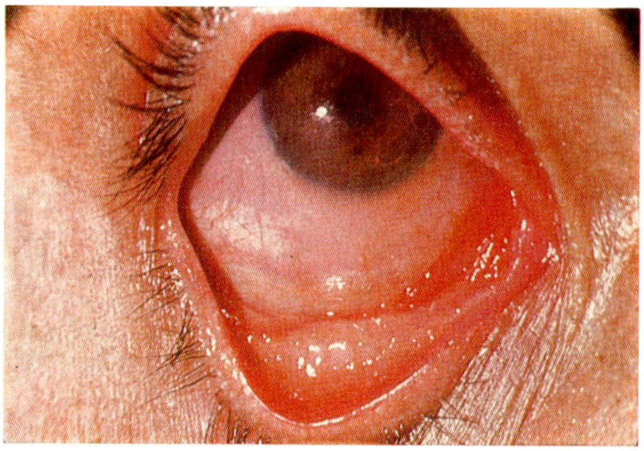

Fig. 6 Conjunctivitis sicca, rose bengal stain (♀ 55 yrs.) (see page 111)

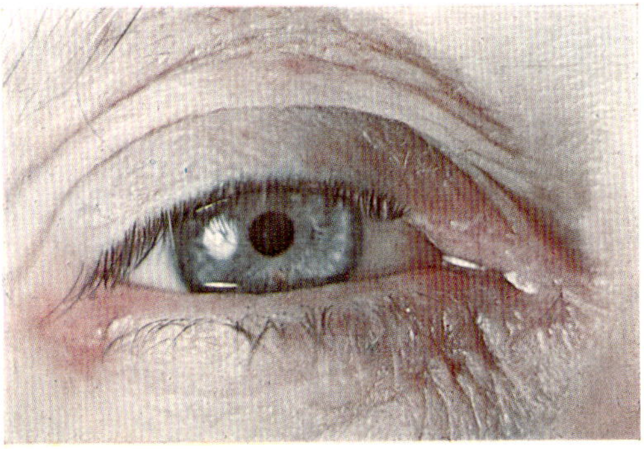

Fig. 1 Angular blepharoconjunctivitis (♂ 41 yrs.) (see page 130)

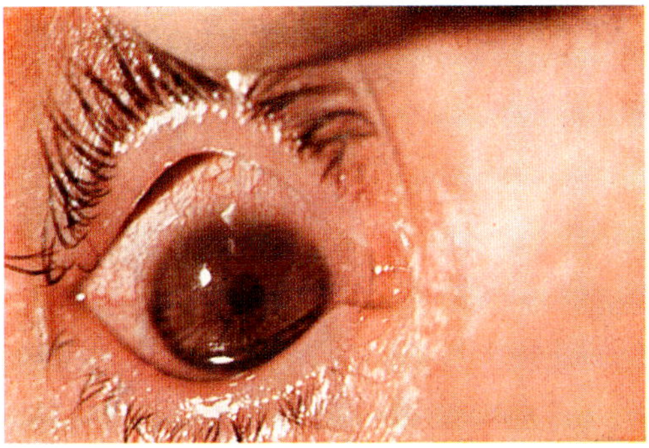

Fig. 2 Trachomatous pannus (♀ 26 yrs.) (see pages 131, 148)

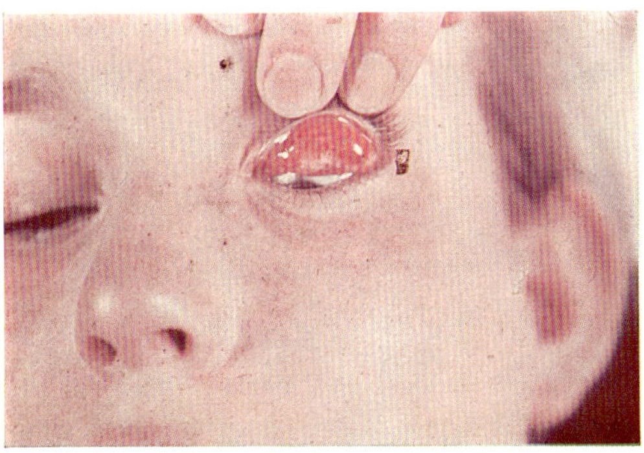

Fig. 3 Parinaud's conjunctivitis (tularemia) with gross follicular conjunctivitis and preauricular lymphadenopathy (see page 131)

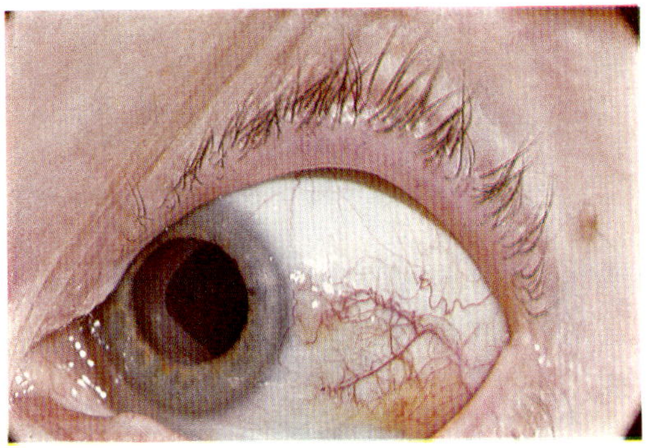

Fig. 4 Conjunctival nodule with vessel dilatation in sarcoidosis (♀ 52 yrs.) (see pages 131, 133)

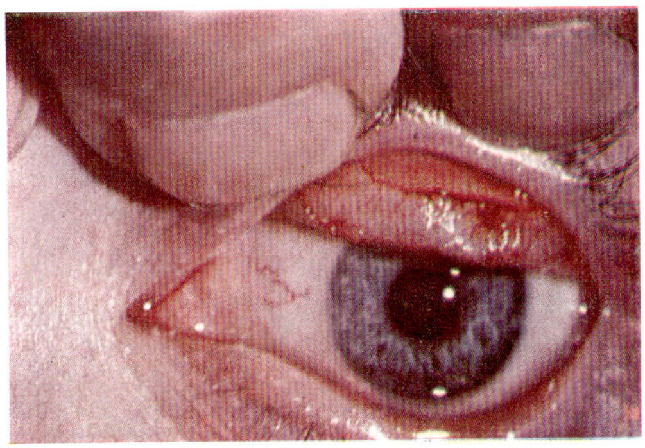

Fig. 5 Secondary amyloidosis of the superior tarsal conjunctiva (♂ 43 yrs.) (see page 136)

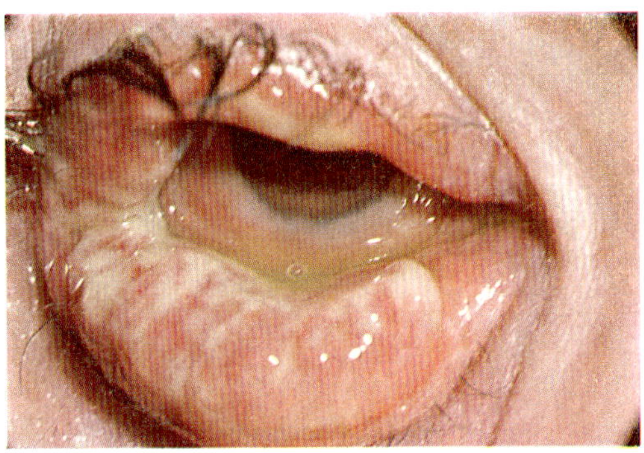

Fig. 6 Inflammatory granulation tissue in pyorhinoblepharostomatitis vegetans (McCarthy's syndrome) (see page 137)

Plate VIII (Chapters 12 and 13)

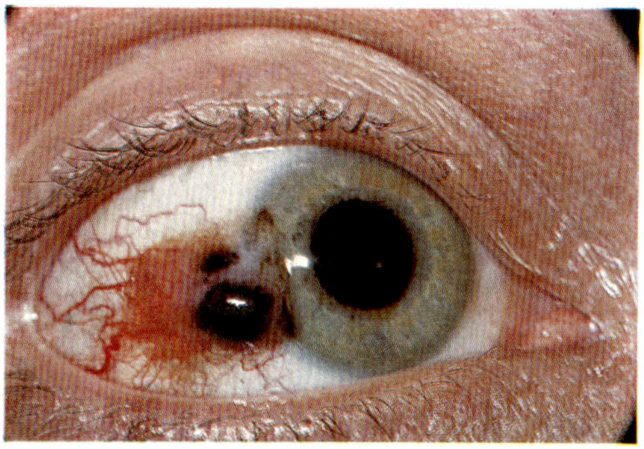

Fig. 1 Conjunctival nevus with malignant melanoma formation (see page 138)

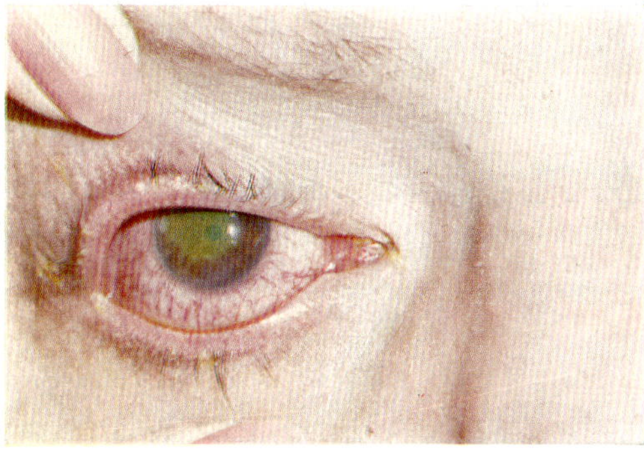

Fig. 4 Hereditary epidermolysis bullosa with fluorescein-stained corneal erosion (♂ 37 yrs.) (see pages 154, 171)

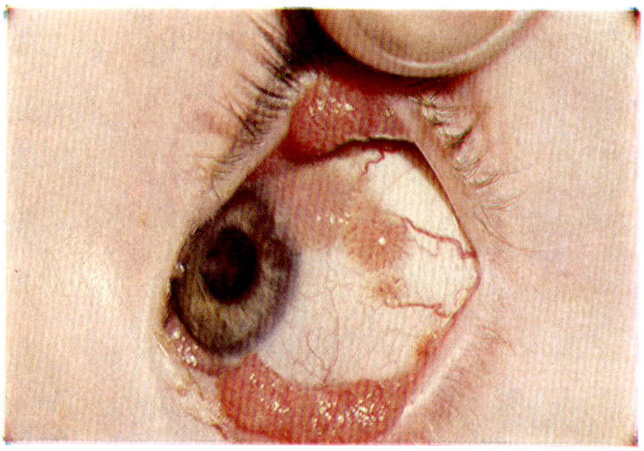

Fig. 2 Conjunctival papillomas (♂ 5 yrs.) (see page 138)

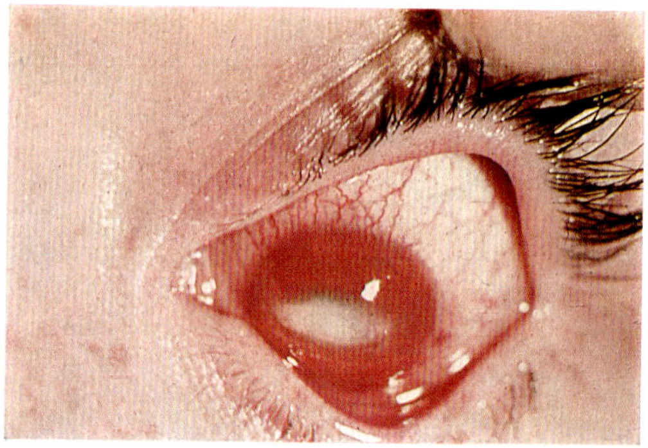

Fig. 5 Interstitial (luetic) keratitis (♀ 13 yrs.) (see page 156)

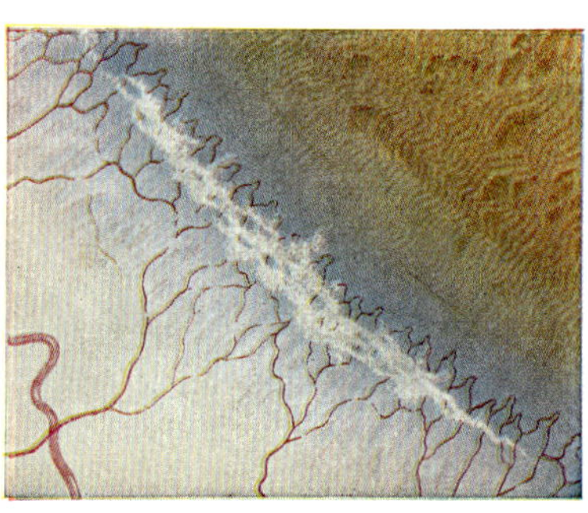

Fig. 3 White limbal girdle of Vogt (from: R. Thiel, Atlas of Diseases of the Eye, 6th ed., Thieme, Stuttgart, 1963) (see page 147)

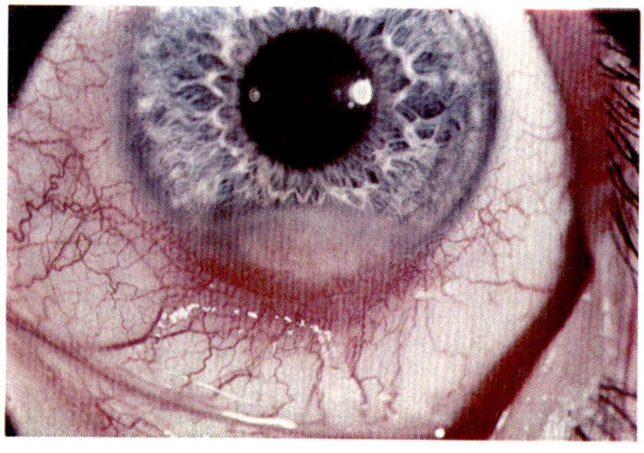

Fig. 6 Sclerosing keratitis (♂ 39 yrs) (see pages 157, 182)

bilateral as often as it is unilateral and may last for years. Corneal clouding, vascularization, stromal thinning, and perforation occur in some cases. Verhoff (1958) described a case which he had followed for 36 years. The disease usually begins in childhood, although a later onset is possible (Nover 1964).

François et al. (1968) investigated the ligneous membrane histologically and showed it to be hyaline plaques rich in mucopolysaccharides.

Vaccinia (see page 95) and **smallpox** (variola, see page 96) can cause membranous conjunctivitis. In variola the systemic findings dominate the clinical picture. Small vesicles form on the lids and conjunctiva. These may lead to corneal ulceration, leukoma formation, and perforation.

Chronic Conjunctivitis

Chronic conjunctivitis with burning, itching, heaviness of the lids, redness, edema and follicle formation should bring to mind noxious external factors such as dust, smoke, nasal-sinus infections, refractive errors, improper glasses, heterophoria, decentered glasses, etc.

Simple chronic conjunctivitis — Follicular conjunctivitis — Vernal conjunctivitis — Leukemic infiltrates — Conjunctivitis sicca — Chronic infectious conjunctivitis.

Nonspecific **chronic conjunctivitis** often causes greater symptomatology than the objective findings warrant. Burning, itching, dryness, heavy lids and easy fatigability all tend to be worse in the evening than in the morning. There may be no obvious cause for the complaints. Frequently, there is a minimal blepharitis. Generally the patients are light-skinned, nervous, neurasthenic individuals. Psychotherapy, change in working environment or mildly astringent eye drops may be helpful.

With time, every chronic conjunctivis develops **follicles** (Plate VI, Fig. 4, page 128 f). In chronic **follicular conjunctivitis** these lymphocytic aggregates are the most prominent finding. The conjunctiva may be slightly swollen and red. Children and juveniles are primarily affected. The follicles can be so densely packed that the conjunctiva takes on a knobby, velvety appearance.

Folliculitis is a symptomatic (burning, itching, foreign body sensation) follicular conjunctivitis.

Folliculosis, which is common in children, gives the same clinical picture but is asymptomatic. Folliculosis is usually associated with benign lymphadenopathy, "adenoid hyperplasia" so common in children. A refractive error may also be present.

With *ectropion* a chronic *conjunctivitis* of the exposed conjunctiva is invariably present.

Vernal catarrh can virtually be diagnosed by the history. Seventy-five percent of patients are young males (6 to 20 years). The conjunctival inflammation, itching, burning, and photophobia are seasonal. The process begins in spring and lasts through the sunny part of the year into fall (Neumann et al. 1959; Morgan 1971; Frankland and Easty 1971).

Hallmarks of the disease include: a homogeneous milky-blue redness of the swollen conjunctiva and large (paving-stone) papillae (Plate VI, Fig. 5, page 128 f). These are particularly prominent in the *palpebral form* of the disease. While the tarsal conjunctiva is primarily involved, the fornices remain free of papillae. A conjunctival smear shows many eosinophils.

In the *bulbar form of vernal conjunctivitis*, yellow-gray to blue gelatinous conjunctival nodules appear at the limbus. They may be single or multiple and varying in size (Fig. 12.12).

The conjunctival papillae (limbal and tarsal) disappear in the winter months. After a varying number of seasons, usually by age 18, the lesions cease to recur. The etiology is thought

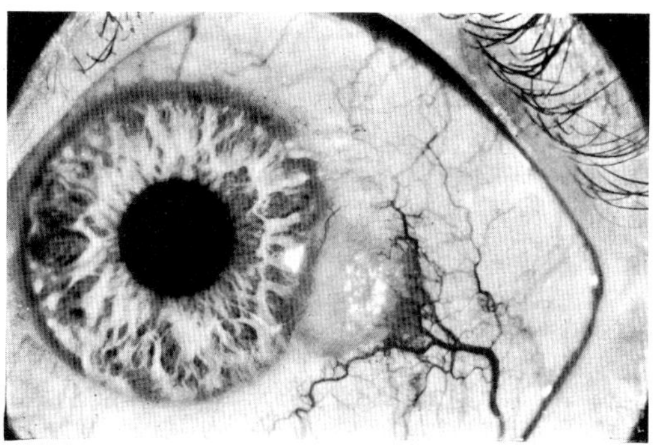

Fig. 12.12 Vernal conjunctivitis (bulbar form) with gelatinous limbal nodule (♂ 10 yrs.)

to be related to heat, sun (greater incidence in warm climates), allergy (eosinophils on conjunctival smear), and individual susceptibility. Since the disease does not occur in high mountain regions, sunlight as such is probably not the etiology (Böke 1963).

Leukemic conjunctival infiltrates: These may appear as numerous follicles or circumscribed pseudotumors.

Keratoconjunctivitis sicca (see page 150) is bilateral and appears as part of Sjögren's syndrome. It usually affects postmenopausal women and causes decreased production of tears, saliva, and mucous membrane secretions. There is a chronic follicular conjunctivitis, especially of the lower lid. The cornea shows punctate staining or filiform keratitis causing injection of the perilimbic vessel. The patient complains of dryness and of a foreign body sensation. Tear secretion is always decreased (Schirmer's test = less than 4 mm in 3 minutes).

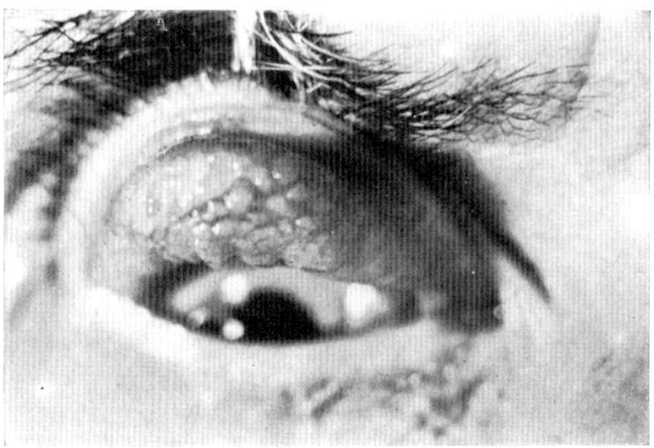

Fig. 12.13 Fresh trachoma follicles (♂ 63 yrs.)

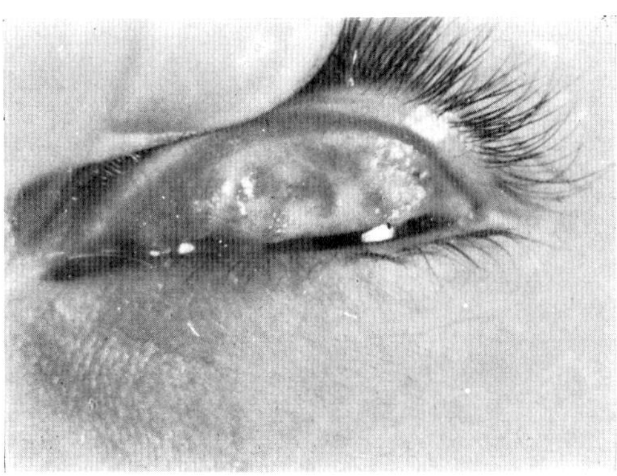

Fig. 12.14 Trachomatous conjunctival scarring (♀ 38 yrs.)

All mucous membranes, especially the mouth, are dry. Achlorhydria, polyarthritis – particularly of the knee – hypotony and hypoglycemia are other findings. Sjögren's syndrome is an autoimmune, collagen disorder (see page 150). Chronic dacryoadenitis (see page 113) in Mikulicz's disease or sarcoidosis (Heerfordt's uveoparotid fever, see page 201) also causes keratoconjunctivitis sicca.

Vitamin A deficiency, with xerophthalmia, hemeralopia and keratomalacia (see page 163) causes the sicca syndrome as well as epidermization, loss of luster and desquamation of the conjunctiva. Bitôt spots (foamy white paralimbic plaques in the interpalpebral fissure area) are classically described in vitamin A deficiency.

Dry eyes may be seen with old trachoma (Fig. 12.14), conjunctival pemphigoid (Fig. 12.11), pemphigus, Stevens-Johnson syndrome, Plummer-Vinson syndrome (dysphagia, hypochromic anemia, xerostomia, hemeralopia) and ariboflavinosis.

Conjunctival xerosis is congenital (François 1963) in familial dysautonomia (Riley-Day) (Liebmann 1956) and congenital anhidrotic ectodermal dysplasia.

Chronic Infectious Conjunctivitis

Angular blepharoconjunctivitis — Trachoma — Parinaud's syndrome — Fungal infections of the conjunctiva — Tuberculosis, lues, leprosy — Sarcoidosis.

Classic **angular blepharoconjunctivitis** is caused by the Morax-Axenfeld diplobacillus (Plate IV, Fig. 2, 128 d; Plate VII, Fig. 1, page 128 g). Staphylococcus will produce the same picture of burning, itching, and angular blepharitis. The skin irritation is caused by a dermalysin produced by the infecting agent.

Trachoma begins insidiously; conjunctival erythema and follicle formation develop (Fig. 12.13). The follicles rupture spontaneously or are easily expressed. They are continuously replaced by new follicles. The inflammation and remissions last for years, or even decades. Conjunctival scarring, shrinkage (Fig. 12.14), and xerosis is the final result.

Scarring often causes the lid to turn inward (entropion). The lashes then rub on the cornea (trichiasis). The cornea stains and superficial

vessels grow down over the cornea from above like a descending curtain *(trachomatous pannus)* (Plate VII, Fig. 2, page 128 g). Conjunctival scars appear as fine white lines. The upper lid droops from the weight (trachomatous ptosis). The etiologic agent is the TRIC virus of trachoma and inclusion body conjunctivitis. Other terms are *Chlamydia, Chlamydozoon* or *Bedsonia*. The incubation time is six to ten days. Prowazek-Halberstadt inclusion bodies, which stain blue with Giemsa stain, may be seen on conjunctival smears in active cases. Trachoma is most common in North Africa, the Middle East, Asia and Eastern Europe. There are small pockets of endemic infection in the southwestern United States. Some 400,000,000 people are infected with trachoma worldwide (one sixth of the world population according to WHO estimate). In areas of North Africa 90 percent of the inhabitants are infected by the age of one year (Strehl 1962).
Differential diagnosis: The follicles in conjunctivitis other than trachoma are more uniform in size and do not rupture or cause scarring. Pemphigoid lacks follicles; conjunctival shrinkage is the predominant symptom.

In **Parinaud's conjunctivitis** (oculoglandular syndrome) (see page 133) the *pre-auricular lymphadenopathy* (up to the size of a chicken egg) is the dominant finding. The affliction is usually unilateral with coarse tarsal follicles and ulceration in the fornices (Plate VII, Fig. 3, page 128 g). Tularemia is the primary cause of Parinaud's conjunctivitis (Wail 1929; Hamburger 1937; Thomas et al. 1952). After an incubation period of two to four days, malaise, headaches, nausea, vomiting and fever develop. The conjunctiva heals after three to four weeks (rarely months) without scarring. Rodents carry the infective agent, which is often contracted by skinning wild rabbits.
Bovine and human tuberculosis (Wessely 1910; Stock 1931; Hartmann 1948) can also cause Parinaud's oculoglandular syndrome. Parinaud's oculoglandular syndrome refers only to a follicular conjunctivitis with pre-auricular lymphadenopathy (Starke 1949) (Fig. 12.15). Other causes include:
Cat-scratch fever: follicular conjunctivitis, phlyctenules, pre-auricular lymphadenopathy and, rarely, keratitis.

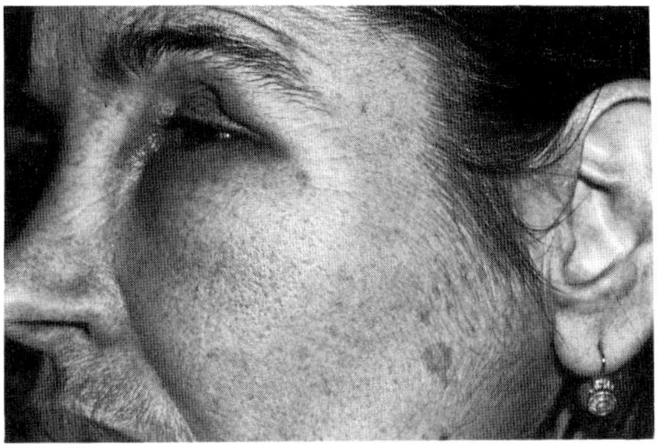

Fig. 12.15 Benign lymphoid hyperplasia with conjunctival follicles and preauricular node swelling (♀ 39 yrs.)

Newcastle disease (fowlpox) causes Parinaud's oculoglandular syndrome, fever, and pulmonary complications.
Lymphogranuloma inguinale is associated with lid edema, follicular conjunctivitis, lymphadenopathy, and rarely iridocyclitis and papilledema.
Coxsackie viruses and *hoof-and-mouth disease* may cause phlyctenule-like nodules, pseudomembranes and ulceration along with pre-auricular lymphadenopathy. *Listeriosis (Listeria monocytogenes, Listerella monocytogenes)* and *Leptothrix* are further causes of the oculoglandular syndrome.

Fungal Conjunctivitis (see page 161)

Tuberculosis, Syphilis, Leprosy

Primary *conjunctival tuberculosis* can cause Parinaud's conjunctivitis (see page 131). Children are particularly prone to forming large (up to the size of a bean) conjunctival ulcers (Damel 1951). Endogenous secondary conjunctival tuberculosis also occurs (Azzolini 1954; Calmettes and Déodati 1950; Galeazzi 1950).
Conjunctival nodules and ulcers are the prominent findings in *tuberculous, lepromatous* and *syphilitic conjunctivitis*.
Pre-auricular lymphadenopathy occurs with primary tuberculous or syphilitic conjunctival infection. Conjunctival nodules in sarcoidosis (Plate VII, Fig. 4, page 128 g) are red-yellow or glassy-white and range in size from that of a pinhead to several millimeters. Conjunctival edema may be present (see page 201).

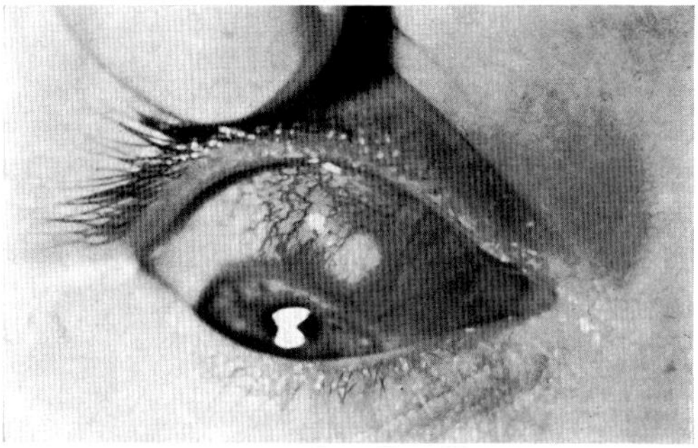

Fig. 12.16 Solitary phlyctenule in scrofulous conjunctivitis

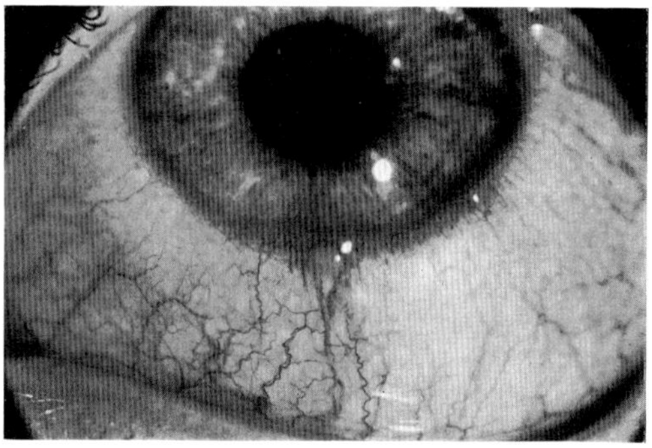

Fig. 12.17 Scrofulous conjunctivitis with small perilimbal phlyctenules (♀ 15 yrs.)

Keratoconjunctivitis with Nodule Formation

In addition to conjunctivitides which secondarily involve the cornea, there are conjunctival inflammations where the cornea is also *primarily affected.*

Scrofulous keratoconjunctivitis – Erythema nodosum – Rosacea keratoconjunctivitis – Lupus erythematosus – Sarcoidosis – Hodgkin's disease – Leprosy – Ophthalmic zoster – Molluscum contagiosum.

Eczematous, phlyctenular scrofulous keratoconjunctivitis (see page 162): The disease may begin in infancy but its usual onset is during the early school years. The patients develop a characteristic facies with rhinitis, nose, mouth and lymph node swelling (the name comes from the resemblance to the pig, i.e., sus scrofa) (Fig. 10.25). A crusty eczema develops around the mouth, nose, ears, scalp, and face. Typical perilimbic phlyctenules form. These are not blisters but rather fleshy nodules. They may be single (Fig. 12.16) or multiple (Fig. 12.17), large or small. The nodules are surrounded by conjunctival and ciliary injection. Phlyctenules are mainly at the limbus but occur anywhere on the bulbar or tarsal conjunctiva. They consist of lymphocytes and crop up for a few days, regress and reappear elsewhere.

The disease is relatively asymptomatic as long as only the conjunctiva is affected. With corneal involvement (see page 162) comes severe photophobia, tearing, and blepharospasm. The blepharospasm causes spastic entropion formation. Lashes rubbing on the cornea provide further irritation until gray, superficial corneal infiltrates and ulcers develop. Perforation occurs only with superinfection. The infiltrate stimulates limbal vessel ingrowth (pannus scrofulosus) (Plate IX, Figs. 4, 5, page 192 a) (see page 162). Generally, healing occurs only after the cornea is totally vascularized. The *"wandering phlyctenule"* is typical of corneal involvement. A perilimbic phlyctenule progressively moves closer to the corneal center, trailing vessel ingrowth behind it. Corneal phlyctenules heal after weeks or months, leaving scars and irregular astigmatism. Conjunctival and corneal phlyctenules tend to be recurrent.

Riehm (1957) found that phlyctenule formation occurred when antigenically damaged, dead or agglutinated tuberculus bacilli enter the blood stream from a primary focus (usually in the lung) and metastasize to the cornea and conjunctiva. Through specific antigens, the degradation process produces inflammation (phlyctenules). Phlyctenule formers tend to be strong reactors on tuberculin skin testing. Age, general health, heredity, and immunologic status play a role (Riehm).

The term *eczematous conjunctivitis* should be limited to cases of true eczema and not include scrofula (Böke 1957).

With improvement in hygiene, scrofula has become rare (Comberg 1955). Marchesani (1947) thought an exudative lymphocytic diathesis to exist which could be set off by tuberculous infection, sun, poor hygiene or malnutrition.

Phlyctenular keratitis, episcleritis, retinal periphlebitis and choroiditis have been reported after BCG immunization (Renard et al. 1959).

Differential diagnosis: Episcleritis nodules are

beneath the mobile conjunctiva; pressure evokes pain. Phlyctenules are also painful. The conjunctival nodules of acne rosacea are chronic, occur in older persons, and are vascularized. Conjunctival sarcoid nodules are acute, chronic, and of variable size.

Erythema nodosum may have an accompanying conjunctivitis with phlyctenules, nodules, and large episcleral lesions (von Röth 1928; Veltišev 1925; Tow 1928; Contino 1953; Kratka 1953). Without therapy these disappear in a few days along with the erythema nodosum (von Röth). Cortisone speeds the healing process (Calamandrei and Ferrata 1951). The picture is scrofulous phlyctenulosis. Isolated cases of iritis with hypopyon are reported (Reis 1906; Katzenelson 1925; Fukazawa 1956). Stajduhar and Pansini (1951) found bilateral disseminated chorioretinal lesions in eleven children from two to twelve years of age. The diagnosis was erythema nodosum of tuberculous etiology.

Rosacea keratoconjunctivitis (see page 162) is common. It resembles scrofulous conjunctivits but appears primarily in *older patients*. A papillary conjunctivitis is present. The phlyctenule-like nodules are vascularized, painless, gray-yellow, and involve conjunctiva and cornea (Plate IX, Fig. 6, page 192 a). The corneal lesions may ulcerate. Dilated tortuous blood vessels frequently extend beyond the infiltrate onto seemingly normal cornea. Calcium deposits form in the old scars. Rosacea keratoconjunctivitis is a chronic, recurrent long-term process. The skin changes should tip one off to the diagnosis.

Lupus erythematosus (see page 92) may involve the cornea or cause a chronic conjunctivitis.

Sarcoid nodules, which are a glassy white, gray to yellow-brown (Plate VII, Fig. 4, page 128 g), may appear anywhere on the skin or conjunctiva. Uveitis (see page 195) and uveoparotid fever (Heerfordt) (see page 202) are more prominent symptoms.

Hodgkin's disease: In lymphoma, myeloma or Hodgkin's disease, there can be gelatinous or firm conjunctival tumefactions.

Leprosy: Nodular conjunctival infiltrates occur (see page 198).

Ophthalmic zoster always involves the first branch of the trigeminal nerve. Lids (see page 95), conjunctiva, cornea, and iris may show vesicle or papule formation. Sequelae include iritis, secondary glaucoma, and zoster myositis.

On rare occasions, **molluscum contagiosum** will infect the conjunctiva or caruncle (Vannas and Lapinleimu 1967).

Conjunctivitis with Pre-Auricular Lymphadenopathy

Paratrachoma (inclusion blennorrhea, swimming pool conjunctivitis), *epidemic keratoconjunctivitis, epidemic hemorrhagic conjunctivitis, mononucleosis, hoof-and-mouth disease, vaccinia, variola.*

Parinaud's conjunctivitis (see page 131) is a symptom complex of follicular conjunctivitis and pre-auricular lymphadenopathy. The latter may become as large as a chicken egg. Causal agents include *tularemia, tuberculosis, cat-scratch fever, lymphogranuloma inguinale, Newcastle disease* (fowlpox), *listeriosis* and *leptothrix. Primary syphilitic* or *tuberculous* conjunctival infection is rarely seen but causes lymphadenopathy. In tuberculosis the lymph nodes may fuse, suppurate, and fistulize to the skin. Any conjunctival *superinfection* (scrofula, eczema, impetigo, after burns, etc.) leads to a painful pre-auricular lymphadenopathy.

Telangiectasia and Vascular Aneurysms (see page 256)

Hereditary hemorrhagic telangiectasia — Aneurysms — Ataxia telangiectasia (Louis-Bar syndrome) — Fabry's syndrome — Endangiitis obliterans — Dysproteinemia — Lymphangiectasia haemorrhagica conjunctivae.

Conjunctival telangiectasias and varices are seen in **hereditary hemorrhagic telangiectasia** (Osler-Weber-Rendu) (Pitter 1941; Miles 1952; Wittmer 1951; Bergmann and Wiedemann 1955; Garner and Grossmann 1956). Recur-

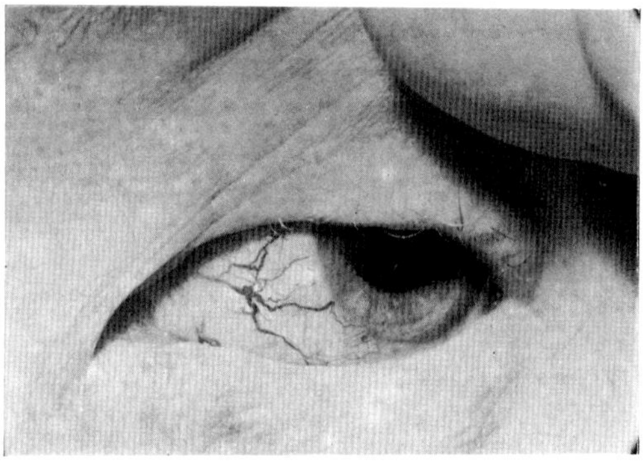

Fig. 12.18 Aneurysmal dilatation of vessels and rarefaction of the conjunctiva following radiation therapy (♀ 52 yrs.)

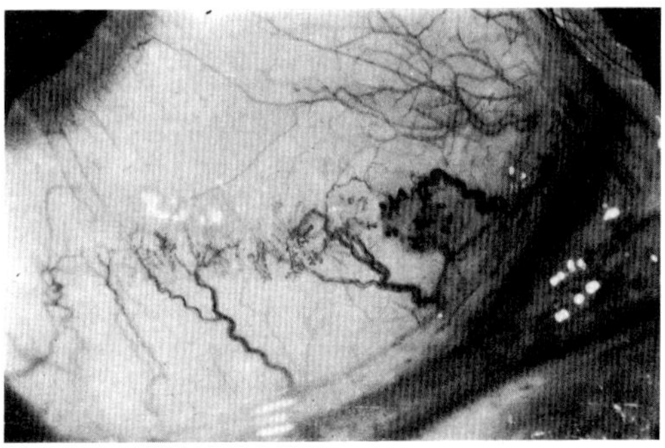

Fig. 12.19 Conjunctival aneurysms (♀ 27 yrs.)

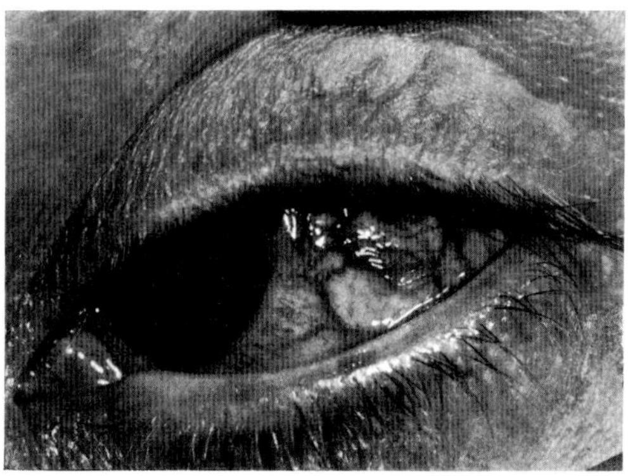

Fig. 12.20 Conjunctival aneurysms and vascular dilatation with metastatic carcinoma to the choroid (♀ 36 yrs.)

rent bleeding may occur from any affected area (including conjunctiva) (François 1938).

Aneurysms of conjunctival vessels occur with diabetes mellitus, chronic congestive glaucoma, after radiation (Fig. 12.18), and as an idiopathic anomaly (Fig. 12.19). Aneurysmal dilatation of conjunctival vessels is found at the base of the pterygium and with underlying choroidal or ciliary body melanomas and metastatic carcinomas (Fig. 12.20).

Ataxia telangiectasia (Louis-Bar syndrome) is one of the phakomatoses. Symptoms include cerebellar ataxia; telangiectasia, especially of the bulbar conjunctiva; café-au-lait spots; nevoid birthmarks; and bronchiectasis. Development and intelligence are usually retarded. The disorder is autosomal recessive. Symptoms are first noted at age three to four. Death is usually caused by recurrent respiratory infections (see page 257).

Angiokeratoma corporis (Fabry's disease) (see page 167 and 257) causes dilated tortuous retinal (Fig. 22.2) and conjunctival vessels as well as cornea verticillata. The disease is an inborn error of metabolism (Ceramide-α-trihexosidase deficiency).

Endangiitis obliterans causes aneurysms and neovascularization (see page 256).

Dysproteinemia (see page 267): Waldenström's macroglobulinemia, cryoglobulinemia, and multiple myeloma are the most significant. There is sludging of blood in *perilimbic vessels*. These become tortuous, dilated, sausage- or pearl-shaped. Retinal vessels are also involved. The veins are tortuous, even sausage-shaped. There are retinal hemorrhages, central retinal vein occlusion, cotton wool spots, exudates and peripheral ciliary aneurysms. Other ocular findings include papilledema and exudative retinal detachment (especially centrally). Clinically, there may be hepatomegaly, splenomegaly, and lymphadenopathy as well as hyperglobulinemia and an elevated erythrocyte sedimentation rate.

Differential diagnosis: The primary consideration would be hematopoietic disorders such as thrombocytopenic purpura, pernicious anemia, iron deficiency anemia, sickle cell anemia, polycythemia, leukemia, and lupus erythematosus. When *unilateral,* central retinal vein thrombosis is the first choice (Berneaud-Kötz 1959; Nover 1952; Knisley 1955; Cagianut and Hoffmann-Egg 1953; Seitz 1969).

Lymphangiectasia Haemorrhagica Conjunctivae

In lymphangiectasia haemorrhagica conjunctivae, conjunctival lymph vessels become permanently or intermittently dilated and filled with blood (Donders 1968; Heydenreich 1956). In a 12-year-old girl reported by Stepanik (1958), the telangiectasias disappeared after a parotid lymphangioma was removed. Conrads and Kühnhardt (1957) believe the telangiectasias are caused by blockage of lymph flow within the conjunctival connective tissue. Abnormal connections between blood and lymph vessels are possible causes.

Physical Damage to the Conjunctiva

Injury — Chemical burns — Thermal burns — Photoelectric ophthalmia — Photodermatitis — X-ray or radium irradiation.

Injury

Any *conjunctival laceration* raises the possibility that the globe is *perforated.*

Chemical and Thermal Burns

Because of the history, chemical (acid, lye [Fig. 13.23], aniline dyes, silver nitrate, potassium permanganate, volatile hydrocarbons) and thermal burns are not a diagnostic problem (see pages 149 and 356).

Ultraviolet Light Keratopathy (see page 354)

Ultraviolet light (lightning, welding arc, snow blindness, sun blindness) causes a superficial punctate keratopathy (see page 149).

Photodermatosis (see page 93)

Photodermatitis can be associated with severe pseudomembranous and ulcerative conjunctivitis (Ullerich et al. 1957):

a) *idiopathic photodermatosis* is caused by an endogenous hypersensitivity to normal amounts of sun light.

b) *exogenous photosensitivity* is based on a phototoxic or photoallergic reaction to some substances.

Of the **idiopathic photodermatoses,** *hydroa aestivale* is the most common. Usually the patient has porphyria (see page 366). Less common diseases are chronic polymorphic light eruption (Hausmann and Haxthausen 1929), light urticaria, spring photodermatitis in children (Burkhardt 1948), actinic, exfoliative cheilitis, and photodermatitis associated with lymphogranuloma inguinale. Light plays a major role in the skin changes of pellagra, various viral exanthems, eczema, psoriasis, Darier's disease, and xeroderma pigmentosum.

Exogenous dermatitic light reaction can be divided into:

1. Phototoxic reactions which occur in any person exposed to both light and phototoxic agents (coal tar [anthracene, benzpyrene], acridine dyes [Trypoflavin, Rivanol, etc.]; eosin, certain plants [Kuske 1940] and animal derivatives).

2. Photoallergy is a light sensitivity by susceptible persons to even small amounts of specific substances. Sulfonamides and phenothiazines are particularly prone to cause this phenomenon. High doses of phenothiazines can also cause retinal pigmentary changes with visual field loss and a disturbance of dark adaptation (Verrey 1956; Rintelen 1956; Wagner 1956).

X-ray and Radium Irradiation

These lead to conjunctival erythema and edema. An overdose causes chronic (months to years) irritation and inflammation of conjunctival vessels. These become tortuous and irregular in caliber (Fig. 12.18). Corneal involvement depends on the amount of radiation. The involvement ranges from superficial punctate staining to diffuse epithelial opacities or chronic non-healing ulcerates.

Scarring with Shrinkage and Drying Out of the Conjunctiva

Xerosis and conjunctival drying — Pemphigoid — Pseudopterygium.

Injury, chemical and *thermal burns* cause symblepharon formation and loss of tear function. *Diphtheria, trachoma, tuberculosis, lues, gonorrhea, pemphigoid, pemphigus, mucocutaneous ocular syndrome* (erythema multiforme, Stevens-Johnson, etc.), cause greater or lesser degrees of scarring and symblepharon formation (see page 147).

Xerosis and Drying of the Conjunctiva

Conjunctival scarring from any cause may lead to pooling and tear stagnation with metaplasia of conjunctival and corneal epithelium *(xerosis)*. Decreased tear production occurs with trachoma, pemphigoid, radiation damage, aging, Sjögren's syndrome and hypovitaminosis A. Vitamin A deficiency is one cause of xerophthalmia (see page 163) with xerosis, Bitôt's spots, night blindness, and keratomalacia. Fluorescein staining in xerosis reveals conjunctival folds running parallel with or concentric to the limbus. Superficial punctate keratopathy may be present.

Benign Mucosal Pemphigoid

In *pemphigoid* the cornea and conjunctiva of older patients is afflicted by vesicles that quickly rupture and form scars (Fig. 12.10). Goblet cells and accessory lacrimal glands are destroyed. The conjunctival scarring leads to xerosis (Fig. 12.11). Entropion and trichiasis occur. The cornea may be completely vascularized.

Differential diagnosis: Blister and membrane formation occurs in erythema multiforme (see page 147). Epidermolysis bullosa, lupus erythematosus, hyperkeratosis connata, porphyria, xeroderma pigmentosum all cause symblepharon formation. Hemorrhagic pseudomembranes suggest diphtheria.

Pseudopterygium (Fig. 10.14, page 88) **and Pterygium**

Burns and other corneal injury stimulate conjunctiva to grow onto the cornea. These *pseudopterygiums* are nonprogressive and do not produce the corneal infiltrate lying in front of the head of a true pterygium (Fig. 12.21). True *pterygia* tend to form in the interpalpebral fissure area.

Conjunctival Pseudotumors

Conjunctival cysts — Leukemic infiltrates — Amyloid deposits — Pinguecula and Bitôt spots — Leukoplakia — Tuberculomas, gumma — Inflammatory granulomata.

Conjunctival cysts are usually traumatic, rarely congenital.

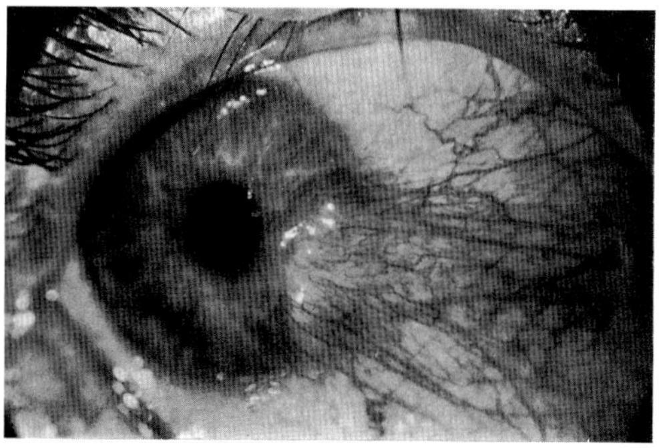

Fig. 12.21 Pterygium (♂ 10 yrs.)

Leukemic infiltrates appear as pseudotumors. **Amyloid deposits** in the cornea are red glassy nodules (Plate VII, Fig. 5, page 128 g). Conjunctival amyloidosis and trachoma are easily mistaken for lymphomatous infiltrates.

Conjunctival tumefaction occurs with any chronic inflammation.

Pinguecula: These are common benign nodules in the interpalpebral fissure area. Histologically, they consist of hyalinized subconjunctival connective tissue. Patients frequently mistake them for neoplasms. **Bitôt spots** simulate tumors (see page 163). These are foamy, white conjunctival lesions in the interpalpebral fissure area.

They are classically associated with, but not limited to, vitamin A deficiency. **Leukoplakia,** or dyskeratosis, is seen primarily in males above the age of 50. It is a precancerous

hyperplasia and metaplasia of the epithelium. The dyskeratotic conjunctival plaques may grow onto the cornea.
Rarely **tuberculomas** or **gumma** appear as solid, yellow, subconjunctival nodules.
Inflammatory granulation tissue. Granulation tissue formation is stimulated by surgery, injury, and inflammations such as chalazion, ligneous conjunctivitis (Fig. 128) and pyorhinoblepharostomatitis vegetans (McCarthy's syndrome) (Plate VII, Fig. 6, page 128 g).

Conjunctival Tumors (see page 175)

Of 1173 conjunctival tumors, Ash (1950) found nevi to be the most common. This was followed in descending order by papilloma and squamous cell carcinoma, pterygium, dermoids, malignant melanomas, basal cell carcinomas, pinguecula, epidermidalization with and without leukoplakia, Bowen's disease, angioma, lymphoma, fibroma and, finally, teratoma.

Dermoids, neurofibromatosis — Nevi, hemangioma — Lymphangioma, melanoma — Papilloma, pre-cancerous — Carcinoma.

Dermoids, neurofibromatosis. *Dermoids* (Fig. 25.3) are firm, yellow to red congenital corneal tumors, usually in the inferior temporal quadrant near the limbus. *Dermoid cysts* may occur in the fornix (Hruby 1941). *Dermolipomas* are soft and normally in the superior temporal (near the lacrimal gland) quadrant. None of these lesions tend to grow.
Oculoauriculovertebral dysplasia of Goldenhar (see page 331) includes hemifacial hypoplasia, auricular or preauricular skin tags, fistulas, epibulbar or subconjunctival dermoids (Fig. 25.3), lipomas and malpositioned teeth (Tost 1969).
Neurofibromas (von Recklinghausen) occur in the conjunctiva and episclera (Fig. 12.22).
Nevi, hemangiomas, lymphangiomas, melanomas: *Nevi, hemangiomas* (Fig. 12.23) and *lymphangiomas* (Fig. 12.24) are benign conjunctival tumors. Glaucoma is a strong possibility whenever a hemangioma involves the area of distribution of the first division of the trigeminal nerve (Sturge-Weber syndrome) (see page 103).

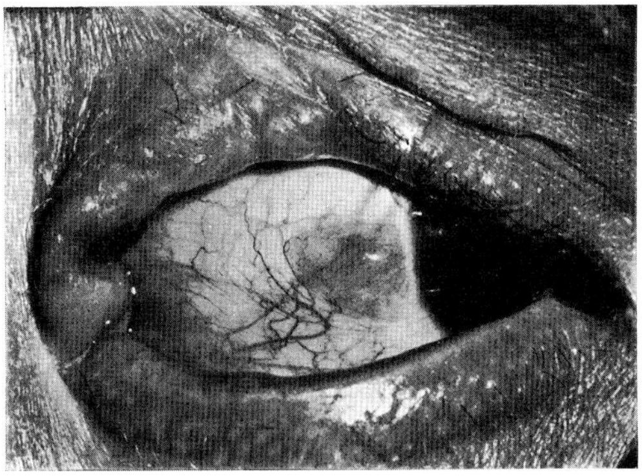

Fig. 12.22 Neurofibroma of the upper lid and conjunctiva (♂ 31 yrs.)

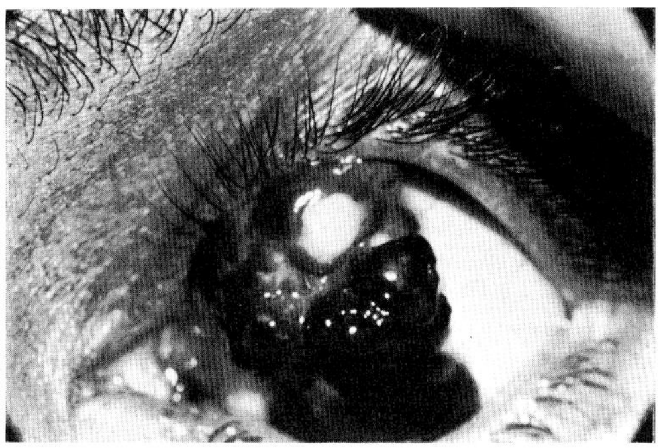

Fig. 12.23 Cavernous hemangioma (♀ 26 yrs.)

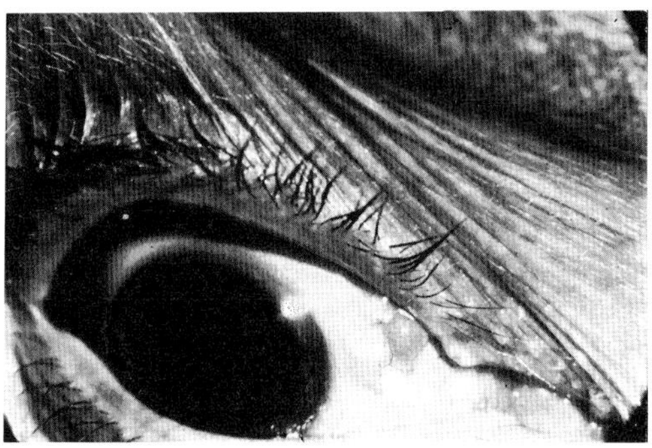

Fig. 12.24 Lymphatic cyst, lymphangioma (♀ 63 yrs.)

Conjunctival and skin telangiectasias are part of the Louis-Bar syndrome. This also includes physical and mental retardation. Ataxia telangiectasia has been found in association with an intracranial aneurysm. It is one of the phakomatoses (Heimann and Terheggen 1969) (see page 296).

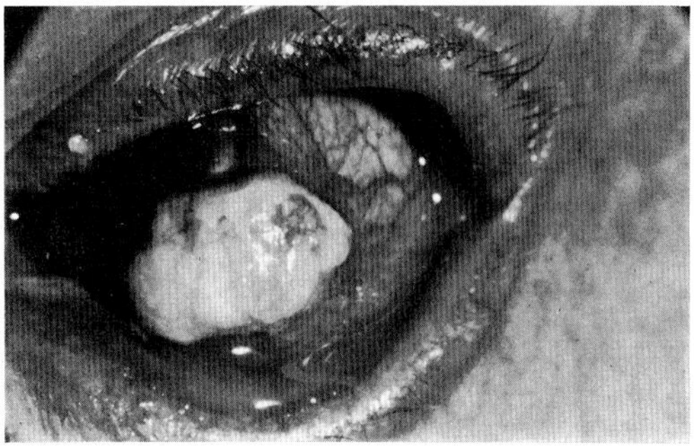

Fig. 12.25 Conjunctival carcinoma (♂ 82 yrs.)

Endangiitis obliterans causes aneurysms and neovascularization (see page 256). A pterygium may simulate a hemangioma (Fig. 12.21). A *pterygium* has a band of dilated vessels extending onto the cornea. Involvement is more common nasally than temporally and, unlike pseudopterygium, a true pterygium is progressive and grows across the cornea with a gray corneal infiltrate just in front of it.

It is clinically impossible to tell if malignant melanoma (Plate VIII, Fig. 1, page 128 h) or melanosis exists histologically in a nevus (see page 104). Conjunctival papillomas (Plate VIII, Fig. 2, page 128 h) are usually small, cauliflower-like, and hemorrhage easily.

Bowen's disease (intraepithelial epithelioma) is a white (leukoplakic) or red tumefaction of the conjunctiva and cornea. It may be cauliflower-like or morbilliform in appearance. The limbus is primarily involved (Fig. 13.52) but the lesion can spread over the entire cornea. Malignant degeneration occasionally occurs. Elderly men are primarily affected (see page 175).

Conjunctival carcinomas (Fig. 12.25). These are almost exclusively squamous cell carcinomas. They may occur in xeroderma pigmentosum.

References

Adamantiades, B.: Sur un cas d'iritis à hypopion récidivant. Ann. Oculist. (Paris) 168 (1931) 271–278

Alkemade, P. P. H.: Phenothiazine-Retinopathy. Ophthalmologica 155 (1968) 70–76

Allen, A. C.: Juvenile melanomas of children and adults and melanocarcinomas of children. Arch. Derm. 82 (1960) 325–335

Allen, A. C., S. Spitz: Malignant Melanoma. Cancer (Philadelphia) 6 (1953) 1–45

Ash, J. E.: Epibulbar Tumors. Amer. J. Ophthal. 33 (1950) 1203–1219

Aust, O.: Beiträge zur Trachomforschung. Albrecht v. Graefes Arch. klin. exp. Ophthal. 123 (1929) 93–139

Ayd, F. I., Jr.: Phenothiozines, skin and eye complications. Intern. Drug. Ther. Newsletter 1 (1966)

Azzolini, U.: Streptomycina e tuberkulosi della congiunctiva. Ter. Antibiot. 3 (1933) 43–45; ref. in: Zbl. Ophthal. 62 (1954) 166

Behçet, H.: Über rezidivierende, aphthöse, durch ein Virus verursachte Geschwüre am Mund, am Auge und an den Genitalien. Derm. Wschr. 105 (1937) 1152–1157

Behr, C.: Über Ophthalmomyiasis interna und externa (Die Fliegenlarvenerkrankung des Auges). Klin. Mbl. Augenheilk. 64 (1920) 161–180

Di Bella, V.: Su di un caso di oftalmia blenorragica con metastasi alle articolazioni. Pediatria 31 (1923) 146–150

Bergmann, G., E. Wiedemann: Beobachtungen in 4 Sippen mit Teleangiektasia hereditaria haemorrhagica. Oslersche Krankheit. Dtsch. Arch. klin. Med. 202 (1955) 26–51

Berneaud-Kötz, G.: Augenbeteiligung bei Dys-Paraproteinämien. Enke, Stuttgart 1959

Böke, W.: Kritische Bemerkungen zum Begriff der Keratoconjunktivitis eccematosa. Klin. Mbl. Augenheilk. 130 (1957) 533–536

Böke, W.: Auge und Allergie. In: Der Augenarzt, Vol. VI, ed. by K. Velhagen. Thieme, Berlin 1963 (pp. 436–492)

Borrie, P.: Eczema of the eyelids. Brit. J. Ophthal. 40 (1956) 742–750

Bourquin, J.: Die angeborene Melanose des Auges. Z. Augenheilk. 37 (1917) 129–174; 294–311

Burckhardt, W.: Photoallergische Ekzeme durch Sulfanilamidsalben. Dermatologica 96 (1948) 280–285

Cagianut, B., L. Hoffmann-Egg: Über Augenhintergrundsveränderungen bei Makroglobulinämien. Albrecht v. Graefes Arch. klin. exp. Ophthal. 153 (1953) 391–406

Calamandrei, G., L. Ferrata: Sulla etiologia della manifestazioni oculari dell' eritema nodosa in base alla efficacia della terapia con ormone corticotropo ipofisario. Atti Soc. Oftal. ital. 12 (1951) 243–244

Calmettes, L., F. Déodati: Tuberculose conjunctivale, guérison par la streptomycine. Bull. Soc. Opht. franç. 1950, 197–199

Comberg, W.: Wege der Prophylaxe in der Augenheilkunde. Prophylaxe 2 (1955) 113–118

Conrads, H., G. Kühnhardt: Zur Pathogenese der Lymphangiectasia haemorrhagica conjunctivae. Klin. Mbl. Augenheilk. 131 (1957) 670–674.

Contino, F.: Manifestazione congiuntivale in corsi di eritema nodoso a tipo epidemico. Riv. ital. Tracoma 5 (1953) 155–161

Corwin, M., W. H. Spencer: Conjunctival melanin depositions. Arch. Ophthal. 69 (1963) 317–321

Cown T. H., M. Bulistocky: The Nevus of Ota or Oculodermal Melanocystosis. Arch. Ophthal. 65 (1961) 483–492

Damel, S. C.: Dos formas de tuberculosis ocular. Tuberculoma perforante de la coroides y tuberculosis primitiva de la conjunctiva. Arch. Soc. oftal. hisp.-amer. 11 (1951) 122–135

Dawson, C. R., J. Schachter, E. M. C. Dunlop, M. H. M. Emarah, A. Freedman, J. A. Garland, I. A. Harper, J. W. Race, M. S. du Toit, J. D. Treharne: Infection by a tric agent and other members of the Bedsonia group, with a note on Reiter's disease. Trans. ophthal. Soc. UK 86 (1967) 291–348

Dawson, C. R., J. Schachter, H. B. Ostler, R. M. Gilbert, D. E. Smith, E. P. Engleman: Inclusion conjunctivitis and Reiter's syndrome in a married couple. Arch. Ophthal. (Chicago) 83 (1970) 300–306

Donders, P. C.: Haemorrhagic lymphangiectasia of the conjunctiva. Ophthalmologica 155 (1968) 308–312

Duke-Elder, S.: Anomalies of pigmentation. System of ophthalmology, Vol. III/2. Kimpton, London 1964 (pp. 794–819)

Duke-Elder, S., A. G. Leigh: Pigmented Tumours. System of ophthalmology, Vol. VIII/2. Kimpton, London 1965 (pp. 1210–1239)

Duke-Elder, S.: Diseases of the outer eye. System of ophthalmology VIII: 1. conjunctiva, 2. cornea and sclera. Kimpton, London 1965

Eickemeyer, K. A.: Zur Ophthalmomyiasis interna. Klin. Mbl. Augenheilk. 130 (1957) 95–102

François, J.: L'angiomatose hémorragique familiale et ses complications oculaires. Arch. d'Ophtal. (Paris) 2 (1938) 425–432

François, J., V. Victoria-Troncoso: La conjunctivite ligneuse. Ophthalmologica 154 (1967) 470–482

François, J., M. Hanssens, V. Victoria-Troncoso: Etude pathologique, histochimique, pathogénique et thérapeutique de la conjunctivite ligneuse. Ophthalmologica 155 (1968) 169–185

François, J., M. Rabaey, L. Evens: Tumeurs melaniques de la conjunctive bulbaire. Ophthalmologica 135 (1958) 1–21

Frankland, A. W., D. Earty: Vernal keratoconjunctivitis: an atopic disease. Trans. ophthal. Soc. UK, 91 (1971) 479–482

Fukazawa, A.: Recurrent uveitis associated with erythema nodosum. J. clin. Ophthal. 10 (1956) 978–982

Galeazzi, C.: Tuberculosi congiuntivale rapidamento guarita con streptomicina. Ann. Ottal. 75 (1949) 64; ref. in: Zbl. ges. Ophthal. 53 (1950) 93

Garner, L. L., E. E. Grossmann: Hereditary hemorrhagic teleangiectasis. Amer. J. Ophthal. 41 (1956) 672–679

Gartmann, H.: Naevus und Melanom. Hautarzt 12 (1961 a) 419–424

Gartmann, H.: Über den zellreichen blauen Naevus. Derm. Wschr. 143 (1961 b) 297–307

Gartmann, H., K. Thurm: Juveniles Melanom der Augenbindehaut. Derm. Wschr. 142 (1960) 805–819

Gilbert, W.: Arbeiten aus der Pathologie der Uveitis mit besonderer Berücksichtigung der Ophthalmia lenta. Albrecht v. Graefes Arch. klin. exp. Ophthal. 152 (1952) 399–412.

Greer, C. H.: Precancerous Melanosis. Proc. roy. Soc. Med. 47 (1954) 730–734

Hamburger, F. A.: Tularaemia oculo-glandularis. Z. Augenheilk. 92 (1937) 249–250

Hartmann, K.: Über ektogene Bindehauttuberkulose durch bovine Tuberkelbazillen und ihre Behandlung mittels Elektrokoagulation. Klin. Mbl. Augenheilk. 113 (1948) 20–28

Hartmann, K.: Über die Erkrankungen des Auges durch Fliegenlarven. Klin. Mbl. Augenheilk. 125 (1954) 227–230

Hausmann, W., H. Haxthausen: Lichterkrankungen der Haut. Sonderband der Strahlentherapie. Urban & Schwarzenberg, Berlin 1929

Heerfordt, C. F.: Über subconjunktivitis epibulbaris gonorrhoica. Albrecht v. Graefes Arch. klin. exp. Ophthal. 72 (1909) 344–366

Heerfordt, C. F.: Über endogene gonorrhoische Hornhaut- und Hautaffektionen. Albrecht v. Graefes Arch. klin. exp. Ophthal. 77 (1910) 145–184

Hegner, A.: Schwere Hornhautnekrosen bei Salvarsanvergiftung. Klin. Mbl. Augenheilk. 59 (1917) 624–636

Heimann, K., G. Terheggen: Augensymptome beim Louis-Bar-Syndrom. 69. Ber. dtsch. ophthal. Ges. 1969, 139–145

Heydenreich, A.: Die Lymphangiectasia haemorrhagica conjunctivae. Klin. Mbl. Augenheilk. 128 (1956) 83–85

Hidano, A., H. Kajima, S. Ideka, S. Mizutani, H. Miyasato, M. Niimura: Natural history of nevus of Ota. Arch. Derm. Syph. (Chicago) 95 (1967) 187–195

Hoffmann, D. H.: Pilzinfektionen des Auges. Fortschr. Augenheilk. 16 (1965) 63–217

Howard, G. M.: The Stevens-Johnson-syndrome. Amer. J. Ophthal. 55 (1963) 893–900

Hruby, K.: Über eine teratoide Geschwulst der oberen Übergangsfalte in Verbindung mit Enophthalmus congenitus und anderen Anomalien. Albrecht v. Graefes Arch. klin. exp. Ophthal. 143 (1941) 456–465

Jaensch, P. A.: Verletzungen, physikalische Schädigungen und Giftwirkungen. In: Der Augenarzt, Vol. V, ed. by K. Velhagen. Thieme, Leipzig 1963 (pp. 837–946)

Jay, B.: Naevi und melanomata of the conjunctiva. Brit. J. Ophthal. 49 (1965 a) 169–204

Jay, B.: The pathology of surface melanomata of the eye. Trans. ophthal. Soc. U. K. 84 (1965 b) 337–356

Jones, B. R., M. K. Al. Hussaini, E. M. C. Dunlop, M. H. M. Emarah, A. Freedman, J. A. Garland, J. A. Harper, J. W. Race, M. S. du Toit, J. D. Teharne: Infection by tric agent and other members of the Bedsonia group; with a note on Reiter's disease. Trans. ophthal. Soc. U. K. 86 (1967) 291–348

Katzenelson, A.: Ein Fall von Hypopyon-Iritis recidivans bei Erythema nodosum. Russk. oftal. z. 4 (1925) 484

Knisley, M. H., L. Warner: Thrombose und Embolie. Schwabe, Basel 1955

Krassai, A.: Über oculare Manifestationen der Bowens Disease. Klin. Mbl. Augenheilk. 154 (1969) 411–422

Kratka, W.: Episcleritis and erythema nodosum. Amer. J. Ophthal. 36 (1953) 510–513

Kreibig, W.: Die Extraktion subkonjunktivaler Loa-Loa-Filarien, ein dringlicher augenärztlicher Eingriff. Klin. Mbl. Augenheilk. 147 (1965) 65–69

Krümmel, H., A. Braus: Myiasis des Auges. Duncker & Humblot, Berlin 1956

Kuske, H.: Perkutane Photosensibilisierung durch pflanzliche Wirkstoffe. Dermatologica 82 (1940) 273–338

Liebmann, S. D.: Ocular manifestations of Riley-Day syndrome. Familial autonomic dysfunction. Arch. Ophthal. 56 (1956) 719–725

Löwenstein, A.: Some aspects of ocular melanotic growth. Brit. J. Ophthal. 33 (1949) 525–543

Lund, H., J. Kraus: Melanotic tumors of the skin. Washington Armed Forces Institute of Pathology 1962

Marchesani, O.: Das Problem der phlyktaenulären Augenkrankheit. Klin. Wschr. 1947, 865–868

Martini, E.: Lehrbuch der medizinischen Entomologie, 3rd Ed. Fischer, Jena 1946

Merté, H. J.: Arbeitsmedizinische Fragen in der Ophthalmologie. Karger, Basel 1969
Merté, H. J.: Arbeits- u. Sozialmedizin. In: Lehrbuch der Augenheilkunde, T. Axenfeld, H. Pau. Fischer, Stuttgart 1973
Meyer, Fr. W.: Keratomalacie bei schwerer Salvarsandermatitis. Albrecht v. Graefes Arch. klin. exp. Ophthal. 143 (1941) 332–336
Miles, N. E.: Hereditary hemorrhagic teleangiectasia. Amer. J. Ophthal. 35 (1952) 543–546
Mooney, D.: Pigmentation after long-term topical use of adrenaline compounds. Brit. J. Ophthal. 54 (1970) 823–826
Morgan, G.: The pathology of vernal conjunctivitis. Trans. ophthal. Soc. UK, 91 (1971) 467–478
Neumann, E., M. J. Gutmann, N. Blumenkrantz, I. C. Michaelson: A review of four hundred cases of vernal conjunctivitis. Amer. J. Ophthal. 47 (1959) 166–172
Nover, A.: Über die als Conjunctivitis lignosa bezeichnete chronische pseudomembranöse Bindehautentzündung. Klin. Mbl. Augenheilk. 145 (1964) 221–233
Nover, A.: Augenveränderungen bei generalisierter hyperergischer Gefäßwandentzündung (Arteriolitis obliterans, Periarteriitis nodosa). Klin. Mbl. Augenheilk. 121 (1952) 297–306
Oppel, O.: Geschwulstähnliche Entartungen der Bindehaut. Klin. Mbl. Augenheilk. 128 (1956) 145–158
Oppel, O.: Augenbeteiligung bei Toxikodermie. Ber. dtsch. ophthal. Ges. 65 (1964) 52–60
Pesch, K. J., A. Wessing: Augenveränderungen beim Lyell-Syndrom. Ophthalmologica 153 (1967) 81–92
Pitter, J.: Eine seltene Lokalisation der Oslerschen Krankheit unter der Bindehaut. Klin. Mbl. Augenheilk. 107 (1941) 76–80
Prizi, O.: Arthritis gonorrhoica nach Blennorrhoea neonatorum. Wien. Klin. Wschr. 37 (1924) 51, 1312–1313
Raïs, H.: Auréomycine et conjunctivite gonococcique. Rev. int. Trachome 29 (1952) 165–170
Reese, A. B.: Praecancerous and cancerous melanosis of the conjunctiva. Amer. J. Ophthal. 39 (1955) 96–100
Reese, A. B.: Tumors of the eye, 2nd. Ed. Harper & Row, New York 1963 (pp. 214–263)
Reich, H., G. Jünemann: Das Debré-Lamy-Lyell-Syndrom. Klin. Mbl. Augenheilk. 157 (1970) 358–365
Reis, W.: Augenerkrankung und Erythema nodosum. Klin. Mbl. Augenheilk. 44 (1906) 203–224
Renard, G., C. Haye, C. Henriot: Contribution à l'étude des accidents oculaires imputés au B. C. G. Rev. Tuberc. (Paris) 22 (1958) 383–392; ref. in: Zbl. ges. Ophthal. 76 (1959) 186
Riehm, W.: Zur Beurteilung der Tuberkulin-Empfindlichkeit bei der scrophulösen Augenentzündung. Klin. Mbl. Augenheilk. 121 (1952) 454–463
Riehm, W.: Die Mitwirkung unspezifischer Reize bei der Pathogenese der scrophulösen Augenentzündung. Klin. Mbl. Augenheilk. 122 (1953) 292–296
Riehm, W.: Erkrankungen des Auges und Allergie. In: Allergie, ed. by K. Hansen. Thieme, Stuttgart 1957 (pp. 954–996)
Rintelen, F.: Diskussionsbemerkung zu: Dégénerescence pigmentaire de la rétine d'origine médicamenteuse (F. Verrey). Ophthalmologica 131 (1956) 296–303
Rodenhäuser, J. H.: Über die Augenpigmentierungen bei Alkaptonurie (Ochronosis oculi). Klin. Mbl. Augenheilk. 131 (1957) 202–215
Röth, A. v.: Bindehautaffektion bei Erythema nodosum. Z. Augenheilk. 66 (1928) 323–327
Roth, J. H.: Luminal poisoning with conjunctival residue. Amer. J. Ophthal. 9 (1926) 533–534
Sallmann, L.: Über die Augenpigmentierung bei endogener Ochronose. Z. Augenheilk. 60 (1926) 164–171
Samuels, B.: Melanosis oculi und sektorenförmige Melanose mit Melanosarkom der Chorioidea. Albrecht v. Graefes Arch. klin. exp. Ophthal. 154 (1953–1954) 361–367
Sautter, H.: Fleckfieber und Auge. Klin. Mbl. Augenheilk. 109 (1943) 24–32
Schlossberger, H.: Experimentelle Bakteriologie und Infektionskrankheiten. Ed. by W. Kolle, H. Hetsch, H. Schlossberger. Urban & Schwarzenberg, München 1952
Schmidt, J. G. H., G. Lischka: Augenveränderungen bei den Syndromen nach E. Fuchs, A. Lyell. Ber. Vers. Rhein.-Westf. Augenärzte 120 (1969) 88–97
Schmidt, J. G. H., G. Lischka: Zur ophthalmologischen Symptomatologie, Therapie und Prognose des Fuchs-Lyell-Syndroms. Klin. Mbl. Augenheilk. 157 (1970) 342–357
Schreck, E.: Veränderungen des Sehorgans bei Haut- und Geschlechtskrankheiten. In: Dermatologie und Venerologie, Vol. IV, ed. by H. A. Gottron, W. Schönfeld. Thieme, Stuttgart 1960 (pp. 831–945)
Seitz, R.: Über die ochronosischen Pigmentierungen am Auge. Klin. Mbl. Augenheilk. 125 (1954) 432–444
Seitz, R.: Erkrankungen der Netzhaut und ihrer Gefäße bei Allgemeinleiden. Almanach für Augenheilkunde. Lehmann, München 1969 (pp. 75–92)
Sidi, E., E. Mawas: Les dermites allergiques des paupières. Bull. Soc. Ophtal. Paris 1953, 246–255
Siegert, E. J.: Zur klinischen und serologischen Diagnostik der gonorrhoischen Iritis. Albrecht v. Graefes Arch. klin. exp. Ophthal. 140 (1939) 303–327
Spitz, S.: Melanomas of childhood. Amer. J. Path. 24 (1948) 491–609
Stajduhar, J., K. Pansini: Die Bedeutung der Veränderungen am Augenhintergrund für die Ätiologie des Erythema nodosum. Ber. dtsch. ophthal. Ges. 57 (1951) 7–11
Starke, H.: Primäre Bindehauttuberkulose. Klin. Wschr. 1949, 151
Stepanik, J.: Periodisch im Schlaf auftretende spontane Blutfüllung der Bindehautlymphräume als Begleitsymptom eines Lymphhämangioms der Parotis. Klin. Mbl. Augenheilk. 132 (1958) 99–103
Stock, W.: Zur Therapie der Konjunctivitis Parinaud. Klin. Mbl. Augenheilk. 87 (1931) 525–526
Strehl, C.: Zum Weltgesundheitstag „Blindheitsverhütung". Klin. Mbl. Augenheilk. 140 (1962) 425–427
Suurküla, J.: Durch Dipterenlarven verursachte Augenkrankheit (Ophthalmomyiasis). Bücherei des Augenarztes, 13. Enke, Stuttgart 1942
Tanner, O. R.: Ocular manifestations of infectious mononucleosis. Arch. Ophthal. 51 (1954) 229–241
Thiel, R.: Die bösartigen Geschwülste der Bindehaut. Bücherei des Augenarztes, 44 (1965) 154–178
Thomas, Ch., J. Cordier, B. Algan: La tularémie oculoganglionnaire. Arch. d'Ophtal. (Paris) 12 (1952) 19–41
Tost, M.: Beitrag zur Dysplasia oculo-auriculo-vertebralis. Klin. Mbl. Augenheilk. 154 (1969) 183–193

Tow, A.: Erythema nodosum and phlyctenular conjunctivitis in a case of hilus gland tuberculosis. Arch. Pediat. 45 (1928) 687–691

Ullerich, K., K. Wulf, A. Wiskemann: Augenaffektionen infolge Lichtsensibilisierung durch eine photodynamisch wirksame Substanz. Klin. Mbl. Augenheilk. 131 (1957) 30–48

Vail, D. T., Jr.: Oculo-glandular form of tularemia. Arch. Ophthal. 2 (1929) 416–430

Vannas, S., K. Lapinleimu: Molluscum contagiosum in the skin, caruncle and conjunctiva. Acta Ophthal. 45 (1967) 314–321

Veltišev, Z.: Erythema nodosum conjunctivae bulbi. Russk. oftal. Z. 4 (1925) 619–621

Verhoeff, F. H.: A case of ligneous conjunctivitis now 36 years in duration. Amer. J. Ophthal. 45 (1958) 246–251

Verrey, F.: Dégénérescence pigmentaire de la retine d'origine médicamenteuse. Ophthalmologica 131 (1956) 296–303

Wagner, P.: Untersuchungen über die Wirkung von Phenothiazinderivaten auf den Augenhintergrund des Tieres. Klin. Mbl. Augenheilk. 129 (1956) 772–781

Wahlberg, K.: Über Arthritis gonorrhoica beim Säugling. Münch. med. Wschr. 72 (1925) 770–771

Wessely, C.: Beitrag zur Kenntnis der Konjunktivaltuberkulose. Vers. Ophthal. Ges. Heidelberg 36 (1910) 81–89

Witmer, R.: Conjunktivaveränderungen beim Morbus Osler. Ophthalmologica (Basel) 121 (1951) 158–159

Wohra, K. C.: Ophthalmia neonatorum. Indian Med. J. 45 (1951) 117–118

13 Cornea

Pathologic Changes in Corneal Size and Curvature

The cornea sits in the sclera like a watch glass. At the limbus it is covered for 1 to 3 mm by conjunctiva and perilimbic vessels. Corneal thickness is 0.8 to 1 mm. Its horizontal diameter is 11.5 mm and the vertical diameter is 10.5 mm. The corneal radius is 7.7 mm.

Large cornea (megalocornea or macrocornea; buphthalmos) — Small cornea (microcornea) and cornea plana — Keratoconus — Keratoglobus — Keratotorus, Terrien's marginal ulceration.

Large Cornea

Megalocornea or **macrocornea** (diameter over 13 mm) is a congenital anomaly sometimes associated with posterior embryotoxon.
Megalocornea is differentiated from buphthalmos by its normal intraocular pressure, flat cornea, normal limbus, regular astigmatism, normal chamber angle, pupil, and bilateral involvement.
Buphthalmos or **hydrophthalmos** (Fig. 19.7) occurs with congenital or infantile glaucoma. The corneal diameter may increase up to 16 mm. There is thinning of the cornea, especially at the limbus, so that it ruptures easily. Tears of Descemet are characteristic (Haab's striae) (Fig. 13.10). If the pressure remains elevated, the cornea becomes edematous (see page 145). Megalocornea and buphthalmos are rarely found within the same family.

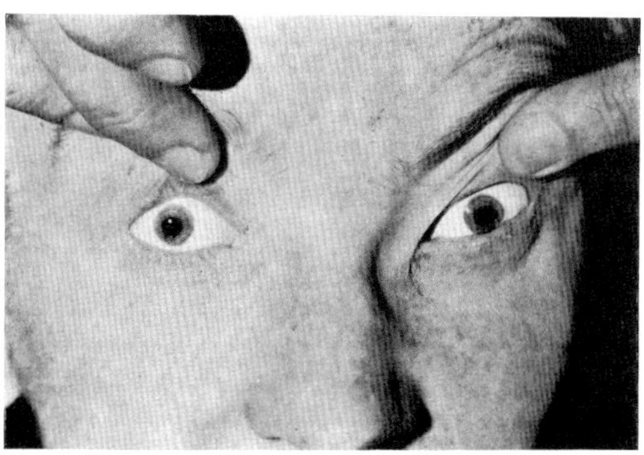

Fig. 13.1 Microcornea (♂ 26 yrs.)

Small Cornea (Diameter under 10 mm [Fig. 13.1])

Microcornea usually occurs as part of microphthalmos (along with nystagmus and amblyopia, and a tendency to develop glaucoma) (see page 228). Microcornea is acquired when the globe shrinks (phthisis bulbi), a phenomenon usually associated with severe corneal clouding. Scar formation may cause a flat cornea.
Cornea plana occurs in otherwise normal eyes; it is hereditary. Frequently there is scleralization of the peripheral cornea giving the appearance of microcornea (Forsius 1961). The border between sclera and clear cornea is indistinct. There is corneal hyperopia.

Keratoconus

Keratoconus (Fig. 13.2) may begin in early childhood but usually presents after puberty. The central cornea is progressively ectatic. Vertical gray "stress" lines appear at the apex of the cone. A pigmented ring runs around the base of the cone (Fleischer ring).
The central cornea becomes scarred and cloudy (Fig. 13.3). Descemet's ridges may form in the area of the cone. The disorder is almost invariably bilateral but may be asymmetric in onset and severity. Women are more often affected than men. Keratoconus has been described in association with retinitis pigmentosa, glaucoma, corneal dystrophies, nuclear cataracts, blue sclera, aniridia, Marfan's syndrome (Günther 1958), vernal catarrh and palmoplantar keratosis.

Keratoconus occurs in about 6 percent of patients with Down's syndrome (Skeller and Oster 1951). Other ocular findings in Down's syndrome include (Woillez and Dansaut 1960): epicanthus with mongoloid slant, keratoconus (often acute), blue iris with Brushfield spots, hyperopia (often with strabismus), and various lens opacities.

Keratoconus has a variable inheritance (Franceschetti et al. 1958).

Blue sclera and lens subluxation (see page 181), found in Ehlers–Danlos syndrome, are potentially associated with keratoconus.

Descemet's membrane may rupture acutely at the apex of the cone, producing sudden, marked corneal edema (*acute keratoconus*, Fig. 13.4) (Rohrschneider and Stohr 1954; Böke and Conrads 1957; Günther 1958 and others). The disk-shaped area of central corneal edema resembles herpetic disciform keratitis. Acute keratoconus is frequent in patients with Down's syndrome (Hofmann 1956). Once the Descemet tears have healed, the corneal edema resolves with residual scarring. The differential diagnosis includes birth trauma (see page 146) and disciform keratitis.

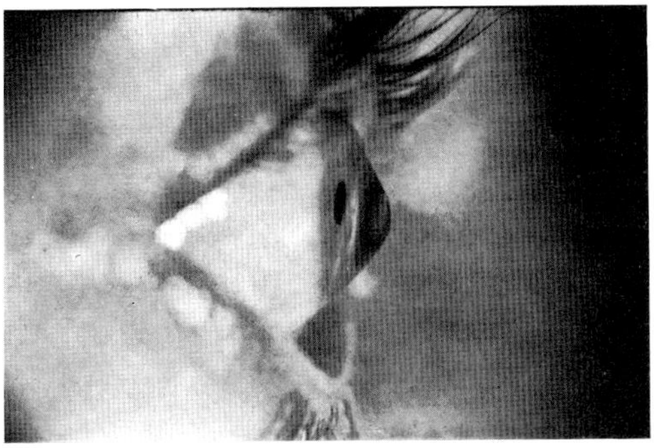

Fig. 13.2 Keratoconus (♀ 49 yrs.)

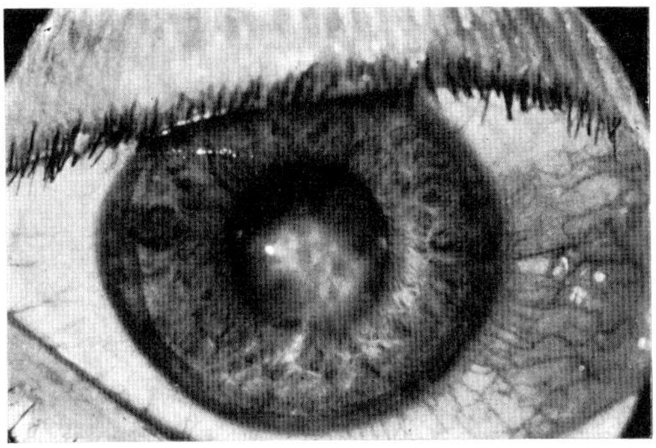

Fig. 13.3 Keratoconus with apical scarring (♀ 25 yrs.)

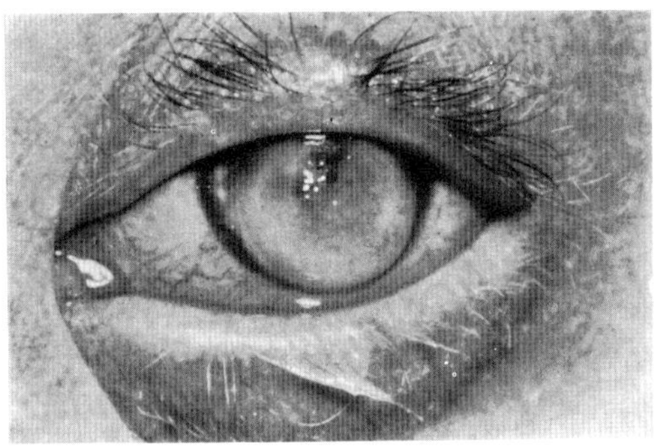

Fig. 13.4 "Acute" keratoconus (♂ 17 yrs.)

Keratoglobus

Keratoglobus (Fig. 13.5) is a bilateral condition beginning in childhood. The entire corneal stroma, especially the periphery, is thin and ectatic. Near the limbus the clear stroma may be one third its normal thickness. The corneal ectasia results in a forward bulging of the entire cornea (Fig. 13.5). Descemet's ruptures occur acutely (acute keratoglobus) (Verrey 1947; Hallerman 1970; Grayson 1963). There is no elevation of intraocular tension and the globe is normal in size.

Keratotorus or Piriform Cornea; Terrien's Marginal Ulceration

Pellucid marginal degeneration (François et al. 1968) is a bilateral, progressive central corneal thinning with protrusion of the cornea inferiorly (Fig. 13.6) to within 1 to 2 mm of the limbus. It is also known as *pear-shaped cornea* (piriform) or keratotorus (Hallermann 1970). The increasing astigmatism causes deterioration of vision. The cornea does not vascularize or develop lipid deposits (François et al. 1968). François et al. found histochemical changes of the mucopolysaccharides. There is a genetic correlation between keratoconus, keratoglobus and keratotorus (Lisch 1970).

Terrien's marginal ulceration occurs at any age, usually after age ten. One third of the affected persons are under the age of forty

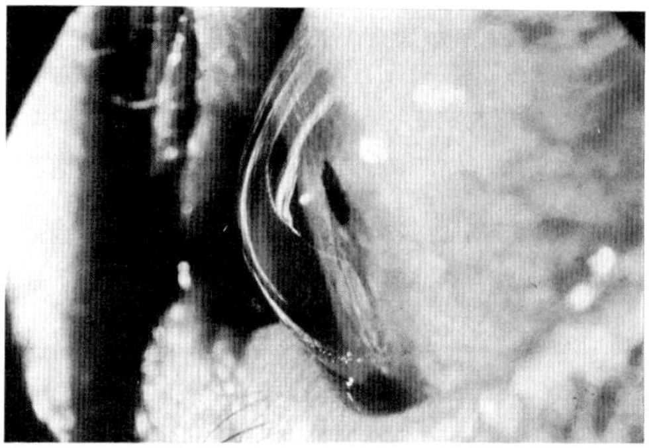

Fig. 13.5 Keratoglobus (♂ 26 yrs.)

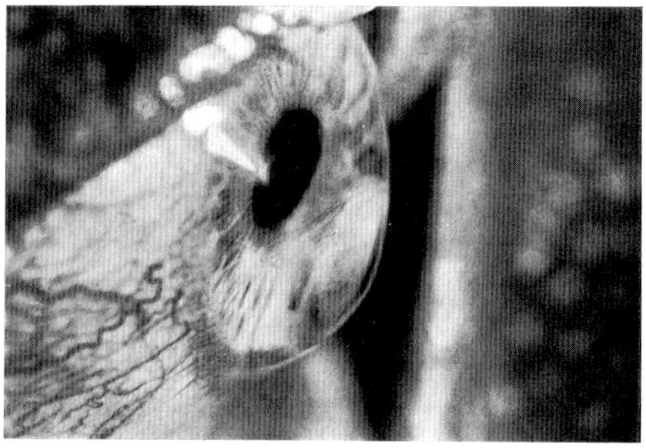

Fig. 13.6 Keratotorus (♂ 51 yrs.)

(Duke-Elder 1965). There is a superficial opacification and vascularization near the limbus in the area of arcus senilis. This is followed by

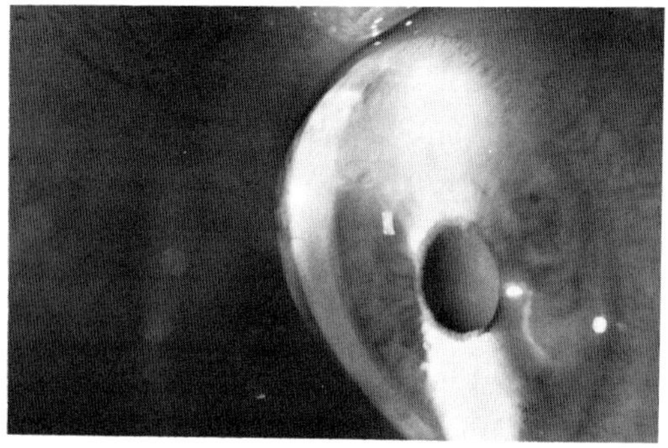

Fig. 13.7 Terrien's marginal ulcer (♀ 42 yrs.)

localized ectasia and thinning which may perforate the cornea (Fig. 13.7). This may be a disturbance of mucopolysaccharides (Nagy 1971).

Posterior Keratoconus

Posterior keratoconus is a congenital, usually central, corneal thinning caused by a reduction in the radius of curvature of the posterior cornea. The anterior corneal curvature remains normal. The cornea may be clear or hazy. Posterior keratoconus may be general or circumscribed (Karlin and Wise 1961; Haney and Falls 1961).

Corneal Reflex Patterns

The cornea is composed of a layer of stratified squamous epithelium, Bowman's membrane, substantia propria with collagen fiber bundles and keratocytes, Descemet's membrane and a single layer of endothelial cells.

When the corneal reflex is dull, the corneal erosions *stain green with fluorescein*. The corneal reflex (placido disk, keratometer) can be (Fig. 13.8):

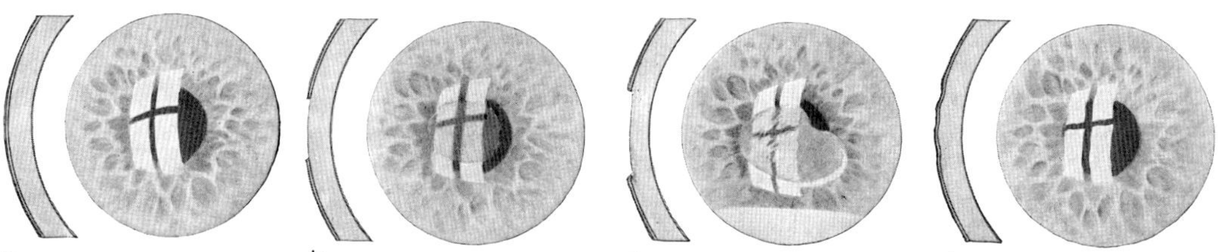

a b c d

Fig. 13.8 Corneal reflex patterns (from R. Thiel: Atlas of Diseases of the Eye, 6th Ed., Thieme, Stuttgart 1963)

a) smooth, glistening = normal cornea
b) smooth, dull (blurred) = epithelial defect = erosion
c) distorted and dull = fresh epithelial and stromal defect (ulcer)
d) distorted, shiny = surface irregularities = irregular astigmatism, stromal scarring = bullous keratopathy

surface stippling = epithelial edema (corneal edema, inflammation, glaucoma attack)
regular astigmatism = congenital anomaly of corneal curvature
irregular astigmatism = acquired, scarring (healed ulcer, injury, etc.).

Changes in Corneal Transparency

The cornea normally contains 72 percent to 82 percent water and is birefringent. There are no blood or lymph vessels. The strong sensory innervation makes the cornea very sensitive to touch and pain.

Infiltrates; scarring — Stromal edema — Corneal edema with glaucoma — Epithelial inclusions — Descemet tears — Superficial striate opacities (alphabet keratitis) — Endothelial deposits — Posterior embryotoxon — Arcus senilis — White limbal girdle (Vogt) — Corneal nerves.

Infiltrates; Scarring

In direct light the cornea has a gray color. Corneal *infiltrates* appear gray to yellow, *scars* are *gray-white*. On transillumination corneal scars and infiltrates appear as dark spots in the red fundus reflex.

Nubecula is minimal scarring, *macula*, a distinct scar; *leukoma*, a white dense scar. Leukomas appear with iris adhesions, elevated pressure, staphyloma or as part of extensive congenital malformations, such as embryopathies (see page 244), prenatal inflammation and dermoids. Sclerocornea is a congenital opacification without vascularization, scarring or inflammation.

Leukoma adherens is caused by a traumatic iridocorneal adhesion. Old leukomas frequently develop hyaline, lipid or calcareous deposits. Irregular, yellow-brown pigment lines develop around the scar.

Coat's rings are small white dots arranged in a ring at the level of or in Bowman's membrane (Bonnet-Gehin and Tavernier 1963).

Peter's anomaly is a central corneal opacity with adherence of pupillary membrane remnants and a defect in Descemet's membrane (Fig. 13.9). The anterior chamber is usually shallow. Microphthalmos or buphthalmos and retinal folds are associated findings (Badtke 1961).

Stromal Edema

Any traumatic or degenerative endothelial damage causes a greater or lesser degree of stromal edema. Epithelial damage produces a minimal amount of stromal swelling. The cornea appears gray in the area of edema. *Descemet's folds* occur with acute swelling and are a reflection of hypotony.

Descemet's folds do not occur with corneal edema caused by glaucoma. With the slit lamp, Descemet's folds are easily recognized as two parallel light reflexes.

Corneal Edema

Corneal edema due to elevated intraocular pressure (acute glaucoma, secondary glauco-

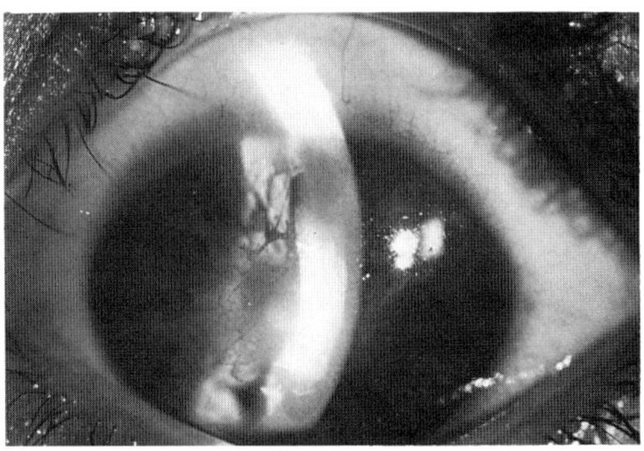

Fig. 13.9 Peter's anomaly with deep paracentral corneal opacity and adherent pupillary membrane (♂ 3½ yrs.)

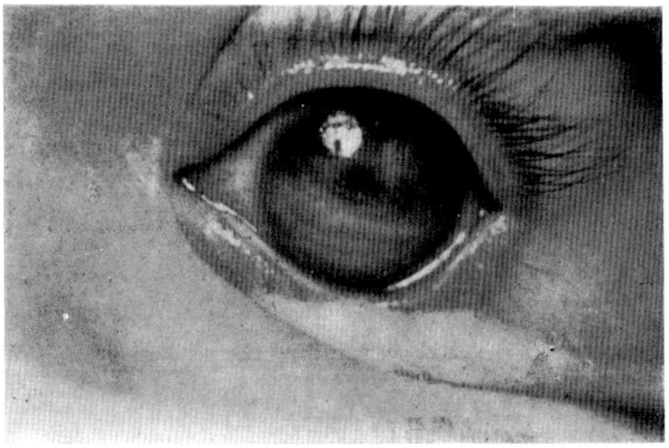

Fig. 13.10 Descemet tears with overlying corneal edema in buphthalmos (♂ 5 months)

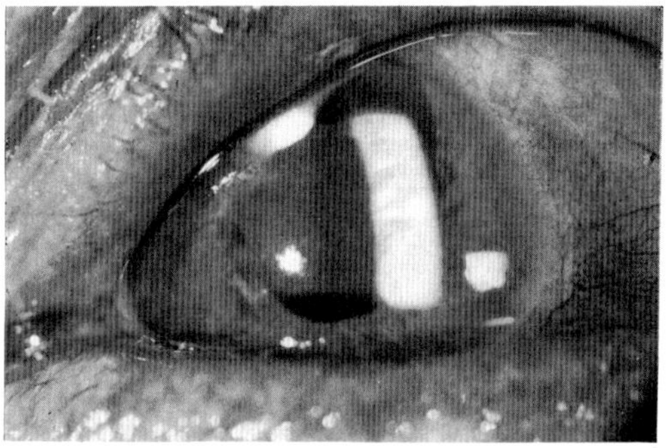

Fig. 13.11 Alphabet keratitis with hypotony from chronic cyclitis (♀ 72 yrs.)

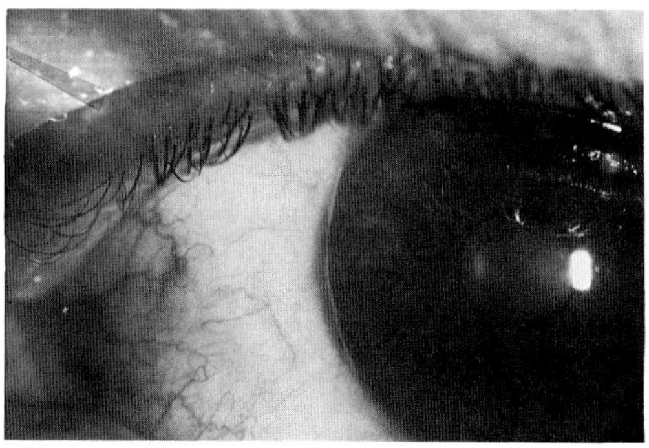

Fig. 13.12 Posterior embryotoxon (♀ 40 yrs.)

ma) does not cause Descemet folds. The cornea becomes dull and loses its normal sheen. On slit lamp examination, the epithelium shows dropletlike swelling which becomes confluent and may rupture. With early epithelial edema the patient subjectively notices colored halos around lights and progressive clouding of vision. Excessive wearing of poor fitting contact lenses can produce a similar epithelial edema.

Epithelial Inclusions

Epithelial implantation (trauma, surgery) into the anterior chamber causes stromal edema in those areas where it grows over the endothelium (Pau and Fernholz 1963, Paufique and Hervoquet 1964). Secondary glaucoma results.

Descemet Tears

On the slit lamp, Descemet tears appear as double contour lines. They are usually old scars, glassy white in appearance, without corneal edema. Descemet tears occur with buphthalmos (Fig. 13.10), keratoconus and trauma, such as in forceps delivery. Descemet's membrane may regenerate abnormally as Descemet ridges or tubules.

Alphabet Keratitis

The etiology of alphabet keratitis (Fig. 13.11) is *hypotony*, following contusion injury, surgery, perforation, iridocyclitis, or phthisis bulbi. There is a crisscrossing of horizontal and vertical lines and gray opacities at the level of Bowman's membrane. Histologically, the corneal epithelium fills in depressions and folds in Bowman's membrane, thereby maintaining a smooth surface.

Endothelial Deposits

When thick, endothelial precipitates (Fig. 16.15) resemble gray opacities. Otherwise, they appear as a fine powder of random cells or fibrin. They may deposit in a line, spindleshape, triangle (apex to center of cornea) or circle (see page 174). The precipitates are often pigmented as with the Kruckenberg's spindle, old iritis and in diabetes mellitus. In time they may be covered by endothelium and new Descemet, giving a glassy appearance.

Posterior Embryotoxon

A prominent ring of Schwalbe visible externally on slit lamp examination occurs in 10 percent of patients (Burian). It is called posterior embryotoxon (Axenfeld) when iris processes adhere to it (Fig. 13.12). Both are a congenital anomaly (Streiff 1949).

Arcus Senilis

Arcus senilis is synonymous with gerontoxon or anterior embryotoxon (see page 164) (Fig. 13.13).

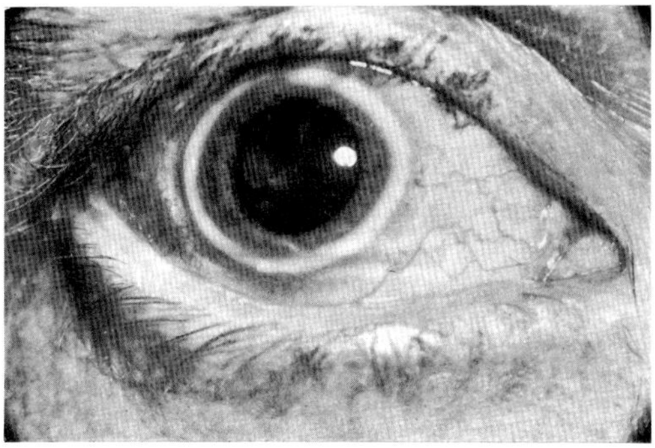

Fig. 13.13 Arcus senilis

White Limbal Girdle (Vogt)

Vogt (1931) described a white girdle at the limbus (Plate VIII, Fig. 3, page 128 h). The lesion is superficial and usually nasal or temporal (Collier 1961).

Corneal Nerves

Increased visibility and thickness of corneal nerves occurs with: neurofibromatosis, ichthyosis, Refsum syndrome, keratoconus, Fuchs' endothelial dystrophy, posterior polymorphous dystrophy, leprosy, and following chloroquine therapy (Pau and Bäumer 1959). It also occurs congenitally.

Corneal Sensitivity

The extreme sensitivity of the corneal surface (blink reflex) is increased or decreased in various diseases. Herpes simplex, neuroparalytic keratitis (loss of trigeminal innervation), and leprosy (see page 94) cause marked corneal anesthesia. A minor decrease in sensitivity is part of any stromal edema (disciform keratitis, acute keratoconus, interstitial keratitis) and with vascularized scars (after burns, trachoma, pemphigus). Corneal hypoesthesia is also seen with: ophthalmic zoster, damage of the trigeminal nerve or gasserian ganglion, superior orbital fissure syndrome, corneal dystrophies (granular, macular, lattice), malaria, psoriasis, hydroa vacciniforme, and diabetes. It occurs postoperatively after cataract extraction, retinal detachment procedures (especially with encircling bands), extensive cyclodiathermy (for glaucoma), keratoplasty, radiation damage, hydrogen sulfide or carbon disulfide injury, or congenitally.

Ciliary Injection

Any keratitis causes a red-blue, pericorneal (ciliary), injection (see page 120) (Plate I, Fig. 1, page 128 a).

Corneal Vascularization (Plate I, Fig. 1, page 128 a)

Deep vessels — Superficial vessels (pannus).

Deep Vascularization

Deep corneal vascularization results from inflammatory corneal edema. The vessels appear abruptly at the limbus and grow into the cornea in a brush-like pattern without anastomoses. They give the cornea a fleshy appearance (see page 155). The most common causes are interstitial keratitis (parenchymatous keratitis), thermal and severe chemical burns (especially lye or strong acids).

Superficial Vascularization (Pannus)

These are a continuation of conjunctival vessels. They are freely anastomosing and are at the level of Bowman's membrane. The most common cause is *trachoma*. The trachomatous pannus (see page 130) (Plate VII, Fig. 2, page 128 g) (epaulet pannus) hangs down from above like a curtain. *Phlyctenules* (see pages 132, 162) (tuberculosis, allergy, staphylococcal) may develop irregular, superficial vascularization (Plate IX, Figs. 4, 5, page 192 a). The residual scars remain for years, develop Fuchs' lines of clearing (Fig. 13.33), brown pigmentation, and irregular astigmatism.
Acne rosacea (see page 162) is associated with superficial and deep vascularization, and corneal infiltrates (Plate IX, Fig. 6, page 192 a). The vessels are tortuous and reach past the corneal infiltrate onto clear cornea.

Thermal and chemical *burns* frequently cause superficial or deep vascularization.
Vitamin B deficiency can cause a superficial, bilateral, perilimbic vascularization (Mann 1945) (Plate X, Fig. 1, page 192 b). Vitamin B_2 deficiency primarily has conjunctival and corneal involvement. Polyneuritis, lid and conjunctival inflammations occur in beriberi. Vitamin B_2 is a complex of riboflavin, nicotinic acid, pantothenic acid (B_{12}) and pyridoxine.

Pellagra is associated with conjunctival and corneal inflammation: superficial punctate keratitis with pannus, photophobia, or disturbance of extraocular muscles.
Ariboflavinosis causes superficial circular vascularization at the limbus. Corneal infiltrates are rare.

Experimentally, similar vascularization is produced by diets deficient in essential amino acids (tryptophan, leucine, phenylalanine). The same clinical picture is found with zinc and salt deficiency (Stern 1950).
A *pterygium* is also vascularized.
A *degenerative pannus* develops after severe ocular inflammation. Absolute glaucoma or trauma are examples.
Metaherpetic or disciform keratitis is associated with a very slowly developing vascularization. A single or few large vessels cross the clear corneal periphery to invade the infiltrate.
Vascularization occurs when an inflammatory lesion is within 3 mm of the limbus. On healing, the vessels become occluded but may still be seen by slit lamp as gray (ghost) lines.

Corneal Erosion

Corneal erosion from physical or chemical damage — Recurrent erosions — Corneal contusion — Superficial punctate keratitis — Filamentary keratitis — Superficial herpetic keratitis.

Corneal Erosion from Physical and Chemical Injury

Corneal erosion from any cause produces severe pain, foreign body sensation, photophobia, lacrimation, and blepharospasm. Ciliary injection and possibly pupillary constriction (iritis) occur. The corneal reflex is not distorted but dull in the area of the erosion. The epithelial defect stains green with fluorescein. The most common etiology is direct foreign body injury. Foreign bodies trapped beneath the upper lid may be at fault (sand, dust, hairs, pieces of insects, etc.). These characteristically cause parallel vertical linear erosions. Calcareous meibomian gland infarcts and trichiasis should be considered. A molluscum contagiosum of the lids can cause recurrent corneal erosions (Nover 1950). Even if no foreign body is found, vertical linear erosions that stain with fluorescein are proof that it was present (usually under the upper lid). With any ocular injury it must be remembered that perforation could occur. The situation is obvious when the anterior chamber is lost, the iris prolapsed, the lens cataractous and swollen, or if hypotony is present. Roentgenograms should be taken even with minimal signs or symptoms if the history (hammering, high speed tools) warrants it.

Recurrent Erosions

Recurrent erosions may occur days, weeks or months after corneal injury. For no apparent reason, the patient awakens during the night or in the morning with severe pain, photophobia, and blepharospasm upen opening his eyes., Presumably the adhesion between epithelium and underlying tissue was insufficient. During the healing phase slit lamp examination reveals small vacuoles between Bowman's membrane and the epithelium.

Tears evaporate at night allowing slight adhesion between corneal epithelium and lid. If the epithelium is not firmly attached to the underlying cornea, it pulls off when the lid is opened. Recurrent erosions occur more frequently if the injury is caused by organic material (leaves, twigs, wood, etc.) (Pau 1963).

Corneal erosions have been found to be hereditary in a large family (Franceschetti 1928) and in two siblings aged 11 and 12 (Remler 1959).

Corneal Contusion

Depending on its severity, contusion injury to the cornea produces corneal *erosion, epithelial* and *stromal edema* (forceps births [see page 158]). Ring-shaped endothelial destruction is also seen. If the injury is more extensive, folds appear in Descemet's membrane. Severe trauma can cause Descemet tears and anterior chamber hemorrhage with hemosiderosis of the cornea (see page 173). Traumatic injuries, just like burns or chemical injury normally are not a differential diagnostic problem.

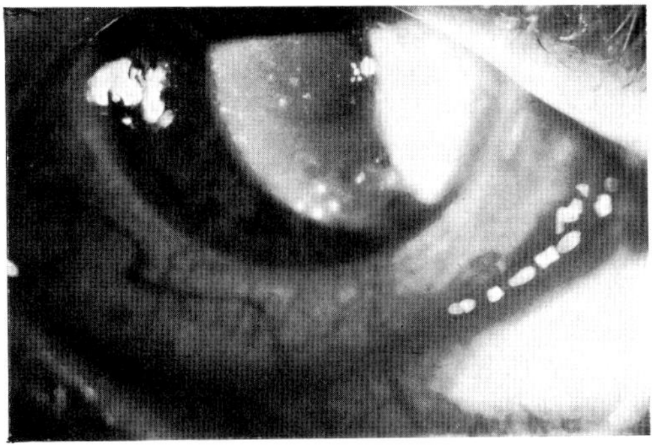

Fig. 13.14 Superficial punctate keratitis (♂ 51 yrs.)

Superficial Punctate Keratitis

Superficial punctate keratitis from physical and chemical injury, occupational disease — Sjögren's syndrome, vitamin B deficiency, avitaminosis A — Keratoconjunctivitis sicca from other causes — Viruses (viral conjunctivitis and superficial punctate keratitis) — Drugs (drug-induced superficial punctate keratitis) — Superficial punctate keratitis in infectious disease.

In superficial punctate keratitis the corneal epithelium develops numerous punctate fluorescein positive erosions (Fig. 13.14) (Jones 1961). Other findings include ciliary injection, conjunctival hyperemia, lid edema, pain, foreign body sensation, tearing photophobia, and blepharospasm.

Superficial Punctate Keratitis from Physical or Chemical Injury

Keratitis from overexposure to ultraviolet light is common. The patient develops symptoms six to eight hours after activities such as welding without protective goggles or looking at a sun lamp, or exposure to bright sun at the beach or in the mountains (snow blindness). The erosions heal within 48 hours. Exposure to *hydrogen sulfide,* which is used in synthetic textile manufacture, causes a superficial punctate keratitis. Mustard gas and *excessive smoke* (as occurred in burning cities during World War II) will cause superficial punctate keratitis.

Radiation to the cornea, as in treatment of ocular tumors, can cause a painful, poorly healing, superficial punctate keratitis with lacrima-

tion and photophobia. The epithelium may be diffusely opaque and nonhealing erosions or ulcerations occur.
The cornea is frequently damaged by *burns* from chemicals or gases (see page 356). The clinical picture reflects the pH value of the acid or alkaline material. Self-defense weapons containing tear gas should be mentioned because they contain organic compounds combined with chloride or bromide groups capable of causing corneal erosions and stromal opacities. Various household sprays, physical impact of spray particles (insecticides, hair spray, deodorants, paint), either chemically or from the impact or both, will cause fine, superficial corneal stippling and erosions (McLean 1967). Mustard gas causes severe burns and blister formation.

The same substances causing conjunctival burns (see page 356) will affect the cornea. Special mention should be made of hydrogen sulfide as an occupational hazard causing punctate keratitis in the synthetic textile fiber industry. Formaldehyde, either as a gas or liquid, causes corneal and conjunctival inflammation with potential ulceration, iritis, and hypotony. Tar, either as steam, dust or solid, can cause skin eczema, melanosis, hyperkeratosis, and carcinoma. Around the eye it causes conjunctival and corneal inflammation with corneal infiltrates.

Acridine, quinine, quinidine, phenothiazine and certain sulfonamides are photosensitizing substances. They cause photoallergy in sensitive persons. Corneal and conjunctival damage may occur. Yellow-brown particles deposit in the cornea in lines and whorls, especially with chloroquine (see page 167).
Occupational diseases causing corneal (conjunctival) inflammation, according to Merté, result from:
Arsenicals – corneal ulcers, conjunctival hemorrhages, necrosis, retinal-optic nerve damage.
Arsenic trichloride – burns, arsenous hydride, pentavalent arsenic bonds (atoxyl) – inflammation to necrosis.
Benzoquinone, aniline derivatives, quinine, quinone, hydroquinone – burns, epithelial abrasion, ulceration, brown discoloration in the palpebral fissure area.
Benzene, toluene, xylene – epithelial damage, neuritis, retinitis.
Nitrobenzene and aminobenzene (methemoglobin formers): nitronaphthalene – severe corneal inflammation with blister formation and ulceration, gray-green superficial corneal staining, band keratopathy with chalky white deposits, and neuritis. Less frequent causes of corneal and conjunctival inflammation include nitrobenzene and dinitrobenzene, dinitrophenol, trinitrophenol (picric acid also causes a yellow discoloration). Aniline (aminobenzene), chloraniline and nitroaniline may also cause band keratopathy. Toluidine, xylidine, toluene, phenyldiamine, paraphenyldiamine, benzidine have a similar effect as aniline. Nitrodekaline causes brown discoloration of the posterior corneal surface and deep brown discoloration of the aqueous.
Halogenated hydrocarbons – chlorbenzene and dichlorbenzene (Globol).
Chrome – recurrent inflammation with erosions, edema, brown discoloration.
Lead – mucous membrane inflammation and optic neuritis.
Carbon disulfide – burns, decreased sensitivity, erosions, ulcerations, optic neuritis.
Hydrogen sulfide – superficial, rarely deep (disciform keratitis) inflammation.

Sjögren's Syndrome, Vitamin A and Vitamin B Deficiencies

Superficial punctate keratitis (sicca keratitis) or sicca syndrome occurs as part of Sjögren's syndrome (see page 130). This is an autoimmune collagen disorder (see page 183). It occurs primarily in postmenopausal females who suffer a severe loss of tear production associated with chronic arthritis (see page 183). The patient complains of dryness, burning and itching, or foreign body sensation in the eyes. There is a superficial punctate keratitis which can be filamentous. In filamentary keratitis, numerous small epithelial shreds or threads are attached to the cornea. Other findings include: dry mouth, nose and throat, achlorhydria, and an elevated erythrocyte sedimentation rate. Rarely there is a low-grade fever and swollen tender parotid. Hashimoto's thyroiditis is another autoimmune disease (see page 183). It may cause myxedema, lid edema and

severe keratitis sicca. Contrary to Sjögren's syndrome, which afflicts mainly postmenopausal women, Hashimoto's thyroiditis with sicca affects younger women.
Ariboflavinosis (see page 148) and *Plummer-Vinson* (iron deficiency) *syndrome* also cause keratoconjunctivitis sicca. Both ariboflavinosis and Plummer-Vinson syndrome are primarily diseases of postmenopausal women. Besides keratoconjunctivitis sicca, Plummer-Vinson syndrome (sideropenic dysphagia) includes generalized mucous membrane dryness, atrophy and hypochromic anemia. *Xerophthalmia* in vitamin A deficiency causes conjunctival xerosis and keratomalacia.

Keratoconjunctivitis Sicca from Other Causes

Other factors producing dry eyes and therefore conjunctivitis sicca (superficial punctate keratitis, filiform keratitis) (Dohlman et al. 1971) (see page 152) are: removal of the lacrimal gland, diseases of the lacrimal gland (Heerfordt's syndrome, sarcoidosis [see page 202], Mikulicz's syndrome), erythema multiforme, and pemphigus, burns, diphtheria, trachoma, etc., cause conjunctival scarring and dry eyes.

Viruses

Varicella (chicken pox) and *herpes zoster* are identical. Both cause superficial punctate keratitis, corneal ulcers, and disciform keratitis.
Zoster may also produce a neuroparalytic keratitis.
Herpes simplex is identified by unilateral involvement, *corneal hypesthesia*, and recurrences set off by generalized stress (systemic infection, trauma, fever, etc.). Superficial herpetic keratitis is categorized as Horner's corneal vesicles which are transient and relatively asymptomatic. The map and star shapes of dendritic keratitis are simply more extensive manifestations of the same process. Herpetic superficial punctate keratitis and herpetic filamentary keratitis also belong here.
If the corneal sensitivity is markedly decreased in a case of superficial punctate keratitis or filamentary keratitis, it is probably due to herpes virus.

Ophthalmologically, the most important **adenoviruses** are type 3 **(pharyngoconjunctival fever)** and type 8 **(epidemic keratoconjunctivitis)**.
Warts (verruca vulgaris) occur at the lid margin causing conjunctival inflammation and keratitis. **Chlamydia** or **Bedsonia**: *Trachoma* (see page 130), inclusion blennorrhea (see page 125), lymphogranuloma venereum, psittacosis, ornithosis, feline pneumonia, parrot conjunctivitis, and, perhaps, Reiter's syndrome (see page 128). Lymphogranuloma causes Parinaud's conjunctivitis, and occasionally corneal involvement: phlyctenules, diffuse infiltrates, marginal ulcers.

Viral conjunctival-corneal inflammations frequently include superficial punctate keratitis (for survey see Bietti 1972). Of the RNA viruses, influenza and para-influenza, measles (probably with an associated vitamin A deficiency), mumps, dengue fever (arbovirus) potentially cause early punctate keratitis or disciform keratitis.

Newcastle disease (fowl pox) causes a unilateral Parinaud's conjunctivitis with preauricular lymphadenopathy and fever. **Foot-and-mouth-disease** (cattle, sheep, hogs) may cause corneal blisters that leave a residual opacification.

DNA viruses include:
Molluscum contagiosum potentially includes infiltrates or ulceration at the corneal margin.

Variola and **Vaccinia** can cause corneal ulcers and infiltrates.
In newborns, **cytomegalovirus** results in fever, splenomegaly, gastroenteritis, pneumonia, and neurologic symptoms. Keratomalacia, dacryoadenitis, scleritis, conjunctivitis, uveitis, and neuroretinitis are less frequent.

After Conjunctival Inflammation

Superficial punctate keratitis may appear after a conjunctivitis (trachoma, scrofula, diphtheria, allergic conjunctivitis). Any conjunctival allergy has some degree of *corneal involvement.* The same substances which are allergenic for lid and conjunctiva are responsible (see pages 92 and 122).

Drugs

Heterocyclic medications, especially pyrazolon derivatives (antipyrine, pyramidon, etc.) cause lid, conjunctival, corneal inflammation, and edema.
It is probably an allergic reaction (see page 122). Toxicity or sensitivity to organic arsenicals may produce severe lid edema, conjunctival and corneal inflammation, ulceration, and transient myopia (see page 26).

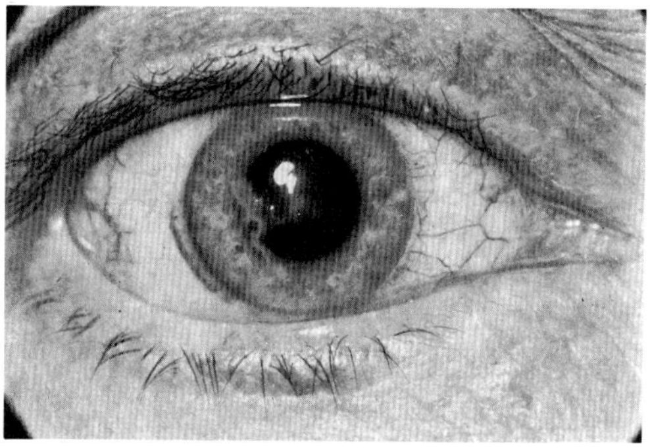

Fig. 13.15 Dendritic keratitis

Infectious Disease

Almost any infectious disease may cause conjunctivitis and keratitis. Iris nodules and retinal hemorrhages can occur. Encephalomyelitic involvement is always possible.

Filamentary Keratitis

The same agents which cause superficial punctate keratitis will produce filamentary keratitis. The primary cause of filamentary keratitis is lost tear production in Sjögren's syndrome, trauma, or after surgical removal of the lacrimal gland.

Recurrent erosions, bullous keratopathy, and viral infection are other common causes. It may occur idiopathically or with epinephrine therapy (Rüger 1970).

Filamentary and punctate keratopathy result from many viral infections, allergies, vitamin A and B deficiency, chemical and physical damage.

Superficial Herpetic Keratitis

In *corneal herpes* one of the most important clinical signs is decreased corneal sensitivity. The superficial epithelium or stroma may be involved. The most common type of herpetic involvement is *dendritic keratitis* (Fig. 13.15). This tends to appear after some systemic stress such as a cold, fever, infectious disease (typhus, malaria) fever therapy, vaccinations, menses, or corneal trauma. It is associated with severe pain and decreased corneal sensitivity. The epithelial defect is linear, branched (dendritic), and stains with fluorescein. Without treatment healing may take weeks or months. In some cases, especially if cortisone is used, the dendritic ulcer expands in size and deep round corneal infiltrates (metaherpetic keratitis) or ulcers develop. The incidence of the disease appears to be increasing (Schenk and Hummer 1958). Men are more often affected than women. Dendritic keratitis can be seen in small children. Occasionally the herpes virus causes *superficial punctate keratitis* or *filamentary keratitis.*

Nummular Keratitis

Epidemic keratoconjunctivitis — Dimmer's nummular keratitis — Causes of nummular keratitis (zoster, varicella, brucellosis).

Epidemic Keratoconjunctivitis

Epidemic keratoconjunctivitis begins with chemosis (especially of the caruncle). There may be an associated pharyngitis. Occasionally, the conjunctiva develops pseudomembranes and small petechial hemorrhages on the upper tarsus. The disease may begin simultaneously in the two eyes. Usually one follows the other in a few days. Inflammation in the second eye is generally attenuated. Yellow serous secretions seal the eye shut at night. Preauricular nodes are always tender and swollen. The incubation period is exactly 8 to 10 days. About five days after the conjunctivitis starts, fine corneal stippling occurs. By the eighth day numerous (10 to 100), fine (0.5 mm in diameter) punctate infiltrates develop under Bowman's membrane (nummular keratitis). Equally large gray corneal scars remain (Fig. 12.7). At first they may cause considerable loss of vision, but disappear for the most part during the next six to twelve months. The condition is highly infectious and often spreads via doctors' offices. The infective agent is adenovirus, type 8 (Jawetz et al. 1957; Hanna et al. 1957; Mitsu et al. 1957; Zintz and Vivell 1959; Wollensak 1956).

Differential diagnosis: First of all, swimming pool conjunctivitis (see page 125) is a possibility. This is considerably milder with no corneal involvement and less conjunctivitis or preauricular adenopathy. Hemorrhages are far more extensive in hemorrhagic conjunctivitis and the incubation period is only 24 hours. Trachoma is more chronic with larger follicles that tend to rupture. There is conjunctival scarring and pannus formation.
Herpetic conjunctivitis usually begins with corneal involvement (dendritic keratitis) or lid vesicles. The caruncle is not swollen and there is no preauricular lymphadenopathy.

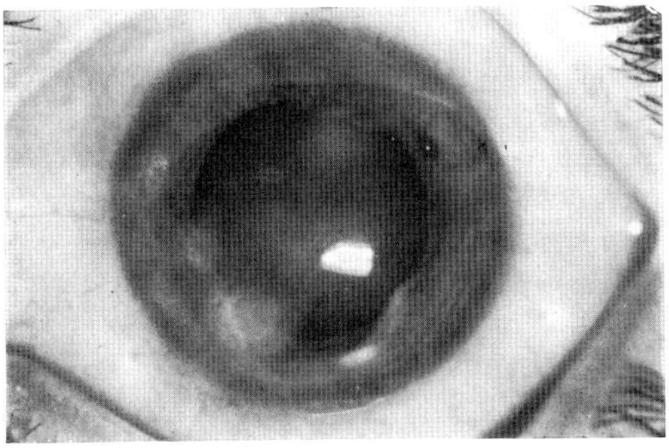

Fig. 13.16 Nummular keratitis (Dimmer) (Photo: Prof. Hofmann, Graz)

Dimmer's Nummular Keratitis

Dimmer's nummular keratitis (Hofmann 1957) (Fig. 13.16) is restricted to agricultural workers.
The disease is almost always unilateral. Its origin is related to injury with grain or grasses which may have occurred months before clinical findings become manifest. The lesions begin beneath Bowman's membrane and slowly move toward the surface. It is only when they penetrate that the patient develops subjective symptoms (photophobia, tear secretion, foreign body sensation). The lesions begin as punctate gray opacities which expand into prominent nodules surrounded by a gray haze. Their diameter is 0.5 to 2 mm. Except for the late generalized irritation, the conjunctiva remains uninvolved. The nodules become more distinct and scar with dellen formation after weeks to months. They rarely vascularize. The disease is active for four to six months and heals over nine to ten months. The average number of lesions is eight to ten but ranges from two to fifty.

Nummular-like Keratitis

Differential diagnosis: Corneal *facettes* giving the picture of nummular keratitis occur most commonly with epidemic keratoconjunctivitis and then Dimmer's nummular keratitis. In epidemic keratoconjunctivitis, the conjunctivitis and preauricular adenopathy dominate clinically. Zoster and varicella can produce nummular keratitis, but the skin involvement aids in the diagnosis. Both viruses also produce corneal hypoanesthesia and iridocyclitis. Scrofula causes severe photophobia in children. As in acne rosacea the corneal lesions are heavily vascularized and should not provide difficulty in differential diagnosis.
Brucellosis (Bang's disease, Malta fever [see page 198]) and onchocerciasis (see page 199) can cause nummular keratitis.

Bullous and Membranous Keratopathies

Erythema multiforme = Oculomucocutaneous syndrome (Fuchs) — Pemphigus, pemphigoid — Epidermolysis bullosa — Photodermatitis — Diffuse bullous keratopathy — Fuchs' endothelial dystrophy — Vitreous adherence, absolute glaucoma.

Erythema Multiforme

A *bullous* or *membranous keratitis* should first of all bring to mind erythema multiforme (oculomucocutaneous syndrome, Fuchs) (see page 168). This is the same disease as Stevens-Johnson syndrome and, in addition to the well-known conjunctival changes, can

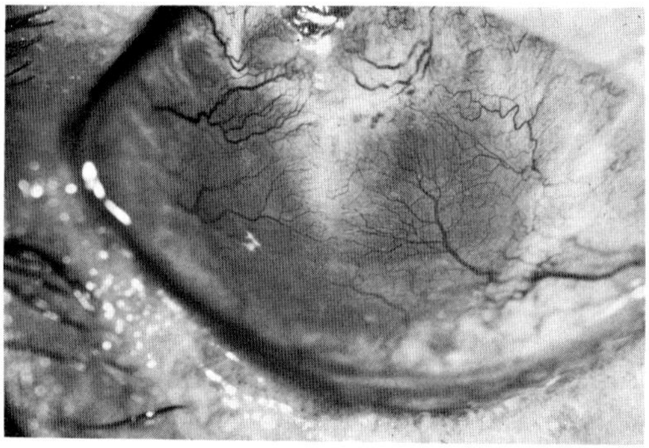

Fig. 13.17 Erythema multiforme with corneal infiltrates, vascularization, scars and symblepharon (♂ 12 yrs.)

cause corneal bullae, pseudomembranes and symblepharon. Late corneal complications include deep stromal infiltrates, vascularization, scarring, and xerosis (Fig. 13.17).

Pemphigus

Pemphigus (Plate VI, Fig. 2, page 128 f) and pemphigoid (see page 97 and 128) (Fig. 13.21) may lead to severe shrinkage, scarring and xerosis of the cornea and conjunctiva.

Epidermolysis Bullosa

In epidermolysis bullosa (see page 97) blisters form after minimal skin trauma. The disease begins in early childhood. Cornea and conjunctiva develop ulcerating blisters, infiltrates which vascularize, scars and symblepharon (Plate VIII, Fig. 4, page 128 h).

Photodermatitis

By photodermatitis (see page 97) we are primarily referring to *xeroderma pigmentosum.* This leads to pigmentation, atrophy, telangiectasia formation, ulceration, and malignant skin changes in those areas exposed to sunlight.

Nodules, ulceration, symblepharon, xerosis, and squamous cell carcinoma may develop at the limbus.

Hydroa vacciniforma can cause corneal epithelial blisters which may ulcerate. Porphyria has to be considered (see page 366).

Diffuse Bullous Keratopathy

Occasionally, a neurotrophic keratitis appears for no known reason and causes bullous keratopathy. This may be unilateral or bilateral and is associated with marked *corneal anesthesia*. The disease ultimately clears but can recur. The cause is unknown.

Fuchs' Endothelial Dystrophy (see page 168)

Cornea guttata (drusen of Descemet's membrane) appear in the central cornea of older persons with Fuchs' endothelial dystrophy. This may lead to stromal and epithelial edema.

Vitreous Adherence, Absolute Glaucoma

Adhesion of vitreous, iris, or lens to the cornea occurs after trauma or surgery. This causes bullous keratitis as does absolute glaucoma (see page 225).

Parenchymatous (Interstitial) Keratitis

Viral parenchymatous keratitis — Luetic keratitis — Nonluetic parenchymatous keratitis (tuberculosis, sarcoidosis) — Parenchymatous keratitis with corneal ulcers — Deep inflammatory keratitis — Sclerosing keratitis — Parenchymatous keratitis in skin diseases — Stromal opacification, after forcepts delivery, in acute keratoconus — Ring abscess of the cornea — Burns.

Viral Parenchymatous Keratitis

Disciform keratitis (primary and metaherpetic) — Ophthalmic zoster — Vaccinia — Measles, rubella, variola, varicella, lymphogranuloma venereum.

Disciform Keratitis

Disciform keratitis (Fig. 13.18) affects the corneal stroma. It may begin deep in the stroma as a primary disciform inflammation or be secondary to recurrent dendritic keratitis (metaherpetic). There is a round opacity, 2 to 4 mm in diameter, lying centrally or paracentrally and inferiorly.

Epithelium overlying the stromal lesion is edematous and precipitates a deposit on the posterior corneal surface. The acute inflammation evolves over months, often leaving permanent scarring and marked vision loss. We differentiate between primary and secondary disciform keratitis. Primary disciform lesions rarely vascularize. Secondary disciform keratitis usually results from recurrent or improperly (steroid therapy) treated dendritic keratitis. These metaherpetic lesions almost invariably vascularize.

Corneal erosions, and poorly healing ulcerations, even perforations, occur with metaherpetic disciform keratitis, especially when steroids have been improperly used.

The endothelial precipitates give rise to the term "posterior herpes."

Ophthalmic Zoster (see page 95).

Varicella and the virus causing ophthalmic zoster are the same. Headache, fever and neuralgias are prodromes of a zoster outbreak. They are followed by skin erythema and edema in the distribution of the sensory nerve.

In ophthalmic zoster numerous small blisters develop on the skin and lids in the area of distribution of the first division of the trigeminal nerve. When the nasociliary nerve is affected in zoster, the eye is involved 50 percent of the time (Holmberg 1951). The most common corneal complication (Scheie 1970) is caused by subepithelial infiltrates which form secondary erosions, superficial punctate or nummular keratitis, or deep corneal infiltrates. The cornea may become edematous with folds in Descemet. Disciform keratitis, neuroparalytic keratitis, corneal ulcer, leukomatous scarring and vascularization are further corneal complications in ophthalmic zoster. Iritis occurs in half the cases. This may lead to segmental iris atrophy, secondary glaucoma and extraocular muscle paresis (total ophthalmoplegia, oculomotor, abducens, trochlear or facial nerve paresis). The paresis tends to resolve over a period of weeks. Retrobulbar neuritis and zoster encephalitis are very rare (Nover 1970). Children may develop zoster meningitis (Inoue and Nakamura 1956) and encephalitis (Schmidt et al. 1955).

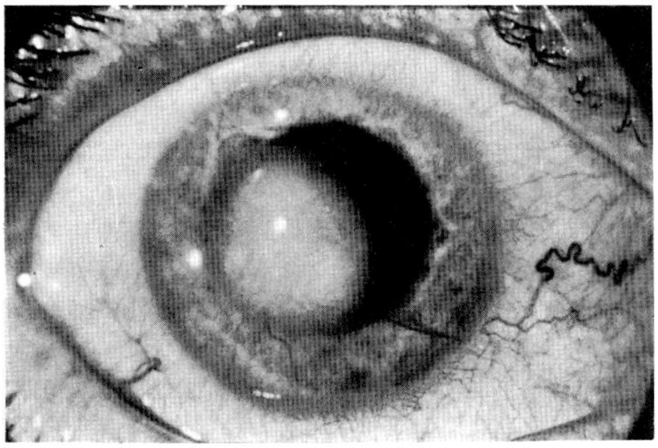

Fig. 13.18 Disciform keratitis (♀ 48 yrs.)

Feyrter (1954) sees zoster as a blood borne infectious disease causing "organ specific" capillary arteritis. Loss of sensation and pupillary reaction (oculomotor nerve) is caused by neuritis of certain nerve roots. The corneal, scleral-uveal necrosis and optic neuritis are caused by capillary involvement by a zoster panarteritis nodosa (Kreibig 1959). Peak involvement is between the ages of 60 and 80, but the disease does occur in infants.

Vaccinia

After vaccination against small pox, vaccinia (see page 95) commonly causes lid ulcers (Fig. 10.28). Localized corneal infiltrates, disciform keratitis and corneal ulcers also occur.

Measles, Rubella, Variola, Varicella, Mumps, Lymphogranuloma Venereum

Corneal involvement in measles, rubella and small pox can occur as superficial or deep infiltrates, possibly disciform, and with ulcer formation. Rarely, varicella causes a similar picture.

Of 2,000 African patients with measles (Wessels and Pratt-Johnson 1956) 2.5 percent became blind from corneal opacities. The lesions were in the deep stroma and caused vascularization and pannus formation. There is danger that the cornea will perforate (Blatz 1956).

Conjunctivitis, keratitis and blepharitis are

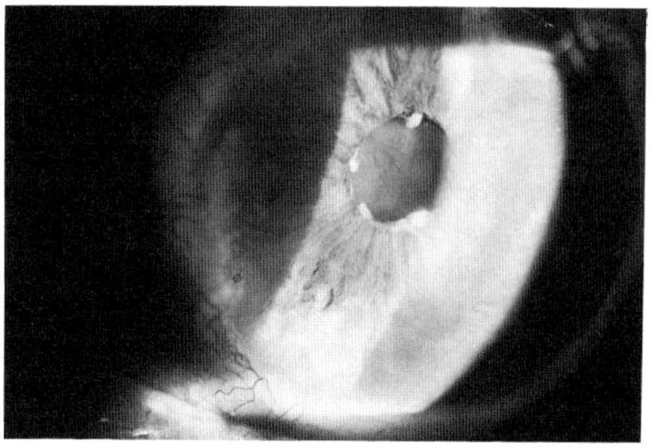

Fig. 13.19 Luetic interstitial keratitis with hyalin accumulation at the pupillary margin (old synechiae) (♀ 42 yrs.)

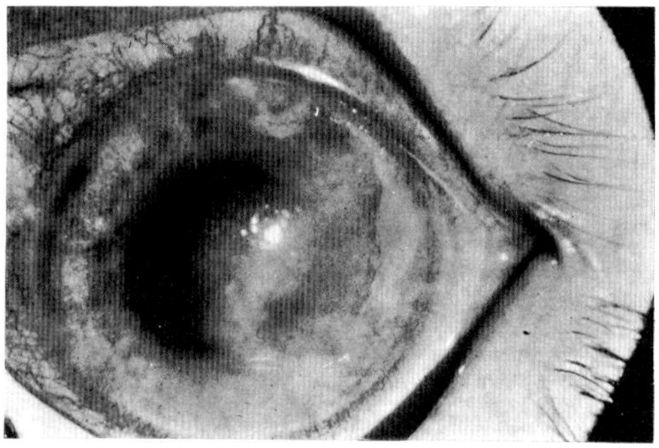

Fig. 13.20 Acute parenchymatous keratitis in congenital syphilis (♀ 35 yrs.)

well known to occur with measles. Less well known are the postinfectious or parainfectious meningoencephalitis. Involvement includes retinitis, papillitis, and optic neuritis as well as optic tract encephalitis. These complications begin between the fourth day and third week of the rash.

Mumps may cause sudden stromal opacification which is transient and clears rapidly. Lymphogranuloma venereum can also cause parenchymatous keratitis.

Parenchymatous (Interstitial) Keratitis

Connatal *luetic parenchymatous keratitis* usually begins between ages of 6 and 18 but may be delayed until after the age of 40 (Fig. 13.19). Marked ciliary injection, with lacrimation, photophobia, pain and corneal haze develops. The haze is more limbal, gray white and diffuse (Fig. 13.20). Deep vessel ingrowth begins from the limbus (Plate VIII, Fig. 5, page 128 h) two to three weeks later. The heavy deep vascularization gives the cornea a red fleshy appearance (salmon patches). After weeks to months (faster with steroid therapy), the cornea clears (Fig. 13.21), again starting at the limbus. Visual recovery varies with the amount of corneal clearing. The second eye becomes involved weeks, months even years after the first. The second eye was affected within one year of the first eye in 91 percent of 302 cases (Creutzburg 1952). Intervals of 25 and even 26 years are reported (Bonnet and Chavanne 1947; Consiglio 1906). Adequate antiluetic therapy will not prevent corneal involvement in the second eye (Fuhs and Böck 1939). Minor trauma may trigger the process. After the cornea clears, empty collapsed blood vessels remain as (ghost) lines in the cornea near Descemet's membrane together with deep scars (Fig. 13.22). The corneal inflammation can be recurrent, especially when immunosuppressive steroid therapy is stopped early. A fibrinous iridocyclitis (Bonnet and Bonnet 1954; Meesmann 1956) with persisting hyalinic gray flaky deposits (Fig. 13.19) in the pupillary region of the iris almost invariably accompanies the acute keratitis. Scleritis also occurs but is rare. Hyaline masses or ridges often persist on the posterior corneal surface (Franceschetti and Balavonne 1953). Secondary glaucoma is common and can cause buphthalmos in affected infants.

Retinitis and anterior chorioretinitis are part of the clinical picture of congenital lues. Heavy brown-black pigmentation occurs anterior to the equator. Salt and pepper fundus changes are classically described (Plate XXVIII, Fig. 4, page 288 d). Retinal periphlebitis has also been reported (Offret and Fargette 1947). Luetic keratitis, especially chorioretinitis, may be accompanied by a brown cupoliform opacification at the posterior surface of the fetal nucleus of the lens (Vogt 1931; Remler 1952). This is stationary and does not cause vision loss. In addition to the eye findings, other signs of congenital lues are invariably present. The Wassermann reaction is positive in 90 to 95 percent of cases (Hoehne 1940; Schmidt 1942). Rhagades are often present at the corners of the mouth (Parrot's stripes). Serous arthritis, saddle nose, and saber shin are further findings.

Hutchinson's triad consists of interstitial keratitis, barrel teeth, and hearing loss.

Nonluetic Interstitial (Parenchymatous) Keratitis

Tuberculosis can cause parenchymatous keratitis consisting of isolated single gray to yellow spot lesions with minimal vascularization. *Sarcoidosis* may cause similar deep vascularized infiltrates (see page 201).

Leprosy (see page 94) (Renard et al. 1963) causes interstitial keratitis and infiltrates along corneal nerves (decreased sensitivity). Later there is pannus formation. Painless, deep, yellow-gray, vascularized infiltrates, which potentially necrose, perforate, and cause staphyloma formation, also occur in leprosy. *Diffuse interstitial keratitis* is reported with mumps, brucellosis, recurrent fever, trypanosomiasis, sleeping sickness, filariasis, and Hodgkin's disease.

Diffuse, deep keratitis involves only the deepest corneal layers and is usually associated with an iridocyclitis. When associated with systemic diseases, the process is presumed to be secondary to an allergic reaction or iridocyclitis.

Cogan I syndrome consists of bilateral nonluetic interstitial keratitis, loss of hearing, and vertigo. As the loss of hearing irreversibly worsens, the ringing in the ears and vertigo improve.

The ocular symptoms are photophobia, lacrimation, pain, and ciliary as well as conjunctival infection. Ring-shaped, yellow stromal infiltrates arise about 1 mm from the limbus and become confluent. The corneal infiltrates may be sufficiently extensive to cause vision loss to light projection only. High steroid dosages quickly improve sight. *Cogan I syndrome* is believed to be a collagen disorder (Bischoff 1972).

Parenchymatous Keratitis and Corneal Ulceration

Corneal ulcers (see page 159) will develop with sufficiently severe interstitial keratitis and superficial erosions. Both conditions may be present for some time before an ulcer appears

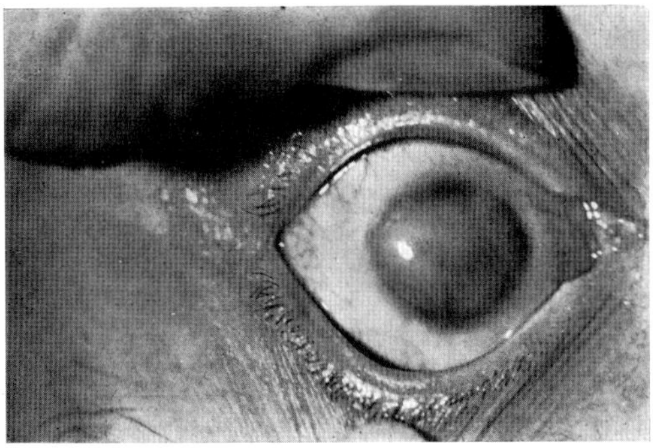

Fig. 13.21 Scarring from luetic interstitial keratitis (♀ 15 yrs.)

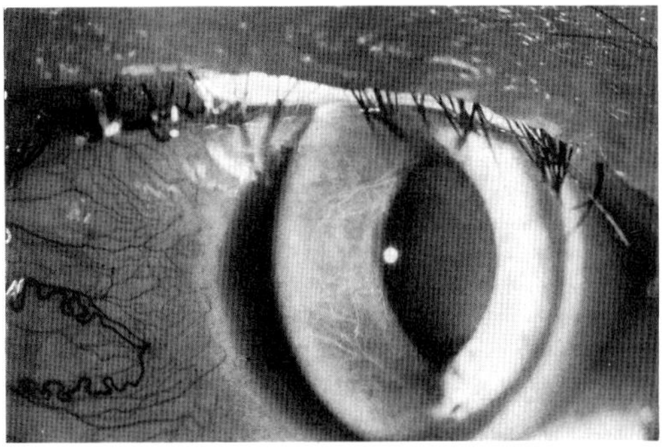

Fig. 13.22 Ghost vessels in the deep corneal layers caused by syphilitic interstitial keratitis

(especially with steroid therapy, topical anesthetic abuse, metaherpetic keratitis, scrofulous keratitis, acne rosacea, etc.).

Deep Punctate Keratitis

This is a descriptive term for deep corneal infiltrates with endothelial precipitates, or even hypopyon formation. They cause pain and lacrimation, and appear as an atypical disciform keratitis with ophthalmic zoster, after local trauma, rarely with mumps or influenza.

Sclerosing Keratitis (see page 182)

Scleritis may cause tongue-shaped, white-yellow infiltrates to extend onto the cornea from the sclera. These are followed by deep vascularization (Plate VIII, Fig. 6, page 128 h). The corneal stroma scars and permanently remains gray-white (sclerotic).

Tuberculosis, sarcoidosis, syphilis, foci or some local process are at fault.

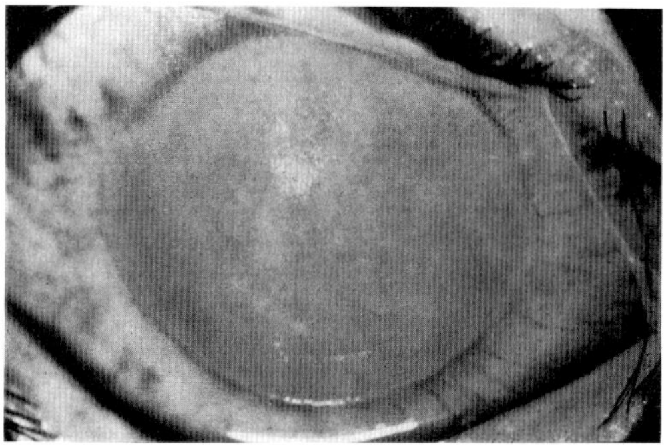

Fig. 13.23 Alkali burn (♂ 18 yrs.)

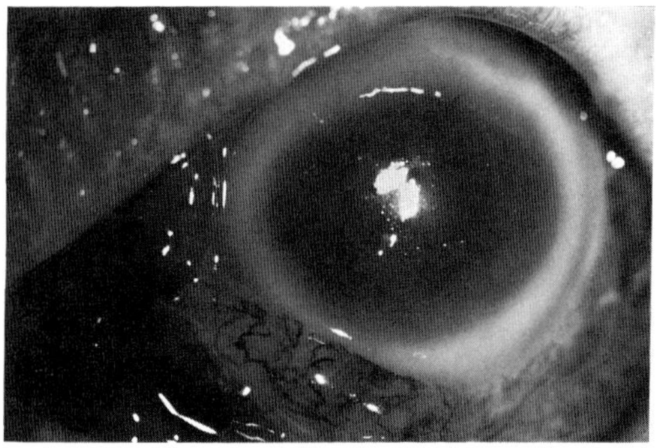

Fig. 13.24 String syndrome (anterior segment ischemia). Dense, gray, peripheral, corneal infiltrates, dirty gray-brown-red iris, fibrin in the anterior chamber, 8 days after an Arruga string operation for retinal detachment (♀ 71 yrs.)

Sclerocornea is a congential opacification and peripheral vascularization of the cornea. There is no sign of inflammation.

Brawny (gelatinous) scleritis (see page 182) is a massive gelatinous swelling of sclera and episcleral tissue around the cornea. It is an autoimmune collagen disorder, frequently associated with rheumatoid arthritis. It occurs in older women and follows a protracted course of remissions and exacerbations. The cornea may be involved in late stages with varying degrees of vascularization.

The underlying pigmented uvea shines through the thinned sclera in the area of healed scleritis. Secondary glaucoma, which is often present, allows staphyloma formation.

Interstitial Keratitis with Skin Diseases

On rare occasions, superficial and deep vascularized infiltrates are observed in psoriasis, palmoplantar keratosis, lichen planus, and molluscum contagiosum.

Incontinentia pigmenti (Bloch-Sulzberger) can have corneal opacities (see page 247).

Corneal Opacification after Forceps Delivery

Part of the forceps may press on the globe causing Descemet tears at birth. Absorption of aqueous results in stromal swelling and acute gray opacification of the cornea. Clinically, this resembles *acute keratoconus* (see page 149). The cornea clears over weeks to months, but double contoured lines remain in the region of the Descemet tears (Fig. 13.10).

Corneal Ring Abscess (Plate IX, Fig. 1, page 192 a)

The ring abscess is a particularly severe interstitial keratitis. A highly infectious object perforates or injures (may be surgical) the cornea. It may also occur with panophthalmitis. After 12 to 24 hours, a gray-yellow infiltrate (1 to 3 mm wide) running parallel to the limbus and a few mm from it develops. The infiltrate goes progressively deeper into the cornea and severe chemosis results. Perforation is common. Ultimately the central cornea becomes opaque. The causal agents are virulent pneumococci, bacillus subtilis, proteus, bacterium pyocyaneum and others. A similar gray-yellow ring infiltrate can occur with anterior segment necrosis, for example, after a "string" encircling procedure (see page 204) for retinal detachment or after circular diathermy was applied to the sclera (Fig. 13.24).

Burns

Chemical (acid, lye, alkali) (Fig. 13.23) or thermal burns turn the stroma gray. When severe enough, the cornea looks like a "boiled fish eye." Corneal thinning or perforation may be seen after one to two weeks if large enough segments of the perilimbic vessels have been sclerosed.

Corneal Ulcers

Most common location of corneal ulcers — Marginal (catarrhal) ulcer — Marginal furrow — Rodent ulcer (Mooren's ulcer) — Ulcus serpens — Gonococcal ulcer — Fungal ulcer — Damage from topical anesthetics and steroids — Ecthyma gangrenosum — Exposure keratitis — Phlyctenular keratitis — Acne rosacea — Metaherpetic keratitis — Neuroparalytic keratitis, congenital anesthesia — Keratomalacia — Trachoma.

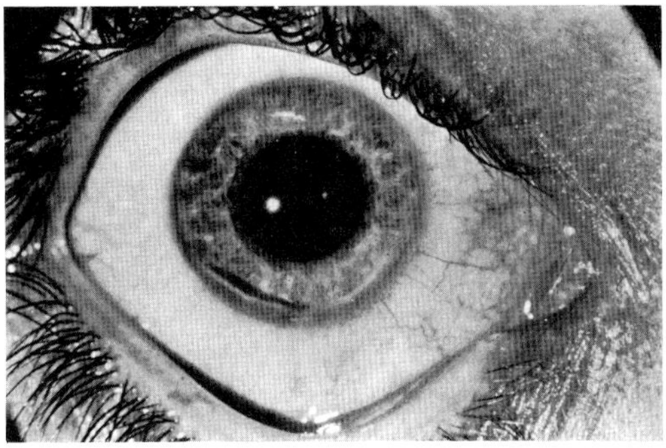

Fig. 13.26 Marginal (catarrhal) ulcer

Most Common Location of Corneal Ulcers (Fig. 13.25)

Marginal (Catarrhal) Ulcer

Marginal ulcers occur in older, postmenopausal individuals. The lesion begins as a gray paralimbic infiltrate (marginal keratitis). This is separated from the limbus by a slight clear zone (Fig. 13.26). There is minor photophobia, lacrimation, and foreign body sensation. At first the infiltrate is small, punctate, confluent, extending up to one fourth of the corneal circumference. Ulceration develops which stimulates vascular ingrowth from the conjunctiva. The ulcers are always peripheral, recurrent, and leave slight gray scars.

On rare occasions, lymphogranuloma venereum will cause perilimbic corneal infiltrates with ulceration and vascularization. Excessive dosages of vitamin A can cause a keratoconjunctivitis with marginal ulceration. Dystrophic corneal ulcers occur with agranulocytosis from any cause (drugs, radiation, tumor infiltration, Fanconi syndrome).

Marginal Furrow (Ectasia)

During the course of years, marked thinning of the paralimbic cornea occurs. This leads to transient ciliary injection which clears after local vascularization (Fig. 13.27). Eventually the

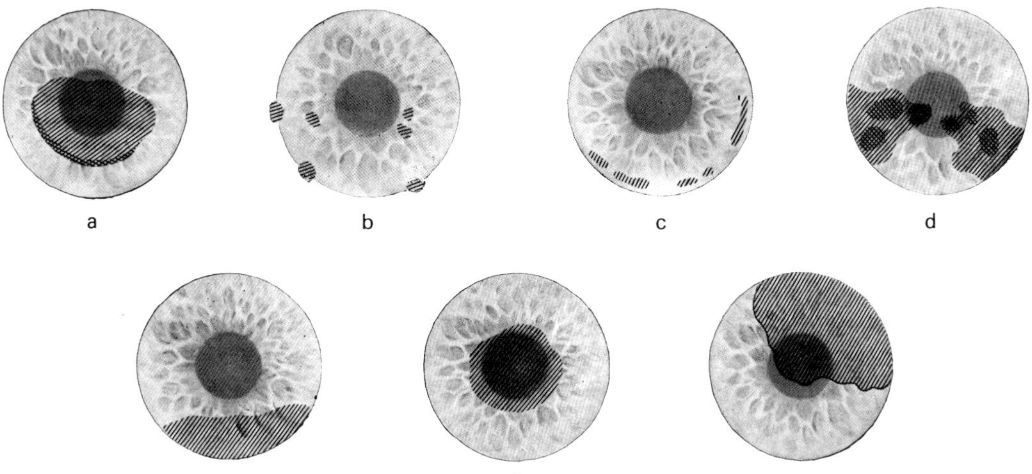

Fig. 13.25 Location and shape of common corneal ulcers (schematic from R. Thiel: Atlas of Diseases of the Eye, 6th Ed., Thieme, Stuttgart 1963). a) Ulcus serpens; b) Ulcera scrofulosa; c) Marginal ulcer; d) Ulcer in rosacea; e) Lagophthalmic ulcer; f) Neuroparalytic ulcer; g) Rodent ulcer

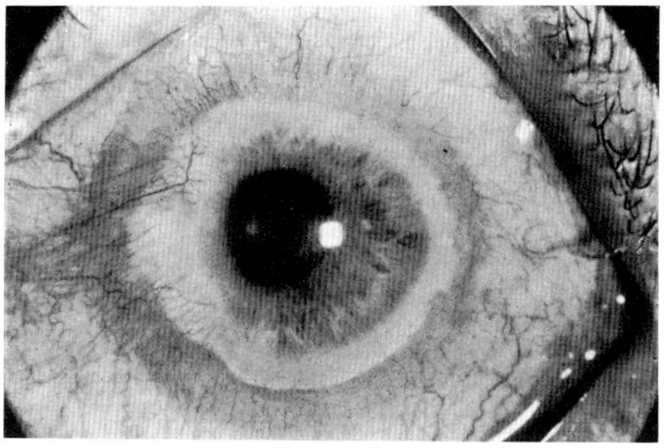

Fig. 13.27 Marginal furrow keratitis (♀ 80 yrs.)

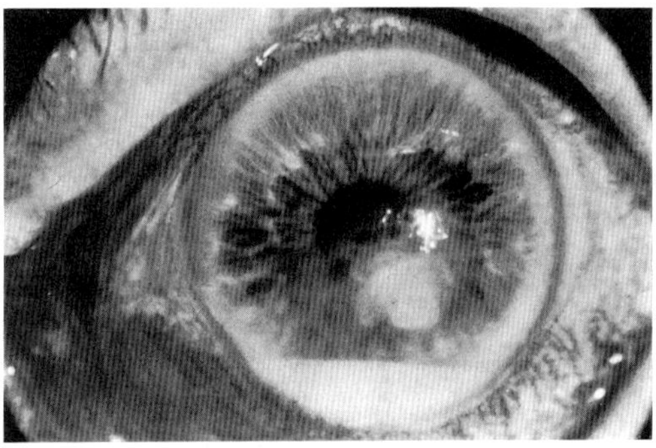

Fig. 13.28 Ulcus serpens with hypopyon (♂ 74 yrs.)

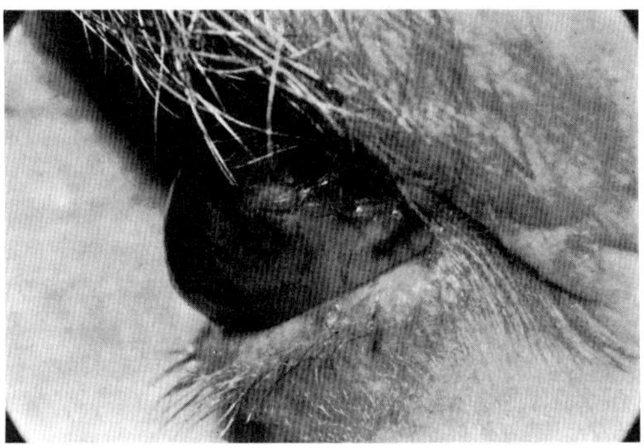

Fig. 13.29 Staphyloma after ulcus serpens perforation

ectasia or thinning can lead to perforations upon minor trauma. Vision is decreased through the induced astigmatism. It is a disease of old men.

Differential diagnosis: Refer to Terrien's marginal degeneration (see page 143).

Rodent Ulcer

Mooren's ulcer (Rodent ulcer, ulcus rodens) begins at the limbus in one sector and is ring-shaped. There is a melting away of the anterior two thirds of the stroma with vascularization of the posterior third (Plate IX, Fig. 2, page 192 a). Stroma and epithelium are undermined on the advancing edge of the ulcer as it spreads toward the corneal center. Over a period of months, the ulcer covers the entire cornea. The process is very painful, there is lacrimation and photophobia. Perforation is rare. The condition is bilateral in 25 to 40 percent of cases. Secondary glaucoma is common. This is probably an autoimmune disorder (Hoffmann 1971).

Ulcus Serpens (Bacterial Ulcer)

(Hypopyon keratitis [Fig. 13.28])

This is the most common corneal ulcer. It is caused by infection after an injury. The gray infiltrate tends to be near the center of the cornea. *Hypopyon* formation is pathognomonic and is caused by the inflammatory iritis. At first the level of the hypopyon shifts easily, but as the reaction becomes more fibrinoid, it turns into a white-yellow mass on the posterior corneal surface (see page 196). Synechiae formation is common. There is marked ciliary injection and dark red conjunctival chemosis. The localized stromal swelling and inflammatory infiltrate may hide the ulcer so that the lesion even protrudes from the corneal surface.

The ulcer is rapidly progressive involving the entire cornea; unless treated, it usually perforates. Panophthalmitis, adherent leucoma, secondary glaucoma, staphyloma (Fig. 13.29) and phthisis bulbi can all result.

Causal agents of ulcus serpens are primarily pneumococcus, and sometimes hemolytic streptococci, Friedlander's bacillus, pseudomonas, staphylococci, diplococci, or other pyogenic organisms.

In addition to trauma, lacrimal sac infections play an etiologic role. Ulcus serpens may appear as a superinfection in metaherpetic keratitis, neuroparalytic keratitis, scrofulous ulcer, etc. The most important differential diagnostic condition is fungal ulcer.

Ulcer Formation in Ophthalmia Neonatorum (Gonococcus)

Severe gonococcal conjunctivitis (see page 124) may compromise the perilimbic vascular supply; superficial erosions, which quickly ulcerate and then perforate, develop. The ulceration may be ring-shaped around the limbus.

Fungal Keratitis

If a corneal ulcer progresses in spite of antibiotic therapy, a fungal etiology has to be considered (Jones; Richards et al. 1969) (candida, aspergillus, penicillium, sporotrichosis, etc.). Antibiotics aid fungal growth on the cornea as well as in culture media (Ley and Sanders 1956). The introduction of antibiotic and steroid therapy appears to be responsible for the increased incidence of mycotic keratitis. Classically, the fungal ulcer has satellite lesions surrounding it (Fig. 13.30). Fine lines may be seen to extend peripherally from the central lesion. These are hyphae which are precursors for satellite colonies (Kaufmann and Wood 1965). The mycotic infiltrate is white to gray-yellow and fluffy, with blurred borders. At first the infiltrate may be round with small extensions, but as it grows, the margins become irregular. The base of a fungal ulcer tends to be a dull gray as opposed to the puslike yellow of bacterial lesions.

Instead of ulcerating, fungi may form firm infiltrates which even extend above the corneal surface. This is particularly true of aspergillus (Hoffmann 1969). Hypopyon formation occurs early in the infection and may be associated with marked Descemet folds. A Wessely ring can form. There is a clear zone between ulcer and ring. The hypopyon, like the iridocyclitis, is fibrinoid and a fibroid clot attaches to the posterior cornea. Without therapy there is little tendency toward healing. The process is chronic and extends over a period of months. Fungal panophthalmitis can necessitate enucleation.

Superficial *aspergillus* and *candida* cause small, yellow-white nodules, primarily at the limbus. These have a nodular dry surface and may be vascularized. Deep infiltrative aspergillus ulcers act like ulcus serpens. Satellite lesions can occur. Blastomycosis, sporotrichosis, mucormycosis and cephalosporin can produce corneal lesions resembling those of ulcus serpens (Hoffmann 1969; François 1968; Jones et al. 1970).

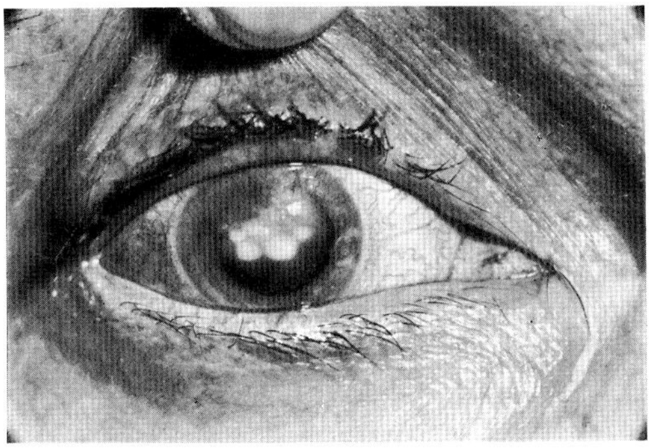

Fig. 13.30 Fungal keratitis demonstrating satellite phenomenon (♀ 55 yrs.)

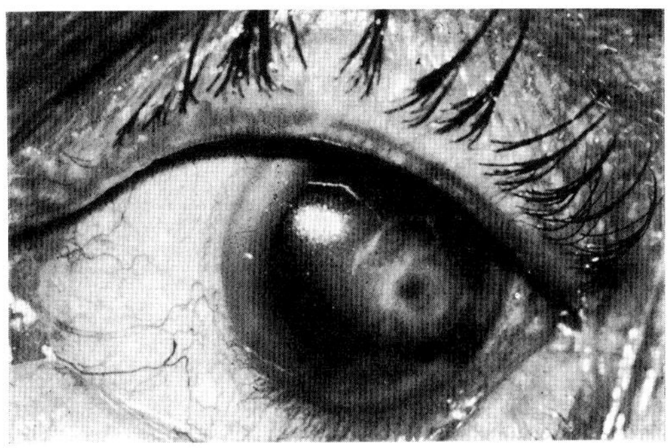

Fig. 13.31 Steroid damage with descemetocele (♂ 54 yrs.)

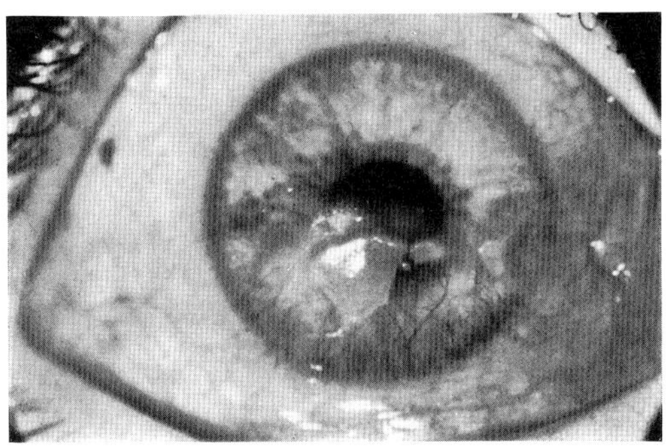

Fig. 13.32 Lagophthalmic keratitis (♂ 19 yrs.)

Almost all mycotic corneal infections are

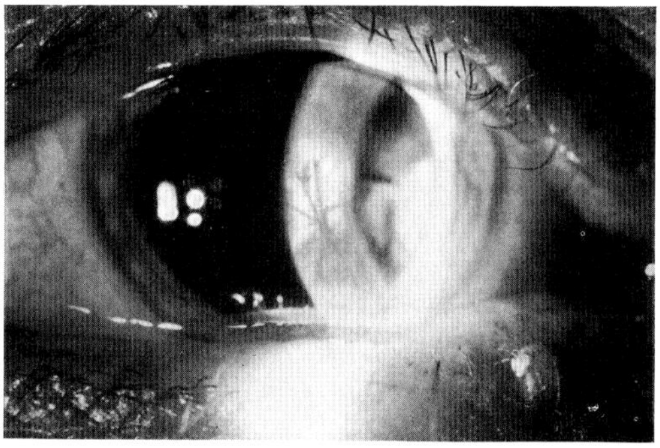

Fig. 13.33 Scrofulous corneal scar with Fuchs' lines of clearing (♀ 51 yrs.)

caused by injury, usually by some vegetable material. Broad spectrum antibiotics have generally been used at some point in the treatment.

Differential diagnosis: Deep corneal scrapings must be made for microscopic examination. Fungi usually stain gram positive. PAS staining is even better. Sabouraud or Kimmig are the best culture media. Negative results do not rule out fungi since these may be deeper within the ulcer (therefore, firm scraping is necessary). Hyphenated forms are the most common corneal fungi (aspergillus, monosporium, cephalosporium) and candida. Dermatophytes are rare (Mclean 1963; Ted Suie and Havener 1963).

Cortisone and Topical Anesthetic Abuse

Chronic use of topical anesthetics (cocaine, pontocaine, ophthaine, etc.) (Plate IX, Fig. 3, page 192 a) (Graeber 1961) or excessive use of steroids can cause corneal erosions with retardation of healing and corneal infiltrates. The infiltrates are yellow-white and progress. The erosions begin superficially, become deeper, and may even perforate (Fig. 13.31). Corneal sensitivity is slightly reduced. The clinical picture resembles neuroparalytic keratitis (see page 163).

Ecthyma Gangrenosum

Bacteremia in debilitated children with an intestinal overgrowth of pseudomonas pyocyanea leads to brown skin lesions and corneal ulceration. This begins at the limbus and can spread over the entire cornea.

Exposure Keratitis (Lagophthalmic Keratitis) (Fig. 13.32)

Improper lid closure, such as occurs after facial paralysis with malignant exophthalmos, cicatrical ectropion or coma, causes corneal exposure. The exposed cornea develops infiltrates, ulcerations, vessel ingrowth, and possibly perforates.

When of long standing, gray prominent scars with epithelial hyperplasia and hyperkeratosis occur. Since Bell's phenomenon turns the eyes up and out during sleep, the lower third of the cornea is most often affected.

Phlyctenular Conjunctivitis
(see page 132)

Phlyctenules occur mainly at the limbus. They may be single or multiple and are nodular aggregates of lymphocytes. Corneal phlyctenules cause stromal infiltration. If within 3 mm of the limbus, they become vascularized (keratitis fascicularis) (Plate IX, Fig. 4, page 192 a). A thick pannus or deep vascularization may develop. The vascularized infiltrates can shift over the entire cornea (wandering phlyctenule) (Plate IX, Fig. 5, page 192 a). With scrofulous phlyctenulosis, tuberculous ulcers can form. Blepharospasm is marked. After healing the residual corneal scars frequently show Fuchs' lines of clearing (Fig. 13.33) along obliterated blood vessels.

Phlyctenular conjunctivitis is an exudative-lymphocytic-allergic diathesis that formerly was thought to be caused predominantly by scrofula. Today it is seen as an allergic reaction against staphylococci and other agents. Scrofula is seen primarily in children between ages six and ten. Diet, hygiene and general health play a role and account in part for the virtual disappearance of the disease in Europe and the United States.

Acne Rosacea Keratitis (see page 133)

Contrary to the benign, although cosmetically

disfiguring, effect on the skin, corneal involvement by acne rosacea can be quite serious. Symptoms are photophobia, tearing, and pain. The corneal nodules are vascularized by tortuous dilated vessels growing as far as and slightly beyond the infiltrate (Plate IX, Fig. 6, page 192 a).

The subepithelial nodules ulcerate and develop lipid or calcium deposition. The disease is recurrent and affects women (between the ages of 40 and 50) more often than men. Scrofula affects primarily children.

Differential diagnosis: Scrofula is seen mainly in children and appears acutely with marked blepharospasm and vascularization of the cornea. *Acne rosacea* keratitis is chronic; the infiltrates increase and vascularize without remission. The disease generally affects elderly persons. *Recurrent marginal ulcers* occurring in older patients are usually unilateral along the limbus and vascularized (Fig. 13.26, see page 159). Marginal ulcers do not migrate or expand toward the center. *Interstitial keratitis* occurs in younger patients and leads to infiltration and deep vascularization of large areas of the cornea. *Herpes* dendrites are not vascularized and corneal sensitivity is decreased. *Trachomatous* pannus lies superiorly, the follicles rupture and there is conjunctival scarring. *Vernal catarrh* has a milky blue edema, large cobblestone papillae on the upper tarsal conjunctiva and limbus. It occurs mainly in young males.

Metaherpetic (Disciform) Keratitis (see page 155)

Improper use of steroid or topical anesthetics can cause ulcer formation.

Neuroparalytic Keratitis (Congenital Anesthesia)

A neurotropic corneal ulcer can appear (as early as 24 hours) after damage to the Gasserian ganglion or the first division of the trigeminal nerve. Such damage can be caused by tumor (pontine-cerebellar angle), trauma, surgical disruption, or alcohol injection of the Gasserian ganglion to treat trigeminal neuralgia. It is primarily a benign lesion with epithelial vesicle formation and can evolve into central, or lower paracentral, epithelial and stromal ulcers (Plate X, Fig. 2, page 192 b). Because of the corneal anesthesia, subjective symptoms are minimal. The ulcer is chronic and a real danger exists for superinfection with secondary infiltrates, iritis, hypopyon, synechiae, and perforation (see ulcus serpens [see page 160]). A trophic ulcer is caused rather by an irritation of the sympathicus than by III/1 anesthesia.

Congenital anesthesia is a lack of sensory innervation of the first branch of the trigeminal nerve. Neuroparalytic keratitis, often with hypopyon, develops within the first year of life and results in central scarring (Pillat 1949; Hewson 1963).

Congenital neuroparalytic keratitis is also seen in familial dysautonomia (Riley-Day syndrome). In this case the congenital lack of tear secretion is an additional factor.

Differential diagnosis: Keratomalacia occurs in malnourished children. Both eyes are affected and other signs of vitamin A deficiency such as hoarseness and brittle nails are present. Exposure keratitis is usually in the lower third of the cornea and associated with lagophthalmos (see page 162).

Xerophthalmia

This occurs in *vitamin A deficiency*. It includes *night blindness, keratomalacia* and *conjunctival xerosis*. Foamy white *(Bitôt) spots* are located in the interpalpebral fissure area.

With xerosis, the conjunctiva is dry, metaplastic, and wrinkled in small folds concentric to the limbus. Skin and other mucous membranes are dry and scaly. Hair and nails lack luster and break easily.

Bitôt spots are located in the interpalpebral fissure area. They are foamy white, not wetted by tears and consist of metaplastic epithelial cells and debris infected with Corynebacterium xerosis.

Pre-xerosis is said to exist when the clinical picture is not fully developed.

Keratomalacia

Keratomalacia (Plate X, Fig. 3, page 192 b) begins as a corneal dryness and haze followed by deep and superficial vascularization. The cornea takes on the appearance of fish scales

or finger nails (necrobiosis or prekeratonecrosis). A danger sign is when stroma becomes visible beneath the epithelium. The stroma may thin rapidly and perforate, allowing iris, even lens, to prolapse. Secondary infection causes panophthalmitis and loss of the eye. Staphyloma, secondary glaucoma, and phthisis bulbi are other sequelae. The disease is invariably bilateral and relatively free of irritation even when the process is severe (Pillat 1930). Xerophthalmia may occur in infants with digestive disorders where vitamin absorption is deficient.
Keratomalacia is also found in hereditary metabolic diseases, such as multiple fibrosis (cystic fibrosis); where vitamin A is malabsorbed (Ullerich and Witte 1961). There is a need for more vitamin A in infectious disease and scrofula. Xeromalacia in adults is usually caused by malabsorption as with alcoholic gastritis, gastroenteritis, the dumping syndrome, digestive disorders and liver disease.

Trachoma

Trachoma (see page 130) causes superior pannus formation. Superficial, poorly demarcated ulcers, which heal with residual scarring, may also occur. If the conjunctival scarring is sufficiently extensive xerosis and corneal scarring with loss of sensitivity result.

Perforating Injuries

Perforating injuries are obvious when iris and lens injury or prolapse result, or when the anterior chamber is lost. They are less obvious when small particles penetrate at high speed. If a worker with high-speed tools claims feeling that something has hit his eye, careful radiologic, ultrasound and ophthalmoscopic examination is indicated.

Arcus Senilis = Gerontoxon (Fig. 13.13), Embryotoxon

Arcus senilis is a common, almost physiologic dystrophy of aging. There is an intracellular deposition of lipids in the cornea. The deposits form a ring about 1.5 mm wide just inside the limbus, but separated from it by a small clear space.
In embryotoxon the same deposits often exist since birth.

Corneal Dystrophies

Classification of hereditary-familial corneal degenerations (after Franceschetti and Forni 1950) (see Gruber 1953) (François 1966; Malbran 1972; Goldberg 1974).

I. Stromal Dystrophies

A. Classic forms
(not congenital, progressive)

1. Dominant heredity
   a) granular dystrophy (Groenouw Type I)
   b) lattice degeneration (Haab-Dimmer)
2. Recessive inheritance
   Macular dystrophy (Groenouw Type II, Fleischer Type I)

B. Congenital (more or less stationary)

1. Recessive	Includes sclerocornea either total or
2. Dominant	only near the limbus, arcus juvenilis, posterior embryotoxon, central cloudy cornea, sickle shaped opacities

C. Diverse Forms

1. Crystalline degeneration (Schnyder)
2. Primary lipid degeneration
3. Primary calcific degeneration (Axenfeld)
4. Cornea farinata (Vogt)
5. Deep filiform dystrophy (Maeder and Danis)

II. Limiting Membrane Dystrophies

A. Anterior limiting membrane

1. Recurrent erosions
(Franceschetti)
2. Juvenile epithelial degeneration (Meesmann's dystrophy)
3. Degeneration of Bowman's membrane with epithelial changes
(Reis, Bücklers, Herrmann and others)
4. Cornea verticillata (Fleischer, Gruber)
5. (Senile) (crocodile shagreen (Vogt, Valerio)
6. Band shaped corneal dystrophy
(Fuchs, Streiff, Zwahlen)
7. Marginal degeneration
(Bietti)

B. Posterior limiting membrane

1. Cornea guttata
(Stähli, Vogt and others)
2. Posterior polymorphous dystrophy
(Koeppe)

III. Combined Forms (stroma and limiting membranes)

1. Diverse (granular degeneration and cornea guttata, band shaped corneal dystrophy and cornea guttata)
2. Edematous corneal dystrophy
a) Combined epithelial-endothelial dystrophy of Fuchs
b) Primary intermittent or essential corneal edema (Aubineau et al.)
c) Posterior polymorphous dystrophy

IV. Corneal degeneration with systemic disease

A. Metabolic disorders

1. Hurler's disease (gargoylism, dysostosis multiplex, lipochondro-osteodystrophy)
2. Hand-Schüller-Christian disease
3. Others (Tay-Sachs, Gaucher's disease, etc.)

B. Disorders of protein metabolism

1. Cystinosis (Bürki)
2. Various etiologies (alkaptonuria, etc.)

C. Dermatologic disorders

Ichthyosis, palmoplantar keratosis,
syringoma of the eyelid, Rothmund's disease, etc.

D. Other systemic diseases (Paget's, porphyria)

The most common corneal dystrophies include:

1. Familial corneal dystrophy
a) Granular corneal dystrophy; b) lattice dystrophy; c) macular dystrophy; d) crystalline corneal dystrophy; e) congenital stationary hereditary dystrophy; f) epithelial corneal dystrophy of Meesmann and Wilke; g) epithelial dystrophy of Kraupa; h) honeycomb, subepithelial corneal dystrophy after Thiel and Behnke; i) dermochondro corneal dystrophy after François; j) cornea verticillata; k) recurrent erosions; l) mosaic degeneration; m) ring shaped dystrophy; n) pre-Descemet's corneal dystrophy; o) senile disciform corneal degeneration; p) corneal guttata; q) Fuchs' endothelial dystrophy; r) blister and dellenform degeneration, polymorphous degeneration of the posterior cornea; s) crocodile shagreen of the posterior corneal surface; t) central cloudy corneal dystrophy.

2. Secondary corneal degenerations
a) Band keratopathy; b) irregular buckling of the posterior corneal surface; c) fat, amyloid, hyaline and calcium infiltrates; d) bullous keratopathy.

3. Storage diseases
a) Hurler's b) cystinosis c) crystal deposition in gout d) hereditary crystaline degeneration (Schnyder).

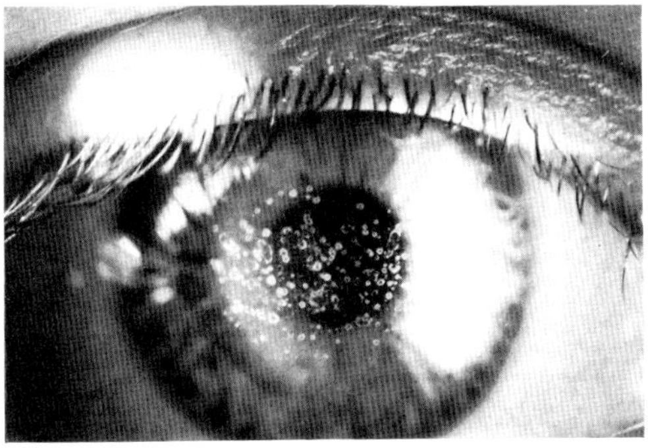

Fig. 13.34 Granular dystrophy (♀ 13 yrs.)

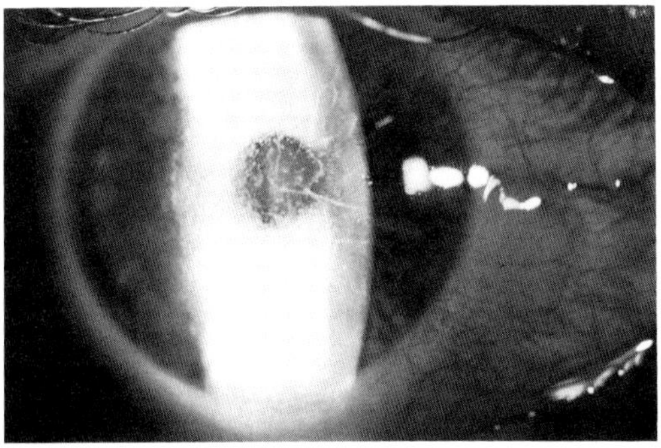

Fig. 13.35 Lattice corneal dystrophy (♂ 42 yrs.)

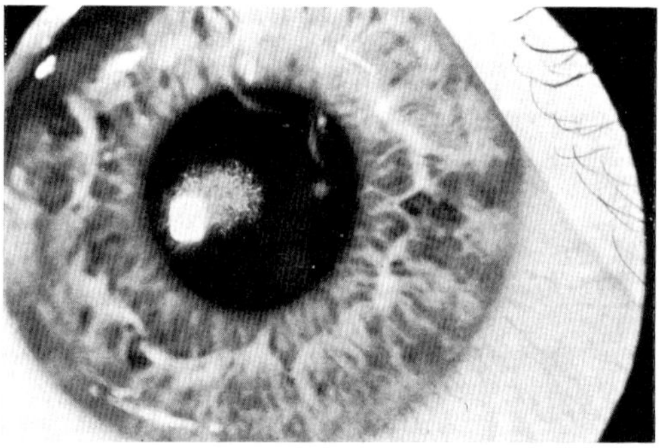

Fig. 13.36 Schnyder's crystalline corneal dystrophy (♀ 7 yrs.)

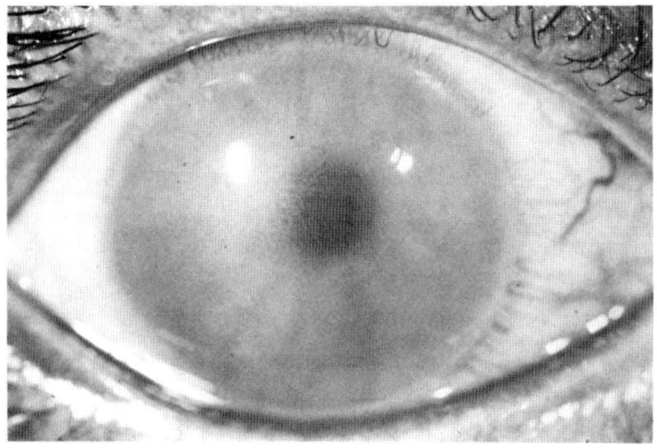

Fig. 13.38 Dense, diffuse, cloudy, bilateral, congenital, corneal dystrophy (♀ 27 yrs.)

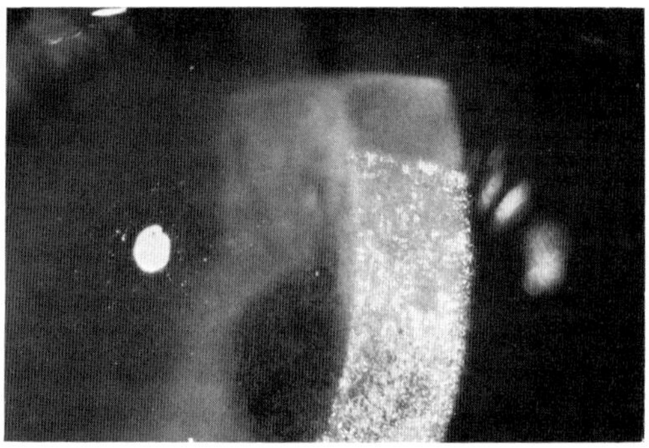

Fig. 13.37 Crystalline corneal dystrophy (♀ 47 yrs.)

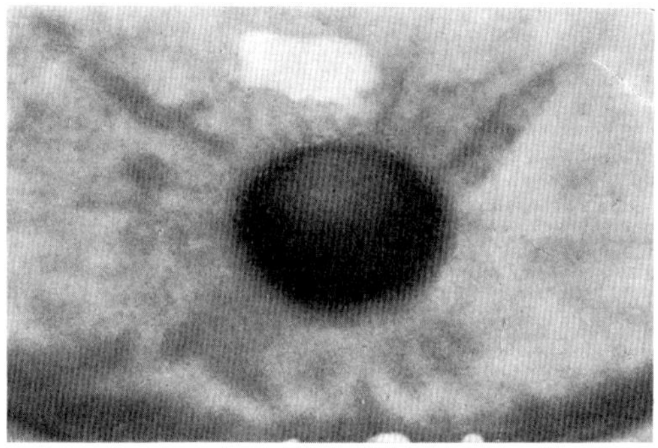

Fig. 13.39 Epithelial corneal dystrophy (Meesmann-Wilke)

1. Familial Corneal Dystrophies

a) *Granular* corneal dystrophy (Groenouw I) (Fig. 13.34) has dominant heredity and appears in the first decade of life. The lesions begin as fine sharply circumscribed subepithelial granules. By age 20 they become larger and are glassy white granules, nodules, rings of varying size, shape and density. Only the center of the cornea is affected. The cornea between lesions is entirely normal. Vision is usually not affected until ages 40 to 50 years.
b) *Lattice dystrophy* (Haab-Dimmer) has a dominant heredity. The lesions become obvious by puberty although minimal changes are seen in early childhood (three to five years). The classic lesions are overlapping linear opacities simulating ghost vessels except for the nodular thickenings irregularly distributed along their course and the fact that they begin and end abruptly within the cornea. The earliest changes are subepithelial but later deep stromal lesions are found.The epithelium is secondarily affected. Lesions tend to be located centrally, while the corneal periphery remains clear. There may be an associated generalized stromal haze (Fig. 13.35). Corneal sensitivity is decreased.
c) *Macular corneal dystrophy* (Groenouw II, Fehr, Fleischer) begins in the first decade of life as minute subepithelial opacities. Later these expand into gray white diffuse lesions of varying size which cause marked decrease in vision. Inheritance is recessive and corneal sensitivity is decreased (Jones and Zimmermann 1959).
d) *Schnyder's crystalline corneal dystrophy* begins in childhood and leads to central or paracentral disk and ring-shaped crystalline deposits in the subepithelium or superficial parenchyma (Figs. 13.36, 13.37). Heredity is dominant.

e) *Congenital, hereditary, dense, diffuse, cloudy corneal dystrophy* manifests centrally as bilateral, symmetrical, diffuse corneal clouding of the deep stroma. Heredity can be dominant or recessive; the congenital endothelial dystrophy (Maumenee 1960) looks quite similar (Fig. 13.38).

f) *Meesmann's dystrophy* (Meesmann and Wilke 1939) is purely epithelial. Heredity is dominant, and glycogen deposits in the epithelial cells. Tiny, white-gray vacuolelike deposits appear in the epithelium, primarily in the interpalpebral fissure area (Fig. 13.39) (Burns 1968; Behnke and Thiel 1965). Lesions are noted as early as age one to two and may be scattered or sectorial in distribution (François 1966, 1972).

g) The *epithelial dystrophy of Kraupa* involves epithelium and superficial stroma. It appears shortly after birth and consists of small epithelial bullae.

h) A dominant *subepithelial honeycomb dystrophy* (Fig. 13.40) was described by Thiel and Behnke (1967). The dystrophy manifests in the second decade of life. Corneal erosions occur at irregular intervals and vision is adversely affected.

In dermo-chondro-corneal dystrophy (François 1966) multiple white, sometimes brown lesions appear subepithelially. These protrude slightly from the corneal surface without causing an inflammatory reaction. Other findings include multiple xanthomalike nodules on the fingers, nose and ears. *Polyepiphyseal osteochondro dystrophy* causes subluxation and contracture (claw hand) of hands and feet (Remky and Engelbrecht 1967).

Cornea verticillata (Fleischer) consists of numerous punctate opacities in the epithelium or Bowman's membrane which form a whorl-like pattern. Similar lesions (Bron 1973) appear in Fabry's disease, and in chloroquine, indomethacin, phenothiazine and Amiodaron deposition. *Fabry's disease* (Fig. 13.41) (Denden and Franceschetti 1969; Font and Fine 1972) is an inborn error of metabolism with glycolipid deposition (see page 366). All blood vessels including those of the retina and conjunctiva become tortuous and develop aneurysms. The most common cause of cornea verticillata is chloroquine deposition (see page 291 and Fig. 13.42). Long term chloroquine therapy (more than 250 mg/day) leads to corneal deposits 33 to 68 percent of the time. Retinal involvement is less common. There is narrowing of retinal vessels, macular edema, optic atrophy and at a late stage, dustlike retinal pigmentation *(Bulls-eye maculopathy)* (Pau and Bäumer 1959; Dannheim and Ortbauer 1965) (see page 291).

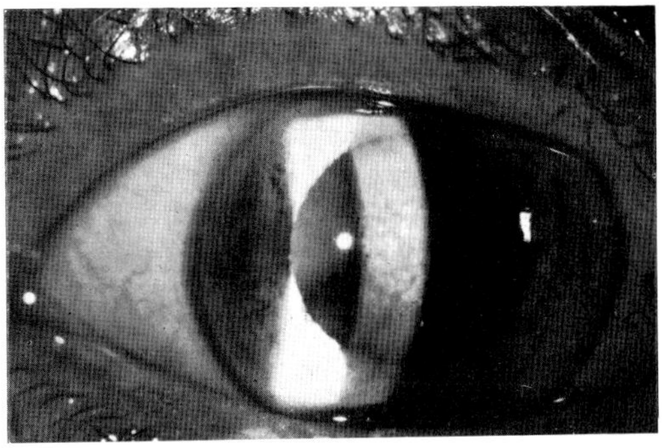

Fig. 13.40 Honeycomb subepithelial corneal dystrophy (♀ 75 yrs.)

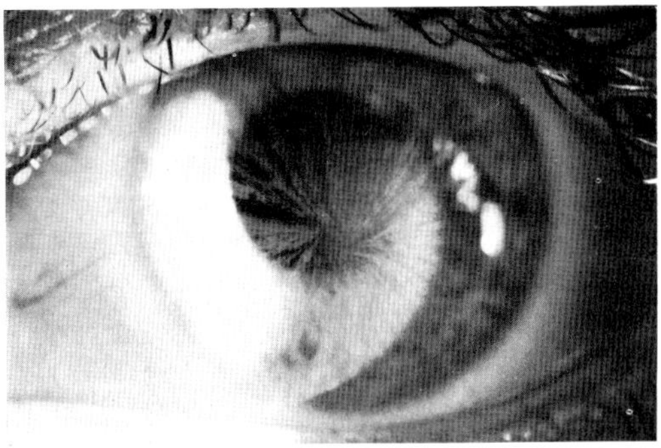

Fig. 13.41 Cornea verticillata in Fabry's disease (♀ 30 yrs.)

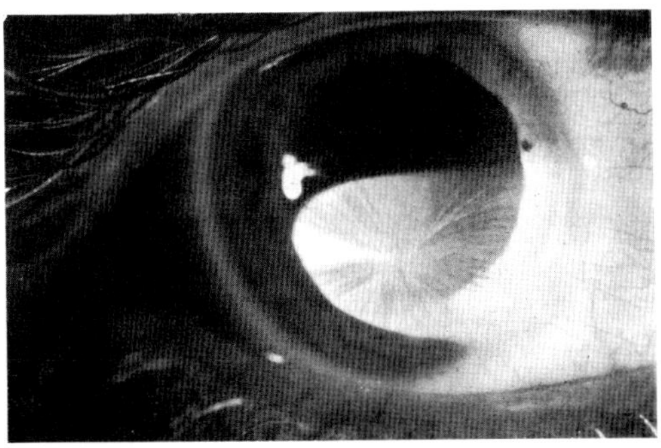

Fig. 13.42 Cornea verticillata caused by chloroquine deposition (♂ 43 yrs.)

Amiodaron use (see page 174) may cause gray-yellow or brown epithelial deposits in the form of cornea verticillata.
Long term indomethacin (Indocin), as with arthritis, can lead to cornea verticillata and retinal damage. ERG and EOG are affected (Burns 1968; Palimeris et al. 1972). Funduscopic changes are similar to those seen with chloroquine.
Neuroleptic phenothiazine preparations cause reversible corneal, conjunctival and retinal deposits (see page 119).

k) *Recurrent erosions* of the corneal epithelium occur spontaneously after minor trauma or may be inherited in a dominant manner (Franceschetti and Klein 1928).

l) *Anterior mosaic degeneration of Vogt (anterior crocodile shagreen).* Gray patches separated by darker areas develop in the corneal center at the level of Bowman's membrane. The dystrophy appears in a juvenile and a senile form. Vision is variably affected.

m) *Reis-Bückler's* ring-shaped dystrophy begins between ages two and five. Gray rings and cottonlike lines develop at the level of Bowman's membrane. These lesions tend to be located centrally in the cornea and with time fuse into maplike shapes. Heredity is dominant. Epithelial changes leading to recurrent erosions ultimately result.

n) *Pre-Descemet corneal dystrophies include: cornea farinata (Vogt)* with small dustlike lesions in the deepest parenchyma. The lesions are bilateral.
Deep punctate dystrophy (Franceschetti and Maeder) consists of numerous sharply delineated white dots that may appear in clumps.
In *deep filiform dystrophy* (Maeder and Danis) varying numbers of small gray-white lines occur at random in the deep stroma of the central cornea.

o) *Senile macular corneal dystrophy* is a form of cornea guttata. Cloudy patches separated by darker lines develop in the deep stroma. Descemet's membrane is gray, thickened and irregular with the appearance of wrinkled cloth. The etiology appears to be the same as cornea guttata (Slezak 1968).

p) *Cornea guttata* are a senile change. Inheritance is irregularly dominant. The lesions are common and best seen by spectral reflection (endothelial mirror) when they appear as gray bedewing or shiny droplike prominences on the posterior corneal surface (Descemet membrane). The central cornea is selectively involved (Wolter and Henderson 1957). Frequently fine pigment granules deposit on the endothelium between the prominences giving the posterior cornea the appearance of beaten metal (Table X, Fig. 5, page 192 b) (see Fuchs' endothelial dystrophy).

q) *Fuchs' endothelial dystrophy* begins as cornea guttata. Secondary changes occur in other corneal layers with an intermediate form between guttata and combined endothelial-epithelial dystrophy. There is a thickening and grayness of the central corneal parenchyma. Later epithelial vacuoles develop which may coalesce and form bullae. The clinical picture is variable. At first corneal edema and epithelial vacuoles are more prominent in the morning than at night. Finally, when the dystrophy is of long standing the epithelial bullae may rupture causing transient erosions with photophobia, foreign body sensation and irritation. The increasing corneal edema and epithelial irregularities lead to decreased vision.

r) Next to cornea guttata the most common endothelial dystrophy is the relatively rare *posterior polymorphous dystrophy* (Koeppe 1916; Forni 1951). The same entity was called blister and dellenform corneal dystrophy by Triebenstein (1925) and Schlichting (1941). Vacuoles, dimples, and even broad bands of varying size covered by endothelium appear at the level of Descemet's membrane. All of the Descemet may be thickened, or changes limited to a gray aureole around groups of vesicles. Histologically the endothelial cells are abnormal, with epithelial characteristics. Irregular layers of basement membrane material is produced which causes the thickened Descemet (Kuwabara 1968; Morgan and Patterson 1967; Tripathi 1975; Grayson 1975; Hanselmayer 1972). There is a strong association with glaucoma.

Posterior polymorphous dystrophy has a dominant inheritance with variable expressivity. Broad iris adhesions and pupillary ectropion are seen in some patients. The lesions have been noted as early as age three but are prob-

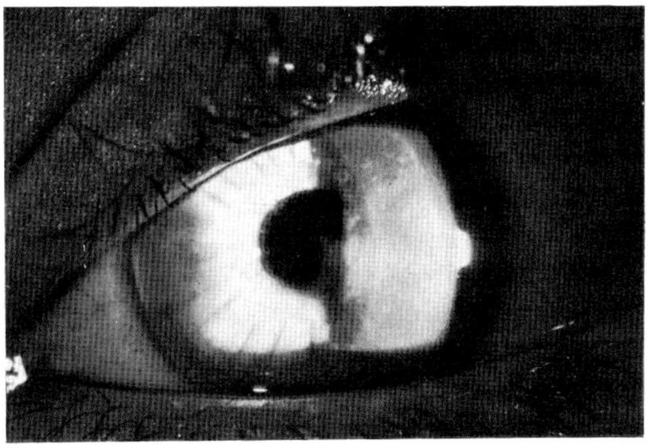

Fig. 13.43 Posterior polymorphous dystrophy of the cornea (♂ 6 yrs.)

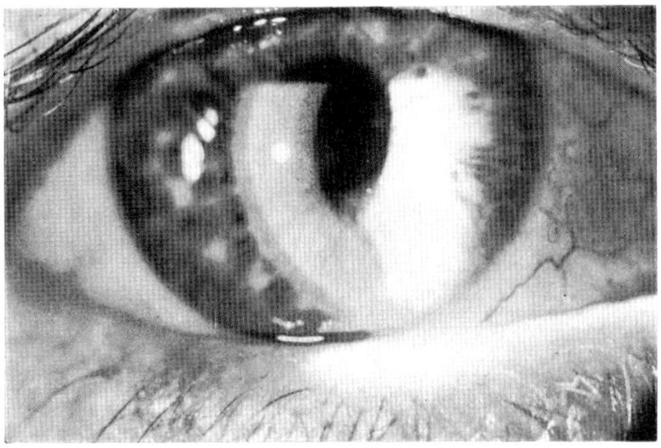

Fig. 13.44 Posterior crocodile shagreen (♂ 57 yrs.)

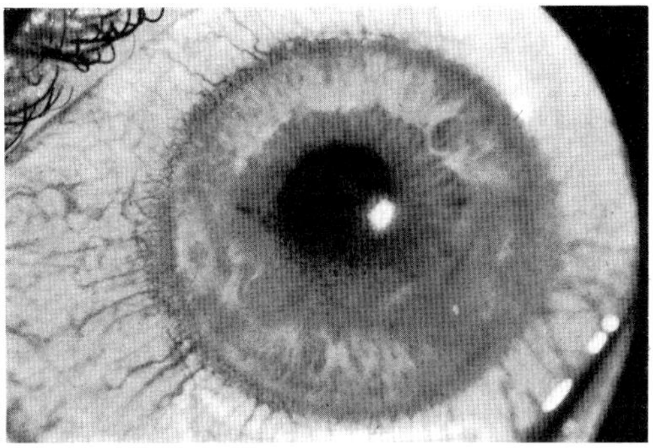

Fig. 13.45 Band keratopathy in Still's disease (♂ 16 yrs.)

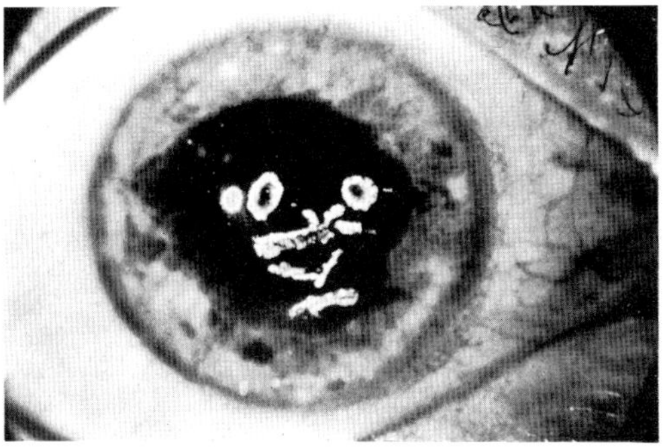

Fig. 13.46 Calcium deposition in a corneal scar (dendritic keratitis) (♀ 39 yrs.)

ably present at birth since cases of neonatal corneal clouding are documented. Some cases of congenital hereditary dystrophy and Chandler's syndrome belong in this category. The dystrophy is usually stationary but combined endothelial-epithelial dystrophy, even band keratopathy occurs. Even without epithelial changes the patients are uniformly photophobic. Vision is usually normal but may be decreased (Fig. 13.43).

s) *Posterior crocodile shagreen* (Vogt): Gray white clouding at the level of Descemet and the posterior third of the corneal stroma is crisscrossed by darker lines giving the appearance of crocodile skin (Fig. 13.44). A similar clinical appearance occurs at the level of Bowman's membrane. The dystrophy occurs in young persons but is primarily a senile change, when the lesions are more fluffy and anterior in the corneal stroma. François speaks of *Central cloudy dystrophy*.

2. Secondary Corneal Degenerations

Band keratopathy (Fig. 13.45) progresses from the corneal periphery to the center in the interpalpebral fissure area. There is opacification and ultimately calcium deposition in the epithelium, Bowman's membrane and superficial stroma.

Band keratopathy is generally secondary to chronic iridocyclitis, sympathetic ophthalmia, deep keratitis, perforating injury, burns, absolute glaucoma or phthisis bulbi. The most common cause of band keratopathy in children is Still's disease (collagen autoimmune disorder) with cataracts, iritis and arthritis (see page 194). High doses of vitamin D, alkali or milk may cause band keratopathy (Crews 1963). Hypercalcemia and hyperparathyroidism as well as chronic external chemical irritation (mercury vapors, calcium bichromate) produce band keratopathy. Band keratopathy

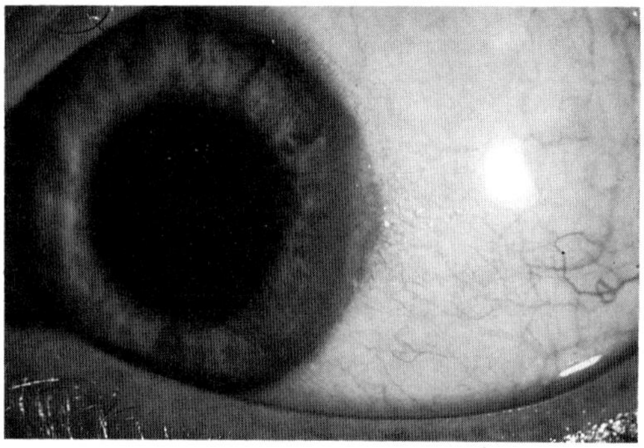

Fig. 13.47 Perilimbal calcium deposited superficially in the cornea and conjunctiva. Renal insufficiency, dialysis patient (♀ 8 yrs.)

is an occupational disease in hatters and furriers owing to irritation and penetration by textile fibers.

Irregular Descemet folds (Vogt). Irregular, delimited gray areas on the posterior corneal surface are seen following keratitis and iridocyclitis. These represent a transition to hyaline precipitates and Descemet ridges.

Corneal scars and leucomas in severely injured eyes (phthisis bulbi, etc.) frequently develop secondary *lipid amyloid* or *hyaline deposits* (Plate XI, Fig, 1, page 192 c). Eyes with absolute glaucoma, chronic intraocular inflammation (iridocyclitis, after multiple or ill-fated surgery, etc.) develop similar infiltrates. Such changes, especially in a phthisical eye, cause secondary corneal dystrophy with epithelial and stromal edema *(bullous keratopathy),* degenerative pannus, (superficial vascularization) and secondary lipid or calcium deposition. Any corneal scar may calcify secondarily (Fig. 13.46). This is especially true of band keratopathy and rosacea keratitis. Chronic overdosing with vitamin D leads to punctate superficial calcium deposits. These stretch across the center of the cornea in a band with a clear zone remaining at the limbus. The lesions are located at the level of Bowman's membranes and require months, even a year, to regress once vitamin D intake is stopped (Gifford and Maguire 1954).

Scleral calcium deposits are a rare complication of hypercalcemia with hypervitaminosis D. With chronic renal insufficiency and in renal dialysis, patients' calcium can deposit in the cornea and conjunctiva near the limbus (Schumacher and Scheller 1969; Fig. 13.47). Besides juvenile and senile arcus, corneal lipid deposition occurs with primary or secondary lipidoses, hypercholesterolemia, hyperlipemia, xanthomatosis, and dermato-chondro-corneal dystrophy.

Bullous keratopathy commonly occurs in blind eyes especially those with absolute glaucoma, Fuchs' endothelial dystrophy, extensive corneal scarring, vitreous touch, opaque grafts or foreign body deposition on the endothelium. The epithelial vesicles may rupture causing painful erosions (see page 168).

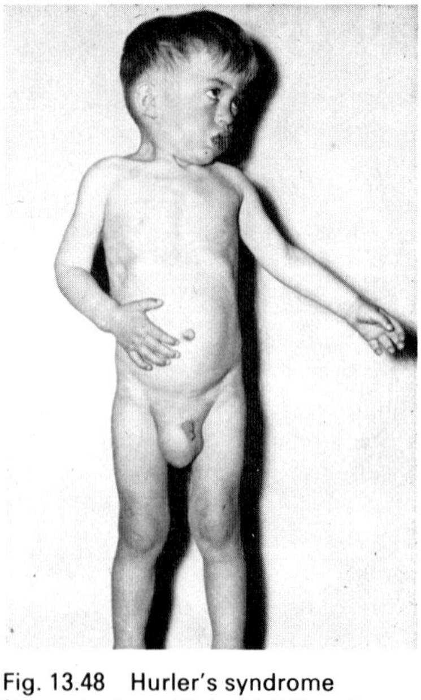

Fig. 13.48 Hurler's syndrome (Dysostosis multiplex) (♂ 3 yrs.)

3. Storage Diseases

Dysostosis multiplex (Pfaundler-Hurler, gargoylism) (Fig. 13.48) has punctate gray-white spots throughout the stroma but concentrated in Bowman's membrane and the superficial layers. This results in corneal clouding which is always bilateral. Corneal clouding is present at birth or appears later. There is an abnormal accumulation and storage of mucopolysaccharides in stromal keratocytes (Badke 1961;

Günther 1958; Pau and Rodeck 1953; Rodger 1969) (see page 365).
Hurler's disease is recessive in inheritance. There is disproportionate dwarfism with an obtrusively large head but short neck and body. The root of the nose is depressed and the nares flare out from the face. The tongue (lingua scrotalis) and lips are thickened abnormally. The characteristic facies gives rise to the name gargoylism. There is kyphoscoliosis similar to rickets. The extremities and fingers are short and plump. The patients have a waddling gait. Liver and spleen are enlarged. Mouth breathing, bronchitis, and pharyngitis are common.
Other mucopolysaccharidoses with corneal haze (see page 365) are: *Morquio's* syndrome and *Scheie* (late Hurler) syndrome. Tapetoretinal degeneration (retinal pigmentary changes, optic atrophy, arteriolar narrowing) with a subnormal or extinguished ERG is not uncommon.
Cystinosis (see page 363) is a rare disease of infants and children with innumerable, small, yellow-white, glistening needle-shaped or punctate crystals deposited in the corneal stroma (Fig. 13.49, Plate XI, Fig. 2, page 192 c). Epithelium and endothelium remain unaffected (Bürki 1954). Histologically the crystals are extracellular in cornea, conjunctiva, episclera and uvea (Bürki 1954; Cogan and Kuwabara 1960; François et al. 1972).

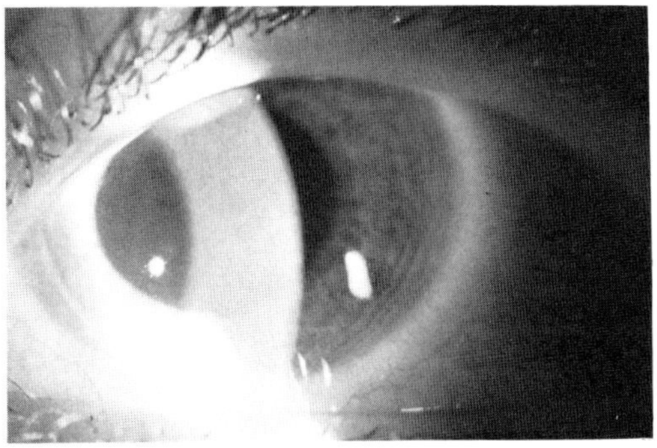

Fig. 13.49 Hurler-Pfaundler syndrome. Small punctate stromal corneal opacities (♂ 25 yrs.)

Lignac-Fanconi syndrome is a form of vitamin D resistant rickets with cystinosis. The patients are photophobic, dwarfed, have severe renal tubular damage, hyperaminoaciduria, glycosuria and hyperphosphaturia. Uric acid crystals can deposit in the cornea in *gout*.
Schnyder's hereditary crystalline corneal degeneration is a hereditary corneal dystrophy with deposition of *cholesterol crystals* in the corneal stroma and a partial absence or interruption of Bowman's membrane (Dellman and Winkelman 1968) (see page 166).

Genodermatoses

Genodermatoses are genetically determined skin disorders which may have associated *dystrophic corneal changes* (Franceschetti and Thier 1971).

Recessive hereditary epidermolysis bullosa — Palmoplantar keratosis — Keratitis follicularis spinulosa decalvans — Ichthyosis vulgaris — Rothmund's syndrome, congenital poikilodermia — Angiokeratoma corporis diffusum (Fabry) — Psoriasis

Recessive Epidermolysis Bullosa

The dominant form of epidermolysis bullosa is usually not associated with corneal changes. *Recessive epidermolysis bullosa* begins immediately after birth. Subepithelial bullae develop which rupture and scar. Nails and terminal phalanges are distorted. *Corneal bullae* rupture and cause recurrent erosions with secondary pannus formation. *Conjunctival bullae* result in *scarring* (Plate VIII, Fig. 4, page 128 h).

Palmoplantar Keratosis

Superficial herpeslike corneal lesions are among the cardinal symptoms in the recessively inherited *Richner-Hanhart* syndrome. Corneal changes are rare in the dominant *Jadassohn-Lewandowsky* syndrome (Pachyonychia congenita) (Schnyder). Dermatologic signs in Richner-Hanhart syndrome include painful keratinized plaques on the knees, hands, feet and elbows as well as subungual keratosis. Usually there is mental retardation. The herpetiform corneal lesions are nonprogressive dystrophic epithelial changes which may be bizarre in shape. Corneal sensitivity is maintained (Franceschetti et al. 1972; Schnyder 1972).

Keratitis Follicularis Spinulosa Decalvans

Keratin barbs in follicles give the skin an abrasive texture. Dystrophic corneal changes and localized alopecia are part of this disorder. Heredity is recessive. Typically the *outer third of the eye brows are missing* (Hertogh's sign). Superficial *dustlike punctate epithelial opacities* and *circular pannus* appear on the *cornea*.
Atypical dystrophic corneal changes are not a regular finding in the other genodermatoses but may appear *spontaneously* (Franceschetti and Thier 1961).

Ichthyosis Vulgaris

Mechanical corneal damage — Dot and maplike epithelial opacities — Linear-netlike deep stromal opacities — Band keratopathy with ichthyosis.

Various corneal changes appear as a rare complication (Cordes and Hogan 1939):

1. Inflammatory form with conjunctival hyperplasia and secondary, mechanical alteration of the cornea.

2. Lid scarring in ichthyosis may cause cicatricial ectropion. Conjunctivitis and keratitis result (Sondermann 1923; Weber 1953).

3. A primary corneal dystrophy equivalent to the skin scales occurs. There are multiple, gray-green, punctate, maplike or nodular epithelial opacities. The underlying stroma is cloudy. The lesions resemble Salzmann's nodular dystrophy,

4. The asymptomatic forms may have punctate, sickle-shaped, or netlike corneal opacities in the deepest stroma, just in front of Descemet's membrane (Franceschetti and Maeder 1954).

5. Primary band keratopathy (Hermans 1956; Franceschetti and Schlappi 1957).

Rothmund's Syndrome

Atrophic dyskeratosis and anomalies of pigmentation ("congenital" poikilodermia) occur in the first year of life. A syndermatotic cataract appears between ages four to six. Other findings include premature graying, alopecia, dystrophy of the nails, abnormal dentition and endocrine disorders.

Werner's syndrome is the progeric atrophic form with spontaneous **ulcerations**. The cataracts appear later but are still juvenile. Heredity of both forms is recessive.

Band keratopathy has frequently been observed in Rothmund's syndrome.

Angiokeratoma Corporis Diffusum (Fabry)

Fabry's disease has *cornea verticillata* (see page 366 and Fig. 13.41) as well as tortuosity, dilatation and even aneurysm formation of bulbar and tarsal conjunctival veins. Dark red to black, pinhead-sized spots and papules develop on the buttocks, navel, breasts, scrotum and extensor surfaces of the extremities. This inborn metabolic error (glycolipid storage) manifests around the seventh to eighth year of life. The corneal deposits are similar to those seen with long-standing chloroquine, indomethacin, phenothiazine and amiodaron use.

Psoriasis

The conjunctiva (Kaldeck 1953; Rössler 1944; Fontana 1953; Schreck 1960) or cornea (Pillat 1934; Vrabec 1952) are rarely involved in psoriasis. Small blisters and plaques appear along with the exacerbations of the skin lesions. Conjunctival veins may be irregular in caliber and dilated.

Corneal Pigmentation

Pigment deposits in scars and with older patients — Hemosiderosis corneae — Kayser-Fleischer ring — Ochronosis — Chloroquine deposits — Phenol, Aniline, quinine — Phenothiazine — Epinephrine preparations — Metal deposition in the cornea (copper, silver, gold, iron, arsenic) — Pigment deposits on the posterior cornea — Melanosis corneae.

Pigment Deposits

Old, formerly vascularized scars frequently become pigmented. Lines or spots of brown pigment are seen in old scrofula scars but also in old traumatic scars and those of interstitial keratitis; ulcus serpens scars can develop brown pigmentation. Superficial corneal pigmentation may be seen running parallel to a pterygium.

Older persons frequently have a bilateral, horizontal, wavy, light brown to yellow line running across the lower third of the cornea (Hudson-Stähli line = linea senilis) (Vogt 1931) (Plate X, Fig. 4, page 192 b). Vogt thought the line to be associated with a break in Bowman's membrane. Tattooing (gold, ink) of leucomas is evident from the history.

Hemosiderosis Corneae

Blood staining of the cornea occurs when an anterior chamber hemorrhage has been present for some time. The process is accelerated and particularly common when there is elevation of intraocular pressure and a severely damaged globe. The staining is disk-shaped, in the center of the cornea (Plate XI, Fig. 3, page 192 c) with a clear band near the limbus (Gramberg-Danielsen 1956). The eye is free of irritation. The epithelium is smooth and only becomes edematous later. To prevent blood staining of the cornea, massive anterior chamber hemorrhages should be irrigated if they have not resolved after one to two weeks.

Blood staining of the cornea in children resolves over a period of months. In adults it takes years or may not occur at all leaving a gray-white disciform opacity.

Kayser-Fleischer Ring (see page 366)

In hepatolenticular degeneration *(Wilson's disease)*, specifically pseudosclerosis (Westphal-Strumpel disease), Kayser and Fleischer described a brown-yellow-green ring (Plate XI, Fig. 4, page 192 c) in Descemet's membrane. The ring, about 2 mm wide, begins directly at the limbus and fades away toward the center. It is deposition of copper (not silver) (Coleman et al. 1963). The Kayser-Fleischer ring appears between ages 11 through 25. Men are more frequently affected than women. Pseudosclerosis due to copper deposition and causing degeneration of the basal ganglia is part of Wilson's disease. Clinical findings include extrapyramidal rigidity, spontaneous tremors and hepatic cirrhosis.

Endogenous Ochronosis

Endogenous ochronosis (see page 364) occurs with *alkaptonuria*. There is a symmetric gray-brown discoloration of the limbal part of the cornea and sclera (Fig. 12.3).

Phenol, Aniline, Quinine

Chronic *phenol*, specifically *carbolic acid damage*, causes a gray-black conjunctival and corneal discoloration in the interpalpebral fissure area. The anesthetic cornea may become gray-white. *Aniline* (Amidobenzole), paraspecifically benzoquinone and hydroquinine cause melanosislike, brown, lid-conjunctival-corneal discoloration (Anderson 1947). Band keratopathy, epithelial damage and corneal ulceration are reported. The corneal nerves appear thickened despite corneal hypoanesthesia. The changes are seen mainly in the interpalpebral fissure area (light reaction). Aniline causes a brown discoloration of the gums, lips and nose, as well as cyanosis, cramps, paresis and speech disturbance.

Chloroquine, Indomethacin, Phenothiazine, Amiodaron-deposits Causing Cornea Verticillata (see page 167)

(Chloroquine and indomethacin deposits, see page 167 and 168).

Bilateral corneal, conjunctival and retinal pigmentation can occur when high dosages of chlorpromazine and *phenothiazines* are given for psychiatric diseases (McClanahan et al. 1966) (see page 168).

Phenothiazine produces yellow-brown pigmentation in the interpalpebral fissure area as linear, brown, superficial, reversible, epithelial deposits similar to cornea verticillata: white-yellow punctate lesions may be seen at the level of Descemet and deep corneal stroma. These appear to be irreversible (Hermans 1972).

Amiodaron *(Cordaron)* a catecholamine used for cardiovascular problems such as angina pectoris can also cause gray-yellow or brown corneal deposits of cornea verticillata. With 600 mg per day, deposits have been observed as early as the ninth day. With 400 mg per day, deposition is less and appears after several months (Verin and Sekkat 1973). The epithelial deposits are intracellular and disappear within a few months (Watillon and Robe-Vanwijck 1972).

Adrenalin Compounds

Chronic topical use of adrenalin preparations, especially epinephrine, causes pigmentation from deposition of black adrenochrome granules on the cornea and conjunctiva. Histochemically the pigment is similar to melanin (Green et al. 1967).

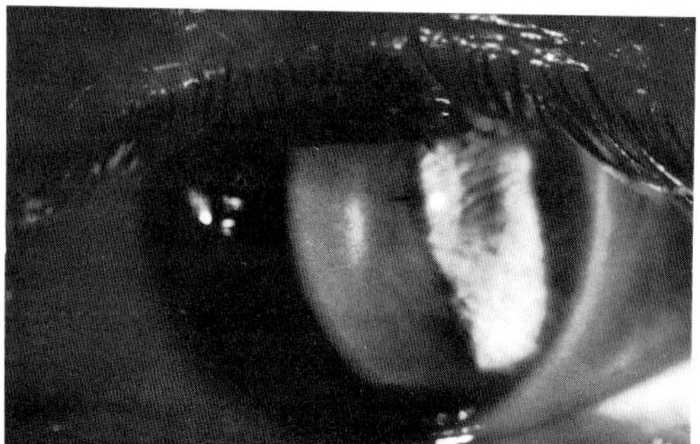

Fig. 13.50 Krukenberg spindle on the posterior corneal surface

Metal Deposition in the Cornea

Discoloration of the cornea from metal deposition occurs with copper (metal fragment in the eye) *(Chalcosis)* and appears blue-green-red; the use of silver compounds either locally, enterally, or parenterally, *(argyrosis)* appears blue-gray; and rarely, after injection of high dosages of gold, *chrysiasis* (yellow-red) occurs. The deposits are fine, glistening dots in Descemet's membrane and sometimes Bowman's membranes in a ring-shaped distribution around the limbus. Gold therapy (rheumatoid disorders, tuberculosis) may lead to asymptomatic gold deposition (chrysiasis). Rarely, corneal ulcers occur (perhaps from haptenes or allergy). In chrysiasis the fine punctate gold crystals are deposited subepithelially in proportion to the intensity of the therapy. The deposition is reversible.

Corneal *siderosis* occurs when iron-containing foreign bodies lodge in the cornea. A brown rust ring develops around the metallic particle. The accumulation of fine pigmented dots in *arsenic melanosis* causes dark pigmented patches on the bulbar conjunctiva and peripheral cornea (Meesmann 1920; Lerner and Fitzpatrick 1953).

Pigment Deposition on the Posterior Cornea

These appear physiologically as fine, brown, individual granules. There is an increase in such deposits with cornea guttata, after surgery (glaucoma, cataract), injury, with diabetes, iritis, and iridocyclitis. Aqueous convection currents allow a characteristic deposition of pigment granules: Türk's line is a vertical line of pigment granules in the lower half of the cornea. Krukenberg's spindle is a deposition of pigment granules in a wide band. These are bilateral, vary in size and run in a band from the corneal center inferiorly. The pigment is not only on top of, but actually within endothelial cells (this occurs with all

long standing precipitates). The eyes are usually normal but Krukenberg's spindle is found with pigmentary glaucoma (Fig. 13.50).
Keratic-gray precipitates in iridocyclitis are usually arranged according to size (Arlt's triangle), the larger being more inferior. They may, as with Fuchs' heterochromia, be random in distribution (see page 192).
Superficial *corneal melanosis* occurs as an extension of conjunctival melanosis. Limbal melanomas may grow onto the cornea.

Pterygium

"True" Pterygium (Fig. 12.21)

True pterygium is a triangular proliferation of conjunctival connective tissue onto the cornea. It is more common nasally than temporally. There is a gray corneal infiltrate just in front of the progressing vascularized head.

"Pseudo" Pterygium (Fig. 10.14)

Pseudopterygium occurs at any age secondary to scarring. True pterygiums appear primarily after the age of twenty. Pseudopterygium with adhesion of conjunctiva to cornea results from scarring after burns or injury. Unlike the true pterygium it is not progressive and does not form a true bridge (a probe cannot be passed underneath it).

Tumors

Corneal tumors (see page 137) include dermoids (Fig. 25.4). There is a high incidence of corneal dermoids in oculo-auricular-vertebral dysplasia (Goldenhar's syndrome) (see page 331), Cri-du-chat (Lejeune) syndrome (see page 329) and with Duane's retraction syndrome. Dermoids usually extend onto the cornea from the limbus. This is also true of *papillomas, lymphomas, lymphangiomas, fibromas, hemangiomas, teratomas* and *epitheliomas. Nevi, Bowen's intraepithelial epitheliomas, carcinomas, melanomas, melanocarcinomas* and *corneal sarcomas* usually originate in the conjunctiva. *Basal cell* carcinomas are seen in xeroderma pigmentosum. Thickening of Descemet's membrane, corneal nerves and corneal clouding occur in neurofibromatosis (von Recklinghausen's syndrome).

Bowen's disease (intraepithelial epithelioma) causes white *(leukoplakic)* or red-gray *(papillomatous)* solid to gelatinous proliferations (Fig. 13.51). They may also be cauliflower or raspberrylike in appearance (see page 138).
The cells are polymorphic. Some cells are large with plump, dark-staining nuclei. A true carcinoma may arise from Bowen's disease (Kreibig 1960; Angervall and Törnquist 1961; Krassat 1969).

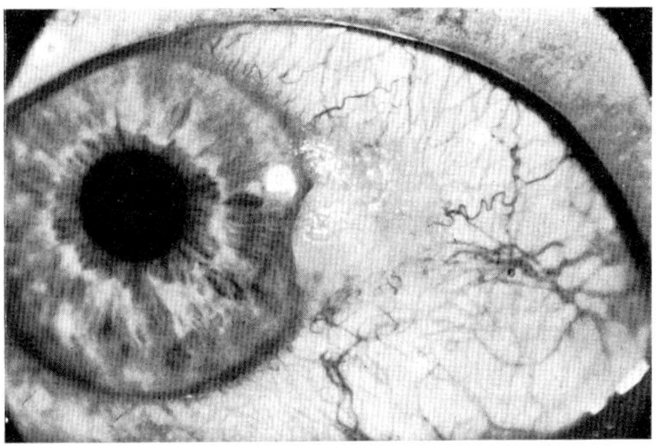

Fig. 13.51 Bowen's disease of the conjunctiva-cornea (♂ 79 yrs.)

References

Anderson, B.: Corneal and conjunctival pigmentation among workers engaged in manufacture of hydroquinone. Arch. Ophthal. 38 (1947) 812–826

Angervall, L., R. Törnquist: Bowen's disease of the cornea and conjunctiva. Acta ophthal. (Kbh.) 39 (1961) 808–816

Ashworth, A. N.: Cortisone in the treatment of syphilitic eye disease. Brit. J. vener. Dis. 29 (1953) 3–7

Ashworth, A. N.: Results of local cortisone therapy in syphilitic interstitial keratitis. Brit. J. vener. Dis. 34 (1958) 83–90

Badtke, G.: Die Mißbildungen des menschlichen Auges. In: Der Augenarzt, Vol. IV, ed. by K. Velhagen. Thieme, Stuttgart 1961

Behnke, H., H. J. Thiel: Über die hereditäre Epitheldystrophie der Hornhaut (Typ Meesmann-Wilke) in Schleswig-Holstein. Klin. Mbl. Augenheilk. 147 (1965) 662–672

Bietti, G. B.: Die Viruskeratitiden. Ber. dtsch. Ophthal. Ges. 71 (1972) 141–171

Bischoff, B.: Ein Beitrag zum Cogan I-Syndrom. Klin. Mbl. Augenheilk. 161 (1972) 551–562

Blatz, H.: Hornhauteinschmelzung nach Masern. Klin. Mbl. Augenheilk. 129 (1956) 762–772

Böke, W., H. Conrads: Zur Histologie der Hornhaut bei akutem Keratokonus. Albrecht v. Graefes Arch. klin. exp. Ophthal. 159 (1957) 277–284

Bonnet, P., J. Bonnet: Iritis bilatérale. Manifestations ganglionnaires et osseuses de la syphilis congénitale. Bull. Soc. Ophtal. (Paris) 67 (1954) 248–251

Bonnet, P., H. Chavanne: Kératite interstitielle hérédosyphilitique bilatérale, les deux localisations étant apparues a 25 ans de distance. Ann. Oculist. (Paris) 180 (1947) 243

Bonnet-Gehin, M., J. Tavernier: Les anneaux cornéens de coats. Ann. Oculist (Paris) 196 (1963) 247–268

Bron, A. J.: Vortex patterns of the corneal epithelium. Trans. ophthal. Soc. UK 93 (1973) 455–472

Bücklers, M.: Die erblichen Hornhautdystrophien. Bücherei des Augenarztes, 3. Enke, Stuttgart 1938

Bürki, E.: Ein weiterer Fall von Cystinosis mit Hornhautveränderungen. Ophthalmologica (Basel) 127 (1954) 309–314

Burns, C. A.: Indomethacin reduced retinal sensitivity and corneal depots. Am. J. Ophth. 66 (1968) 825–835

Burns, R. P.: Meesmann's corneal dystrophy. Trans. Amer. ophthal. Soc. 66 (1968) 530–635

Cogan, D. G.: Nonsyphilitic interstitial keratitis and vestibuloauditory symptoms. Arch. Ophthal. 42 (1949) 42–49

Cogan, D. G., T. Kuwabara: Ocular pathology of cystinosis. Amer. Arch. Ophthal. 63 (1960) 51–57

Coleman, S. L., T. E. Sanders, B. D. Field: Hepatolenticular Degeneration. Amer. J. Ophthal. 56 (1963) 297–299

Collier, M.: Epilepsie tardive et syndrome droit hémihypertrophie dyskeratose folliculaire de Darier naevus de la queue du sourcil fibres a myéline de la rétine. Bull. Soc. Ophtal. (Paris) 72 (1959) 530–537

Collier, M.: La dégénérescence limbique en ceinture blanche de Vogt. Arch. Ophtal. 21 (1961) 329–353; 454–479

Consiglio.: Langes Intervall bei Keratitis parenchymatosa zwischen dem rechten Auge und dem linken. Z. Augenheilk. 15 (1906) 177

Coppieters, R., L. Evers: Cystinosis, Amer. J. Ophthal. 73 (1972) 643–650

Cordes, F. G., M. J. Hogan: Ocular ichthyosis. Report of a case. Arch. Ophthal. (Chicago) 22 (1939) 590–594

Creutzburg.: Beitrag zur Frage der einseitigen Keratitis parenchymatosa e lue connata. Ophthal. Kongreß, D. D. R. 2, 1952

Crews, S. J.: Toxic effects on the eye and visual apparatus resulting from the systemic absorption of recently introduced chemical agents. Trans. ophthal. Soc. U. K. 82 (1963) 387–406

Dannheim, R., R. Ortbauer: Komplikationen am Auge bei Behandlung mit Chloroquin (Resochin). Klin. Mbl. Augenheilk. 146 (1965) 708–713

Delleman, J. W., J. E. Winkelman: Degeneratio corneae cristallinea hereditaria. Ophthalmologica 155 (1968) 409–426

Denden, A., A. Th. Franceschetti: Cornea Verticillata: Ein Symptom des Morbus Fabry-Anderson. Ber. dtsch. ophthal. Ges. 69 (1969) 145–149

Dohlman, C. H., P. Wright et al.: Symposium on the dry eye. Trans. ophthal. Soc. UK 91 (1971) 105–165

Duke-Elder, St. Sr.: System of Ophthalmology. In: The anatomy of the visual system, Vol. II. Kimpton, London 1961

Duke-Elder, St. Sr.: System of Ophthalmology. In: Normal and abnormal development, Vol. III. Kimpton, London 1961

Duke-Elder, St. Sr.: System of Ophthalmology. In: Congenital deformities. Kimpton, London 1964

Duke-Elder, St. Sr.: System of Ophthalmology. In: Diseases of the outer eye, Vol. VIII/2. Kimpton, London 1965

Duke-Elder, St. Sr.: System of Ophthalmology. In: The physiology of the eye and of vision, Vol. IV. Kimpton, London 1968

Eggers, C.: Dystrophia cornealis posterior polymorpha. Ophthalmologica 154 (1967) 1–5

Fazakes, A.: Oculomykosen und ihre Behandlung. Klin. Mbl. Augenheilk. 127 (1955) 701–721

Feyrter, F.: Über den Zoster. Hautarzt 5 (1954) 391–397

Font, R. L., B. S. Fine: Ocular pathology in Fabry's disease, Amer. J. Ophthal. 73 (1972) 419–430

Fontana, G.: Alterazioni vascolari del limbus sclerocorneale nella psoriasi. G. ital. Oftal. 6 (1953) 316–321

Forni, S.: Dégénérescence polymorphe familiale de la membran limitante postérieure de la cornée. Arch. Ophtal. (Paris) 11 (1951) 162–166

Forsius, H.: Studien über Cornea plana congenita bei 19 Kranken in 9 Familien. Acta ophthal. 39 (1961) 203–221

Franceschetti, A.: Hereditäre rezidivierende Erosion der Hornhaut. Z. Augenheilk. 66 (1928) 309–316

Franceschetti, A.: Clinical and social aspects of heredity in ophthalmology. Acta XVI Concilium Ophthalmologicum (Britannia) 157 (1950)

Franceschetti, A., C. Balavione: Réseau hyalin rétrocornéen après keratie parenchymateuse. Ophthalmologica (Basel) 125 (1953) 344–345

Franceschetti, A., S. Forni: Clinical and social aspects of heredity in ophthalmology. Acta XVI Concilium Ophthalmologicum, Britannia 1950

Franceschetti, A., G. Maeder: Dystrophie profonde de la cornée dans un cas d'ichtyose congénitale. Bull. Soc. Ophtal. (Paris) 67 (1954) 146–150

Franceschetti, A., V. Schläppi: Dégénérescence en bandelette et dystrophie prédescemétique de la cornée, dans un cas d'ichtyose congénitale. Dermatologica (Basel) 115 (1957) 217–223

Franceschetti, A., C. J. Thier: Über Hornhautdystrophien bei Genodermatosen unter besonderer Berücksichtigung der Palmoplantarkeratosen. Albrecht v. Graefes Arch. klin. exp. Ophthal. 162 (1961) 610–670

Franceschetti, A., K. Lisch, D. Klein: Zwei eineiige Zwillingspaare mit konkordantem Keratokonus. Klin. Mbl. Augenheilk. 133 (1958) 15–30

Franceschetti, A., D. Klein, S. Forni, J. Babel: Discussion on the clinical and social aspects of heredity in ophthalmology. Trans. ophthal. Soc. U. K. 70 (1951) 23–24

Franceschetti, A. Th., U. W. Schnyder, W. R. Felgenhauer: Die Cornea beim Richner-Hanhart-Syndrom. Ber. dtsch. ophthal. Ges. 72 (1972) 109–114

François, J.: Heredo-familial corneal dystrophies. Trans. ophthal. Soc. U. K. 86 (1966) 367–416

François, J.: Les mycoses oculaires. Masson, Paris 1968

François, J., M. Hanssens, L. Stockmans: Dégénérescence marginale pellucide de la cornée. Ophthalmologica (Basel) 155 (1968) 337–356

François, J.: Heredofamiliäre Hornhautdystrophien. Ber. dtsch. ophthal. Ges. 71 (1972) 171–222

Fuhs, H., J. Böck: Indikationen und Erfolge der Fiebertherapie bei Lues (unter besonderer Berücksichtigung ophthalmologischer Belange). Klin. Mbl. Augenheilk. 104 (1939) 129–145

Gifford, E. S., E. F. Maguire: Bandkeratopathy in Vit. D intoxication. Am. Arch. Ophthalm. 52 (1954) 106

Goldberg, M. F.: Genetic and metabolic eye disease. Little, Brown and Comp. Boston 1974

Graeber, W.: Der Anästhetikumschaden der Hornhaut. Klin. Mbl. Augenheilk. 139 (1961) 369–377

Gramberg-Danielsen, B.: Die scheibenförmige Durchblutung der Cornea. Klin. Mbl. Augenheilk. 129 (1956) 828–831

Grayson, M.: Acute Keratoglobus. Amer. J. Ophthal. 56 (1963) 300–302

Green, W. R., G. J. Kaufer, S. Dubroff: Black cornea, a complication of topical use of epinephrine. Ophthalmologica 154 (1967) 88–95

Gruber, M.: Beitrag zur Kenntnis der Morphologie der familiären Hornhautdegeneration. Ophthalmologica 125 (1953) 380–389

Günther, G.: Keratoplastik in zwei Fällen von akutem Keratokonus mit histologischem Beitrag zur Pathologie der Hornhaut. Klin. Mbl. Augenheilk. 133 (1958) 40–50

Hallermann, W.: Über atypischen Keratokonus und andere konstitutionell-progressive Hornhautektasien. Klin. Mbl. Augenheilk. 156 (1970) 161–173

Haney, W. P., H. F. Falls: The occurence of congenital ceratoconus posticus circumscriptus. Amer. J. Ophthal. 52 (1961) 53–57

Hanna, L., E. Jawetz, Y. Mitsui, P. Thygeson, S. J. Kimura, A. Nicholas: Continuing studies on the association of adenovirus type 8 with epidemic keratoconjunctivitis. Amer. J. Ophthal. 44 (1957) 66–74

Hanselmayer, H.: Zur Histopathologie der hinteren polymorphen Hornhautdystrophie nach Schlichting. Graefes Arch. 184 (1972) 345–347

Hermans, G.: Les phenothiazines. Bull. soc. Belge d'Ophtalm. 160 (1972) 51–69

Hermans, R.: Opacité en bandelette de la cornée et ichtyose. Bull. Soc. belge Ophtal. 113 (1956) 317–327

Hewson, E. G.: Congenital trigeminal anaesthesia. Brit. J. Ophthal. 47 (1963) 308–311

Heydenreich, A.: Chemisch-toxische Schäden der Augen. Klin. Mbl. Augenheilk. 149 (1966) 145–165

Hoehne, H.: Über Keratitis parenchymatosa. Klin. Mbl. Augenheilk. 105 (1940) 656–693

Hoffmann, D. H.: Pilzerkrankungen der Hornhaut. In: Almanach für die Augenheilkunde, ed. by J. Küchle. Lehmann, München 1969 (pp. 49–57)

Hofmann, H.: Akuter Keratokonus bei mongoloider Idiotie. Klin. Mbl. Augenheilk. 129 (1956) 756–762

Hofmann, H.: Keratitis nummularis Dimmer. Albrecht v. Graefes Arch. klin. exp. Ophthal. 159 (1957) 117–158

Hofmann, H.: Ein Beitrag zum Ulcus rodens. Klin. Mbl. Augenheilk. 159 (1971) 460–467

Hogan, H. J., L. E. Zimmermann: Ophthalmic pathology, 2nd. Ed. Saunders, Philadelphia 1962

Holmberg, A.: Two cases of isolated ophthalmoplegia interna in herpes zoster ophthalmicus. Acta ophthal. (Kbh.) 29 (1951) 483–486

Inoue, K., M. Nakamura: Eye symptoms complicated with encephalitis after herpes zoster. J. clin. Ophthal. (Tokyo) 9 (1955) 1131–1133; ref. in: Zbl. ges. Ophthal. 67 (1956) 138

Jacobs, E. C.: Oculo-ovo-genital-syndrome: a deficiency disease. Ann. intern. Med. 35 (1951) 1049–1054

Jawetz, E., P. Thygeson, L. Hanna, A. Nicholas, S. Kimura: Antibodies to APC-Virus type 8 in epidemic keratoconjunctivitis. Proc. Soc. exp. Biol. (N. Y.) 92 (1956) 91–95; cited by Zbl. ges. Ophthal. 69 (1957) 330

Jones, B. R.: The differential diagnosis of punctata keratitis. Trans. ophthal. Soc. U. K. 80 (1961) 665–675

Jones, B. R., A. B. Richards et al.: Symposium on direct fungal infection of the eye. Trans. ophthal. Soc. UK 89 (1969) 727–818

Jones, S. T., L. E. Zimmerman: Macular dystrophy of the cornea (Groenouw Type II). Amer. J. Ophthal. 47 (1959) 1–16

Kaldeck, R.: Ocular psoriasis. Arch. Derm. Syph. (Chicago) 68 (1953) 44–49

Karlin, D. B., G. N. Wise: Keratoconus posticus. Amer. J. Ophthal. 52 (1961) 119–121

Kaufmann, H. E., R. M. Wood: Mycotic keratitis. Amer. J. Ophthal. 59 (1965) 993–1000

King, H. J., J. W. McTigue: The cornea world congress. Butterworth, London 1965

Koeppe, L.: Angeborene Dellenbildung der Hornhauthinterfläche. Graefes Arch. 91 (1916) 363

Krassai, A.: Über oculare Manifestation der Bowens disease. Klin. Mbl. Augenheilk. 154 (1969) 411–422

Kraupa, E.: Pflege der Augen. Z. Augenheilk. 82 (1934) 353

Kreibig, W.: Die Zostererkrankung des Auges. Klin. Mbl. Augenheilk. 135 (1959) 1–31

Kreibig, W.: Morbus Bowen und Auge. Klin. Mbl. Augenheilk. 137 (1960) 721–728

Küchle, H. J.: Über Cortisonschäden am Auge: In: Entwicklung und Fortschritt in der Augenheilkunde, ed. by Sautter. Enke, Stuttgart 1963 (pp. 458–476)

Lerner, A., T. Fitzpatrick: The control of melanogenesis in human pigment cells. In: Pigment cell growth, ed. by M. Gordon. Academic Press, New York 1953 (pp. 319–333)

Ley, A. P., T. E. Sanders: Fungus Keratitis. Arch. Ophthal. 56 (1956) 257–264

Lisch, H.: Torische Vorwölbung der Hornhaut. Klin. Mbl. Augenheilk. 157 (1970) 523–528

Malbran, E. S.: Corneal dystrophies: A clinical pathological and surgical approach. Amer. J. Ophthal. 74 (1972) 771–809

Mann, I.: Ariboflavinosis. Amer. J. Ophthal. 28 (1945) 243–247

Maumenee, A. E.: Congenital hereditary corneal dystrophy. Amer. J. Ophthal. 50 (1960) 1114

McClamahan, W. S., J. E. Harris, W. H. Knoblauch, L. M. Tredici, R. L. Udasco: Ocular manifestations of chronic phenothiazine derivate administration. Arch. ophthal. 75 (1966) 319–395

McLean, J. M.: Ocolomycosis. Amer. J. Ophthal. 56 (1963) 537–549

McLean, A. L.: Spray Keratitis. Trans. Amer. Acad. Ophthal. Otolaryng. 71 (1967) 330–340

Meesmann, A.: Ein Fall von Arsenmelanose. Klin. Mbl. Augenheilk. 64 (1920) 548

Meesmann, A.: Ophthalmologie für die Praxis. Herdförmige lymphocytäre Uveitiden. Med. Klin. 1956, 1146–1148

Meesmann, A., Fr. Wilke: Klinische und anatomische Untersuchungen über eine bisher unbekannte, dominant vererbte Epitheldystrophie der Hornhaut. Klin. Mbl. Augenheilk. 103 (1939) 361–391

Merté, H. J.: Arbeitsmedizinische Fragen der Ophthalmologie. Karger, Basel 1969

Merté, H. J.: Arbeits- und Sozialmedizin. In: Lehrbuch der Augenheilkunde, ed. by T. Axenfeld, H. Pau. Fischer, Stuttgart 1973

Mitsui, Y., E. Jawetz: Isolation of adenovirus type 8 from a case of epidemic keratokonjunctivitis in Japan. Amer. J. Ophthal. 43 (1957) 91–93

Mitsui, Y., J. Hanabusa, R. Minoda, S. Ogata: Effect of inoculating adenovirus type 8 into human volunteers. Amer. J. Ophthal. 43 (1957) 84–90

Moll, H.: Erblindung nach Masern. Arch. Kinderheilk. 155 (1957) 186–191

Morgan, G., A. Patterson: Pathology of posterior polymorphous degeneration of the cornea. Brit. J. Ophthal. 51 (1967) 433–437

Nagy, M.: Die Terriensche Krankheit – ein Syndrom. Klin. Mbl. Augenheilk. 159 (1971) 350–356

Nover, A.: Rezidivierende Keratitis durch Molluscum cantugiosum des Unterliedes. Klin. Mbl. Augenheilk. 117 (1950) 302–304

Nover, A.: Zoster und Auge. Klin. Mbl. Augenheilk. 156 (1970) 305–317

Offret, G., L. Fargette: Chorio-rétinite et périphlébite rétinienne hérédosyphilitique. Arch. Ophtal. (Paris) 7 (1947) 609

Palimeris, G., J. Koliopoulos, P. Velissaropoulos: Ocular side effects of Indomethacin. Ophthalmologica 164 (1972) 339–353

Pau, H.: Ätiologische Betrachtungen zur rezidivierenden Erosion. Klin. Mbl. Augenheilk. 142 (1963) 388–394

Pau, H., A. Bäumer: Resochineinlagerungen in der Cornea. Klin. Mbl. Augenheilk. 135 (1959) 362–377

Pau, H., J. Gernholz: Epithelimplantation in die Vorderkammer nach perforierender Verletzung und Staroperation. Klin. Mbl. Augenheilk. 142 (1963) 465–482

Pau, H., H. Rodeck: Die Pfaundler-Hurlersche Krankheit. Klin. Mbl. Augenheilk. 122 (1953) 141–158

Paufique, L., F. Hervouët: L'invasion épithéliale de la chambre antérieure après opération de cataracte. Ann. Oculist. (Paris) 197 (1964) 1–29; 106–129

Payrau, P., Y. Pouliquen, J. P. Faure, G. Offret: La transparence de cornée. Masson, Paris 1967

Pillat, A.: Über Präxerosis und Xerosis corneae als selbständige Krankheitsbilder der Mangelerkrankung des Auges beim Erwachsenen. Albrecht v. Graefes Arch. klin. exp. Ophthal. 124 (1930) 486–506

Pillat, A.: Zur Frage der Miterkrankung der Hornhaut bei Psoriasis (Keratitis psoriatica). Klin. Mbl. Augenheilk. 93 (1934) 751–765

Pillat, A.: Epithelschädigung der Hornhaut bei angeborener Trigeminushypoplasie. Wien. Klin. Wschr. 61 (1949) 605

Reese, A. B.: Tumors of the eye. 2nd Ed. Harper & Row, New York 1963

Remky, H., G. Engelbrecht: Dystrophia dermo-chondrocornealis (François). Klin. Mbl. Augenheilk. 151 (1967) 319–331

Remler, O.: Über die sogenannte braune schalenförmige Linsentrübung. Klin. Mbl. Augenheilk. 121 (1952) 647–653

Remler, O.: Über familiäres Auftreten von rezidivierender Hornhauterosion und ihre therapeutische Beeinflussung. Klin. Mbl. Augenheilk. 135 (1959) 263–270

Renard, G., P. Dhermy, P. Harter, N. van Ba: Les atteintes du globe oculaire au cours de la lèpre. Arch. Ophtal. 23 (1963) 249–273

Rieger, R.: Erbpathologie des Auges. In: Der Augenarzt, Vol. I, ed. by K. Velhagen. Thieme, Leipzig 1958

Rodger, F. C.: Metabolic and nutritional eye diseases. Thomas, Springfield, Ill. 1969

Rohen, J.: Handbuch der mikroskopischen Anatomie des Menschen. In: Haut- und Sinnesorgane, Vol. III/4, ed. by Möllendorf Bargmann. Springer, Berlin 1964

Rohrschneider, W., C. Stöhr: Akuter Keratokonus. Klin. Mbl. Augenheilk. 125 (1954) 305–315

Rössler, F.: Ein Fall mit Psoriasis der Conjunctiva. Dermatologie a. d. Ophthal. Ges. in Wien (22. 2. 1943). Klin. Mbl. Augenheilk. 110 (1944) 645

Rüger, K.: Keratitis filiformis nach L. Glaukosan. Klin. Mbl. Augenheilk. 157 (1970) 825–827

Scheie, H. G.: Herpes zoster ophthalmicus. Trans. ophthal. Soc. UK 90 (1970) 899–930

Schenk, H., E. Hummer: Statistische Untersuchungen herpetischer Hornhauterkrankungen aus 3 Dekaden der Jahre 1926–1955. Albrecht v. Graefes Arch. klin. exp. Ophthal. 160 (1958) 368–377

Schenk, H., R. Kunze: Cortisonschaden am Auge. Klin. Mbl. Augenheilk. 136 (1960) 663–672

Schlichting, H.: Blasen- und dellenförmige Endotheldystrophie der Hornhaut. Klin. Mbl. Augenheilk. 107 (1941) 425–435

Schmidt, W.: Über das serologische Verhalten der Keratitis parenchymatosa in verschiedenen Lebensaltern. Klin. Wschr. 1 (1942) 132–134

Schmidt, R. P., E. Roseman, A. J. Steigman: Cranial nerve paralysis in herpes zoster encephalitis of childhood. Clinical and electroencephalographic observations. J. Pediatr. 46 (1955) 215–218; ref. in: Zbl. ges. Ophthal. 65 (1955) 169

Schnyder, U. W.: Erbliche Palmoplantarkeratosen und Corneaveränderungen. Ber. dtsch. ophthal. Ges. 72 (1972) 106–109

Schreck, E.: Dermatologie und Venerologie, Vol. IV, ed. by H. A. Gottron. Thieme, Stuttgart 1960 (p. 836)

Schumacher, H., H. Scheler. Metastatische Kalzifizierung an Kornea und Konjunktiva bei chronischer Niereninsuffizienz. Klin. Mbl. Augenheilk. 154 (1969) 815–819

Siemens, H. W.: Keratosis follicularis spinulosa decalvans. 14. Kongr. Dtsch. Dermat. Ges. Dresden, 1925. Arch. Derm. Syph. (Berlin) 151 (1926) 384–386

Sjögren, H.: Some problems concerning keratoconjunctivitis sicca and the sicca syndrome. Acta ophthal. 29 (1951) 33–47

Skeller, E., J. Oster: Eye symptoms in mongolism. Acta ophthal. (Kbh.) 29 (1951) 149–161

Slezak, H.: Eine besondere Form der senilen Hornhautentartung (senile scheibenförmige Hornhautendotheldegeneration). Ber. dtsch. ophthal. Ges. 68 (1968) 216–220

Sondermann, G.: Über Augenstörungen bei Ichthyosis congenita. Klin. Mbl. Augenheilk. 70 (1923) 180–184

Stern, J. J.: The ocular manifestation of riboflavin deficiency. Amer. J. Ophthal. 33 (1950) 1127–1136

Stocker, F. W., L. B. Holt: Rare form of hereditary epithelial dystrophy. Arch. Ophthal. 53 (1955) 536–541

Streiff, E. B.: Dysplasie marginale postérieure de la cornée dans le cadre de malformations irido-cornéennes. Ophthalmologica (Basel) 118 (1949) 815–827

Suie, Ted, W. H. Havener: Mycology of the eye: A review. Amer. J. Ophthal. 56 (1963) 63–77

Thiel, H. J.: Die hereditäre Epitheldystrophie der Hornhaut (Meesmann-Wilke). Fortschritte in der Ophthalmologie. 26 (1972) 75–146

Thiel, H. J., H. Behnke: Eine bisher unbekannte subepitheliale hereditäre Hornhautdystrophie. Klin. Mbl. Augenheilk. 150 (1967) 862–874

Triebenstein: Veränderungen an der Hornhauthinterfläche. Klin. Mbl. Augenheilk. 74 (1925) 777

Ullerich, K., A. Witte: Die zystische Pankreasfibrose (Mucoviscidosis) als Ursache einer Keratomalazie. Klin. Mbl. Augenheilk. 139 (1961) 59–72

Vérin, Ph., A. Sekkat: Eine neue medikamentös bedingte Augenerkrankung: Die Amiodaron-Thesaurismose. Klin. Mbl. Augenheilk. 162 (1973) 675–680

Verrey, F.: Kératoglobe aigu. Ophthalmologica (Basel) 114 (1947) 284–288

Vogt, A.: Lehrbuch und Atlas der Spaltlampenmikroskopie des lebenden Auges. Vol. II/2. Springer, Berlin 1931

Vrabec, F.: Description histologique d'un cas du psoriasis à localisation conjunctivale, cornéenne et cutanée. Ophthalmologica (Basel) 124 (1952) 105–108

Watillon, M. et A. Robe-Vanwijk: Les médicaments cardiovasculaires. Bull. Soc. Belge d'Ophtalm. 160 (1972) 185–192

Weber, G.: Über einen Fall von Ichthyosis congenita mit Lidschrumpfung. Derm. Wschr. 128 (1953) 1144–1149

Wessels, J. H. W., J. A. Pratt-Johnson: Measles: a common cause of blindness in Sekhukuniland. Med. Proc. 2 (1956) 587–589

Woillez, M., Ch. Dansaut: Les manifestations oculaires dans le mongolisme. Arch. Ophtal. (Paris) 20 (1960) 810–828

Wollensak, J.: Die Keratoconjunctivitis epidemica. Klin. Mbl. Augenheilk. 147 (1965) 465–479

Wolter, J. R., J. W. Henderson: Cornea guttata. Klin. Mbl. Augenheilk. 131 (1957) 725–737

Zintz, R., O. Vivell: Untersuchungen zur Klinik und Ätiologie der epidemischen Keratokonjunktivitis. Klin. Mbl. Augenheilk. 135 (1959) 521–533

14 Sclera

Size and Shape of the Globe

Hyperopia, myopia — Buphthalmos — Scleral staphyloma.

Myopia, Hyperopia

High myopia is associated with an elongated, tubular globe; hyperopia and microphthalmos with a short globe. Malignant myopia causes elongation of the globe and scleral thinning. Ophthalmoscopically, ectatic areas (staphyloma posticum verum) may be seen at the posterior pole (macular region).

Buphthalmos

Buphthalmos or hydrophthalmos (Fig. 19.4) results when the intraocular pressure is elevated at birth or in the first two years of life, while the cornea and sclera are still expansile. The sclera stretches more in the anterior than in the posterior portion of the globe.

Scleral Staphyloma (Fig. 14.1)

Circumscribed, partial ectasias (scleral staphylomas) result when there is localized scleral thinning or weakness. This is usually caused by inflammation, trauma or degeneration. Normal intraocular pressure then causes a staphyloma to form. The process is accelerated if the intraocular pressure is elevated.
Intercalary staphylomata are located in the region of the canal of Schlemm anterior to the ciliary body. Ciliary staphylomas form at the ciliary body. Equatorial staphylomata occur at the points of exit of vortex veins.
Staphylomas are blue-brown-black (visible uvea) scleral bulges which vary enormously in shape and size. When glaucoma is also present, the sclera frequently becomes progressively more ectatic and the globe increases in size. In cases of hydrophthalmos, excessive myopia, and staphyloma, minor trauma may perforate the thinned sclera. Staphylomas transilluminate readily, differentiating them from choroidal tumors.

Color of the Sclera

Scleral melanosis — Ochronosis — Xeroderma pigmentosum — Scleral scars — Blue sclera.

Color: White-blue in youth, white-yellow with age. A yellow sclera is the first sign of icterus.

Scleral Melanosis

There are brown, occasionally irregular, map-like pigmented patches which may be progressive or stationary. The condition is hereditary in some cases.

Ochronosis

In ochronosis there are gray-brown round spots in the sclera (see page 137; Fig. 12.3). The condition is particularly prominent in areas exposed to light. In two-thirds of the cases of ochronosis with alkaptonuria, the earliest signs were pigmentation in the interpalpebral fissure area (Sallmann 1926). The pigment deposits become visible in the third or fourth decade and increase with age. Histologically, pigment plaques (homogentisic acid) are scattered in the cornea, sclera and conjunctiva (Seitz 1954; Rodenhäuser 1957).

Rare findings include atypical pigmentary degeneration of the retina, sheathing of retinal arterioles and optic atrophy. Arthritis, calculi (prostate, kidney), and cardiac dysfunction also occur. Alkaptonuria may be present in infancy.

Xeroderma Pigmentosum

Pigmentation of all areas of skin exposed to sunlight begins in xeroderma pigmentosum by age two to three. Erythema, inflammation, dark brown pigment spots, skin atrophy, leukoplakia and scarring occur. Eye findings include cicatricial ectropion of the lids, conjunctivitis, blepharitis, conjunctival telangiectasia and scarring. Corneal ulcers and conjunctival squamous cell carcinoma may develop. Corneal infiltrates and ulcers tend to vascularize. Basal cell carcinomas extending into cornea and sclera may cause loss of the eye (Thiel 1949) or iris atrophy (Huerkamp 1951).

Scleral Scars

Localized *blue-black discoloration* of the sclera (scleral thinning allows uveal pigment to be seen) occurs with any *chronic scleritis*, especially *scleromalacia perforans*. *Scleral staphylomas* are frequent sequelae of such inflammations (Fig. 14.1). Owing to marked scleral thinning and loss of birefringence (Pau 1955) there is a blue-black discoloration, e.g., visible ciliary body pigment.

Senile equatorial scleromalacia is an age-dependent thinning and black discoloration of the sclera in front of or between the insertions of the rectus muscles (Fig. 14.2, page 183).

The black-blue patches are oval or elongated, a few millimeters wide. The thinned sclera allows uveal pigment to shine through.

Blue Sclera

Blue sclera (Lobstein-van der Hoeve syndrome) (Plate XI, Fig. 5, page 192 c) results less from scleral thinning than from colloidal chemical changes. Rudemann feels that there is an embryonic arrest in the development of scleral collagen fibers. Ptosis, hydrophthalmos, megalocornea, keratoconus, lamellar cataracts and hypoplasia of the iris stroma are associated findings. In the dominant, hereditary, connective tissue disorder osteogenesis imperfecta (Lobstein's osteopsathyrosis idiopathica, van der Hoeve's syndrome, fragilitis osseum hereditaria, Vrolik's syndrome, Eddowes' syndrome, Adair Dighton's syndrome – Badtke 1961) there is fragility of bones (osteopsathyrosis), hyperextensibility and subluxation of joints, and deafness owing to otosclerosis (van der Hoeve and de Kleyn). Penetrance is 94 percent for blue sclera, 55.9 percent for bony fragility and 23.7 percent for deafness (Fuss 1935).

Blue sclera occurs with *incontinentia pigmenti* (Bloch-Sulzberger syndrome), craniofacial dysostosis (Crouzon), Albright's hereditary osteodystrophy (pseudohypoparathyroidism), Hallermann-Streiff syndrome (mandibulo-oculo-facial dyscephaly) and Turner's syndrome (XO genotype).

Ocular findings in the *Ehlers-Danlos syndrome* sometimes include blue sclera, keratoconus and subluxation of the lens (Thomas et al. 1954). The same is true of Marfan's syndrome.

Inflammation

Episcleritis — Scleritis — Sclerosing keratitis — Granulomatous scleritis — Brawny scleritis, annular scleritis, progressive sclerokeratitis — Massive granuloma, posterior scleritis — Scleromalacia perforans — Necrotizing nodular scleritis — Collagen (autoimmune) disorders — Porphyria — Metastatic scleritis — Tuberculosis, lues, leprosy, zoster.

Episcleritis

Episcleritis (Plate XI, Fig. 6, page 192 c) is differentiated from scleritis by the formation of superficial nodules (nodular episcleritis). The conjunctiva overlying the nodule is mobile. Marked conjunctival as well as ciliary injection is common. *Episcleritis periodica fugax* denotes diffuse inflammatory swelling of the episclera and conjunctiva at various locations. This lasts for several days and may be recurrent.

Episcleritis is painful and mildly recurrent, but heals completely after several weeks. Photophobia, lacrimation and ulceration, which are not found with episcleritis, easily differen-

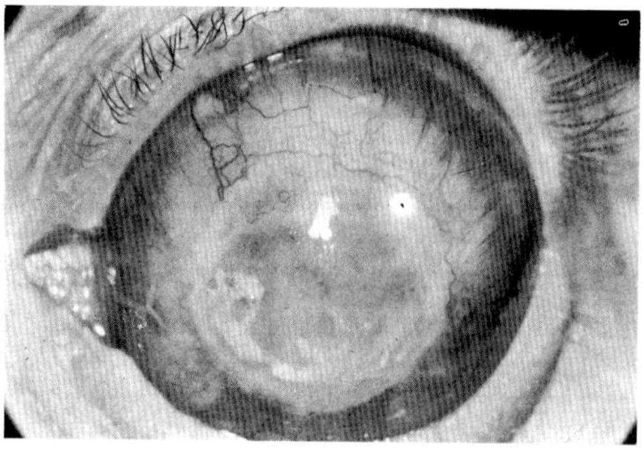

Fig. 14.1 Scleral staphyloma following scleral keratitis

tiate it from phlyctenulosis. Acne rosacea conjunctivitis may simulate scleritis (see page 162). Localized inflammation and pressure sensitivity is an important differential diagnostic point from conjunctivitis.

Scleritis

The choroid is often secondarily involved in *scleritis*. Clinically, anterior and posterior scleritis can be differentiated. Deep anterior scleritis causes diffuse, dark red, violaceous, blue-red scleral thickening appearing as a painful nodule (Plate XII, Fig. 1, page 192 d) or confluent nodules (scleritis annularis) involving all visible sclera.

There is a deep violaceous ciliary injection. Compared to episcleritis which lasts for weeks at most, scleritis often lasts for months and heals as a slate-gray, blue, transparent, sometimes thin, ectatic staphyloma or scar (Fig. 14.1). Peripheral choroiditis, iridocyclitis and secondary glaucoma are common.

Etiology of *scleritis* and *episcleritis* includes: rheumatoid disorders, focal processes, erythema nodosum (see collagen disorders, autoimmune diseases), syphilis, tuberculosis (abortive metastasis of antigenically damaged bacilli) and gout. Gout has recurrent nightly attacks of pain. Leptospirosis (see page 198) and Reiter's syndrome (see page 128) are also associated with episcleritis. Hematogenous dissemination in gonorrhea may cause scleritis and episcleritis.

Sclerosing Keratitis

When scleritis occurs sufficiently close to the limbus, the cornea may transform into a white sclera-like tissue (see page 157; Plate VIII, Fig. 6, page 128 h).

Granulomatous Scleritis

Granulomatous scleritis in collagen or autoimmune disorders includes *brawny scleritis* where the edematous episclera encroaches on the peripheral cornea as *annular scleritis*, causing *progressive sclerokeratitis*. The sclera can be many times its normal thickness which is known as *"massive granuloma of the sclera"* (Wolter and Landis 1958; Wollensak 1968). A massive granuloma of the sclera may appear as *posterior scleritis with exophthalmos*. Other granulomatous scleritides are: *scleromalacia perforans* and *necrotizing nodular scleritis*.

Brawny scleritis (progressive sclerokeratitis, progressive scleroperikeratitis) is an annular, gelatinous (Plate XII, Fig. 2, page 192 d), almost cystic red-brown edematous scleritis with dilatation of conjunctival vessels. The process is often bilateral and occurs mainly in older patients (over 60 yrs.). The brawny connective tissue swelling may force the edematous episclera onto the cornea (sclerokeratitis). Superficial, sharply demarcated corneal edema can occur along with iridocyclitis, corneal ulceration and vascularization. The disease has a protracted painful course usually leading to blindness or loss of the eye. It is considered one of the collagen diseases.

Massive granuloma of the sclera: With brawny scleritis the sclera may swell to many times its normal thickness, which is then called "massive granuloma of the sclera" (Wollensak 1968).

A massive granuloma of the posterior sclera *(posterior scleritis or sclerotenonitis)* is not directly visible and can only be diagnosed by the accompanying symptomatology: marked pain on moving the eye, exophthalmos, chemosis, and lid edema (Goder 1969). Severe cases include choroiditis, exudative retinal detachment, retrobulbar neuritis and posterior staphyloma formation.

Remissions and exacerbations of massive granulomas lead to chorioretinal and optic nerve involvement and possibly to blindness.

The *differential diagnosis* from orbital cellulitis is important. Orbital cellulitis is a progressive, severe systemic illness with fever, which is not the case in scleritis and tenonitis.

Inflammatory orbital granulomas produce displacement of the globe. In primary myositis (see page 53) the mobility of the globe is much reduced. Endocrine ophthalmopathy is usually bilateral with other typical signs (see page 339).

Scleromalacia perforans (van der Hoeve) has a predilection for women over 50 years. Gray-yellow nodules form and fuse into oval punched-out scleral holes with a few remaining scleral fibers (Plate XII, Fig. 3, page 192 d). This occurs virtually without reaction or pain.

The necrosis exposes the underlying uvea causing secondary uveitis and potentially panophthalmitis (Plate XII, Fig. 4, page 192 d). Scleromalacia perforans mainly affects older women suffering from primary chronic polyarthritis. Subjective complaints are minimal. As long as there are no intraocular complications, vision remains normal. François et al. (1969) point out that the fibrinoid necrosis of collagen fibers and their ground substances in scleromalacia perforans could be considered an antigen-antibody reaction. Episcleritis followed by scleromalacia perforans with secondary iritis is sometimes part of the clinical picture of primary chronic polyarthritis (Witmer 1970).

Necrotizing nodular scleritis (necroscleritis nodosa): There is marked pain, inflammation and erythema with formation of small yellow necrotic *nodules*. These may become confluent and slough, leaving a bare uvea.

Collagen disorders: Included in this category are, among others, periarteritis nodosa, dermatomyositis, scleroderma, lupus erythematosus, temporal arteritis, acute rheumatism and rheumatic arthritis. With each of these disorders there is a unique fibrinoid necrosis of collagen fibers. The group of primary chronic arthritis, which preferentially afflict menopausal women (2.5:1 compared to men), should be considered a collagen or autoimmune disease.

Ocular findings with *primary chronic arthritis* include: *necrotizing scleritis, scleromalacia perforans* and *massive granuloma of the sclera*. Massive granuloma of the sclera is also called *brawny scleritis, annular scleritis,* and when it occurs in the posterior part of the globe, *posterior scleritis*. Two to three percent of all cases of primary chronic polyarthritis are accompanied by uveitis.

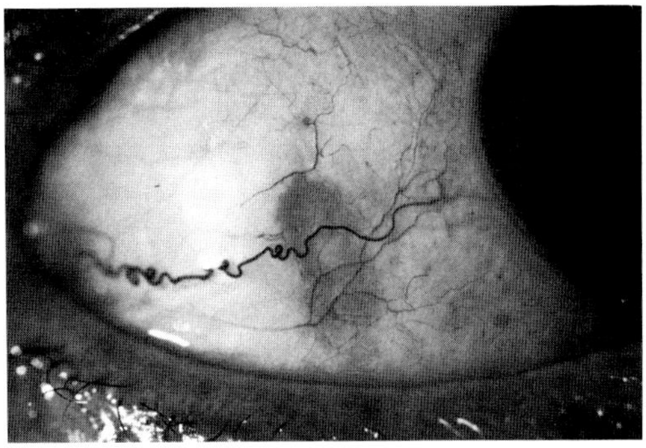

Fig. 14.2 Senile equatorial scleral malacia directly in front of the horizontal ocular muscles in the palpebral fissure area (♀ 73 yrs.)

Still's and *Felty's* syndromes (see page 197) are special categories of rheumatoid disease.

Still's syndrome is the *primary chronic polyarthritis of childhood;* febrile polyarthritis dominates. Spleen and lymph nodes are enlarged. Leukopenia and potential dysproteinemia occur. Rheumatoid factor is missing in 80 percent of cases. *Felty's syndrome* is the same disease in adults. Here the rheumatoid factor is present 95 percent of the time. Fever is not seen in Felty's syndrome.

Sjögren's disease is considered one of the rheumatoid disorders. Sjögren's disease includes the sicca syndrome with punctate and filamentary keratitis, parotid swelling (lymphocytic infiltration), preauricular lymphadenopathy and often polyarthritis.

A number of diagnostic tests are helpful in establishing a diagnosis of rheumatoid disease: antistreptolysin, anti-staphylysin reaction, C-reactive protein determination, serum complement (complement is consumed in antigen-antibody reactions), and rheumatoid factor or antinuclear factors.

Panchondritis (Hoffman 1959) is a rare rheumatic disease included among the collagen disorders. *Episcleritis* occurs. Other antigenic disorders often classified as *collagen diseases* include:

1. *panarteritis,* specifically *periartertitis nodosa*
2. hypersensitivity angitis
3. *Wegener's granulomatosis*
4. Goodpasture's syndrome

Renal involvement and hypertension, causing typical fundus changes, is common with panarteritis (Böck 1959).

Wegener's granulomatosis extends into the orbit from the sinuses causing necrotizing granulomas and exophthalmos. Necrotizing ulcers may appear on the sclera, conjunctiva and at the limbus (limbal ulcers). More common, though still rare, ocular findings include conjunctivitis and iritis, ptosis, lid edema, lid necrosis, keratitis, retinal folds and optic atrophy. Wegener's granulomatosis (see page 338) is an inflammatory granulomatous process of the nose, sinuses, trachea, pharynx and inner ear. High, almost septic fever, generalized arteritis, multiple vascular granulomas, and nodular glomerulonephritis are further manifestations. Death is predictable within three months to four years. This may be an allergic-immune reaction similar to periarteritis nodosa. The most important components are necrotizing inflammations and a tendency to tumefaction (Kyrieleis 1968).

Porphyria

Scleromalacia is seen in *porphyria* (see p. 366).

Metastatic Bacterial Scleritis

Infectious scleritis due to metastasis of bacteria (episcleritis metastatica furunculiformis) is rare. Episcleral nodules form which quickly necrotize and become abscessed (Plate XII, Fig. 5, page 192 d). The abscess usually ruptures externally and heals quickly leaving dark scleral scars. Scleral perforation with panophthalmitis is rare.

Staphylococcus aureus and occasionally streptococci are the usual agents (Otto and Hild 1957).

Tuberculosis, Lues, Leprosy, Zoster

Tuberculomas with yellow nodules, *luetic* episcleral nodules or *gumma* of the sclera extending to the uvea, and *lepromatous* episcleritis are rare.

Ophthalmic zoster can cause scleritis. There may be a secondary uveitis.

Tendonitis

Tendonitis occurring at the insertion of the rectus muscles is not uncommon. It appears as a painful erythema. There is usually a transition to episcleritis.

Dilatation of Episcleral Vessels

Episcleral vessels can be dilated and engorged with blood (caput medusae). This occurs with pulsating exophthalmos as in arteriovenous anastomosis (carotid rupture in the cavernous sinus) (Plate XXXI, Fig. 6, page 288 g), and in some cases of absolute glaucoma. Takayasu's disease, or pulseless disease, also causes dilatation of episcleral vessels (see page 271).

Cysts

Scleral cysts are very rare. They are usually traumatic implantation cysts and are rarely congenital.

Tumors

Tumors of the sclera are rare. They may be lymphomas, lymphadenomas, fibromas or hemangiomas. Hemangiomas in the trigeminal distribution (Sturge-Weber syndrome) are associated with glaucoma (see page 224). Choroidal melanomas (20 percent), retinoblastomas (10 percent), or epibulbar tumors (carcinomas, melanoblastomas) can grow into the sclera.

Injuries

Severe blunt trauma (fists, balls, cowhorns, edges of tables, etc.) causes a typical scleral rupture in the region of Schlemm's canal $1-1\frac{1}{2}$ mm from the limbus. Expulsion of intraocular contents (lens, iris, vitreous) is common. Conjunctival edema may obscure the rupture. The "mushy", soft globe indicates the diagnosis.

References

Badtke, G.: Die Mißbildungen des menschlichen Auges. In: Der Augenarzt, Vol. IV, ed. by K. Velhagen. Thieme, Stuttgart 1961

Boeck, J.: Ocular changes in periarteriitis nodosa. Amer. J. Ophthal. 42 (1956) 567–576

Duke-Elder, St. Sr.: Diseases of the sklera. System of ophthalmology, Vol. VIII/2. Kimpton, London 1965 (p. 995)

Forni, S.: Cornée et selérotique. I & II. Fortschr. Augenheilk. 5 (1956); 8 (1958)

François, J., V. Victoria-Troncoso, M. Hanssens, J. Bacskulin: Scléromalacie perforante et collagénose. Ophthalmologica 159 (1969) 71–95

Fuss, H.: Über abnorme Knochenbrüchigkeit. Arch. klin. Chir. 182 (1935 a) 425–442

Fuss, H.: Die erbliche Osteopsothyrose. Dtsch. Z. Chir. 245 (1935 b) 279–293

Goder, G.: Scleritis posterior pseudo-tumorosa. Klin. Mbl. Augenheilk. 155 (1969) 200–214

Günther, G.: Erkrankungen der Lederhaut. In: Der Augenarzt, Vol. II, ed. by K. Velhagen. Thieme, Stuttgart 1959 (p. 847)

Hewson, G. E.: Scleral tumors. In: Tumoren des Auges und seiner Adnexe, ed. by J. François. Karger, Basel 1966 (pp. 51–57)

Hoeve, van der, J., A. de Kleyn: Blaue Sclera, Knochenbrüchigkeit und Schwerhörigkeit. Albrecht v. Graefes Arch. klin. exp. Ophthal. 95 (1918) 81–93

Hoffmann, D. H.: Doppelseitige Episkleritis bei Panchondritis. Klin. Mbl. Augenheilk. 135 (1959) 844–846

Huerkamp, B.: Irisschwund bei Xeroderma pigmentosum. Klin. Mbl. Augenheilk. 119 (1951) 286–292

Kyrieleis, E.: Augenbeteiligung bei Wegenerscher Granulomatose. Klin. Mbl. Augenheilk. 153 (1968) 651–655

Oberhoff, K.: Sklera. In: Handbuch der speziellen pathologischen Anatomie und Histologie, ed. by O. Henke, B. Lubarsch. Springer, Berlin 1937

Otto, J., E. Hild: Über die Episkleritis metastatica furunculiformis. Klin. Mbl. Augenheilk. 131 (1957) 541–544

Pau, H.: Die Doppelbrechung von Sklera und Cornea. Albrecht v. Graefes Arch. klin. exp. Ophthal. 156 (1955) 415–426

Rodenhäuser, J. H.: Über die Augenpigmentierungen bei Alkaptonurie (Ochronosis oculi). Klin. Mbl. Augenheilk. 131 (1957) 202–215

Ruedemann, A. D.: Osteogenesis imperfecta congenita and blue sclerotics. A clinico-pathologic study. Amer. Arch. ophthal. 49 (1953) 6–16

Sallmann, L.: Über die Augenpigmentierung bei endogener Ochronose. Z. Augenheilk. 60 (1926) 164–171

Schieck, E.: Die Erkrankungen der Sklera. In: Kurzes Handbuch der Ophthalmologie, Vol. IV, ed. by E. Schieck, A. Brückner. Springer, Berlin 1931

Seitz, R.: Über die ochronosischen Pigmentierungen am Auge. Klin. Mbl. Augenheilk. 125 (1954) 432–440

Thiel, R.: Xeroderma pigmentosum. Dtsch. Ophthal. Ges. 1949, 346

Thomas, Ch., J. Cordier, B. Algan: Les altérations oculaires de la maladie de Ehlers-Danlos. Arch. Ophthal. (Paris) 14 (1954) 691–697

Witmer, R.: Augenveränderungen bei Autoimmunerkrankungen. Ber. ophthal. Ges. Heidelberg 70 (1970) 301–306

Wollensak, J.: Klinik und Pathogenese der nekrotisierenden Skleritis. Klin. Mbl. Augenheilk. 153 (1968) 775–788

Wolter, J. R., C. B. Landis: Zur Klinik der Pathologie des massiven Granuloms der Sklera. Klin. Mbl. Augenheilk. 132 (1958) 59–70

15 Anterior Chamber

Depth

Deep anterior chamber — Flat anterior chamber.

Deep Anterior Chamber

(with open angle)

The anterior chamber is especially deep with posterior subluxation of the lens (see page 252) and aphakia. Iridocyclitis usually results in deepening of the anterior chamber. A deep anterior chamber with increased protein in the aqueous and a soft globe occurs with choroidal detachment after damage to the posterior pole (vitreal, retinal hemorrhages, retinal detachment, perforating injuries, etc.).

Flat Anterior Chamber

(with narrow angles)

An attack of acute angle closure glaucoma must be considered (see page 223), as must chronic angle closure glaucoma. Other causes include lenticular swelling, anterior luxation or subluxation of the lens and choroidal detachment with a flat anterior chamber (after cataract, retinal detachment or glaucoma surgery).

Increased Protein and Cells in the Anterior Chamber

As in any iritis a primarily *cell-free opalescence* (Tyndall effect) occurs with *serous iritis*, after blunt trauma or vitreous loss. There is the danger of secondary glaucoma.

Increased *opalescence* with cells, leucocytes, lymphocytes, macrophages, endothelial, etc. along with an increase in fibrin (flakes, threads, nets) (Fig. 16.25) results in *fibrinous iritis*. Marked increase in leucocytes, e.g., with infection, causes *hypopyon*, i.e., layering out of pus (Fig. 16.28) (ulcus serpens, hypopyon iritis, endophthalmitis). *Tumor cells* may be found in the anterior chamber with retinoblastoma, metastatic carcinoma, and lymphosarcoma (Remky 1961). These cells may cause a pseudouveitis with hypopyon formation.

An *increase in erythrocytes* (hemorrhage) causes a hyphema which may settle with a horizontal level line (trauma, rubeosis iridis, hemorrhagic glaucoma). "Spontaneous" anterior chamber hemorrhage in children occurs with juvenile xanthogranulomatosis, leukemia and retinoblastomas. Rarely, angiomas and lymphosarcomas cause spontaneous anterior chamber hemorrhage.

Nitrobenzol poisoning can turn the aqueous a deep brown-red.

Posterior Corneal Precipitates

Such precipitates are the deposition of individual inflammatory products. These may consist of the smallest protein particles and form a fine network of star-shaped opacities on the posterior cornea, e.g., with heterochromic precipitates.

The precipitate may be larger and appear as individual deposits which are *round, oval* or *confluent*. The posterior cornea can be *covered by a fibrin sheet*. The larger precipitates are found more inferiorly. They assume a triangular configuration with the apex pointing towards the corneal center. Fine punctate precipitates can be physiologic and appear as a vertical line (Ehrlich-Türk) in the lower half of the cornea.

Overwhelmingly the *precipitates* are *gray-white*, but can be yellow, lardaceous (leucocytes, tumor cells), pure white (heterochromic precipitates, fibrin, lens material) or *glassy* (old precipitates covered by endothelium and new Descemet).

Old precipitates are permeated with fine *pigment granules* (from iris pigment epithelium), and have an irregular, tatty border.

Precipitates on the posterior corneal surface appear with uveal inflammation (iridocyclitis, chorioretinitis), with inflammation of the cornea (luetic interstitial keratitis, tuberculosis, disciform herpes), corneal dystrophies (cornea guttata or Fuchs' endothelial dystrophy) and injury. Pigment deposits on the posterior corneal surface occur with cornea guttata, diabetes, old precipitates, pigment dispersion syndrome and pigmentary glaucoma. Tumor precipitates (retinoblastoma, metastatic carcinoma) occur.

Nitrobenzene causes a brown discoloration of the aqueous and posterior cornea.

Reference

Remky, H.: Tumorzellen im Kammerwasser. Klin. Mbl. Augenheilk. 138 (1961) 643—649

16 Iris

Uvea

The *uveal* tract consists of the iris, ciliary body and choroid.

Iris Defects

Congenital aniridia — Congenital iris coloboma — Acquired iris coloboma — Torn sphincter — Iridodialysis — Iridoschisis — Essential, progressive iris atrophy — Mesodermal dysgenesis.

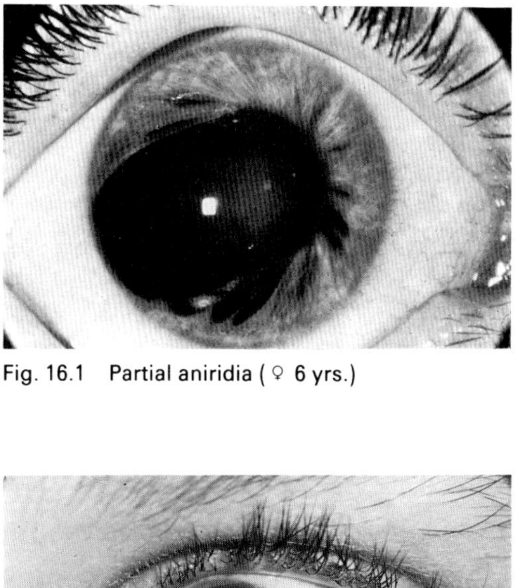

Fig. 16.1 Partial aniridia (♀ 6 yrs.)

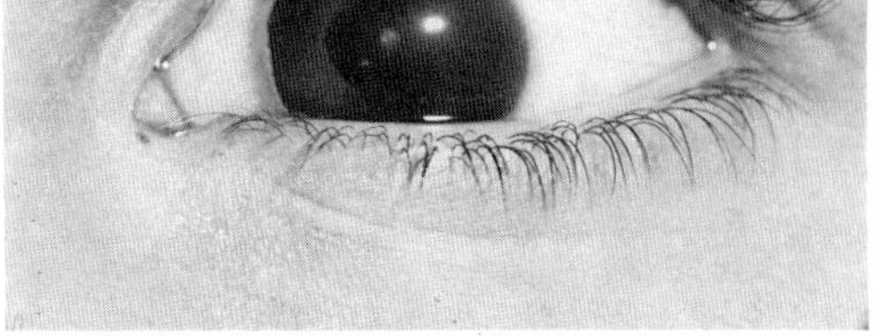

Fig. 16.2 Partial aniridia. The stromal iris leaf is barely present nasally. The pigmented iris leaf is largely intact. (♂ 11 yrs.)

Congenital Aniridia

This is an autosomal dominant or recessively inherited disorder with total (aniridia) or partial (reduced amount of iris, coloboma, stromal hypoplasia) lack of iris (Figs. 16.1, 16.2) (Drenkhahn and Behnke 1961). Aniridia is commonly associated with a vascularized corneal pannus, lens opacities (cortical, anterior and posterior pole, fetal nucleus), ectopia lentis, lens coloboma, microphakia, amblyopia, absence or hypoplasia of the macula, optic nerve hypoplasia, nystagmus and strabismus. Microcornea, microphthalmos and ptosis occur less frequently.

Thalidomide taken 35 to 39 days after the last menstrual period may produce aniridia in the embryo (see page 244).

Congenital Iris Coloboma, Iris Hypoplasia

A congenital iris coloboma (Fig. 16.3) normally points inferiorly (embryonic fissure). The pupillary border is maintained along the edges of the coloboma. Congenital iris colobomata are usually associated with a ciliary body and choroidal coloboma. A coloboma may be incomplete (Fig. 16.4) with only the mesodermal stromal leaf missing. The pigmented leaf is then visible as a brown discolored area. This occurs frequently with *hypoplasia* inferiorly in the region of the former embryonic fissure.

Iris coloboma and microphthalmos are often inherited together in a dominant manner. Stromal hypoplasia may be total or circumscribed. Incomplete closure of the fetal fissure results in *iris, ciliary body and choroidal colobomata.* The defects lie inferiorly and slightly nasally (typical coloboma, as opposed to atypical coloboma which appears at any other position [Badtke 1961]).

Various *embryopathies* (see page 244) with malformation of the extremities, heart, ears and kidneys caused by exogenous agents also show ocular damage. Thalidomide is an unfortunate but perfect example. Ocular malformations include sixth and seventh nerve paresis, strabismus, microphthalmos, cataract, iris and choroidal coloboma.

On rare occasions tuberous sclerosis is associated with iris and choroidal colobomata. This is one of the *phakomatoses.* Sebaceous adenoma, retinal and intracranial hamartomas occur along with seizures and mental retardation (see page 296).

Trisomy D (13–15) (Patau, Smith, Therman, Inhorn and Wagner [see page 329]) may have microphthalmos, iris coloboma, partial aniridia, cataracts and connective tissue hypoplasia. The infants usually survive for only a few weeks. Cogan and Kuwabara (1964) found intraocular cartilage in each of the six eyes they examined. Other anomalies include cerebral defects, harelip, cleft palate, polydactyly, congenital heart defects, etc. (Schade 1963; Hoepner and Yanoff 1972).

Iris coloboma also occurs with Trisomy 17–18 (see page 329).

Acquired Iris Colobomata

In acquired, traumatic or surgical iris colobomata the borders of the coloboma are sharp without a pigmentary ruff.

Sphincter Tears

Traumatic tears of the sphincter of the iris (Fig. 16.5).

Iridodialysis

Traumatic disinsertion of the iris root, called iridodialysis (Fig. 16.6), may at times cause monocular diplopia. The presence of an iridodialysis may only be indicated by a pupillary deformity at the appropriate location.

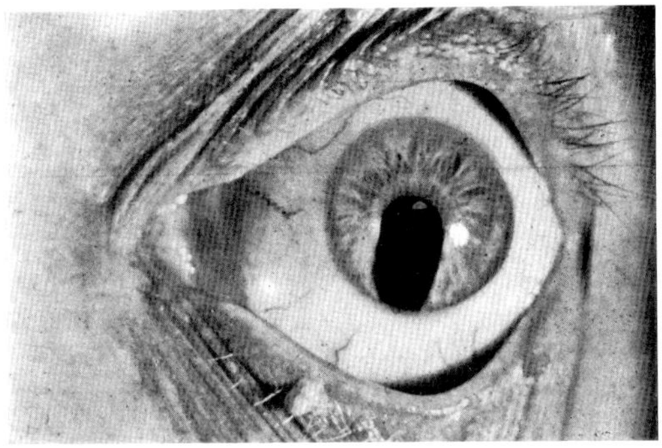

Fig. 16.3 Congenital iris coloboma

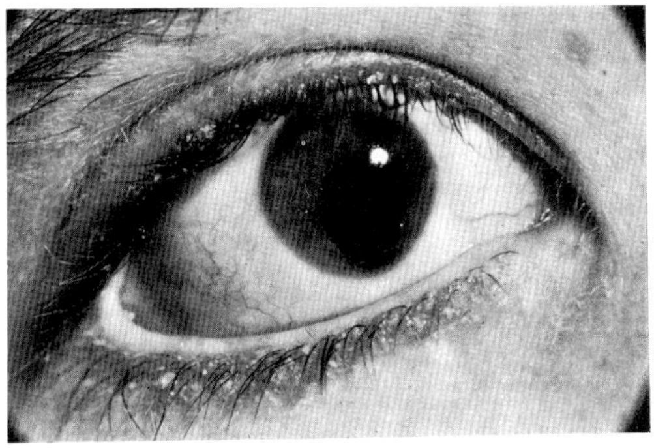

Fig. 16.4 Bridge coloboma, squamous blepharitis, antimongoloid slant (♂ 14 yrs.)

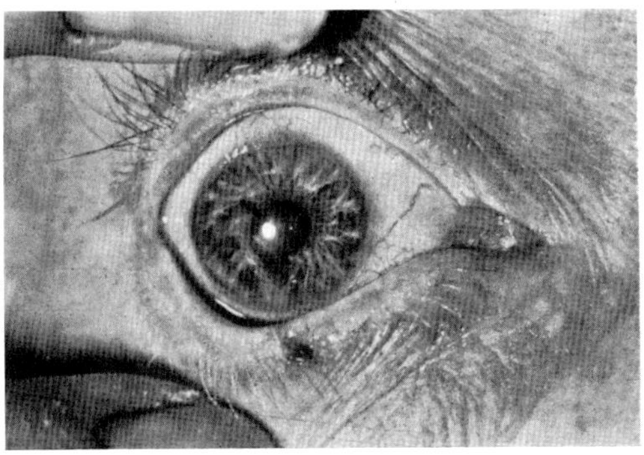

Fig. 16.5 Traumatic tear in the iris sphincter at 6 o'clock position (♂ 52 yrs.)

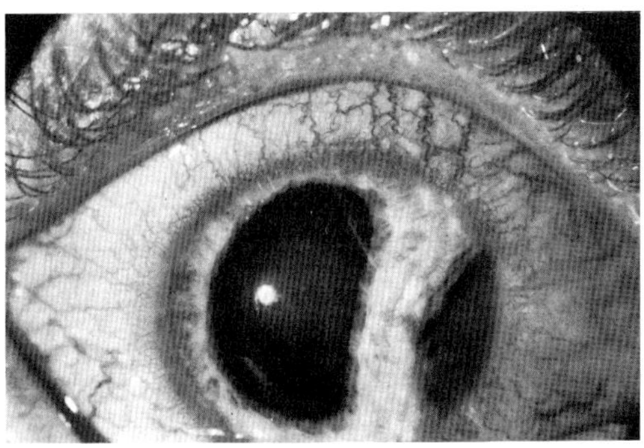

Fig. 16.6 Iridodialysis (♀ 21 yrs.)

Iridoschisis (Splitting)

Iridoschisis (splitting of the iris) is a separation and dissolution of the anterior stromal leaf occurring mainly in persons over the age of 60. Tattered stromal fibers float in the anterior chamber and may touch the posterior cornea or deposit as gray remnants in the inferior chamber angle. Of significance is that the pupil always remains centered. It reacts normally or becomes fixed in miosis. The process is usually bilateral and normally begins in the inferior nasal quadrant in the region of the embryonic fissure. Atrophy of the pigmented iris leaf may occur after the stromal changes. Glaucoma is common (Bonnet and Vianey 1970). A picture resembling iridoschisis occurs with iritis and anterior synechiae. Occasionally the pigmented iris leaf may be detached with an otherwise normal appearing iris stroma. On dilatation the entire pigment leaf, possibly with holes, is exposed (Figs. 16.7, 16.8).

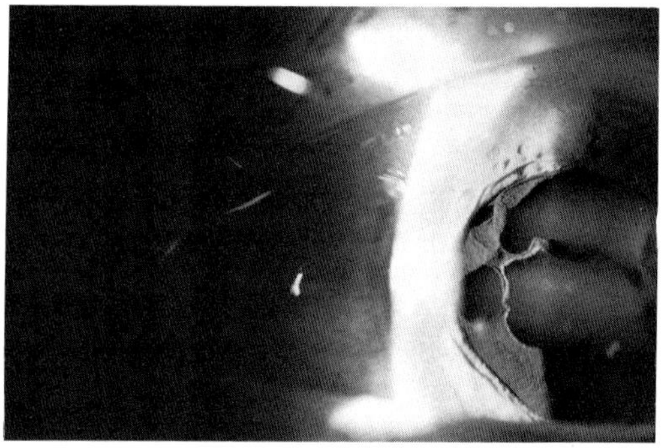

Fig. 16.7 Iridoschisis between the stromal and (seen with mydriasis) pigmented iris leaf (♂ 26 yrs.)

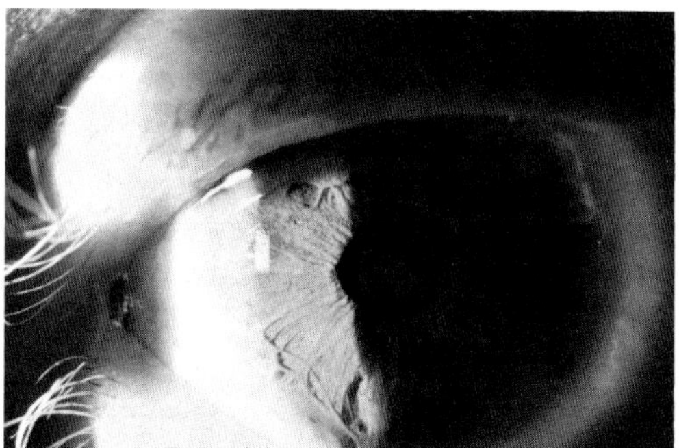

Fig. 16.8 Iridoschisis: Lysis of the anterior stromal leaf with free stromal fibers (below) (♀ 47 yrs.)

Essential Progressive Iris Atrophy

In essential progressive iris atrophy there is an ever increasing loss of mesodermal stroma *(dystrophia mesodermalis progressiva iridis)* which later carries over to the pigment leaf. The pupillary sphincter remains unaffected for a long time. The progressive development of anterior synechiae distorts the pupil more and more. A therapeutically recalcitrant secondary glaucoma is almost always present. Cataracts are common. The disease may appear in children but most commonly manifests between ages 20 and 50.

Mesodermal Dysgenesis (Rieger's Dysgenesis Mesodermalis Iridis et Corneae)

Rieger's syndrome (Plate XIII, Fig. 1, page 192 e) includes slit-like pupils, hypoplasia of the stromal leaf with exposure and hole formation in the pigment leaf of the iris. Mesodermal dysgenesis may, therefore, demonstrate pseudopolycoria and corectopia. Iris processes from the peripheral and even central iris stretch across the chamber angle onto the cornea. The chamber angle anomaly is causally related to a glaucoma difficult to control. Ectodermally determined true, partial anodontia may be present. It is questionable as to what degree this is a congenital anomaly or whether there is a progressive mesodermal distrophy with connective tissue in the chamber angle and growth of corneal endothelium onto the iris (Pau et al. 1962). *Progressive mesodermal iris atrophy* differs from *progressive ectodermal iris atrophy* in Fuchs' heterochromia complicata (see page 192, Plate XIII, Fig. 5, page 192 e).

The *differential diagnosis* includes congenital corectopia or polycoria as well as atypical iris coloboma or aniridia. Progressive iris atrophy is seen after trauma, with glaucoma (especially chronic narrow angle or hemorrhagic), and with iritis (for example, zoster). There is progressive iris atrophy of the pigmented leaf *(dystrophia epithelialis progressiva iridis)* in

Fuchs' heterochromia complicata since this is not an inflammation. Iridoschisis may simulate iris atrophy. Radiation damage and Takayasu's syndrome are other causes of iris atrophy.

Displacement; Distortion of the Pupil

Polycoria – Ectopia pupillae – Ectropion – Entropion of the pigment border – Persistent pupillary membrane.

Polycoria

True polycoria is rare, but when present there are two or more pupils each of which has its own sphincter muscle and pupillary reaction. Usually polycoria is a *false* one, i.e., holes in the iris. These result from atrophic processes with glaucoma, progressive iris atrophy, mesodermal dysgenesis (Plate XIII, Fig. 1, page 192 e), persistent pupillary membranes, etc.

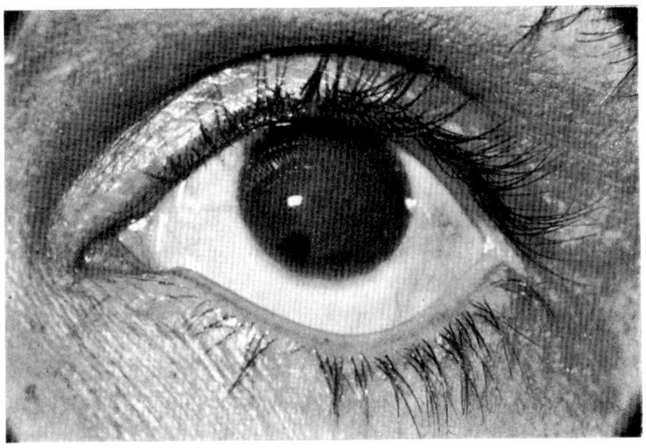

Fig. 16.9 Ectopic pupil (♂ 30 yrs.)

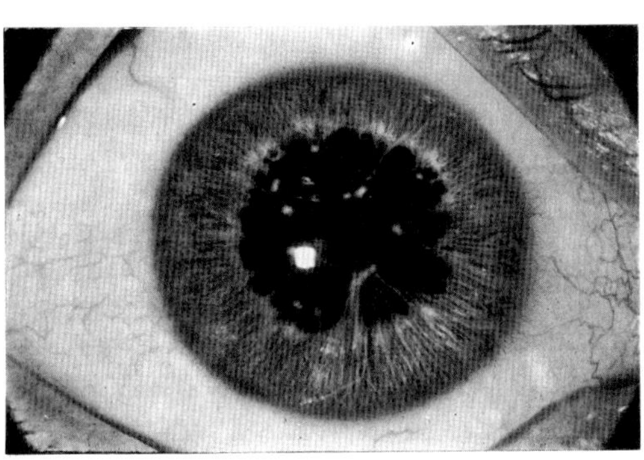

Fig. 16.10 Persistent pupillary membrane

Ectopic Pupil

Congenital ectopic pupil (corectopia, slit pupils [Fig. 16.9]) is usually caused by connective tissue or vascular strands extending from the iris to the pars plana, ciliary body or vitreous. The pupil is constricted. Microphakia is common, microphthalmos less so. Corectopia may occur secondarily with pupillary ectropion or persistent attacks of glaucoma.

Ectropion; Entropion of the Pigmented Border

Congenital anomalies of the pupillary border pigment ruff, such as ectropion or flocculi, are rare. Entropion formation is even more rare. Acquired entropion occurs when posterior synechiae form while the pupil is dilated. As the pupil constricts the adhesions cause inversion of the pupillary border and stroma. Ectropion (supertractio iridis) (Plate XIII, Fig. 2, page 192 e) results from scarification with shrinkage of the anterior iris surface pulling pigment from the posterior leaf forward. Pupillary ectropion occurs with rubeosis iridis, mesodermal dysgenesis (Rieger), epithelial downgrowth or implantation cysts, perforating injury, Cogan-Reese syndrome (Scheie, Yanoff 1975), chronic inflammation and secondary glaucoma. In long-standing glaucoma the corneal endothelium may grow onto the surface of the iris and lay down new Descemet material (Wolter and Fechner 1962). The same thing may occur with progressive mesodermal dystrophy (Pau et al. 1962).

Persistent Pupillary Membrane

A persistent pupillary membrane (Fig. 16.10) is recognized by the fact that it arises from the iris collarette and not the pigmented pupillary ruff (which is not present at birth). The persisting remnants of the fetal pupillary membrane appear as strands or nets and may insert on the lens. Similarly, posterior synechiae developed in utero also insert at the iris collarette.

Iris Color

Albinism — Heterochromia — Diabetes — Senile changes — Vascularization of the iris.

The color of the iris is a function of its pigment content. Blue, for example, indicates reflected light with lack of pigment. Because of the lack of pigment, the iris is blue at birth and remains so until the end of the second year of life.

Lack of Pigment (Albinism)

(see page 364)

With total albinism (Plate XIII, Fig. 3, page 192 e) eyelashes and brows are nearly white. The iris is gray-white and transmits the red of the fundus reflex. The pupil appears red even in normal daylight since light enters the eye not only through the pupil but also through the iris and sclera. *Total, partial* and *isolated ocular albinism* is almost always associated with macular hypoplasia and greater or lesser degrees of amblyopia. Astigmatism is common. Since the iris fails in its function as a diaphragm to keep out light, photophobia is marked. The macular hypoplasia and poor vision result in pendular nystagmus which varies with fixation: coarse, fine, irregular, rotary, etc. The *Chédiak-Higashi syndrome* includes oculocutaneous albinism with photophobia and nystagmus, lymphadenopathy, hepatosplenomegaly, anemia and a sensitivity to ultraviolet light. The leukocytes contain large cytoplasmic glycolipid inclusions and are an ineffective defense against infection. Inheritance is recessive with death usually occurring before age 10.
The *Waardenburg syndrome* includes blepharophimosis, lateral displacement of the puncta, heterochromia iridis and potential albinism of the fundus. Heredity is dominant, though irregularly so.

Heterochromia

The iris may be pigmented to greater or lesser degrees. This can be due to actual melanosis or more circumscribed pigment patches or nevi. *Heterochromia* is a difference in iris color of the two eyes.

Heterochromia simplex — Heterochromia complicata (Fuchs) — Siderosis — Secondary heterochromia — Pigment dispersion and crystals in the iris — Circumscribed light patches — Wölfflin's iris nodules, Brushfield's spots — Nevi, unilateral melanosis.

Heterochromia simplex (Plate XIII, Fig. 4, page 192 e) is sympathetic damage in early childhood. The affected eye is lighter than the other and exhibits Horner's syndrome complex (miosis, ptosis, enophthalmos).
Simple hereditary heterochromia also exists. Heterochromia iridis occurs in status dysraphicus and in Waardenburg's syndrome. The latter includes blepharophimosis, white forelock, and lateral displacement of the lacrimal puncta.
Heterochromia complicata = *Fuchs' heterochromia* (Plate XIII, Fig. 5, page 192 e).
There is increasing atrophy of the pigmented iris leaf with transparency of the pupillary margin (progressive ectodermal iris atrophy). The iris stroma is also slightly depigmented. Precipitates form on the posterior corneal surface and in the vitreous. A progressive posterior subcapsular cataract develops (permeability cataract, *cataracta complicata*). Eventually there is secondary glaucoma.
The corneal precipitates are fine, star-shaped, single or multiple granules, irregularly distributed over the entire posterior corneal surface. They are usually pigment-free. The term "heterochromic cyclitis" is not correct, since this progressive ectodermal iris atrophy with transudation of protein is not a real inflammation. Heterochromia complicata is primarily unilat-

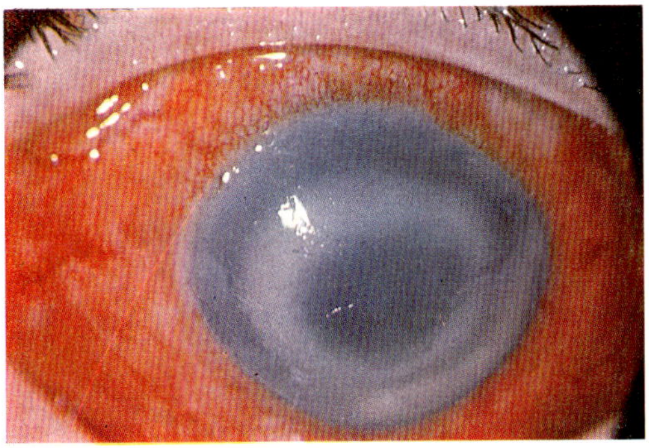

Fig. 1 Ring abscess of the cornea (♀ 63 yrs.) (see page 158)

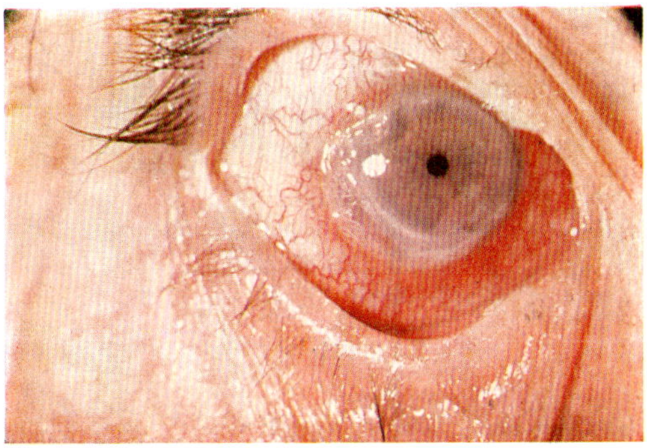

Fig. 2 Deep inferior and lateral paralimbic defect of rodent ulcer (♂ 57 yrs.) (see page 160)

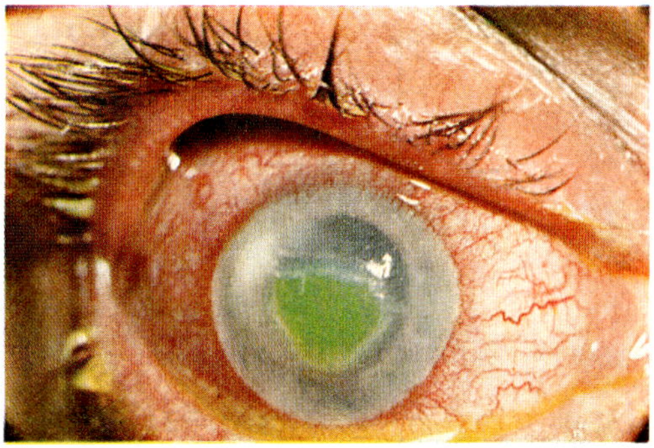

Fig. 3 Topical anesthetic abuse causing corneal edema and erosion (see pages 122, 162)

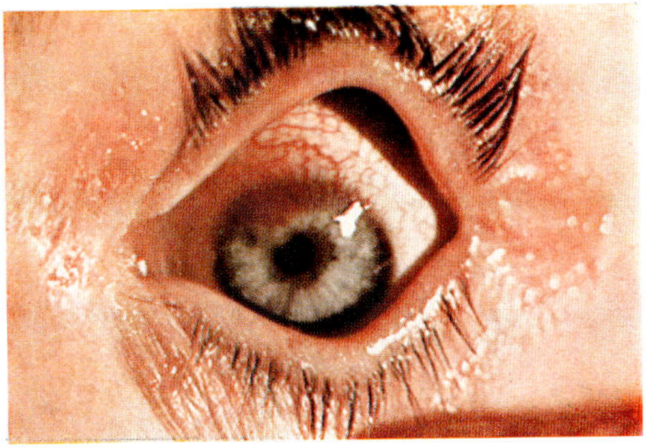

Fig. 4 Scrofulous keratitis with vascularized phlyctenules (♀ 12 yrs.) (see pages 132, 148, 162)

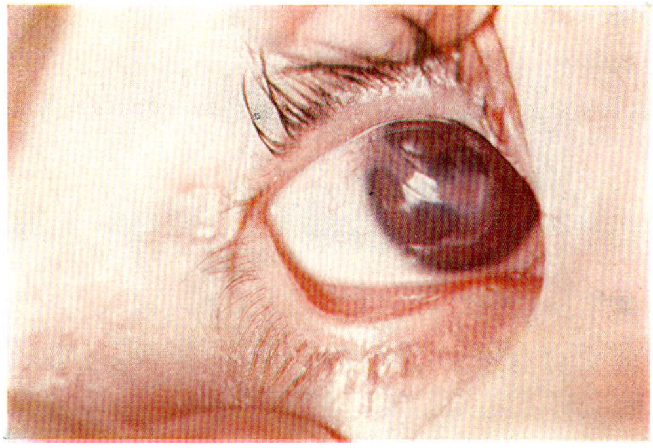

Fig. 5 Scrofulous keratitis with a wandering phlyctenule (from superior temporally to the center) (♀ 4 yrs.) (see pages 132, 148, 162)

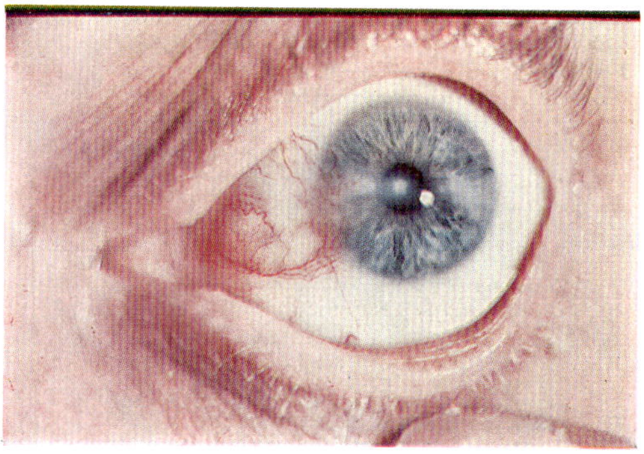

Fig. 6 Acne rosacea keratitis with early vascularization of a nasal infiltrate (♀ 52 yrs.) (see pages 133, 148, 163)

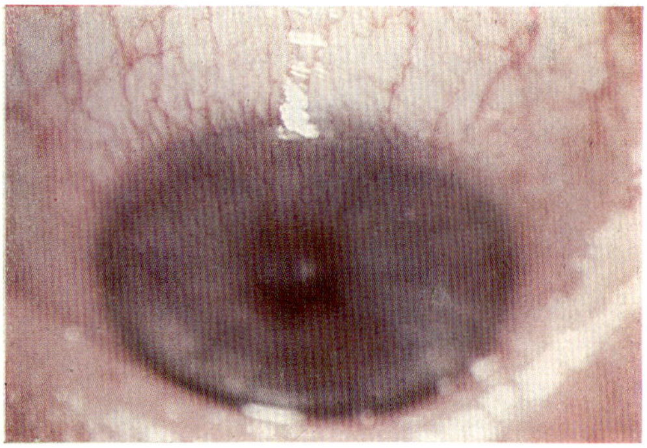

Fig. 1 Superficial circular vascularization in vitamin B deficiency (see page 148)

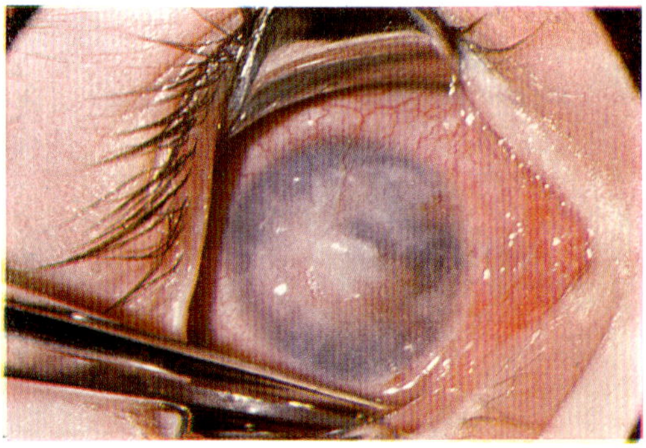

Fig. 3 Keratomalacia with vascularization of the deiccated cornea (♂ 1½ yrs.) (see page 163)

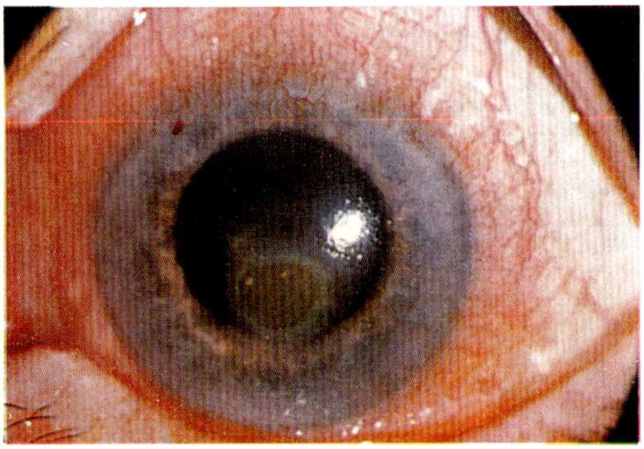

Fig. 2 Fluorescein staining of a paracentral erosion in neuroparalytic keratitis after electrocoagulation of the gasserian ganglion (♀ 74 yrs.) (see page 163)

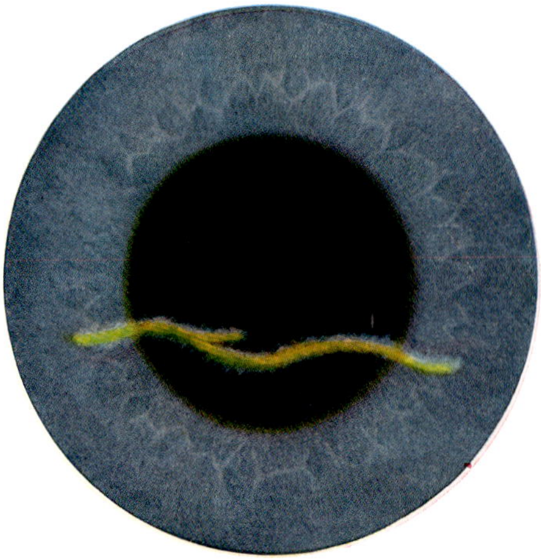

Fig. 4 Hudson-Stähli line (linea corneae senilis) (from: R. Thiel: Atlas of Diseases of the Eye, 6th edition, Thieme, Stuttgart, 1963) (see page 173)

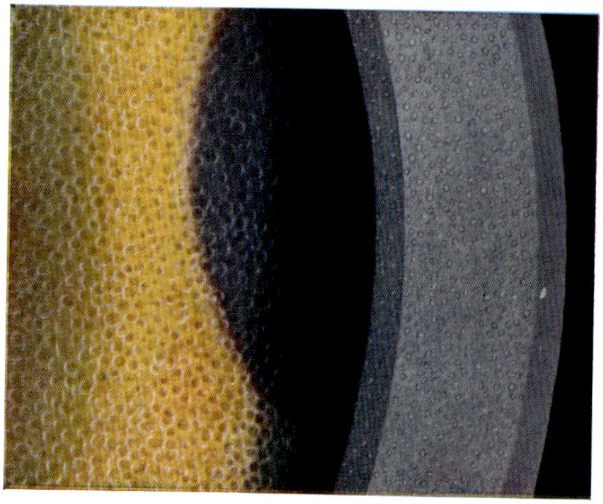

Fig. 5 Cornea guttata (from R. Thiel: Atlas of Diseases of the Eye, 6th edition, Thieme, Stuttgart, 1963) (see page 168)

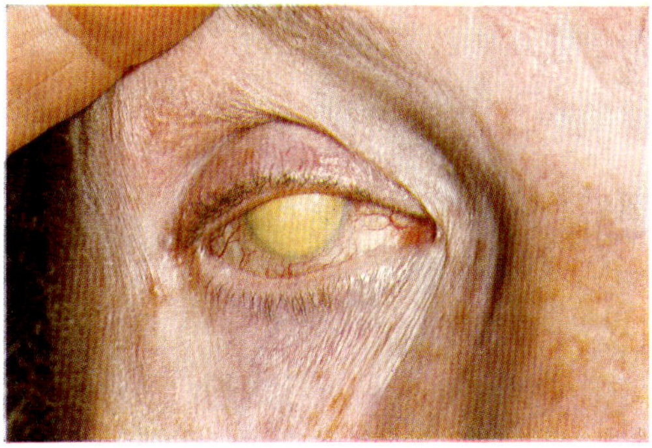

Fig. 1 Lipid deposition in an old corneal scar (♀ 65 yrs.) (see page 170)

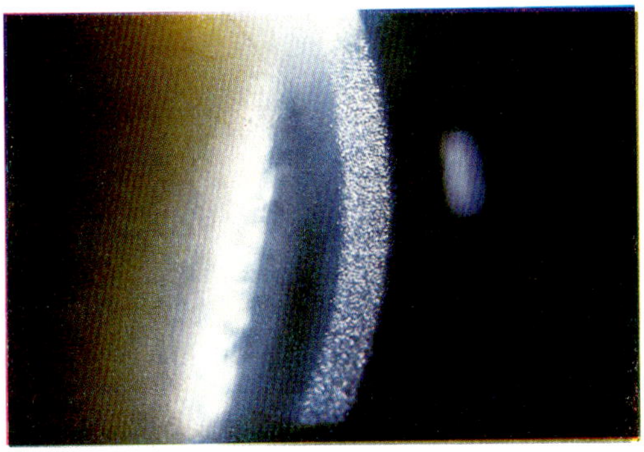

Fig. 2 Cystinosis with a dense accumulation of small crystals in the corneal stroma (♀ 4 yrs.) (see pages 171, 363)

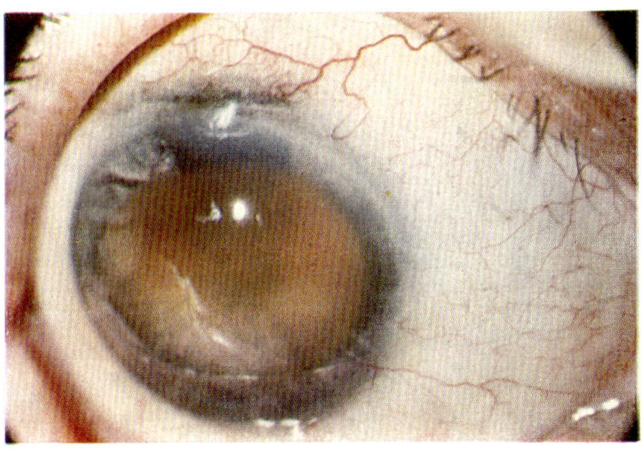

Fig. 3 Blood staining hemosiderosis of the cornea with a clear zone at the corneal periphery (♂ 57 yrs.) (see page 173)

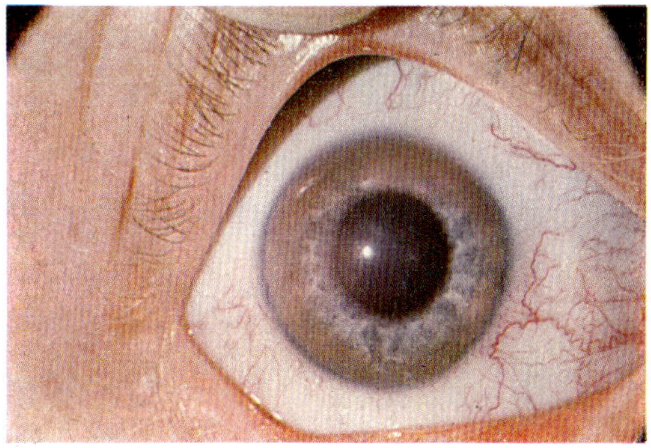

Fig. 4 Kayser-Fleischer ring (see pages 173, 366)

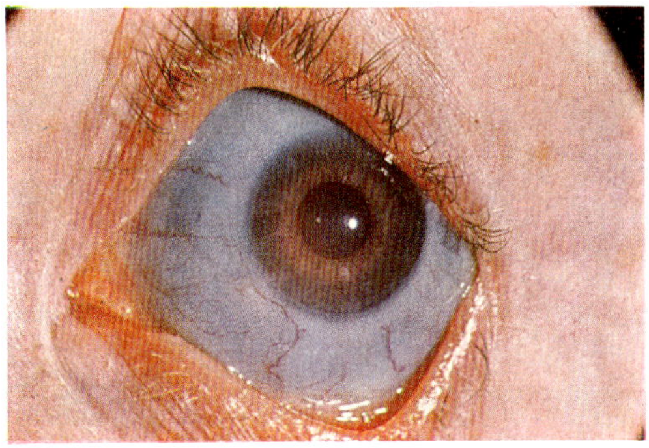

Fig. 5 Blue sclera in osteogenesis imperfecta (see page 181)

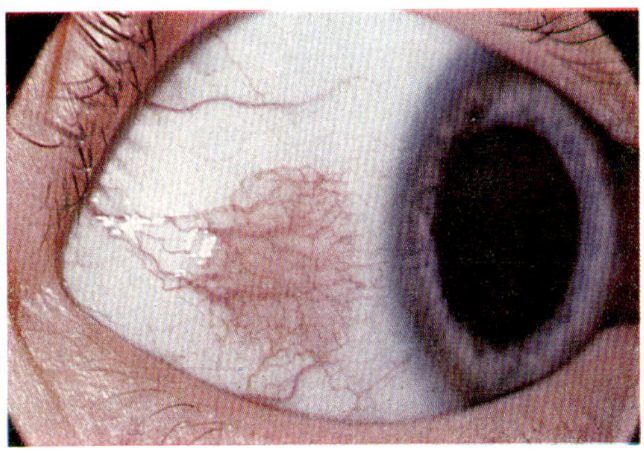

Fig. 6 Episcleritis with dilatation of the mobile episcleral vessels (♂ 6 yrs.) (see page 181)

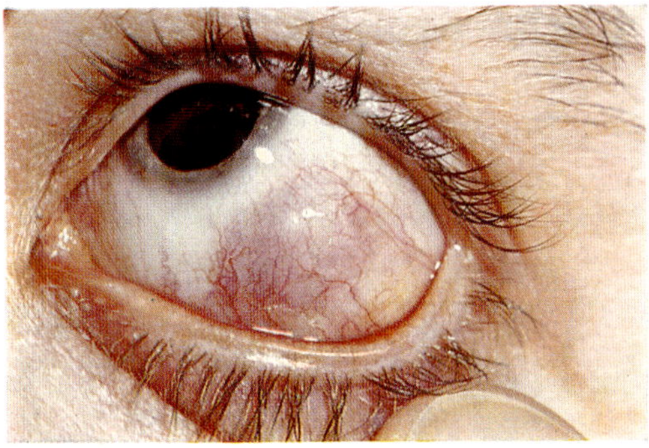

Fig. 1 Scleritis, diffuse violaceous swelling (♀ 35 yrs.) (see page 182)

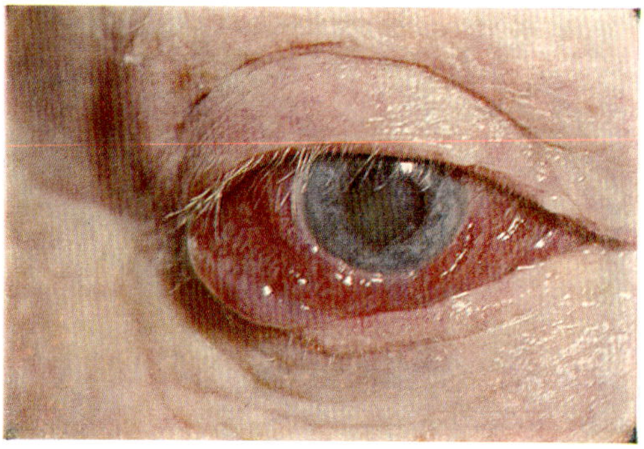

Fig. 2 Brawny scleritis with conjunctival chemosis and annular thickening of the sclera (♀ 81 yrs.) (see page 182)

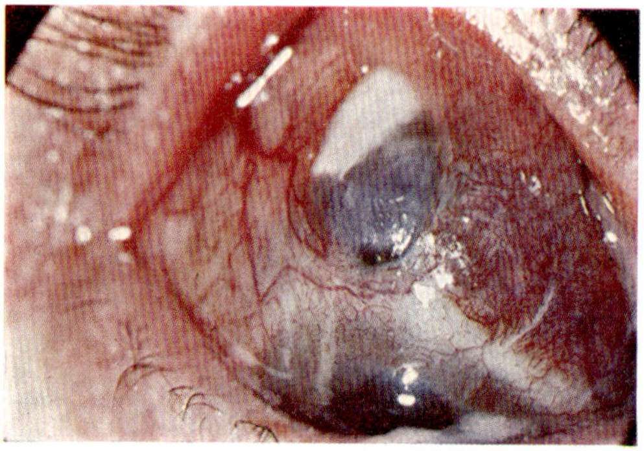

Fig. 3 Scleromalacia perforans; punched out scleral defect reaching to the uvea (♀ 63 yrs.) (see page 183)

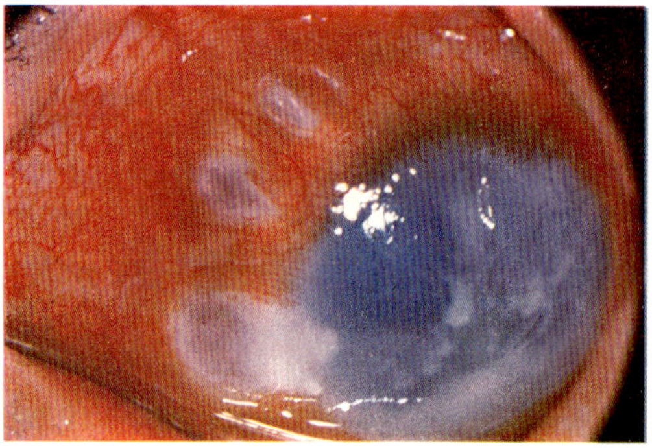

Fig. 4 Scleromalacia perforans with panophthalmitis and three scleral perforations near the limbus (see page 183)

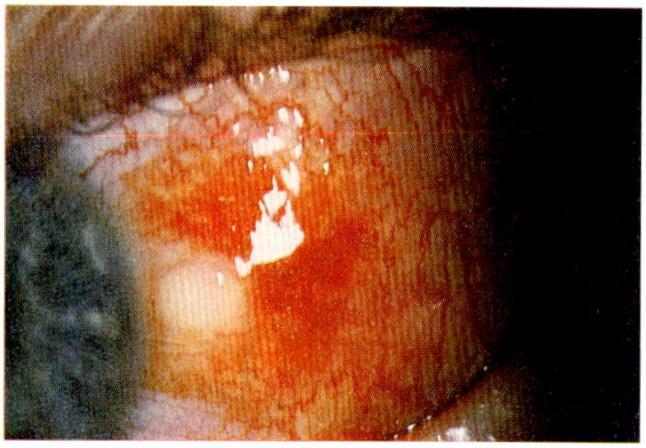

Fig. 5 Metastatic (infectious) scleritis (♀ 5 yrs.) (see page 184)

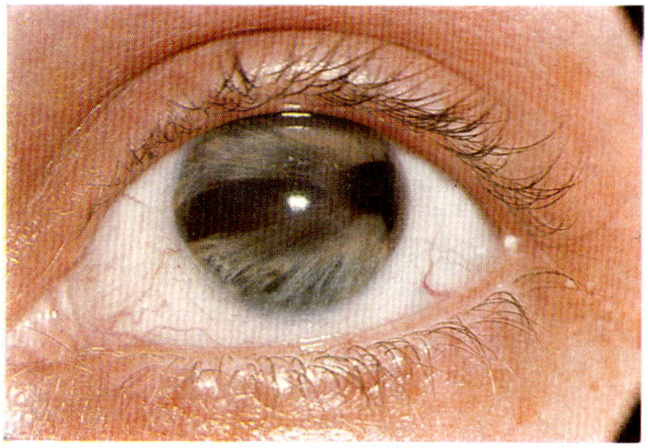

Fig. 1 Dysgenesis mesodermalis iridis et corneae (Rieger's syndrome) with polycoria (♀ 29 yrs.) (see pages 190, 191)

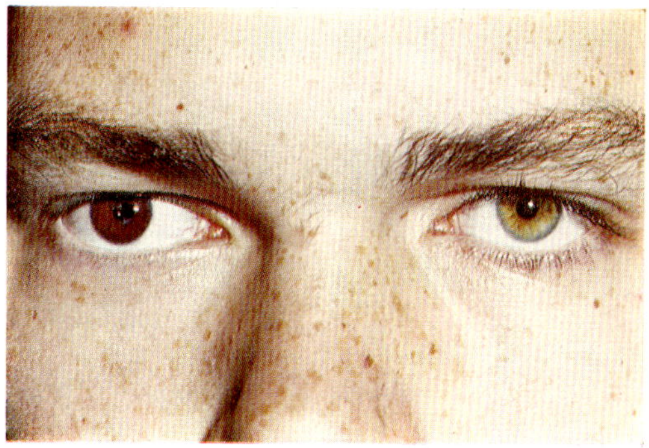

Fig. 4 Simple heterochromia, the right eye is brown, the left iris is blue (♂ 16 yrs.) (see page 192)

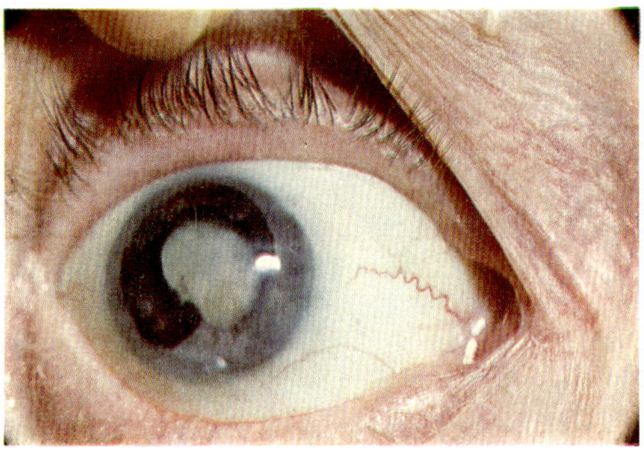

Fig. 2 Pupillary ectropion and a mature cataract Retraction of the iris stroma pulls the pigment epithelium onto the anterior surface of the iris (♀ 59 yrs.) (see page 191)

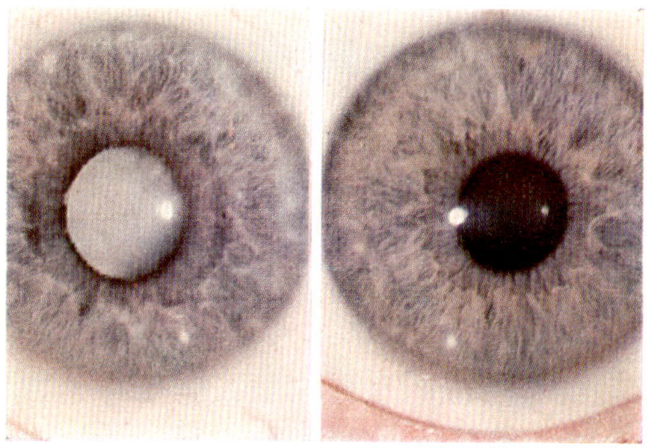

Fig. 5 Fuchs' heterochromia complicata, right = iris atrophy cataract, left = normal (♀ 37 yrs.) (see pages 190, 192)

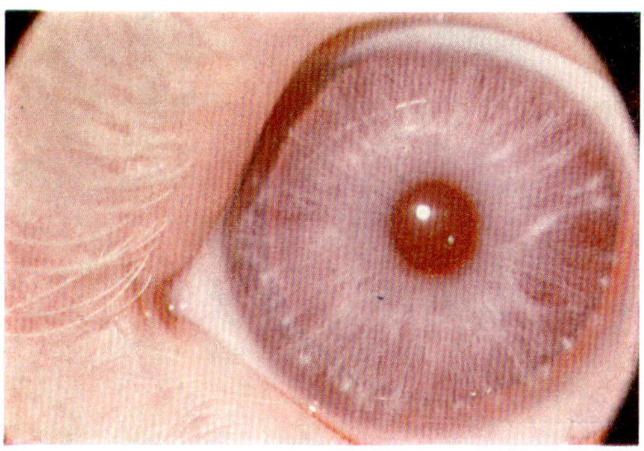

Fig. 3 Brushfield spots in an albino (♂ 8 yrs.) (see pages 99, 192, 364)

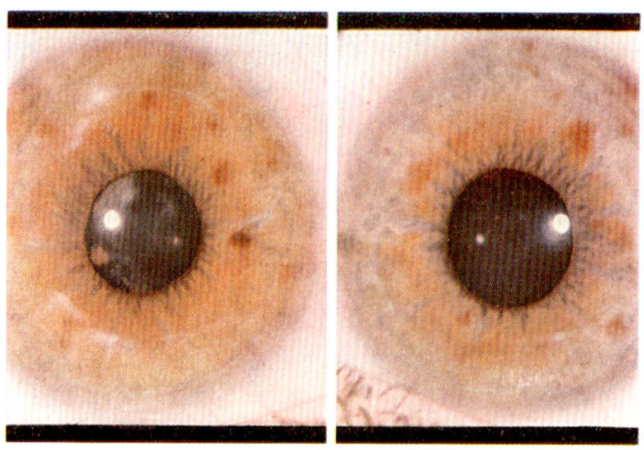

Fig. 6 Siderosis of lens and iris on the left. The right side is normal (see pages 193, 360)

Plate XIV (Chapter 16)

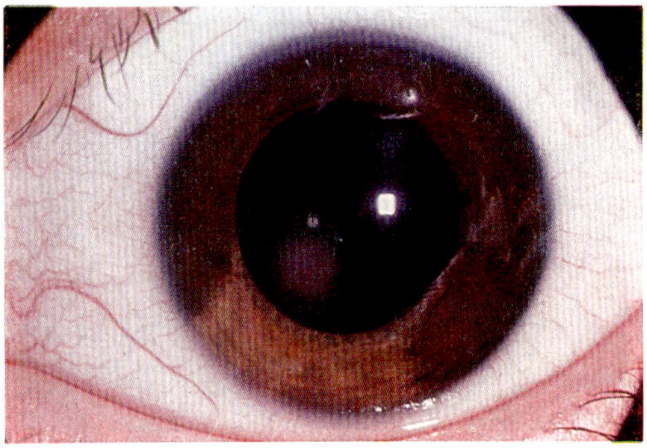

Fig. 1 Melanosis iridis (♀ 20 yrs.) (see page 194)

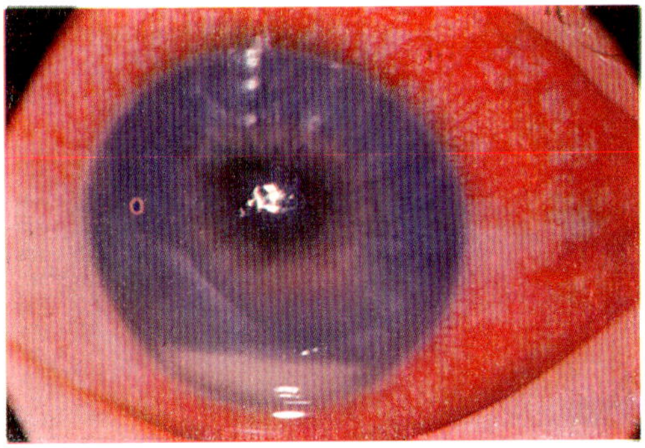

Fig. 2 Infectious iritis with hypopyon (see page 202)

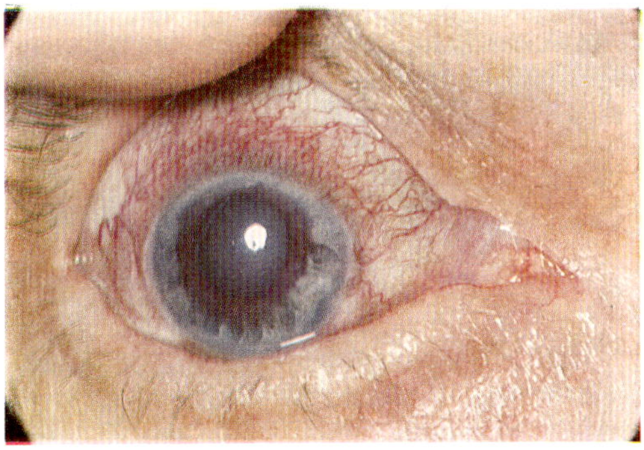

Fig. 3 Rubeosis iridis after central vein thrombosis (see pages 194, 204, 227)

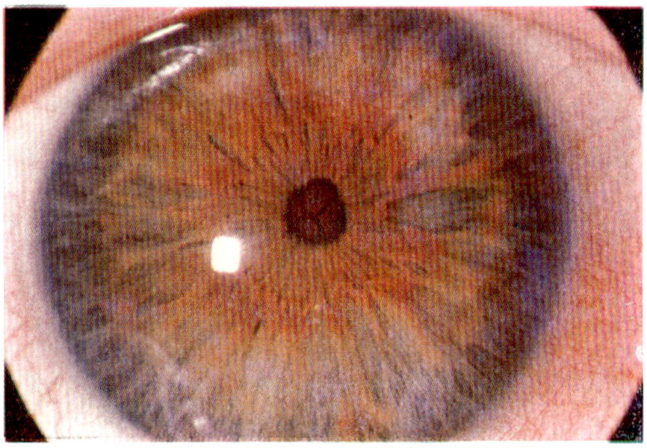

Fig. 4 Miotic cysts at the pupillary border after phospholine iodine therapy (see page 206)

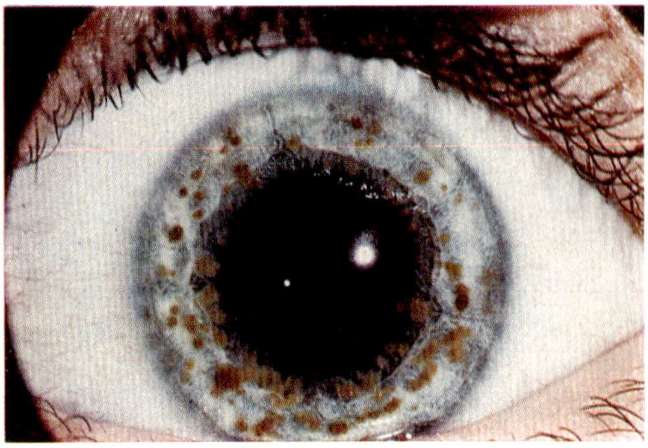

Fig. 5 Nevi in neurofibromatosis (♂ 12 yrs.) (see page 207)

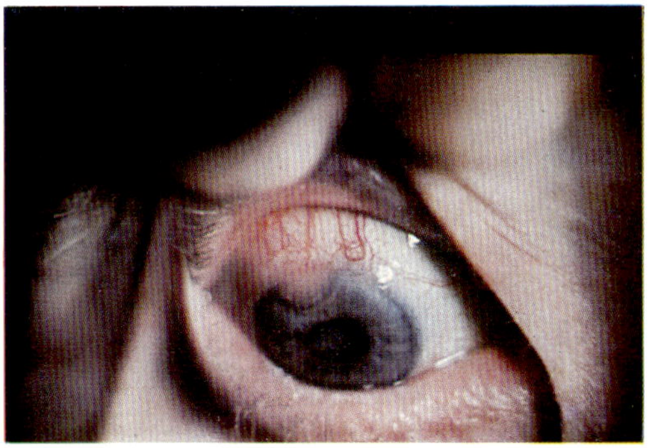

Fig. 6 Bronchial carcinoma metastatic to the iris (♀ 62 yrs.) (see page 32)

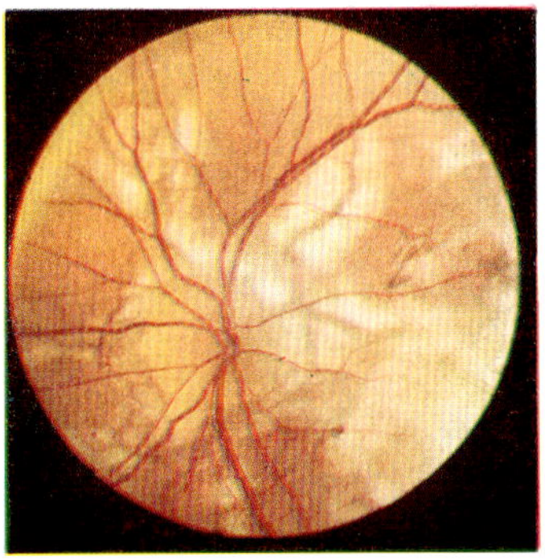

Fig. 1 Blood vessellike peripapillary bands, (angioid streaks) optic disc drusen (♂ 45 yrs.) (see pages 213, 219)

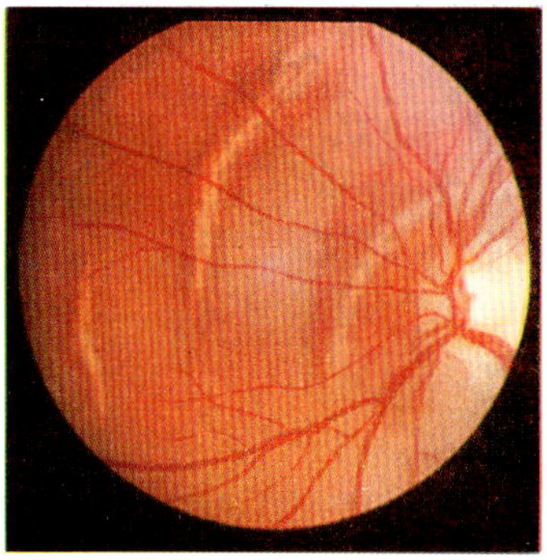

Fig. 4 Old choroidal rupture; the hemorrhage has reabsorbed exposing underlying sclera (♂ 24 yrs.) (see pages 214, 285)

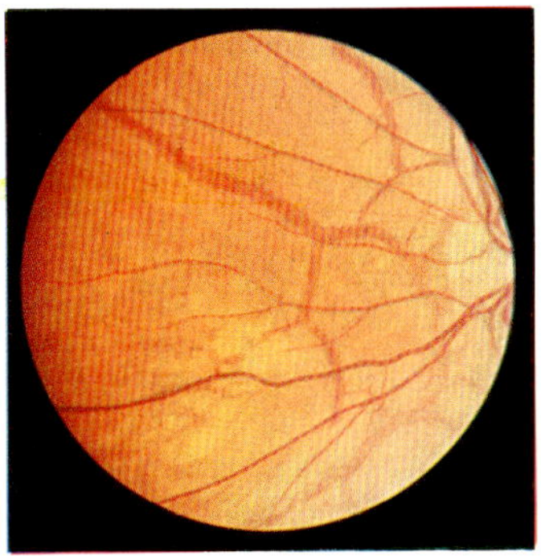

Fig. 2 Vessellike radiating angioid streaks (♀ 40 yrs.) (see pages 213, 219)

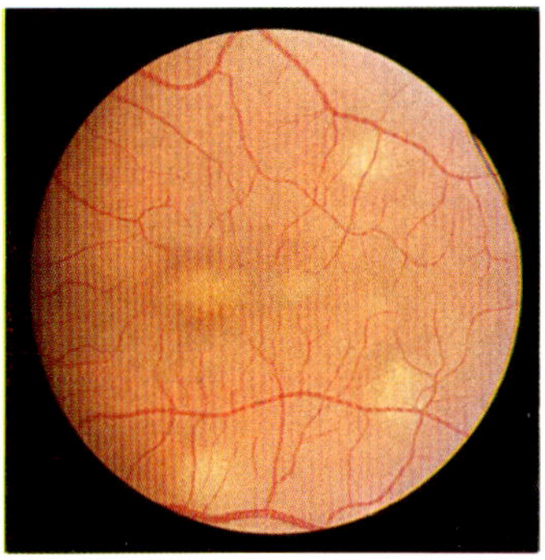

Fig. 5 Fresh disseminated chorioretinitis with blurred, round-oval, yellow-gray lesions (♀ 46 yrs.) (see page 215)

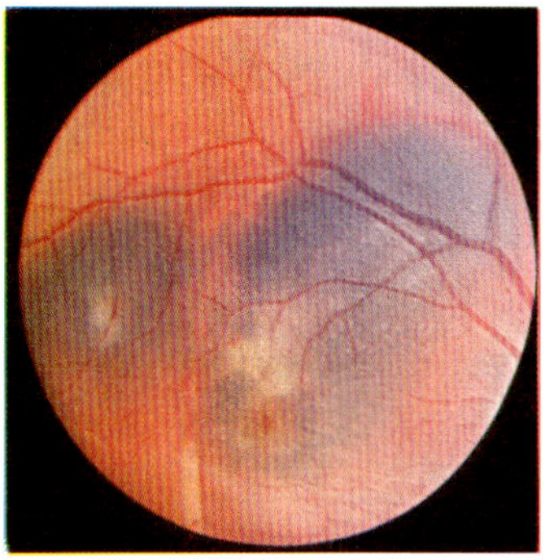

Fig. 3 Fresh choroidal rupture (subretinal hemorrhage) (♂ 22 yrs.) (see page 214)

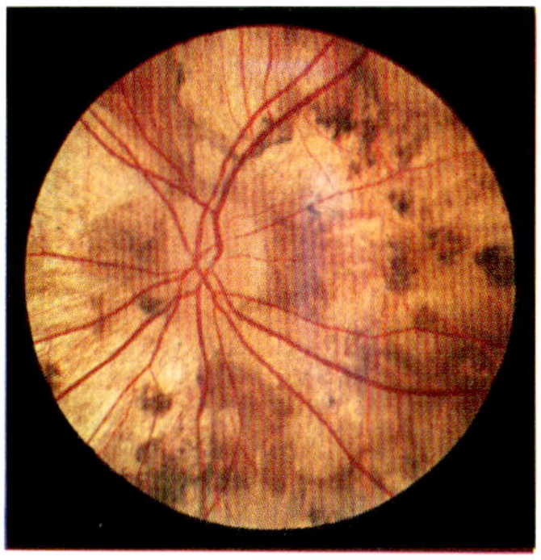

Fig. 6 Old disseminated chorioretinitis with sharply delineated areas of pigmentation and depigmentation (♀ 43 yrs.) (see page 215)

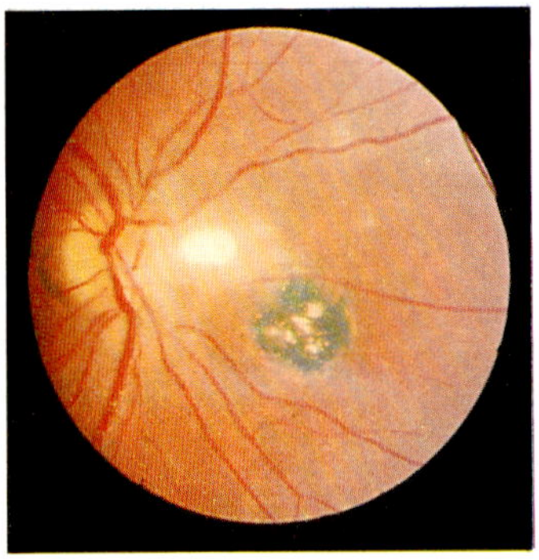

Fig. 1 Juxtapapillary chorioretinitis (Jensen) (gray-blurred fresh lesion and pigmented old lesion) (♀ 21 yrs.) (see pages 215, 294)

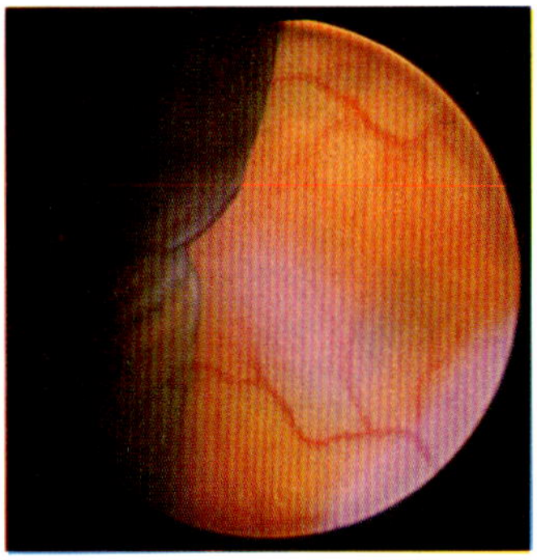

Fig. 2 Choriodal detachment (spongiosis) with loss of the anterior chamber after cataract surgery (♀ 66 yrs.) (see pages 218, 228)

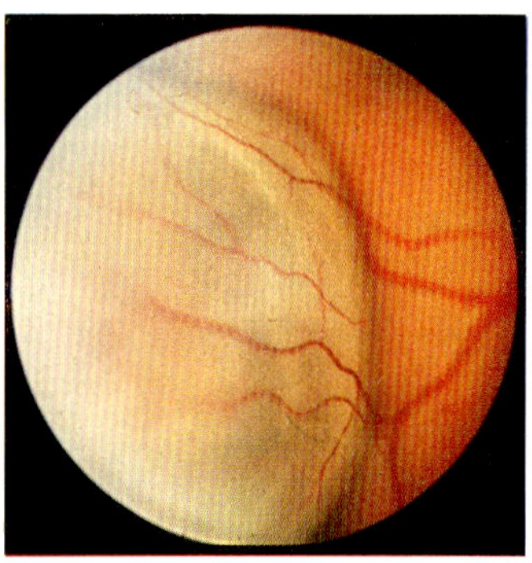

Fig. 3 Choroidal melanoma (♀ 62 yrs.) (see page 220)

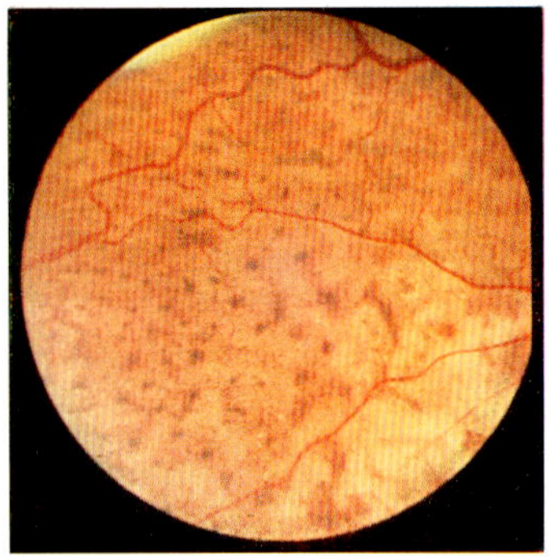

Fig. 4 Bronchial carcinoma metastatic to the choroid causing punctate pigmentation – depigmentation following irradiation (♀ 40 yrs.) (see page 220)

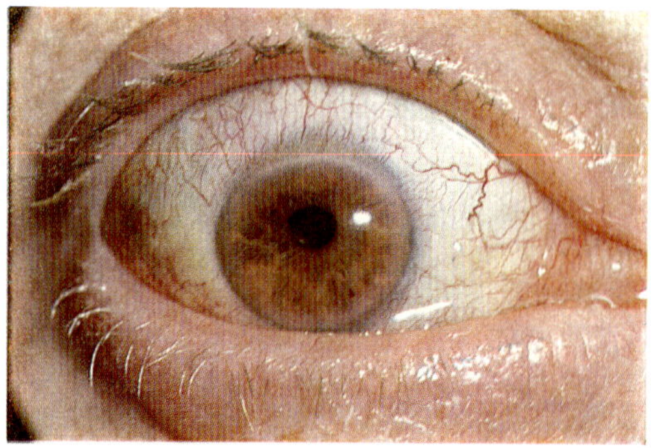

Fig. 5 Mild ciliary injection with chronic glaucoma (♂ 62 yrs.) (see pages 32, 224)

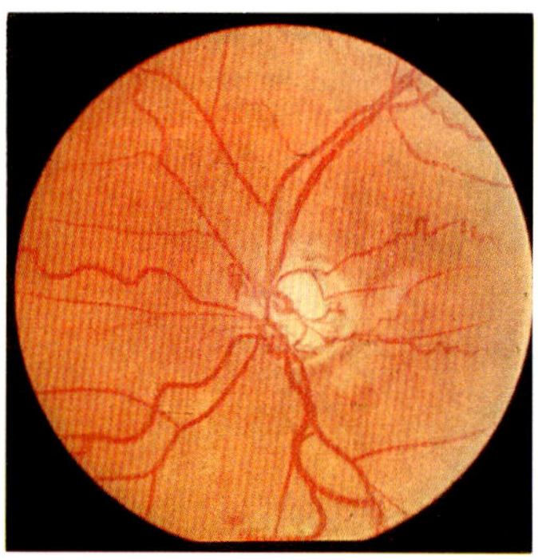

Fig. 6 Glaucomatous cupping and optic atrophy; bayonet deformity of the vessels (♂ 72 yrs.) (see pages 224, 305)

eral, being bilateral in only 10 percent of patients. Anterior or posterior synechiae are almost never present. New vessel formation in the chamber angle is almost always present when the condition is of long standing. The occurrence of a hyphema with anterior chamber paracentesis is allegedly pathognomonic of heterochromic cyclitis (Amsler et al. 1955). Fluorescein effusion from iris vessels into the aqueous is accelerated (Fig. 16.11, Amsler et al. 1955).

In Fuchs' heterochromia complicata and in congenital or early damage to the sympathetic innervation, the lighter eye is the diseased one.

Siderosis of the iris (Plate XIII, Fig. 6, page 192 e) is a brown discoloration from an intraocular iron foreign body. Other findings of ocular siderosis include brown flecks under the anterior lens capsule in the lens epithelium and retinal pigment dispersion similar to what is seen in retinitis pigmentosa. ERG and EOG are altered when damage is sufficiently extensive. Posterior subcapsular cataracts also occur.

Secondary heterochromia may occur with iris atrophy from any cause: trauma, post iritis, glaucoma, post radiation, and essential progressive iris atrophy. Pulseless disease also causes stromal iris atrophy (see page 271, 315).

Pigment Dispersion: Pigment granules of varying size will deposit on the iris surface. This may be physiologic or appear after glaucomatous attacks and with diabetes.

Fine **crystals** can deposit in the iris with both cystinosis and gout.

Longstanding phenothiazine therapy causes deposition of small brown-yellow granules in the cornea, stroma, anterior lens capsule, retina, conjunctiva and iris (Edler 1966).

Localized areas of depigmentation are seen with focal iris atrophy after circumscribed iritis, zoster, or acute glaucoma. Owing to loss of pigment epithelium the iris transilluminates in these areas. Takayasu's (pulseless) disease (see page 271) can cause iris atrophy and neovascularization of the iris root. Norrie's disease may have iris atrophy as well as a retrolental connective tissue mass (see page 235, 329). Any iris tumor can cause circumscribed loss of pigmentation; increase, on the other hand, is rare (see page 207). White congenital scars are a further cause of areas of depigmentation (Fig. 16.12).

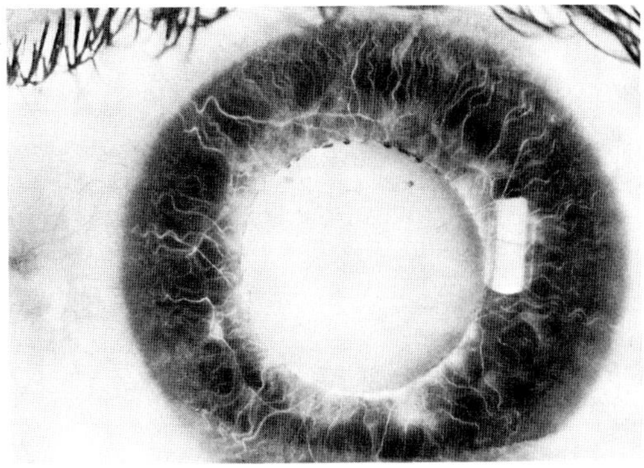

Fig. 16.11 Fuchs' complicated heterochromia. The fluorescein angiogram shows leakage of iris vessels (after 20 seconds)

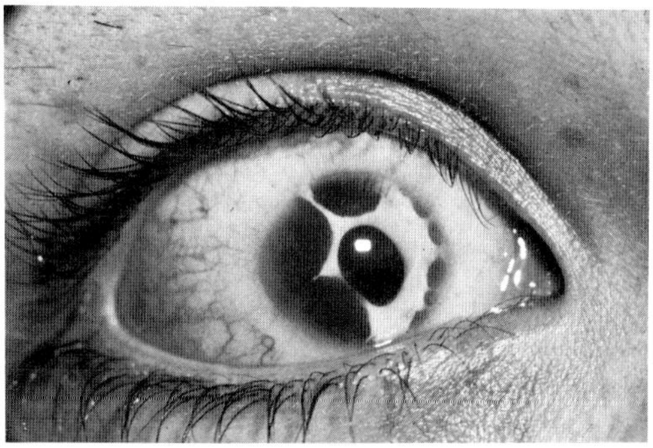

Fig. 16.12 Congenital replacement of the iris by white scars. With glaucoma (♀ 17 yrs.)

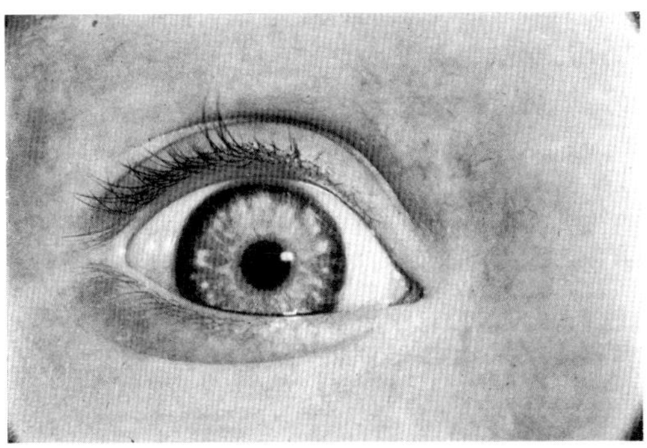

Fig. 16.13 Brushfield spots (♀ 9 months)

Wolfflin's iris nodules are small white spots in the iris periphery in normal blue-eyed individuals. The same spots appearing in mongoloids are known as *Brushfield's spots* (Fig. 16.13) and are present at birth in Down's syndrome (Purtscher 1958/59). They occur in 20 to 25 percent of normal blue-eyed persons versus 85 to 90 percent of Down's patients. The spots are nodular accumulations of dense connective tissue. Mongolism is associated with coronal, zonular and suture cataracts.

Nevi, unilateral melanosis: Nevi, i.e., variable pigmentation of the iris, may be present to the extent of causing unilateral melanosis (Plate XIV, Fig. 1, page 192 f) which presents as a dark brown iris unilaterally. The nevus of Ota causes nevoid hyperpigmentation of the entire area of distribution of the first branch of the trigeminal nerve (see page 100). Neurofibromatosis may be associated with numerous nevi of the iris (see page 103).

Discoloration by iritis: A dirty green-red color, particularly easy to see in light-colored irises.

Pinpoint Transillumination with Diabetes

Owing to *lacy degeneration* of the iris pigment epithelium in diabetes, pinpoints of light are visible through the iris on retroillumination. The pupillary ruff may be pale and spongy with sieve-like holes. The pupillary border may be hyalinized with thick pseudocysts. The pupil responds poorly to dilating drops. Pupillary dilatation or surgical intervention may result in massive release of pigment that appears as a brown cloud in the anterior chamber. The most feared iris complication of diabetes is rubeosis.

Senile Changes

Noninflammatory pigmentary dispersion frequently occurs with age. The pupillary ruff is depigmented and pigment granules deposit on the surface of the iris (in the iris stroma), chamber angle, and posterior cornea. Atrophy of the iris pigment leaf is particularly noticeable on retroillumination. With age, the iris stroma becomes less distinct and the surface relief of the anterior stroma less crisp.

Vascularization

Vascularization of the *chamber angle* and *iris* occurs in longstanding anterior uveitis. Networks of new vessels form along with increased iris atrophy and intraocular hypotension; hypertension is rare. Anterior synechiae may develop. Neovascularization with sarcoidosis, syphilitic granuloma, or foreign bodies is more localized.

Vascularized tumors of the iris (including leiomyomas and angiomas) are rare. Spontaneous hyphemas occur. When present in children juvenile xanthogranulomatosis has to be considered (see page 207).

Rubeosis iridis (see page 204; Plate XIV, Fig. 3, page 192 f) is seen most commonly with central retinal vein thrombosis. Diabetic retinopathy is the next most common concurrent disorder, with retinal periphlebitis, old retinal detachment, central retinal artery emboli (Davenport 1959), arteriosclerotic hemorrhages and severe perforating injuries being less common. *Rubeosis iridis* begins as fine, newly formed capillary nets near the pupillary border. This is followed by capillary formation at the iris periphery and then over the entire iris, with pupillary ectropion. Ultimately the chamber angle is involved with complete peripheral synechiae. The intraocular pressure is almost always highly elevated. The entire process takes about three months with central retinal vein thrombosis and may extend over several years in diabetes. The newly formed vessels arborize on the iris surface and are not radial in the iris stroma.

Iritis and Iridocyclitis (Anterior Uveitis)

Signs of inflammation — Complications with iritis and iridocyclitis — Serous iritis — Fibrinous iritis — Nodular iritis — Purulent iritis — Hemorrhagic iritis — Iritis with a deep anterior chamber — Cyclitis — Differential diagnosis.

Signs of Inflammation in Iritis and Iridocyclitis

Calor — Rubor — Tumor — Dolor — Loss of function — Increased protein in the anterior chamber and vitreous.

Calor: Increased temperature with inflammation accentuates normal aqueous convection currents. The warm iris causes the aqueous to rise with all its constituents near the surface of the iris. Once there, it streams downwards near the cooler posterior corneal surface. Inflammatory precipitates deposit in a triangular fashion (Arlt's triangle) on the posterior cornea because of this convection current. The larger deposits lie more inferiorly. In the acute stage of ciliary injection, the temperature is elevated at the limbus.

Rubor: Ciliary, pericorneal injection. In a pale iris, hyperemia causes a reddish-gray discoloration. A brown iris does not reveal this change. Iris nodules, if present, may be reddish, yellow-brown or gray-white, glassy, or milky-blue in appearance.

Tumor: Edema of the iris (partly caused by histamine release) can narrow the pupil mechanically (increased tissue volume). The surface relief of the iris is faded and less distinct. Gray iris deposits and nodular granulomata (tuberculosis, syphilis, sarcoid, focal inflammation) may or may not be vascularized.

Dolor: Sharp eye pain radiating to the brow and head may occur, especially with accommodation and pupillary constriction (light reflex). The pain achieves the intensity of a neuralgia. Concurrent meningeal irritation, when present, is a further cause of pain. Secondary glaucoma always has to be considered. Photophobia and lacrimation are less prominent in anterior uveitis.

Loss of function: Miosis, i.e., edematous swelling of iris stroma and vagal irritation from histamine release, results in loss of function. Posterior synechiae (adhesion between iris and lens) (Fig. 16.16) can progress to pupillary seclusion (Fig. 19.4). Vision is decreased by cells and protein in the aqueous or vitreous, and by

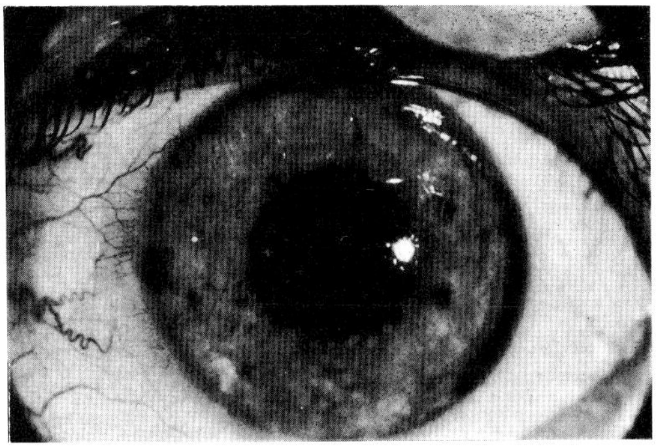

Fig. 16.14 Large precipitates on the posterior corneal surface (Arlt's triangle)

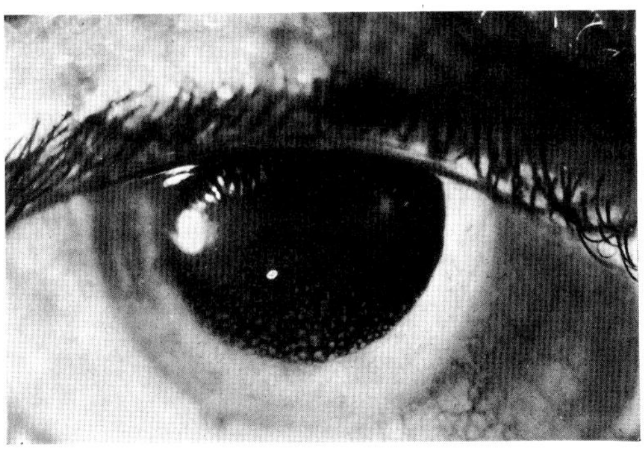

Fig. 16.15 Fine precipitates on the posterior corneal surface (Arlt's triangle) (♀ 36 yrs.)

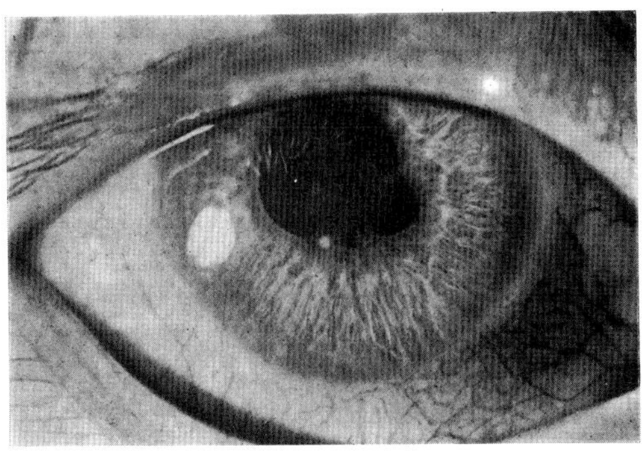

Fig. 16.16 Posterior synechiae

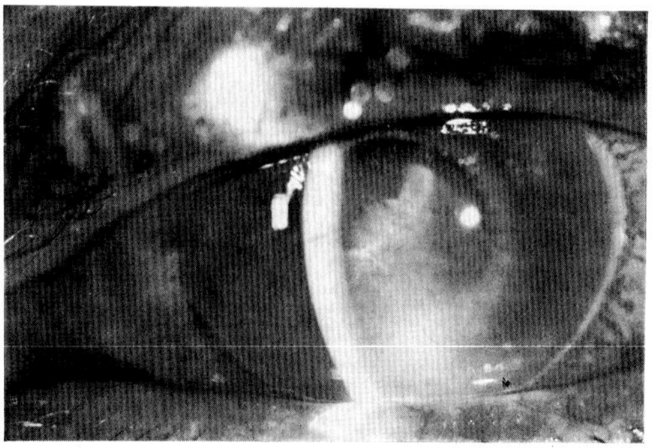

Fig. 16.17 Fibrin in the anterior chamber in acute iritis

membranous fibrin deposits on the anterior surface of the lens.

Increased protein content of aqueous and vitreous causes varying degrees of Tyndall's effect (aqueous or vitreal flare).

Cells (lymphocytes, leucocytes, macrophages, erythrocytes) and *fibrin* (Fig. 16.17) deposit on the posterior corneal surface (Fig. 16.14 and 16.15).

In *cyclitis*, cells and protein increase in the vitreous. Depending on the severity of the ciliary reaction, vitreal opacities may be dustlike, fibrillar, floccular or may form white, pigmented or hemorrhagic sheets.

In transmitted light these opacities appear as dark shadows which move with the globe. On direct illumination they are white, gray or bloody. Since the fundus is poorly visible the color of the disc seems darker and a misdiagnosis of "neuritis" is often made.

Acute choroiditis and *retinitis* can cause *vitreous opacities*. The cellular-fibrinous opacities appear as gray clouds or sheets especially in juxtapapillary chorioretinitis.

Longstanding anterior as well as posterior uveitis can lead to liquefaction of the vitreous and posterior vitreous detachment.

Complications of Iritis and Iridocyclitis

Corneal involvement — Scleral involvement — Secondary glaucoma — Hypotony — Cataract — Fundus changes — Acute glaucoma attacks.

Corneal involvement: Chronic iritis leads to corneal involvement through direct endothelial damage or indirectly from precipitation of protein particles. Stromal, even epithelial, edema results with ingress of aqueous. *Fibrin deposition* in *Arlt's triangle* can also cause localized stromal edema (Fig. 16.18). Varying degrees of deep stromal vascularization may occur if edema remains permanent. Old endothelial precipitates can be covered by the endothelium and take on the appearance of "glassy precipitates."

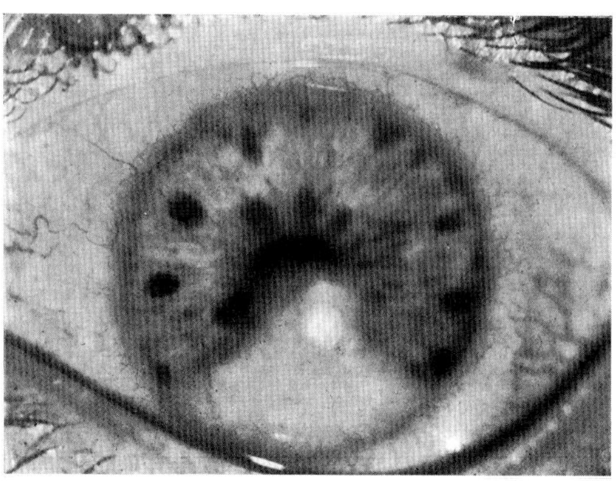

Fig. 16.18 Fibrin deposition on the posterior corneal surface (Arlt's triangle) (♂ 28 yrs.)

Chronic iritis, especially in children (Still's disease), will lead to *band keratopathy* (see page 169).

Involvement of the sclera: Scleritis or episcleritis may accompany recurrent iritis. The thinned sclera can become *staphylomatous*.

Secondary glaucoma: Gelatinous and membranous exudates deposit in the chamber angle during acute iritis. Furthermore, the iris is edematous and Schlemm's canal may fill with blood. Chronic iritis usually causes narrowing of the chamber angle. (Hypotony, which is common with acute iritis, causes a deepening of the anterior chamber.) Pigment deposits in the angle and new vessels may form. When a flat anterior chamber persists for longer than two weeks (usually from proliferation, rubeosis iridis, mesodermal dysgenesis [Rieger 1935], injury), goniosynechiae with secondary glaucoma result from organization of the inflammatory exudate. Pupillary seclusion by posterior synechiae prevents aqueous circulation and may result in iris bombé with secondary angle closure.

Hypotony: When intraocular pressure fails to recover, the ciliary body is irreparably atrophied, and phthisis bulbi may result.

Cataract: Chronic anterior or posterior uveitis disrupts the permeability of the lens resulting in *cataracta complicata*, i.e., permeability cataract formation (Fig. 21.5).

Fundus changes: Iridocyclitis is frequently accompanied by fundus changes.

The optic disc may be slightly prominent and blurred owing to vascular dilatation, venous stasis or edema of the nerve head (*papilledema e vacuo* = "with hypotony"). Optic atrophy can result. In uveitis white-gray, round nodules may appear along retinal arteries (segmental reversible arteritis) (Kyrieleis) (see page 259). Similar lesions also occur along the veins. The macula reflex in chronic uveitis may be irregular owing to *cystic macular changes* (Plate XXV, Fig. 2, page 288 a) or localized serous detachment. Both result in decreased acuity and a central scotoma.

Acute glaucoma attack: Corneal edema, flat anterior chamber and *middilated pupil* (iritis = constricted pupil) are important differential diagnostic points in acute *angle closure glaucoma*.

Types of Iritis

Serous Iritis

Minimal aqueous clouding, few cells, ciliary injection, a tendency for synechia formation and early onset of secondary glaucoma. Most common causes: ophthalmic zoster (see page 95), lues, tuberculosis, Still's disease.

Fibrinous Iritis

Marked aqueous clouding with an abundance of cells and fibrin (Fig. 16.17). Early, massive synechia formation (posterior synechiae). Marked ciliary injection with pain and decreased vision.

Causes: foci from tonsils, teeth, sinuses, lung etc., *rheumatism, syphilis, tuberculosis, gonorrhea, toxoplasmosis.*

Still's disease, Felty's syndrome — Ankylosing spondylitis — Reiter's syndrome — Vogt-Koyanagi syndrome, Harada's uveoencephalitis — Leptospirosis — Brucellosis — Rickettsial (recurrent) fever, typhus, malaria, leprosy, plague — Viral infections — Fungal infections — Parasites: nematodes, tape worms, larvae, amebic dysentery — Ophthalmia nodosa — Gout — Congenital iritis — Incontinentia pigmenti — Intraocular tumors, retinal detachment, hemorrhage — Phacogenic iritis — Diabetic iridocyclitis — Gonococcal iritis — Sympathetic ophthalmia — Erythropoietic disorders.

Still's Disease, Felty's Syndrome

Chronic infantile polyarthritis (Still-Chauffard syndrome) causes bilateral, slowly progressive, almost irritation-free chronic or subacute iridocyclitis often accompanied by cataract formation and band keratopathy (Fig. 13.46). Chronic (ankylosing) polyarthritis, lymphadenopathy, splenomegaly, leukopenic anemia, elevated erythrocyte sedimentation rate and increased streptolysin appear between ages 2 and 14. A lack of calcium results in osteoporosis.

Anterior uveitis with arthropathy is more common, especially in girls, than the full-blown picture of Still's disease.

In adults the clinical picture of *Still's* disease is known as *Felty's syndrome*. Felty's syndrome appears mainly in older women. Besides iridocyclitis there is chronic arthritis, leukopenia, hypersplenism, and dysproteinemia. Still's disease and Felty's syndrome are autoimmune collagen disorders.

Ankylosing Spondylitis

Ankylosing spondylitis *(Marie-Strümpell-Bechterew disease)* (autoimmune collagen disease, see page 183) primarily affects men. Iridocyclitis, which may be recurrent, bilateral

and alternating occurs in 30 to 50 percent of cases.
The iritis is usually serofibrinous with a strong tendency for synechiae formation. Hypopyon and even hyphaemas occur. Secondary glaucoma and cataracts are common.

Reiter's Syndrome

Oculo-urethral-synovial syndrome *(Reiter-Fiessinger-Leroy disease)* (see page 128) affects primarily men between the ages of 20 and 40. Acute iritis, episcleritis, urethritis and arthritis occur. Gastro-intestinal disturbances (bloody-mucoid diarrhea), fever and skin exanthemas (macular-vesicular-pustular dermatitis) and lymphadenopathy complete the clinical picture. In 15 percent of cases there is a fibrinous iridocyclitis, potentially with keratitis and optic atrophy.

Vogt-Koyanagi Syndrome, Harada's Uveoencephalitis

Iridocyclitis in the *Vogt-Koyanagi syndrome* has an acute onset but chronic course. In 50 percent of cases there is an inner ear disturbance ranging from hyperacusis to deafness. Eighty percent of affected patients show white eyelashes (poliosis), eyebrows and hair as well as vitiligo of lids and other areas of the skin. Fever and mild meningeal irritation (headache, meningismus) are common. Lymphocytes appear in the spinal fluid.

In *Harada's disease,* besides uveitis, prominent findings include acute inflammatory retinal detachment which becomes chronic (70 percent), choroidal detachment, and sometimes papilledema or retrobulbar neuritis.

Systemic manifestations are the same as in the Vogt-Koyanagi disease. Both Vogt-Koyanagi and Harada's disease are included in the *uveocutaneous meningoencephalitis* syndrome.

Leptospirosis

Leptospirosis (Leptospira icterohemorrhagiae, L. grippotyphosa, L. canicola, L. pomona, L. batavia) has an incubation period of 2 to 14 days after which fever, conjunctivitis, muscle and nerve pain occur. The clinical picture varies: meningitis, influenza, typhoid, etc. Weeks later a subacute, chronic, potentially recurrent, serofibrinous iridocyclitis appears as a late complication. Serous meningitis or encephalomyelitis may do the same. The characteristic *thick vitreous membranes* with precipitates resembling snowflakes can remain for years. Other ocular findings include: conjunctivitis, scleritis, icterus, optic neuritis, and extraocular muscle paresis (Hager et al. 1962).

Miscellaneous Agents

Brucellosis, rickettsia (Rocky Mountain spotted fever, Japanese river fever), typhus, malaria occasionally cause iridocyclitis. *Leprosy* is associated with serofibrinous, nodular or pussy iritis. Iritis with *recurrent fever* (spirochetes) may creep up slowly or be abrupt in onset. Hypopyon formation is possible. Retinitis or optic neuritis is rare. Ocular manifestations which occur in 3 to 4 percent of cases of *plague (Pasteurella pestis)* include: metastatic ophthalmia, exudative retinitis, uveitis, iridocyclitis, ulcerating keratitis, conjunctivitis.

Viruses

Viruses frequently cause superficial inflammation and hemorrhage. This may lead to circumscribed areas of depigmentation-vitiligo. Etiologic agents include: *zoster, herpes simplex, pox, varicella,* and practically any viral infection.

Fungal uveitides are extremely rare, occurring almost exclusively in chronically ill individuals debilitated by tuberculosis, endocarditis, leukemia, etc.

Parasitic Diseases

Nematodes: Parasitic effects of worms (nematodes) on the eye (Carter 1958; Lemos da Silva 1957; Schoop et al. 1961):

Rarely *Ascarides* will damage the eye directly. The parasites enter the nose, lacrimal sac or canaliculus via the gut and esophagus. Indirect damage from toxins, blood and lymph loss is more common. Amaurosis, photophobia, hemianopia, accommodative spasm, mydriasis and miosis occur.

Oxyuris (pinworm = *Enterobius vermicularis*) sometimes causes blepharitis and ocular muscle disturbances.

Trichuris produce the same symptoms as *Ascarides* and *Oxyuris*. Severe changes may exist in *Ankylostomiasis:* lid and facial edema, dilated pupil, lacrimation and occasionally retrobulbar neuritis with juvenile cataract.

Trichinosis begins three to six days after eating infected meat. Symptoms include: diarrhea, muscle pain, non-specific generalized complaints, bilateral lid edema and chemosis (Spaeth 1942; R. Schmidt 1944; Holler and Schmidt 1941; Lehrfeld and Breisacher 1940). The pale yellow chemotic conjunctiva may protrude between the lids. Subconjunctival hemorrhages may occur. The infection spreads bilaterally to the extraocular muscles causing diplopia, painful restriction of ocular movement (Krämer 1899; Groenouw 1920; Blank 1920) and exophthalmos. Retinal edema and hemorrhage (Nicolesco 1938; Spaeth 1942; R. Schmidt 1944), anterior and posterior uveitis and optic neuritis have been observed. Involvement of intraocular muscles causes mydriasis and accommodative paresis.

Of the filaria, *Filaria bancrofti* is the most significant. The microfilaria circulate in the bloodstream and either directly or through toxins cause lid edema, retinal hemorrhages or exudative iritis. *Filaria loa* appears subconjunctivally, from where it can be removed. *Filaria loa larvae* are very mobile and found in the lids, anterior chamber, vitreous and beneath the retina.

Filaria conjunctivae and *F. volvulus* affect the ocular adnexa.

Onchocerciasis (river blindness) is endemic to Africa and tropical areas of central America. This chronic infection lasts for years and is caused by the filaria *Onchocerca volvulus* transmitted by a biting fly, genus *Simulium*. Pinhead to egg-size nodules and erysipelas-like skin changes occur. The symptoms in onchocerciasis (Robles' disease) are caused by the large number of microfilariae. Associated are painful conjunctivitis, keratitis (each dead microfilaria causes an infiltrative reaction, these become confluent), punctate keratitis, sclerosing keratitis, iritis, iridocyclitis, cataract, chorioretinitis, posterior pole pigment dispersion and atrophy, and optic atrophy (Budden 1957; Rodger 1958, 1960; Rones 1960; Branley 1956; Symposium Society of France 1958).

In the chronic stage the conjunctiva falls into folds. Risk to the eye is greater the closer the typical skin nodules are to it (Appelman and Michiels 1956).

Rarely, nematode infection of the eye occurs with larvae of *Gnathostoma spinigerum, Ascaris lumbricoides*, ancylostomata *(Necator americanus, Ancylostoma duodenale), Loa loa, Wuchereria bancrofti*, Thelaziidae, and *Dranuncula medinensis*. They lead to conjunctivitis, endophthalmitis, retinal and vitreous hemorrhages. The larvae may be visible in the eye or conjunctiva (Schoop et al. 1961).

Toxocara canis infection (see page 283), while rare, is the most common intraocular nematode in nontropical, hygienically advanced areas of North America.

Tapeworms: Of the Cestoda, the encysted tapeworm larva of *Taenia (Cysticercus)* is more commonly found within the eye than *Echinococcus* (Maag 1958); the cysticercus was intravitreal in 41 percent, subretinal in 32 percent and subconjunctival in 16 percent as well as in the anterior chamber and orbit (Talkovskij 1951). Iridocyclitis, retinal hemorrhages and retinal detachment (Goerger 1957) as well as papilledema and optic atrophy result. In the vitreous the cysticercus looks like a white-green bubble with an iridescent border (crystalline deposits).

The dog tapeworm *(Taenia echinococcus)* cysticercus may develop into a giant cyst, potentially with sister lesions. The orbit is preferentially involved, leading to exophthalmos. The enlarged cysticercus of the dog tapeworm is found more commonly in the orbit and adnexa than in the eye itself (Maag 1958). Papilledema and optic atrophy may result (Walsh 1957). When intraocular it looks like a tumor.

Fly larvae: Entry of fly larvae into the eye (ophthalmomyiasis interna) elicits a reaction ranging from uveitis (exudative, purulent, or granulomatous) to panophthalmitis. The larvae are 0.5 to 5 mm in size and appear in the anterior chamber, vitreous, retina or choroid. Vitreous opacities, hemorrhages, and retinal detachment develop. The lens may subluxate.

Tropical amebic dysentery may demonstrate iridocyclitis, even chorioretinitis.

Ophthalmia Nodosa

Caterpillar, blackberry and other sharp, spiny hairs have barbs on their shaft which are directed backwards. When these hairs fall into the eye they can work their way into the cornea (Schirmer 1954; Flieringa 1956) or deeper, setting off a chronic granulomatous uveitis in the iris, ciliary body and choroid (Weve 1931; Dreyer 1953; Gundersen et al. 1952).

Uveitis with Gout

Gout can result in painful attacks of iridocyclitis, with episcleritis and conjunctivitis. Occasionally uric acid crystals deposit in the iris. This may cause nightly bouts of ciliary neuralgia with miosis. Serum uric acid is elevated.

Connatal Uveitis

In connatal uveitis posterior synechiae form between lens and iris collarette. Other findings may include persisting pupillary membrane, anterior polar cataract, microphthalmos or buphthalmos.

Incontinentia Pigmenti

The eye is affected in one-quarter of the cases of *incontinentia pigmenti* (Bloch-Sulzberger syndrome) (Franceschetti and Jadassohn 1954). Principal findings are a fetal or infantile uveitis (potentially with metastatic ophthalmia or persistent hyperplastic primary vitreous) and pseudoglioma. Optic atrophy and papillitis are rare. Strabismus is common (Wollensak 1959).

Tumors, Hemorrhages

Retinoblastoma may masquerade as panophthalmitis or endophthalmitis and has to be considered with any intraocular inflammation in children.

Subclinical, chronic or acute iritis can result from *necrosis of intraocular tumors* with *longstanding retinal detachment* or old intravitreal *hemorrhages* (periphlebitis, diabetes, traumatic).

Phakogenic Ophthalmia

Released lens protein (after surgery, perforating injury, leakage through a permeable lens capsule [hypermature cataract]) can cause a severe, chronic, plastic iritis. The keratic precipitates are lardaceous and, at times, confluent. Lens material deposits in the chamber angle. Secondary glaucoma is common.

In terms of the differential diagnosis it is important that postsurgical infection appears within a few days after the operation. Phakogenic uveitis requires 10 days to several weeks. With infection there is rapid, massive effusion of fibrin and leukocytes into the anterior chamber as well as chemosis. Phakogenic uveitis builds up gradually.

The differential diagnosis from sympathetic ophthalmia is more difficult. When light projection is still present in face of a ruptured lens capsule and plastic iritis, as much lens material as possible should be removed surgically. Contrary to sympathetic ophthalmia, a phakogenic reaction will then subside almost immediately.

Swollen lens protein and fibrin may be mistaken for a hypopyon. In addition to lens protein an adjuvant is needed to produce phakogenic ophthalmia (foreign protein, bacterial toxin, allergies) (H. Müller 1952).

Diabetic Iridocyclitis

Diabetic iridocyclitis appears many years after the onset of diabetes. There is vacuolation of the iris pigment epithelium with pigment dispersion in the anterior chamber.

Gonococcal Iritis

This occurs as an acute serofibrinous iridocyclitis with hematogenous spread of the gonococci. It is almost always found in association with gonococcal arthritis.

Sympathetic Ophthalmia (see page 360)

Sympathetic ophthalmia may occur after any perforating injury (surgical, foreign body, sharp objects, ruptured globe, perforating ulcer or tumor). The injured eye develops a chronic endophthalmitis and iridocyclitis, and sometimes chorioretinitis and optic neuritis. This occurs especially with uveal damage. Onset is subdued with a slow increase in aqueous cells, protein and fibrin. At first, the corneal precipitates are fine and punctate, later becoming coarse, confluent, and lardaceous. The iris is hyperemic with prominent individual blood vessels. Neovascularization may be present. Posterior synechiae, membranes and vessels attach to the lens capsule (seclusio, occlusio pupillae). Rarely cataracts, secondary glaucoma and phthisis bulbi will result.

Inflammation may begin in the second, previously sound (sympathizing) eye between 14 days and several years after the injury. The usual time period is 45 to 60 days. There is pain, lacrimation, photophobia and disturbance of accommodation. The sympathizing eye develops a chronic uveitis similar to that of the first eye and ranges from a light serous iritis to the most severe fibrinous iridocyclitis with all the complications potentially afflicting the first eye. Improvement with treatment may be transient and the uveitis continue to flare up. Histologically, nests of lymphocytes infiltrate the uvea, especially the choroid. Epithelioid and giant cells are also found.

After perforation of the globe, sympathetic ophthalmia must be considered with any chronic intraocular inflammation. The diagnosis is assured if uveitis also begins in the second previously uninvolved eye.

Differential diagnosis: The Vogt-Koyanagi (Harada) disease has a strong clinical similarity to the picture of sympathetic ophthalmia. Onset, however, is more acute and poliosis, vitiligo, and other generalized symptoms are not part of sympathetic ophthalmia. (Phakogenic ophthalmia, see page 200.)

The history of perforation makes a fibrinous iritis from other causes unlikely. Keratic precipitates in sympathetic ophthalmia are lardaceous and the exudates tend to form vascularized membranes covering the anterior lens surface.

Erythropoietic Disorders

Iridocyclitis also occurs in diseases of the blood-forming elements: *lymphoma, lymphosarcoma, leukemia, reticuloendotheliosis* and *reticulum cell sarcoma*. There may be a nodular or generalized thickening of the iris. Rarely there is aqueous clouding with keratic precipitates and even pseudohypopyon formation.

Nodular Iritis

Symptoms are minimal ciliary injection, with minor complaints and little aqueous flare. Gray-blue, blue-white or yellow-brown nodules varying from pinhead to pea size (Fig. 16.19) develop in the iris. The nodules may vascularize, stimulating formation of posterior synechiae in their vicinity.

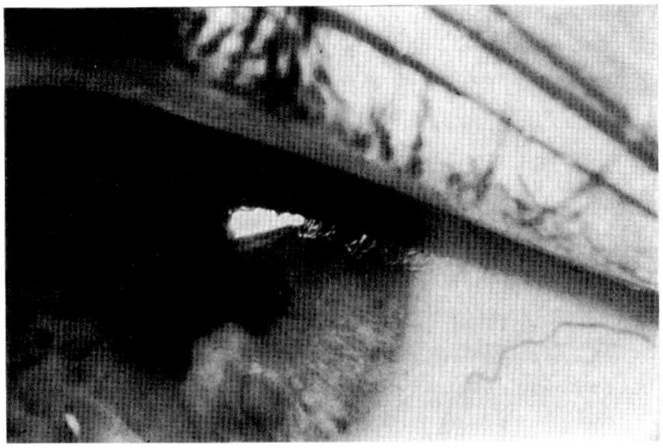

Fig. 16.19 Nodular iritis (sarcoidosis)

Tuberculosis — Sarcoidosis — Heerfordt's syndrome — Syphilis — Various causes.

Tuberculosis

A true uveitis based on metastatic bacilli to the uvea is rare. It occurs mainly in children and tends to involve one eye only. The atypical form is usually bilateral, begins between ages 30 and 40 and afflicts women more than men.

Contrary to previous thought the clinical appearance, e.g., iris nodules in chronic recurrent iridocyclitis (choroiditis not included), is of no value in making an etiologic diagnosis. Threshold sensitivity determination to tuberculin demonstrated a statistically greater sensitivity for persons suspected of ocular tuberculosis than the control group (Härtl and Thiel 1950). Antibody determination (Middlebrook-Dubois method) was overwhelmingly positive in cases of sarcoidosis, eczematous keratitis and various forms of scleritis (Doden and Heymann 1959).

Comparison of antibody concentrations in serum and aqueous of uveitis patients has been made. Elevated levels of specific local antibodies in the eye are of etiologic significance (Goldman and Witmer 1954; Remky 1958). Since the uveitis fails to respond to anti-tubercular medications, Zintz and Wegner (1953) conclude that witholding chemotherapy in cases of "tuberculous uveitis" is not an error.

Tuberculosis was once thought to account for a significant percentage of uveitis (Doden 1964). At the present time it is hardly ever a consideration (Doden, personal communication).

Sarcoidosis

Synonyms: Besnier-Boeck-Schaumann disease, Boeck's disease, benign sarcoidosis, miliary lupus, lupus pernio, benign lymphogranulomatosis, tuberculous giant cell hyperplasia, Boeck's sarcoidosis, epithelioid granulomatosis.

Klein et al. (1955) estimate ocular involvement in sarcoidosis to be between 30 and 40 percent. Present opinion is that sarcoidosis has a tuberculous etiology (Wegner and Wurm 1957).
Sarcoid nodules can appear on the lids as easily as anywhere else in the skin. They may be typical granulomas or isolated red-brown nodules. Conjunctival nodules are more common (page 131). These are red-yellow or glassy white, pinhead to pea-sized (Ullerich 1952, Krümmel 1953). They may calcify with time. Ulceration is less common (Lapri 1957). Deep vascularized corneal infiltrates may be seen with sarcoidosis. Involvement of the lacrimal glands (uveoparotid fever) causes lack of tear secretion and keratitis sicca.

The uvea is classically affected in the sarcoid form of iritis and iridocyclitis. Granulomatous iritis should stimulate a search for other signs (lymph nodes, lung) of sarcoidosis.
Wegner found sarcoidosis in 15 percent of all chronic uveitis patients at the eye sanatorium in Höchenschwand. The disease is usually bilateral and pleomorphic. Gray-yellow, partially translucent, potentially vascularized, at times numerous, sometimes solitary, even giant nodules are found on the iris.
Of 172 patients with sarcoidosis Wegner found 161 with iridocyclitis. Among these 35 had choroiditis, 11 Heerfordt's syndrome (uveoparotid fever) and 8 Mikulicz's syndrome (bilateral symmetrical lacrimal and parotid gland swelling). Heerfordt's syndrome, some cases of Mikulicz's syndrome, and sarcoidosis are all considered part of epithelioid cell granulomatosis (Ullerich 1952). Heerfordt's syndrome, which is a febrile inflammation of uvea and parotid (uveoparotid), is classified as an oculoglandular form of sarcoidosis (vide infra).

Slightly prominent exudates or disseminated foci may be seen in the choroid in sarcoidosis. Retinal findings, usually in association with an iridocyclitis, resemble periphlebitis. Small retinal veins show sheathing and gray-white infiltrates along the vessel walls (candlewax drippings).
Orbital sarcoidosis most often involves the lacrimal glands and results in Mikulicz's syndrome. There is a loss of tear secretion which leads to keratoconjunctivitis sicca. A tumor-simulating granuloma sometimes, although rarely, appears in the orbit.

Of diagnostic value in sarcoidosis are: the negative tuberculin reaction, lung and hand X-rays, hyperproteinemia, hypercalcemia, and skin-lymph node-conjunctival biopsy.

Heerfordt's Glandular Fever

Uveoparotid fever is considered a manifestation of sarcoidosis. Iridocyclitis is combined with inflammation of the salivary glands and sometimes the lacrimal glands. Keratitis, episcleritis, extraocular muscle paresis, facial nerve paresis and a mild fever are other symptoms.

Syphilis

Acquired lues, especially in the secondary stage, causes macules (roseolae) and papules. In the iris these appear as circumscribed, superficial, hyperemic, pink spots. More appropriately these are described as fleshy vascularized nodules. The roseolae disappear in a few days without visible scarring. Vascularized nodules become gray-yellow, frequently leaving sharply demarcated atrophic spots in the iris. Lardaceous, gray-white keratic precipitates deposit on the posterior cornea in the typical triangular fashion.
A cellular exudate also develops in the vitreous. During the tertiary stage gummas may form in the ciliary body and adjacent iris. These appear as expansive, tumor-like, white-yellow, knobby vascularized nodules projecting into the anterior chamber or vitreous.
Luetic foci of choroidal inflammation usually cause pigment clumping. The lesions are generally in the retinal periphery but may be central or juxtapapillary.

Various Causes

Nodular iritis is seen in *leprosy, sympathetic ophthalmia* and *ophthalmia nodosa.*

Purulent Iritis (Uveitis)

Marked ciliary injection, usually with chemosis, and pain are characteristic. At first, pus accumulates in the anterior chamber as a hypopyon (Plate XIV, Fig. 2, page 192 f) with a fluid level. Later it may fill the entire anterior chamber. Simultaneously there may be an outpouring of fibrin (Fig. 16.15). The iris is obscured and appears red-gray. Purulent iritis is usually seen only with endophthalmitis or panophthalmitis.

Bacterial infection — Metastatic ophthalmia — Fungal infection — Ulcus serpens — Recurrent hypopyon iritis.

Causes

Bacterial infection usually occurs after perforating injury, perforated corneal ulcer, iris prolapse and late postoperative infection, or infected filtering bleb.

Metastatic ophthalmia: Embolization by highly virulent bacteria causes metastatic ophthalmia (Fig. 16.20). This usually occurs in debilitated patients (diabetes, cachexia, etc.).

Sources for septic emboli include boils, cellulitis, puerperal sepsis, osteomyelitis, meningitis, encephalitis, endocarditis, pyelonephritis, peritonitis, pneumonia, typhus, scarlet fever, etc. The disease occurs at any age, is rarely bilateral and has been described in infants where it occurred in utero (Linnen 1950).

Fungal infection: Fungal *endophthalmitis* is severe, generally leading to loss of the eye (Hoffmann 1965, François 1968). The diagnosis is usually made histologically. The most common agents are: *Actinomyces* (gram positive bacteria), *Aspergillus, Candida, Cryptococcus* and *Blastomyces*. Histoplasmosis is a presumed agent causing recurrent iridocyclitis and small yellow nodules in the fundus which later atrophy.

Ulcus serpens: *Ulcus serpens* commonly causes hypopyon even without perforation (Fig. 13.28).

Recurrent hypopyon iritis: The picture of *recurrent hypopyon iritis* (Behçet syndrome) or *ophthalmia lenta* (Gilbert) is one of constantly recurring accumulation of pus in the anterior chamber along with circumscribed mucous membrane ulcers and low grade fever. The hallmark of the Behçet-Gilbert-Adamantiades disease is the acute, recurrent, unilateral or bilateral hypopyon iritis in a relatively irritation-free eye (Fig. 16.21). Small gray-yellow ulcers (aphthae) appear on the mucous membranes (mouth, pharynx, genitalia). Pyoderma and erythematous skin lesions are possible. There is a low grade fever with elevation of the erythrocyte sedimentation rate. Recurrent angiopathies resembling thrombophlebitis, periangiitis or central vessel emboli affect the fundus (Plate XXIV, Fig. 2, page 224 h). Hypopyon may appear with *erythema nodosa* iritis. There is perhaps a certain relationship between Behçet's disease and pyoderma, acute and chronic polyarthritis, joint effusion, Reiter's syndrome and ankylosing spondylitis. Neuro-Behçet includes meningitis, encephalitis and paresis (Lemke 1965).

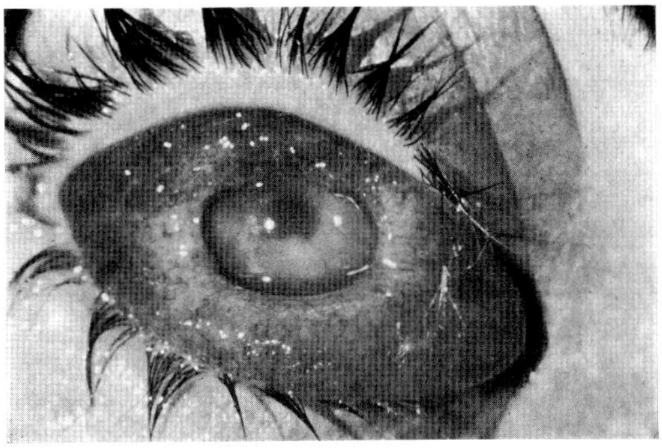

Fig. 16.20 Endophthalmitis and panophthalmitis

Toxic Iritis with Deep Anterior Chamber

So-called toxic iritis with a deep anterior chamber and *marked increase in aqueous protein* is usually caused by choroidal detachment. The globe is mushy soft and the anterior chamber very deep. The iris is displaced backwards in a step-wise fashion as is the lens.

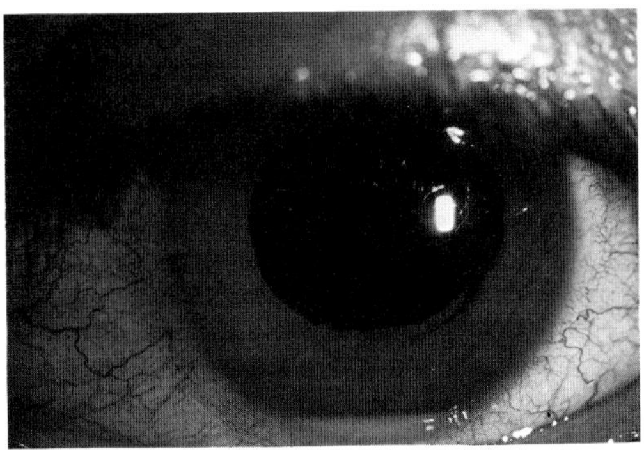

Fig. 16.21 Recurrent hypopyon iritis (Behçet) with a two millimeter hypopyon and cells in the anterior chamber without fibrin (♂ 16 yrs.)

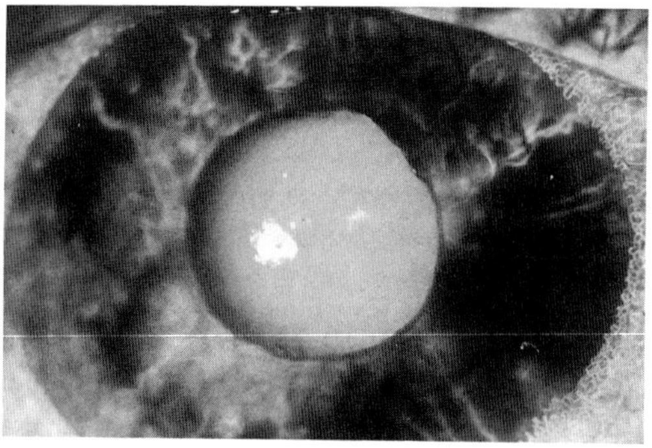

Fig. 16.22 Diabetic rubeosis iridis. Fluorescein angiography shows new vessel formation with protein leakage.

There is an outpouring of protein in the aqueous with few cells.

Etiology probably centers around damage in the posterior segment (retinal detachment, vitreous hemorrhage usually with diabetes, arteriosclerosis, injury) (see page 218). A similar picture (few cells, marked flare) occurs with leakage of lens proteins through the intact lens capsule (cataracta hypermatura) (Fig. 16.22). Rarely, diabetes will cause a marked increase in aqueous protein with few cells.

In the "string syndrome" after encircling operations or circular diathermy, a chemosis and excess protein exudation into the anterior chamber may develop in some cases combined with necrosis of the iris and ciliary body (Boniuk and Zimmermann 1961, Manson 1966) (Fig. 13.24, page 158).

Hemorrhagic Iritis

Hemorrhagic iritis with hyphema — Rubeosis iridis.

Hemorrhagic iritis with anterior chamber **hyphema** is rare. It may be seen with ophthalmic zoster, herpetic infection and rubeosis. It is common postoperatively.

Despite ciliary injection, aqueous clouding, pain and a tendency for posterior synechiae formation, **rubeosis iridis** (see page 194; Plate XIV, Fig. 3, page 192 f) is only reflexly related to iritis.

At first, a net of numerous small capillaries develops at the pupil and peripheral iris. Later, thicker, red, new vessels form on the iris. Goniosynechiae develop. Fluorescein angiography demonstrates a leakage into the aqueous (Fig. 16.22). In diabetes, rubeosis of the iris occurs in combination with stage II or stage III diabetic retinopathy. After diabetes, central retinal vein occlusion is the most common cause of rubeosis iridis. Other causes include: hemorrhagic retinopathy in hypertension or arteriosclerosis, pulseless disease, carotid occlusion (ischemic retina), pulsating exophthalmos (see page 340), central retinal artery emboli, periphlebitis, Coats' disease, retinal detachment, absolute glaucoma, Leber's miliary aneurysms, sickle cell retinopathy, hemangioma of the retina or iris, retrolental fibroplasia, retinoblastoma, pseudoglioma of the vitreous (see page 234), iris melanoma, and carcinomas metastatic to the iris.

Within weeks or months, rubeosis almost always results in uncontrollable secondary glaucoma. Rubeosis may regress significantly if it is possible to control the glaucoma surgically.

Iridocyclitis

To a greater or lesser extent iritis is usually accompanied by cyclitis (see page 211)

Inflammatory exudate from the ciliary body enters the vitreous where it appears as clouds of fine cellular, punctate, or floccular opacities. It may aggregate in opaque sheets. The optic disc may appear blurred and swollen with iridocyclitis (not a true papilledema or optic neuritis). Severe cyclitis may lead to hypopyon formation, even phthisis bulbi. Severe cyclitis in young persons, especially males, is often associated with a maculopathy (see page 282).

Differential Diagnosis of Iridocyclitis

A variety of diagnostic tests can be used to establish an *etiologic diagnosis* in uveitis (Witmer 1965, Campinchi et al. 1973): skin tests (tuberculin, toxoplasmin, histoplasmin, brucellin, Kolim, Kveim), X-ray (sinuses, teeth, lung, joints), laboratory tests (hematologic, erythrocyte sedimentation rate, serum electrophoresis and immunophoresis, fasting blood sugar).

Serologic tests aiding in the etiologic diagnosis of iridocyclitis (Witmer 1965) include: VDRL, Middlebrook-Dubois hemagglutination test for tuberculosis, anti-streptolysin-O titer, latex agglutination, agglutination for leptospirosis, brucellosis, typhus, paratyphus, viruses, Rickettsia, dye tests, complement, and indirect hemagglutination for toxoplasmosis. If higher antibody levels for tuberculosis, toxoplasmosis, streptococci or leptospirosis are found in the aqueous rather than in the serum, these may be manufactured locally (uveal tract).
Even with the most extensive investigation, the etiology of most endogenous ocular inflammations remains undiscovered (Siegert 1961).

Iris Cysts

Spontaneous iris cysts — Epithelium implantation cysts — Miotic cysts.

Iris cysts (Thiel 1960) may be idiopathic, appearing spontaneously in the iris stroma or pigment epithelium. Stromal cysts are lined by multilayered epithelium or single-layered endothelium. Pigment epithelium cysts develop from the pigment epithelium. Cysts of the pigmented pupillary border can be dominantly *inherited* (Fig.16.23) (Meyer 1969). Small pigment cysts may be pedunculated or float free in the anterior chamber (Fig. 16.24 a, b) or vitreous.

Epithelial implantation cysts (Fig. 16.25) occur after penetrating injury (including surgery) where surface epithelium is carried (or grows) into the anterior chamber. *Epithelial downgrowth* over the posterior cornea, iris, or vitreous face invariably leads to secondary glaucoma.

When iris cysts form, they are only partially delimited by the iris. Pseudodetritus is visible in serous cysts with translucent walls. If epidermis or eyelashes are implanted, laminated pearly cysts develop (Fig. 16.26).

Miotic cysts: Brown pigmented cysts at the pupillary border appear with chronic use of strong miotics (prostigmine, phospholine io-

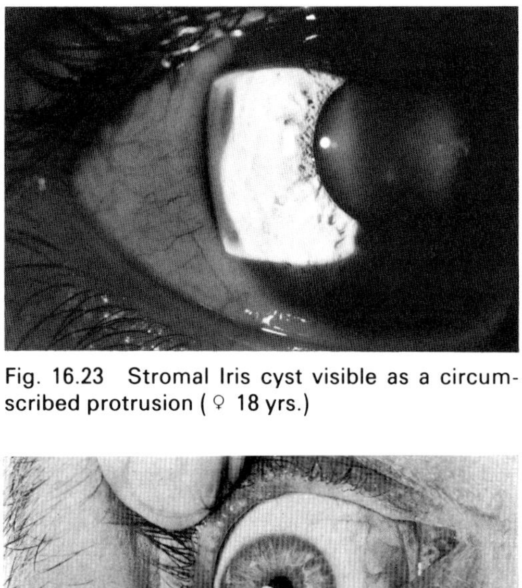

Fig. 16.23 Stromal Iris cyst visible as a circumscribed protrusion (♀ 18 yrs.)

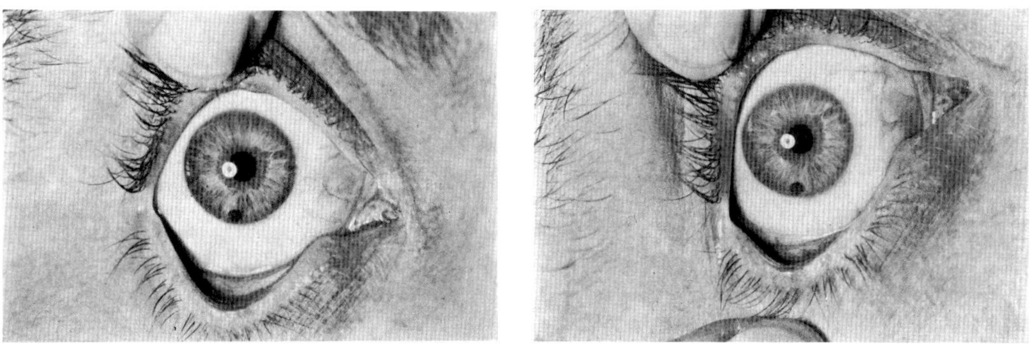

a b

Fig. 16.24 Free, spontaneous, pigmented cyst in the anterior chamber: a) at six o'clock; b) at eight o'clock (head tilted to the right)

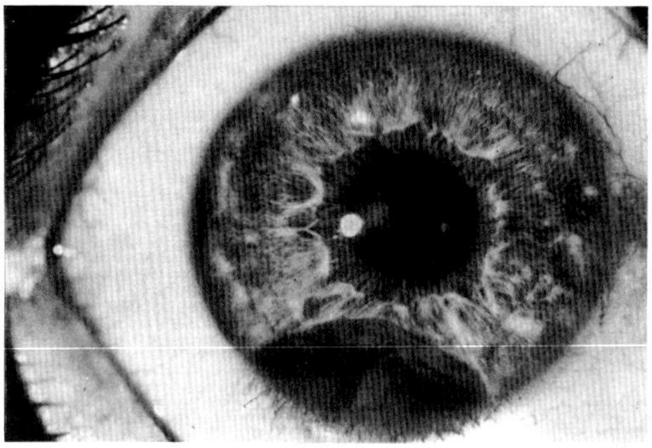

Fig. 16.25 Implantation cyst (♂ 40 yrs.)

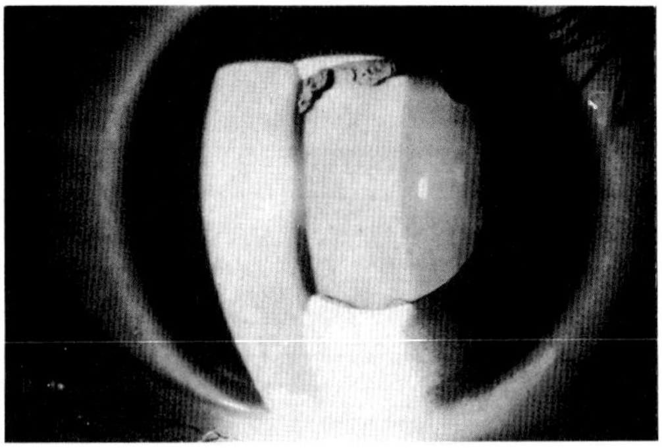

Fig. 16.27 Flocculi at the pupillary border

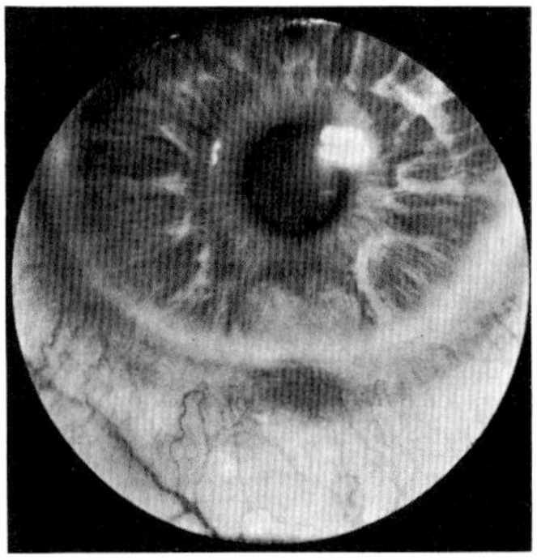

Fig. 16.26 Pearl cyst in 6 o'clock position (♂ 62 yrs.)

dide, DFP) (Plate XIV, Fig. 4, page 192 f). These may occlude the pupil to the point of blindness. The cysts tend to resolve once the medication is stopped. Miotic cysts resemble the *cystic pigment epithelial floccules* at the pupillary ruff (Fig. 16.27) which may be dominantly inherited (Meyer 1969).

Trauma

Perforating injury — Blunt trauma.

Perforating Injuries

Penetration and retention of a foreign body containing iron can lead to *siderosis* of the *iris*, i.e., a brown-yellow discoloration. Foreign bodies containing copper cause a blue-gray discoloration known as *chalcosis iridis*. Both iron and copper produce chronic irritation.

Glass and stone foreign bodies may be retained without any irritation once the original injury has healed. Caterpillar hairs cause the foreign body granulomatous uveitis of ophthalmia nodosa. Iridocyclitis with *depigmentation* of the iris occurs after *bee* or *wasp stings* into the eye.

Sympathetic ophthalmia (see page 200)

Phakogenic ophthalmia (see page 200)

Blunt Trauma

Blunt trauma causes contusion injuries: hemorrhage, traumatic mydriasis, iridoplegia, sphincter tears, iridodialysis, and traumatic heterochromia. Iridodonesis is present with subluxation of the lens.

Tumors

Nevi — Melanoma — Leiomyoma — Brushfield's spots — Nevoxanthoendothelioma — Metastatic tumor — Differential diagnosis of tumors — Pseudotumor.

Nevi

Iris nevi are common, occurring in 65 percent of the population. Neurofibromas in von Recklinghausen's disease look like multiple brown-yellow nevi (Plate XIV, Fig. 5, page 192 f) of varying size.

Various possible ocular manifestations of von Recklinghausen's neurofibromatosis are (Verbeck 1969):

a) plexiform neuroma with ptosis, plexiform neuroma of the lids, elephantiasis of the lids
b) conjunctival nevi, conjunctival tumors
c) iris nodules, pedunculated iris tumors
d) pupillary ectropion
e) retinal, choroidal tumors; melanosis
f) tumors of the optic nerve, optic disc prominence, papilledema, optic atrophy
g) enlarged optic foramina, i.e., widened optic canal
h) retrobulbar tumors
i) exophthalmos, pulsating exophthalmos
j) defects in orbital bone
k) abducens-facial nerve paresis
l) enlarged sella turcica
m) corneal vascularization, tumors on the cornea, gray enlargement of corneal nerve endings, corneal nevi
n) congenital cataracts
o) buphthalmos, absolute glaucoma.

Nevus and Melanoma

An important differential diagnostic point between iris nevi and melanoma (melanoblastoma, Fig. 16.28) is that the pupil may not react normally in the area of the melanoma. This is a stiff, brown-black infiltrating tumor. If the diagnosis is in doubt an excisional biopsy should be performed. When the tumor is limited to the iris, local excision is adequate. If the ciliary body is involved, cyclectomy or enucleation becomes necessary. With a large melanoma, episcleral vessels may form a caput medusae.

Leiomyoma

Leiomyomas of the iris are rare and appear as slowly growing, yellow-gray nodules eventually causing pupillary ectropion. Cataract, recurrent anterior chamber hemorrhages and secondary glaucoma are common.

Brushfield's Spots

The otherwise physiologic, peripheral, circumscribed, gray stromal iris thickenings appear with greater number and frequency in Down's syndrome (see page 329) (Skeller and Oster 1951; Zimmerman 1965).

Nevoxanthoendothelioma

Juvenile xanthogranulomas of the iris are usually unilateral and appear mainly in the first years of life. Spontaneous anterior chamber hemorrhage is common. This aids in the differential diagnosis from a hemangioma or melanoma. There may be a diffuse discoloration of the iris or localized yellow-brown nodules. Circumscribed heterochromia occurs with time. Often an unmanageable secondary glaucoma leads to buphthalmos and blindness. Nevoxanthoendotheliomas also appear on the cornea, conjunctiva, skin and in the orbits (Holland 1966; Jünemann 1969; Zimmerman 1965; Saraux et al. 1967).

Metastatic Tumors

Carcinomas are practically the only tumors metastasizing to the iris (Plate XIV, Fig. 6, page 192 f). They are rare and usually appear

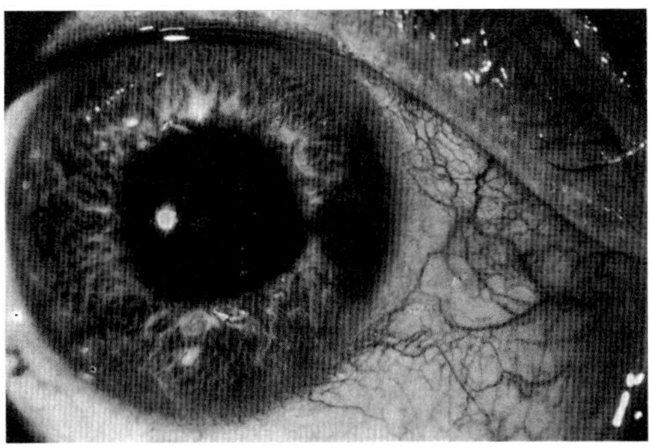

Fig. 16.28 Melanoma of the iris (♂ 62 yrs.)

in combination with choroidal metastasis reaching the iris via the bloodstream. Clinically they appear as gray-yellow or reddish, single or multiple nodules. They are rarely bilateral. Increased anterior chamber protein, even hemorrhages, occur. Tumors metastatic to the ciliary body usually cause iritis and progressive iris displacement.
Sixty to seventy percent of metastatic iris tumors are primary in the breast. Other possibilities include: primary carcinomas of the bronchi, stomach, colon, thyroid, prostate, uterus and adnexa, and testes.

Differential Diagnosis (Tumors, Pseudotumors)

With iris tumors, consideration must be given to melanomas, inflammatory granulomas (as with syphilis, tuberculosis, sarcoidosis, and foreign bodies), leukemic and lymphatic (Pfanz 1957) infiltrates, pseudotumors and cysts. Occasionally retinoblastoma (see page 294) forms nodular seeds on the iris. These appear as gray-yellow, avascular, single or multiple nodules on the iris surface. The iris vessels are dilated. Tumor cells can deposit on the posterior cornea or layer out as a pseudohypopyon in the anterior chamber.

References

Amsler, M., F. Verrey, A. Huber: L'humeur aqueuse et ses fonctions. Masson, Paris 1955

Appelmans, M., J. Michiels: Onchocerkose oculaire dépistée chez uns Européen trois ans après le retour d'Afrique. Bull. Soc. belge Ophtal. 113 (1956) 494–500

Badtke, G.: Die Mißbildungen des menschlichen Auges. In: Der Augenarzt, Vol. IV, ed. by K. Velhagen. Thieme, Stuttgart 1961

Blank, G.: Über Trichinose. Dtsch. Arch. klin. Med. 132 (1920) 179–203

Böke, W.: Die Manifestationsformen der Boeckschen Sarkoidose am Sehorgan. Klin. Mbl. Augenheilk. 139 (1961) 1–25

Boniuk, M., L. E. Zimmerman: Necrosis of the iris, ciliary body, lens and retina following scleral buckling operations with circling polyethylene tubes. Trans. Amer. Acad. Ophthal. Otolaryng. 65 (1961) 671–693

Bonnet, M., E. Vianey: Contribution a l'étude de l'iridoschis. Arch. ophtal. (Paris) 30, (1970) 7–34, 129–140

Branley, M. A.: Über die Onchozerkosis (Morbus Robles). Klin. Mbl. Augenheilk. 128 (1956) 1–15

Brushfield, T.: Mongolism. Brit. J. Child. Dis. 21 (1924) 241–258

Budden, F. H.: Natural history of onchocerciasis. Brit. J. Ophthal. 41 (1957) 214–227

Campinchi, R., J. P. Faure, E. Bloch-Michel, J. Haut: Uveitis, immunology ,and allergic phenomena. Thomas. Springfield, Ill., 1973

Carter, R. C.: Intraocular nematodiasis. Amer. J. Ophthal. 45 (1958) 853–869

Choyce, D. P.: Personal experience of onchocerciasis in central America, Africa and the British Isles with a note on O. cervicalis in horses. Trans. ophthal. Soc. U. K. 84 (1965) 371–406

Cogan, D. G., T. Kuwabara: Ocular pathology of the 13–15 trisomy syndrome. Amer. Arch. Ophthal. 72 (1964) 246–253

Danis, P.: L'angiome de la chorioide. Arch. Ophtal. (Paris) 12 (1952) 487–509

Davenport, R. C.: Facets of glaucoma. Trans. ophthal. Soc. U. K. 79 (1959) 3–14

Doden, W.: Die Tuberkulose des Auges und seiner Adnexe. In: Handbuch der Tuberkulose, Vol. IV, ed. by J. Hein, H. Kleinschmidt, E. Uehlinger. Thieme, Stuttgart 1964 (pp. 539–576)

Doden, W., G. Heymann: Tuberkulose-Antikörper bei Gesunden, Tuberkulösen und bei Kranken mit chronisch entzündlichen Augenleiden. Ber. dtsch. ophthal. Ges. 62 (1959) 307–309

Drenkhahn, F. O., H. Behnke: Die Variabilität der klinischen Ausprägung des Irisdefektes in zwei Familien mit erblicher Aniridie. Klin. Mbl. Augenheilk. 138 (1961) 545–557

Dreyer, C.: Ophthalmia nodosa. Acta ophthal. (Kbh.) 31 (1953) 429–436

Duke-Elder, S.: Diseases of the uveal tract. System of ophthalmology IX. Kimpton, London 1966

Edler, K.: Ocular changes associated with chlorpromazine therapy. Acta ophthalm. (Kbh) 44 (1966) 405–409

Flieringa, H. J.: A modified method of goniotomy. Ophthalmologica (Basel) 132 (1956) 187–190

Franceschetti, A., W. Jadassohn: A propos de l'incontinentia pigmenti délimitation le deux syndromes differentes figurant sous le même terme. Dermatologica (Basel) 108 (1954) 1–28

François, J.: Les Mycoses oculaires. Masson, Paris 1968

Goerger, F.: Sur un cas de cysticercose intraoculaire. Ann. Oculist (Paris) 189 (1957) 988–992

Goldmann, H., R. Witmer: Antikörper im Kammerwasser. Ophthalmologica (Basel) 127 (1954) 323–330

Groenouw, A.: Beziehungen der Allgemeinleiden und Organerkrankungen zu Veränderungen und Krankheiten des Sehorgans. Graefe-Saemisch, Hdb. III. 3rd Ed. Part 2, Chap. 22 (1920) 846

Groenouw, A.: Beziehungen der Allgemeinleiden und Organerkrankungen zu Veränderungen und Krankheiten des Sehorgans. In: Handbuch der gesamten Augenheilkunde, 3rd Ed., Vol. II/22, ed. by A. Graefe, Th. Saemisch. Springer, Berlin 1920 (p. 846)

Gundersen, T., P. Heath, L. K. Garron: Ophthalmia nodosa. Amer. J. Ophthal. 35 (1952) 555–565

Hager, G., H. Mochmann, E. Burmeister: Augenerkrankungen bei und nach Leptospirosen. Klin. Mbl. Augenheilk. 140 (1962) 845–854

Härtl, H. G., R. Thiel: Zur Ätiologie der chronisch-rezidivierenden Erkrankungen des Uvealtraktus. Die Bedeutung der Intracutanimpfung mit gereinigtem Tuberkulin (GT). Bücherei des Augenarztes, 20. Enke, Stuttgart 1950 (pp. 144–162)

Hoepner, J., M. Yanoff: Ocular anomalies in trisomy 13–15. Amer. J. Ophthal. 74 (1972) 729–737

Hoffmann, D. H.: Pilzinfektionen des Auges. Fortschr. d. Augenheilk. 16 (1965) 63–217

Holland, G.: Augenveränderungen beim juvenilen Xantho-Granulom. Klin. Mbl. Augenheilk. 149 (1966) 353–358

Holler, G., P. Schmidt: Ein kasuistischer Beitrag zur Klinik und Therapie der Trichinose. Med. Klin. 37 (1941) 984–988; 37 (1941) 1012–1015.

Ignatio-Lopez, M.: Un caso de Wohlfahrtiosis conjunctival. Arch. Soc. oftal. hisp.-amer. 12 (1952) 1045–1056

Jünemann, G.: Zur Differentialdiagnose und Therapie des Naevoxanthoendothelioms der Iris. Ber. dtsch. ophthal. Ges. 69 (1969) 136–139

Klein, M., R. J. Calvert, W. E. Joseph, E. Smith: Rarities in ocular sarcoidosis. Brit. J. Ophthal. 39 (1955) 416–421

Krämer, A.: Die tierischen Schmarotzer des Auges. In: Handbuch der gesamten Augenheilkunde, 2nd Ed., Vol. X, ed. by A. Graefe, Th. Saemisch. 1899 (pp. 193–208)

Krümmel, H.: Epitheloidzellige Granulomatose (Boecksches Sarkoid) an der Bindehaut. Ophthalmologica (Basel) 126 (1953) 193–208

Lehrfeld, L., C. F. Breisacher: A case of trichinosis presenting chemosis of the bulbar conjunctica. J. Amer. med. Ass. 115 (1940) 1794

Lemke, L.: Zur Differentialdiagnose der rezidivierenden Hypopyon-Iritis. Acta ophthal. 43 (1965) 487–495

Lemos, da Silva, J. L.: Die parasitäre Wirkung der Würmer im menschlichen Sehapparat. Anh. bras. Oftal. 19 (1956) 244–260; ref. in: Zbl. Ophthal. 71 (1957) 255–256

Lepri, J.: Reticuloendotheliosen bei gleichzeitiger konjunktivaler Injektion. Klin. Mbl. Augenheilk. 130 (1957) 163–175

Linnen, H. J.: Beiderseitige metastatische Ophthalmie bei einem 7 Tage alten Säugling als Fogle einer intrauterin erworbenen Entzündung? Klin. Mbl. Augenheilk. 117 (1950) 120–127

Maag, B.: Bericht über einen wurmartigen Parasiten im Glaskörper des menschlichen Auges. Klin. Mbl. Augenheilk. 133 (1958) 713–718

Manson, N.: The "string syndrome" Brit. J. Ophthal. 48 (1964) 70–74

Mattson, R.: Über glaukomatozyklitische Krisen. Acta ophthal. 32 (1954) 523–533

Merté, H. J.: Über glaukomatozyklitische Krisen. Klin. Mbl. Augenheilk. 135 (1959) 434–435

Meyer, H. J.: Dominant vererbte Pupillarpigmentzysten. Klin. Mbl. Augenheilk. 154 (1969) 158–166

Müller, H.: Tierexperimentelle Untersuchungen zur Ophthalmia phakogenetica. Albrecht v. Graefes Arch. klin. exp. Ophthal. 153 (1952) 1–35

Nicolesco, P., Strat, Iamandi: Diagnostic étiologique de la septicémie trichinosique. Kongr.-Zbl. ges. inn. Med. 94 (1938) 292

Pau, H., W. Graeber, W. Holtermann: Die fortschreitende Atrophie des Irisstromas mit Lochbildung und Proliferation des Hornhautendothels. Klin. Mbl. Augenheilk. 141 (1962) 568–582

Pfanz, W.: Über lymphatische Tumoren am Sehorgan. Klin. Mbl. Augenheilk. 131 (1957) 439–447

Posner, A., A. Schlossman: Syndrome of glaucomatocyclitic crises. Amer. J. Ophthal. 31 (1948) 735–736

Posner, A., A. Schlossman: Further observations on the syndrome of glaucomato-cyclitic crises. Trans. Amer. Acad. Ophthal. Otolaryng. 57 (1953) 531–536

Purtscher, E.: Knotenförmige Verdichtungen im Irisstroma bei Mongolismus. Albrecht v. Graefes Arch. klin. exp. Ophthal. 160 (1958/59) 200–215

Remky, H.: Zur Klinik der serologisch diagnostizierten Augentuberkulose. Klin. Mbl. Augenheilk. 133 (1958) 518–529

Rieger, H.: Beiträge zur Kenntnis seltener Mißbildungen der Iris. Albrecht v. Graefes Arch. klin. exp. Ophthal. 133 (1935) 602–635

Riegere, H.: Erbfragen in der Augenheilkunde. Albrecht v. Graefes Arch. klin. exp. Ophthal. 143 (1941) 277–299

Rodger, F. C.: Posterior degenerative lesion of onchocerciasis. Brit. J. Ophthal. 42 (1958) 21–37

Rodger, F. C.: The pathogenesis and pathology of ocular onchocericiasis. Amer. J. Ophthal. 49 (1960) 104–135, 327–337; 560–594

Rohrschneider, W.: Typische und atypische Tuberkulose der Uvea. Klin. Mbl. Augenheilk. 126 (1955) 529–534

Rones, B.: Ochronosis oculi in alkaptonuria. Amer. J. Ophthal. 49 (1960) 440–446

Saraux, H., A. Brini, P. Dhermy, J. C. Brugier: Le xantho granulome juvénile. Ann. Oculist (Paris) 200 (1967) 1036–1065

Schade, H.: Chromosomenanomalien beim Menschen. Med. Welt 1963, 48, 49, 51

Schirmer, R.: Beitrag zur Raupenhaarerkrankung der Hornhaut. Klin. Mbl. Augenheilk. 124 (1954) 202–205

Schmidt, R.: Über Augenveränderungen bei Trichinose. Klin. Mbl. Augenheilk. 110 (1944) 73–79

Schoop, G., W. A. Lieb, J. Lamina, J. Hiemich: Die Parasiten des Auges. Tierexperimentelle Untersuchungen über die Trichinose des Auges. Klin. Mbl. Augenheilk. 139 (1961) 433–465

Siegert, P.: Probleme der Ätiologie endogener Augenentzündungen. Klin. Mbl. Augenheilk. 138 (1961) 621–631

Skeller, E., J. Øster: Eye symptoms in mongolism. Acta ophthal. 29 (1951) 149–161

Slezak, H.: Zur Klinik, Pathogenese und Differentialdiagnose der peripheren Uveitis. Albrecht v. Graefes Arch. klin. exp. Ophthal. 174 (1967) 9–33

Spaeth, H.: Die Trichinose. Dtsch. Med. Wschr. 68 (1942) 912–916

Talkovskij, S. J.: Helminthosen in der Augenheilkunde. Sovet Med. 15 (1951) 17–21. Ref. Zbl. ges. Ophthalm. 58 (1952/53) 28

Thiel, R.: Sekundärglaukom nach Epithel- oder Endotheleinwanderung in die Vorderkammer. Klin. Mbl. Augenheilk. 137 (1960) 705–720

Ullerich, K.: Der Augenbefund der epitheloidzelligen Granulomatose. Albrecht v. Graefes Arch. klin. exp. Ophthal. 153 (1952) 289–311

Verbeck, B.: Augenbeteiligung bei Neurofibromatose v. Recklinghausen. Klin. Mbl. Augenheilk. 155 (1969) 751–764

Walsch, F. B.: Clinical Neuro-Ophthalmology. Williams & Wilkins, Baltimore 1957 (p. 530)

Wegner, W., K. Wurm: Der Morbus Boeck der Augen. Bücherei des Augenarztes, 27. Enke, Stuttgart 1957 (pp. 116–131)

Weve, H.: Über die durch die Nesselhaare der Goldafterraupe (Euproctis chrysorrhoea) erzeugte Augenentzündung (Ophthalmia nodosa seu pseudotuberculosa). Arch. Augenheilk. 104 (1931) 192–221

Witmer, R.: Klinik und Diagnostik der Uveitis in heutiger Sicht. Klin. Mbl. Augenheilk. 138 (1961) 609–621

Witmer, R.: Klinik der Uveitis, Labordiagnostik. Ophthalmologica (Basel) 149 (1965) 390–404

Wollensak, J.: Charakteristische Augenbefunde beim Syndroma Bloch-Sulzberger (Incontinentia pigmenti). Klin. Mbl. Augenheilk. 134 (1959) 692–706

Wolter, J. R., P. U. Fechner: Glass membranes on the anterior iris surface. Amer. J. Ophthal. 53 (1962) 235–243

Zimmerman, L. E.: Ocular lesions of juvenile xanthogranuloma. Amer. J. Ophthal. 60 (1965 a) 1011–1035

Zimmerman, L. E.: Ocular lesions of juvenile xanthogranuloma. Trans. Amer. Acad. Ophthal. Otolaryng. 69 (1965 b) 412–442

Zintz, R., W. Wegner: Über die Behandlung der tierexperimentellen und menschlichen Augentuberkulose mit Neoteben. Dtsch. med. Wschr. 1953, 433–435

17 Ciliary Body

Cyclitis

Besides the common *iridocyclitis* (see page 204) a pure cyclitis with little or no iris involvement is possible.

Cyclitis is present when filamentary or dust-like vitreous opacities and cells appear without any sign of retinitis. Usually the vitreous liquefies at the same time so that the patient becomes aware of mobile opacities. These may be seen with the ophthalmoscope. The ciliary exudates can reach the anterior chamber through the pupil. Here they may precipitate in classic fashion (Arlt's triangle) on the inferior half of the cornea. An important differential diagnostic point is that there are no posterior synechiae with cyclitic precipitates. As a consequence of cyclitis, aqueous production may decrease. This may be so severe as to cause phthisis or cataracts. The etiologies of cyclitis are those already discussed for iridocyclitis. Primary considerations include localized involvement with tuberculosis, syphilis, leptospirosis, sarcoidosis, sympathetic ophthalmia, focal infection, etc. Similar to chorioretinitis, cyclitis may cause a segmental, reversible retinal vasculitis.

Peripheral Uveitis

Chronic inflammation of the ciliary body leads to *peripheral uveitis*. This is usually bilateral with vitreous membranes forming at the pars plana and ora serrata. The peripheral opacities are seen on direct ophthalmoscopy using scleral depression. A serous, infiltrative and exudative form can be differentiated. Precipitates may appear in the chamber angle and on the posterior cornea.

Anterior choroiditis also causes dust-like vitreous opacities; a peripheral chorioretinal lesion is seen at the same time.

The *differential diagnosis* (Slezak 1967) includes *Leber's retinal degeneration* with multiple ciliary aneurysms in the retinal periphery (see page 257). These may form pockets of opaque circumscribed retinal detachments in the far periphery. These are multiple, round aneurysms of retinal arterioles. *Hereditary hyaloideo-retinal degeneration* (Wagner) is associated with white preretinal membranes at the equator which have multiple perforations. These membranes do not extend to the ora serrata. Otherwise the vitreous remains clear. *Peripheral vitreoretinal adhesions* and adhesions parallel to the ora are free of inflammation.

Glaucomatocyclitic Crisis: The Posner-Schlossman Syndrome

This involves attacks of open angle glaucoma in an eye with mild cyclitis and fine corneal precipitates but free from irritation (Mattson 1954; Merté 1959) (see page 228).

References

Mattson, R.: Über glaukomatozyklitische Krisen. Acta ophthal. 32 (1954) 523–533

Merté, H. J.: Über glaukomatozyklitische Krisen. Klin. Mbl. Augenheilk. 135, (1959) 434–435

Slezak, H.: Zur Klinik, Pathogenese und Differentialdiagnose der peripheren Uveitis. Albrecht v. Graefes Arch. klin. exp. Ophthal. 174 (1967) 9–33

18 Choroid

Choroidal Coloboma

Choroidal colobomata result from incomplete development of the eye. These lie inferior nasally, corresponding to the embryonic fissure (typical choroidal coloboma) (Fig. 18.1). Atypical colobomata appear in any position. Choroidal colobomata appear as white areolas with pigmented borders. They may extend to the optic nerve and can be divided (bridge coloboma) by normal choroid. The inferior conus of the optic disc is sometimes a rudimentary choroidal coloboma. Iris colobomata may also be present. Besides a hereditary etiology they may be associated with mandibulo-ocular (see page 332) or mandibulo-facial dysostosis (see page 331) and multiple congenital defects (embryopathy). Toxoplasma scars (see page 283) may simulate a coloboma (especially macular coloboma).

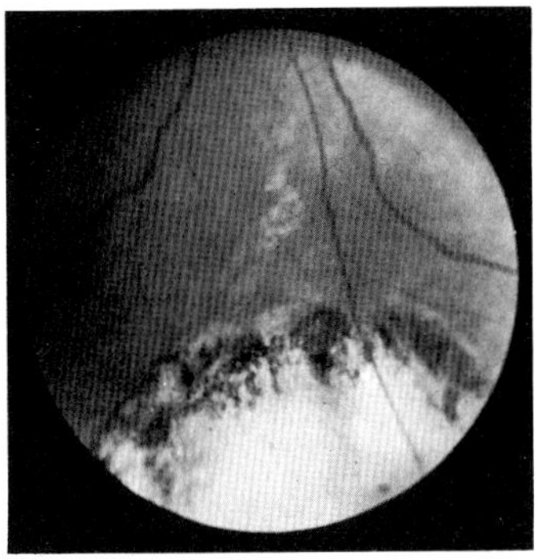

Fig. 18.1 Large inferior choroidal coloboma

Alterations in Pigment Content

Increased Pigmentation

Pigmented races, pigmented nevi, melanoma — Choroiditis, contusion injury, hemorrhage — Peripheral "paving-stone" degeneration — Light diathermy, cryo-effects — Angioid streaks.

Pigmented Races

Pigmented nevi must be observed for possible malignant melanoma (see page 220) (especially when there is otherwise a paucity of pigment in the retinal pigment epithelium). Malignant melanomas eventually become diffuse, prominent and lead to secondary retinal detachment. Pigmentation (and depigmentation) occurs following any choroiditis (diffuse, disseminated, juxtapapillary), contusion injury, or even hemorrhage. Peripheral *"paving-stone"* degeneration is common in myopes and usually consists of depigmented patches with a pigmented border. They may, however, be pigmented.

Macular burns (see page 354) following observation of a solar eclipse, *atom bomb blasts*, or *photocoagulation* cause pigmented chorioretinal scars. *Diathermy* and *cryotherapy* produce similar (usually peripheral) lesions.

Angioid streaks (Knapp) (see page 219) are increasingly pigmented bands. These form circumferentially around the papilla or radiate from it (Plate XV, Figs. 1, 2, see page 192 g). Late macular hemorrhage and scarring occurs.

Decreased Pigmentation

Excessive myopia — Albinism — Drusen — Choroidal rupture — Choroiditis and chorioretinitis — Choroidal sclerosis — Senile macular degeneration — Essential progressive choroidal atrophy.

Excessive myopia: Fundus findings in high myopia (see page 25) are caused by stretching of tissues (Plate XXI, Fig. 5, page 224 e). Thinning of the pigment epithelium results in a pale fundus. Choroidal vessels are visible and sclera can be seen in vessel-free areas. Atrophy or absence of the choroid produces a white ring or crescent-shaped conus around the optic disc. White or yellowish, sharply delineated cracks (lacquer cracks) of varying width in Bruch's membrane (lamina elastica) result from stretching. The white sclera and red choroidal vessels are easily visible and cause vision loss, even central scotomata. Small round macular hemorrhages beneath the pigment epithelium appear suddenly, especially in older patients with high myopia. These develop a black pigmentation (Fuchs' spot) (Plate XXII, Fig. 1, page 224 f). Posterior staphylomas, a localized scleral ectasia at the posterior pole, are common.

The myopic crescent is part of high myopia. It is white when only sclera remains and mottled when only the pigment epithelium is missing over thinned choroid. Because of the posterior distention of the globe, the optic nerve enters at an oblique angle causing the optic nerve head to appear more oval. The oblique insertion of the nerve causes a supervolution of the retina at the disc, i.e., the choroid stops at the disc but the retina overlaps it before the nerve fibers bend backwards to enter the optic nerve. The retinal vessels appear stretched. Sclerotic areas of retinal degeneration appear in the retinal periphery. These lead to retinal tears with detachment.

"Paving-stone degeneration" consisting of areas of depigmentation (and hyperpigmentation) occur between the equator and ora serrata. Here there is localized atrophy of the choroid so that underlying sclera is directly visible. High myopes develop liquefaction of the vitreous early in life.

Albinism: With albinism there is a lack of pigment in the fundus (Plate XXI, Fig. 3, page 224 e). The foveola is usually aplastic, resulting in amblyopia and nystagmus (see page 64).

Drusen appear in the fundus as small, gray-yellow to yellow, sharply delineated lesions often with a small ring of pigment around them. Drusen are excrescences of hyaline material on Bruch's membrane formed by the pigment epithelium. They are an abiotrophy appearing near the equator in older persons. They can, however, occur at any location, often in combination with *senile pigment dispersion* and *deposition*. Tay's guttate choroiditis consists of large drusen in the macular and paramacular region. Doyne's honeycomb choroiditis gives a similar picture. It is not clear whether these are a form of central tapetoretinal degeneration or, more likely, giant central drusen of a familial nature. Senile drusen do not cause vision loss, scarring, or become confluent.

Choroidal rupture: Choroidal rupture with severe trauma exposes crescents of white sclera (Plate XV, Figs. 3, 4, page 192 g) situated concentrically around the papilla. When the rupture is recent, hemorrhages which are absorbed after two to three weeks are seen at the site of the choroidal rupture (Plate XV, Fig. 3, page 192 g).

Choroiditis, chorioretinitis: Every chorioretinitis results in scarring with varying degrees of pigmentation and depigmentation (Plate XV, Fig. 6, page 192 g; Plate XVI, Fig. 1, page 192 g).

Sclerosis of choroidal vessels causes atrophy of the overlying pigment epithelium with circumscribed or diffuse pigment dispersion. The space between choroidal vessels may be hyperpigmented (fundus tabulatus). The choroidal vessels become increasingly gray-white-yellow with a narrow blood column. When totally obliterated they appear as white strands. These changes may be diffuse or localized, often sectorially, to the retinal center or periphery (Fig. 22.25). The affliction is usually bilateral and symmetric; rarely is it unilateral. Premature choroidal sclerosis is seen with tapetoretinal degeneration (see page 286) and progressive choroidal atrophy (see page 219, 288), Generalized choroidal sclerosis also occurs (Sorsby and Davey 1955).

The nonhemorrhagic or "dry" form of senile macular degeneration (chorioretinopathy) begins as a central pigmentary disturbance. This may evolve into a "wet" or hemorrhagic disciform degeneration (Kuhnt-Junius) with central hemorrhages, exudates and connective tissue scarring (see page 281, Fig. 22.26).

Round depigmented chorioretinal lesions preferentially located near the optic disc are seen in **Aicardi's syndrome.** The optic nerve head may be colobomatous and the eye microphthalmic (Tillmann and v. Bermuth, Fig. 18.2). Aicardi's syndrome also includes agenesis of the corpus callosum, infantile spasms, severe mental retardation and EEG anomalies. Vertebral and rib anomalies may be present. Cases reported so far have been limited to females.

Essential progressive choroidal atrophy: Progressive depigmentation and choroidal atrophy occurs in choroideremia (Plate XXVII, Fig. 5, page 288 c), central progessive choroidal atrophy (Fig. 22.25) and gyrate atrophy of the choroid and retina (see page 288).

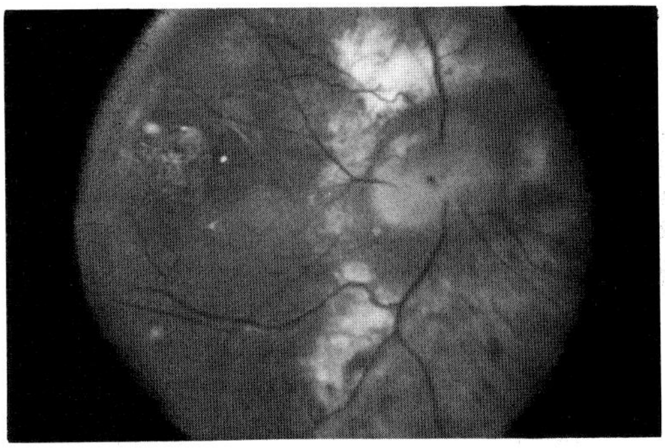

Fig. 18.2 Aicardi's syndrome: Coloboma of the optic nerve and macula with round confluent depigmented peripapillary retinal and choroidal lesions (♀ 6 yrs.)

Choroiditis (Posterior Uveitis)

Subjective complaints with choroiditis — Disseminated chorioretinitis — Juxtapapillary chorioretinitis of Jensen — Diffuse chorioretinitis — Central serous chorioretinitis — Presumed histoplasmic chorioretinitis — Toxoplasmosis — Chorioretinitis and exudative detachment — Subretinal striae — Sympathetic ophthalmia — Fungal infections — Onchocerciasis — Secondary anatomical changes with uveitis — Establishing the diagnosis.

Subjective symptoms with choroiditis: vision loss with central lesions, photopsias (seeing sparks), flimmering vision with central or paracentral inflammation that is fresh, dark spots (positive scotomata) which disappear later and become negative scotomata. When the process occurs centrally metamorphopsia and micropsia may be reported. Color vision may be variably affected, usually with a blue-yellow or, more rarely, red-green disturbance.

Disseminated chorioretinitis: There are yellow-gray edematous lesions with blurred margins (Plate XV, Fig. 5, page 192 g). They may be $\frac{1}{2}$–$1\frac{1}{2}$ disc diameter in size becoming smaller and more sharply delineated as they heal. Scarring occurs after three weeks, leaving white depigmented (sclera), or red (thinned choroidal vessels), or bizarre black-brown pigmented lesions (Plate XV, Fig. 6, page 192 g). The inflammation may recur intermittently or fresh lesions appear at the border of the old scars so that ultimately the entire fundus has map-like scarring. Etiologically, the primary choices are focal involvement such as syphilis, tuberculosis and sarcoidosis.

Tuberculosis. Pulmonary and extrapulmonary tuberculosis rarely involves the eye. Miliary tuberculosis and tuberculous meningitis, however, develop small, gray-white, blurred retinal and choroidal lesions scattered throughout the fundus.
Such lesions were seen in 80 percent of miliary tuberculosis and 41 percent of tuberculous meningitis owing to a primary intracranial lesion (Custodis and Heinemann 1949; Heinemann 1949).
Optic disc changes (Cramer 1952: 73 percent), such as papilledema, papillitis and post inflammatory optic atrophy are described in miliary tuberculosis (Böke 1955; Blagojevic and Arambrasic 1956) (see page 309).
Sarcoidosis can cause disseminated lesions or slightly prominent exudates (see page 201).

Juxtapapillary chorioretinitis of Jensen: In fresh juxtapapillary chorioretinitis (Jensen) (see page 294), also known as neurofibrillitis retinae (van der Hoeve), a gray 1 to 2 disc diameter size lesion, called choroiditis ad papillam (Schreck), occurs near the optic disc. After $1\frac{1}{2}$ to 4 months, this turns into a black-white-red scar (Plate XVI, Fig. 1, page 192 h). Recurrence near the old lesion is common. Vitreous exudates and corneal precipitates occur. Rarely, branch artery occlusion, emboli and periphlebitis develop. Peak incidence of involvement is around age thirty. Typically, permanent, arcuate scotomata develop owing to

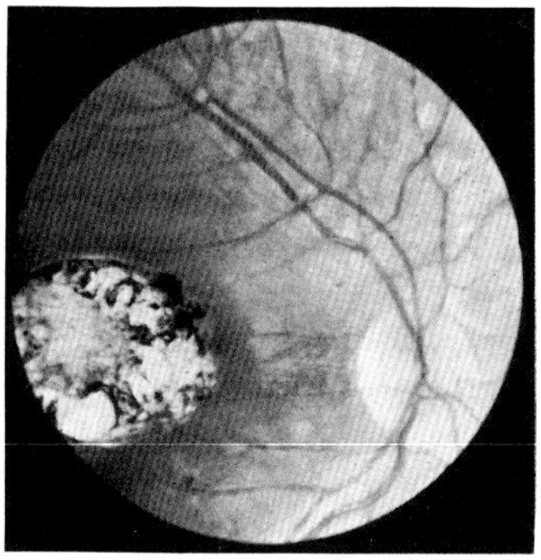

Fig. 18.3 Macular scar in congenital toxoplasmosis (♀ 9 yrs.)

involvement of nerve fiber bundles (Fig. 3.12). The lesions may appear elsewhere in the fundus. Originally these were incorrectly thought to represent solitary tubercles. Involvement prior to age 10 (2.3 percent) is more rare than between ages 10 and 20 (20.4 percent) (Waubke 1959).

Diffuse chorioretinitis (neuroretinal-choroiditis) (see page 293) causes a diffuse gray discoloration of the retina, often with neuritis and marked vitreous clouding. Scarring occurs after a few weeks and results in a "pepper and salt" fundus (Plate XXVIII, Fig. 4, page 288 d). Diffuse chorioretinitis is similar to anterior choroiditis in that they both have peripheral pigment clumping. The etiology can be congenital or acquired syphilis, focal inflammation, tuberculosis or a general virus infection (measles, rubella, mumps, vaccination etc.).

Central serous chorioretinitis (see page 283) shows all transitional forms to *central serous retinopathy* (Plate XXVI, Fig. 5, page 288 b) with detachment of the retinal pigment epithelium. By history, central serous chorioretinitis begins with a positive central scotoma appreciated as a gray, round or oval central spot. Hypermetropia owing to elevation of the retina develops along with metamorphopsia and micropsia. Accommodation may also be disturbed. There is a round to oval central subretinal exudate $\frac{1}{2}$–2 disc diameters in size. Within this area a small "leak" is seen on fluorescein angiography (Fig. 22.28). Small, white-yellow precipitates may be seen in the subretinal space. Middle-aged men are affected most often. One-fourth of the cases recur.

Presumed histoplasmic chorioretinitis

Central and juxtapapillary subpigment epithelial neovascularization and hemorrhages leading to scarring and severe vision loss in young people are presumed to be caused by histoplasmosis. In Europe, if there is no evidence of histoplasmosis, the entity is known as central hemorrhagic chorioretinitis (Plate XXVI, Fig. 6, page 288 b) (Rieger 1951; Pau 1968), or focal hemorrhagic chorioiditis (Schildberg and Wessing 1975), or presumed ocular histoplasmosis (Schlaegel 1975).

Toxoplasmosis

Toxoplasmic chorioretinitis — Postnatal chorioretinitis — Diagnosis of toxoplasmosis — Differential diagnosis.

Toxoplasmic chorioretinal scars (see retina, Fig. 22.27) are sharp, "punched out" lesions. By birth the intrauterine central chorioretinitis has usually healed. This was first shown to be caused by toxoplasmosis by Janku (1923) and is seen with congenital toxoplasmosis in 75 percent of cases. Usually there is a round to horizontal oval central gray-white scar exposing the sclera. It is 1 to 3 disc diameters in size and surrounded by black pigment clumps (Fig. 18.3). These macular scars were formerly thought to be macular colobomata (Hogan 1958; Rougier and Garin 1955; Perkins 1973; Ryan and Smith 1974).

In addition to the central chorioretinal scar, other ocular findings in congenital toxoplasmosis include evidence of intrauterine iridocyclitis (François 1954: 17 percent), and at times iris bombé or phthisis bulbi. Such a congenital uveitis may flare up later causing acute or chronic inflammation (Straub 1955).

The picture of *postnatally acquired toxoplasmosis* is relatively uncharacteristic and may include fever, maculopapular exanthem, pneumonia, hepatosplenomegaly, lymphadenopathy, intestinal disorders, encephalitis and nonspecific chorioretinitis (Wahle 1958). Fresh toxoplasmosis causes gray, blurred retinal lesions with vitreous haze. After several weeks a heavily pigmented scar remains. The Sabin-Feldman dye titer, skin reaction and complement fixation are strongly positive.

Diagnosis of toxoplasmosis: The most reliable diagnostic test for ocular toxoplasmosis is a comparison of aqueous and serum dye test titers on the basis of gamma globulin distribution between the two body fluids (Remky 1968).

The protozoa are transmitted transplacentally during pregnancy, causing a variety of fetal damage including microphthalmos, cataracts and strabismus as well as hydrocephaly, neurologic changes, intracranial calcifications (especially of the choroidal plexus), electroencephalographic alterations, psychomotor retardation and alterations in the cerebrospinal fluid (François 1954).

Aside from toxoplasmosis, the *differential diagnosis* of strongly pigmented/depigmented chorioretinal scars includes *histoplasmosis* (see page 283). Asbury (1966) found choroidal scars after toxoplasmosis in 3.2 percent and with histoplasmosis in 1.6 percent of patients.

Chorioretinal scars also occur with *Toxocara canis* (see page 283), tuberculosis, syphilis and fungal infections. Colobomata, even atypical ones, are more uniform in location and appearance and readily diagnosed when associated with a family history, iris or lens involvement.

Choroiditis and exudative retinal detachment: *Choroiditis*, for example Harada's disease (see pages 198, 277), may cause an *exudative retinal detachment*.

Subretinal striae: *Subretinal striae* are variously pigmented gray-white nodules or connective tissue strands between the choroid and retina. These changes appear after reattachment of a long-standing retinal detachment of a primary, secondary or inflammatory nature.

Sympathetic ophthalmia (see page 360): The danger of sympathetic ophthalmia exists when a chronic, insidious, uveal inflammation, especially iridocyclitis, occurs after accidental or surgical perforation of the globe. Acute endophthalmitis does not cause sympathetic ophthalmia. Sympathetic ophthalmia usually appears 4 to 8 weeks after the perforating injury. It may, however, occur as early as ten days or be delayed for many years.

The clinical picture is that of an insidious iridocyclitis also involving the uninjured (sympathizing) eye. The range of accommodation and dark adaptation are reduced. This is followed by a progressive plastic iritis with increased aqueous protein, corneal precipitates, posterior synechiae and inflammatory vitreous exudate. Small, multiple, yellow choroidal nodules with blurred margins appear, especially peripherally. Secondary glaucoma develops because of the posterior synchiae and pupillary occlusion. Cataracts are also present. In the final stages there is phthisis and blindness, often of both eyes.

Histologically there is a dense lymphocytic infiltration of the uvea (iris, ciliary body and choroid), along with epithelioid and giant cells. According to Redslob (1956), 43 percent of children with sympathetic ophthalmia before the age of fifteen required enucleation. The pathogenesis of sympathetic ophthalmia is still unclear. Possibly unknown agents (viral?) spread from one eye to the other. Whether the mode of spread is along the optic nerves, hematogenous, or lymphatics is as unknown as the causal agent or toxins which selectively affect the uvea. The most popular current thought is that sympathetic ophthalmia is an autoimmune process. Other theories include an allergic or anaphylactic reaction.

Rare Causes of *Posterior (and Anterior) Uveitis*

Fungi (blastomycosis, histoplasmosis, coccidiomycosis, sporotrichosis, candida) occur primarily after perforating injuries but may be endogenous, probably hematogenous (Nover 1950; Heinsius 1950).

Onchocercosis (see page 199) primarily causes chorioretinitis with secondary glaucoma and cataracts. Nummular keratitis may develop (Neumann and Gunders 1963).

Secondary anatomic changes with uveitis: Eyes enucleated because of chronic *uveitis* persisting for years may have giant drusen, calcification and ossification of the uvea.

Establishing the diagnosis (see page 204): In uveitis, examination for infectious foci, serologic reactions (with the exception of syphilis), blood cultures for bacteria or fungi, serum electrophoresis, and cutaneous sensitivity testing are usually uninformative.

Choroidal Detachment, Spongiosis Choroideae

Choroidal detachments have to be differentiated into those with a flat and those with a maintained anterior chamber (Pau 1957). With the exception of spontaneous detachments, hypotony is almost always present. The choroid has a forward bulge, especially temporally and nasally in the vicinity of vortex veins but less so above and below (Plate XVI, Fig. 2, page 192 h). The detachment may reach forward to the lens. It has practically no folds and is immobile. Choroidal detachments are slate gray and transilluminate. Pigmented demarcation lines appear when the detachment is of long duration.

Choroidal detachment with loss of the anterior chamber — Choroidal detachment with a deep anterior chamber — Spontaneous serous anterior choroidal detachment — Differential diagnosis of choroidal detachment.

With loss of the anterior chamber: Choroidal detachment with loss of the anterior chamber usually occurs after damage to the anterior segment of the globe (cataract surgery, iridencleisis, perforating keratoplasty, injury or uveal ulcer, trephination, etc.). The detachment usually appears a few days after surgery and resolves over two to three weeks. Very rarely, it persists for months or years, even causing vision loss. Postoperative choroidal detachment is particularly common when there is a persistent fistula, but often appears without one. A similar picture occurs with a partial expulsive hemorrhage.

With a deep anterior chamber: In choroidal detachment with a deep anterior chamber the iris is bent backwards like a bayonet. The aqueous has a gray-yellow discoloration with markedly increased protein content, but few cells. Damage to the posterior pole (retinal detachment, injury, hemorrhage) is the usual etiology.

Harada's disease and sympathetic ophthalmia may have choroidal detachment along with the inflammatory retinal detachment (see page 198). Traction from organizing inflammatory tissue may cause choroidal detachment in phthisical eyes.

Spontaneous serous anterior choroidal detachment: Spontaneous serous detachment of the anterior choroid occurs. This has the appearance of a ring-shaped tumor. Recurrent *exudative ciliary body and choroidal detachment* was called *cyclitis anularis exsudativa pseudotumorosa* by Schreck (Gamringer et al. 1959; Wollensak 1962).

Differential diagnosis of melanoma or choroidal detachment: With choroidal detachment there is hypotony and the mass transilluminates. Ultrasound readily differentiates between choroidal detachment and tumors (Oksala 1958).

Expulsive Hemorrhage

Expulsive hemorrhage occurs when the globe is opened surgically (cataract, glaucoma surgery, perforating injuries). Severe pain and vomiting occur. Expulsive hemorrhage is more common in older patients (hypotony, arteriosclerosis, diabetes, lues, glaucoma, myopia, old uveal inflammation or injuries). The brittle, arteriosclerotic choroidal or ciliary arteries rupture and the subsequent hematoma pushes choroid-retina, vitreous, lens, and iris out of the eye. The expulsive hemorrhage occurs at the time of surgery in one-third of all patients, three to six hours later in one-third and between seven hours and nine days in the final third of cases (Pau 1958).

Hereditary Progressive Choroidal Atrophy

(Krill 1972, Franceschetti et al. 1974)

Essential progressive choroidal atrophy — Choroideremia — Central progressive choroidal atrophy — Gyrate atrophy of the choroid and retina — Angioid streaks.

Essential progressive choroidal atrophy: This includes choroideremia, gyrate atrophy and central progressive choroidal atrophy. These are forms of tapetoretinal degeneration (see page 288).

Choroideremia (Plate XXVII, Fig. 5, page 288 c) is a hereditary (sex-linked recessive) bilateral, choroidal and retinal degeneration (tapetoretinal, see page 288). Night blindness and visual field constriction develop in childhood in affected males. White (sclera) lesions with red choroidal vessels are found in the mid-periphery. The atrophy progresses both centrally and towards the periphery. A central, normal red island is maintained the longest. Correspondingly, central vision remains intact. The optic disc becomes atrophic and retinal vessels narrow. The electroretinogram (ERG) b-wave disappears. Choroideremia is a progressive atrophy of the choriocapillaris and outer retinal layers (Sorsby et al. 1952; Pameyer et al. 1960).

Central progressive choroidal atrophy begins peripapillary and in the macula. It spreads to the periphery. Choroidal vessels are often sclerosed in the atrophic area. The disease may begin in childhood or old age. Retinal (tapetoretinal) degeneration is common (see page 288). The *differential diagnosis* includes: bilateral progressive macular degeneration, myopic degeneration, arteriosclerotic and senile atrophy, and inflammatory scarring. These conditions are rarely as bilaterally symmetric in their progression or degree of atrophy as those with exposure of white, underlying sclera. Inverse retinitis pigmentosa should be considered.

With *gyrate atrophy of the choroid and retina* there is a progressive circumscribed choroidal degeneration. Heredity may be dominant or recessive. Hemeralopia with visual field loss begins in childhood. The atrophy originates in the mid-periphery as islands or sectorial lesions (Fig. 18.4) with sharp borders. The atrophic patches progressively enlarge and become confluent. Choroid and pigment epithelium disappear. At times, choroidal vessels in the white (sclera) atrophic patches are sclerosed. The normal areas slowly diminish. Net-like or arborizing pigment flecks appear in the atrophic areas. Optic disc and retinal vessels may be normal or, as in tapetoretinal degeneration, there may be waxy pallor of the disc with narrowed retinal vessels (see page 288). High myopia is common. Cataracts develop with time.

Angioid streaks (Knapp, see page 282; Plate XV, Figs. 1, 2, page 192 g) occur in pseudoxanthoma elasticum (Grönblad-Strandberg syndrome), rarely in the Ehlers-Danlos syndrome, Paget's disease, sickle cell anemia, hypertensive cardiovascular disorders and senile elastosis of the skin. Angioid streaks appear as red stripes around the optic disc or radiating out from it. The lesions are in Bruch's membrane (Domke and Tost 1964) and may take on a gray-brown pigmentation. In the macular region, hemorrhages and connective tissue scars very similar to senile macular degeneration (disciform macular degeneration) develop. Systemic involvement in pseudoxanthoma elasticum includes skin changes (pseudoxanthoma elasticum Darier), hemorrhages, arterial calcification and aneurysm formation. Heredity is recessive but may be dominant.

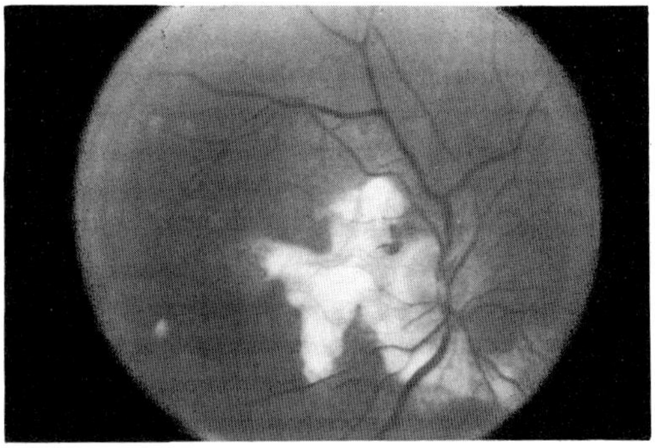

Fig. 18.4 Gyrate atrophy (♂ 51 yrs.)

Differential diagnosis: Pigmented demarcation lines from choroidal detachment are peripheral and parallel to the ora. Connective tissue bands in old unoperated retinal detachments are white-yellow with areas of heavy pigmentation. Patchy areas of pigmented lines can appear following irradiation of a metastatic carcinoma. Choroidal ruptures and tapetoretinal degeneration should present no diagnostic problem.

Choroiditis striata (Kraffel 1955), peripapillary helicoid chorioretinitis (Franceschetti 1962), geographic choroidopathy (Hamilton and Bird 1974) is a progressive bilateral peripapillary chorioretinal atrophy (Fig. 18.4) extending spokelike towards the periphery. The disease is nonhereditary, arises in middle age and is caused by progressive degenerative alterations of choroidal vessels.

Tumors and Pseudotumors

Choroidal angioma — Choroidal melanoma — Carcinomas metastatic to the choroid — Pseudotumors of the choroid — Differential diagnosis of choroidal tumors.

Choroidal angiomas: Choroidal *angiomas* appear as prominent gray-white, tan, green or irregularly pigmented juxtapapillary lesions (Plate XXVIII, Fig. 6, page 288 d) (Chisholm and Blach 1973). Patients may have similar vascular tumors on the face. The *differential diagnosis* from choroidal melanoma may be very difficult. The diagnosis can rarely be made with certainty, even with fluorescein angiography (see below). Both lesions grow slowly with overlying serous retinal detachment.

Choroidal angiomas in the Sturge-Weber syndrome (see page 226) may be associated with congenital glaucoma and buphthalmos.

Choroidal melanomas (melanoblastoma, melanosarcoma) appear mainly in patients over fifty years of age. They are slate-gray, isolated, nodular tumors elevating the overlying retina or ciliary body (Plate XVI, Fig. 3, page 192 h). The overlying retina is frequently detached. Eventually secondary glaucoma develops. Central areas of the tumor may become necrotic and calcify. Hemorrhage, inflammation with hyphema, hypopyon and vitreous clouding occur. In 50 percent of cases, patients die from metastases. The choroid is a more common site of intraocular melanoma than the iris or ciliary body (Thiel et al. 1961: 88 percent to 5 percent to 7 percent).

On occasion a choroidal melanoma may be metastatic from elsewhere (skin, conjunctiva, breast, ovary, etc.). The question always remains: Which is the true source?

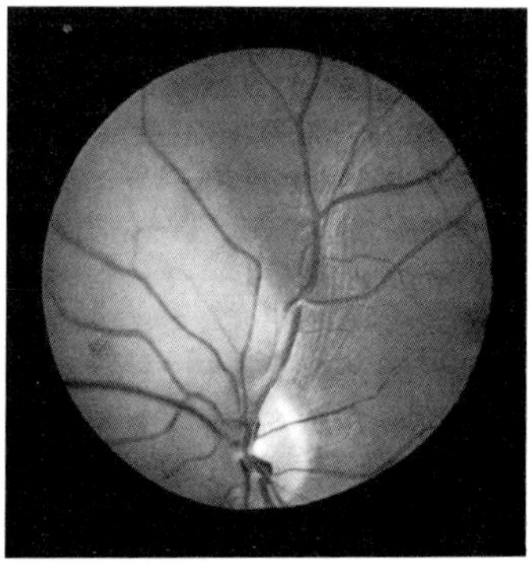

Fig. 18.5 Choroidal metastases in a patient operated for carcinoma of the breast 2½ years earlier. Gray-yellow, dense lesion elevating the retina below and nasal to the optic disc (♀ 42 yrs.)

Metastatic choroidal carcinomas are slightly prominent, diffuse gray to yellow lesions similar to acute choroiditis (Plate XVI, Fig. 4, page 192 h). The lesions become confluent and grow rapidly. Generally there is a detachment of the overlying retina through which the prominent underlying tumor may or may not be visible. After irradiation, and at times without, the retina develops a cystic, mottled, gray, motheaten appearance. The primary tumor is a mammary carcinoma in 60 to 70 percent of cases followed by bronchial, gastric, colonic, renal, adrenal, thyroid, thymus, hepatic, pancreas, prostate, gonadal, and uterine tumors and chorioepithelioma. The latent period between appearance of the primary tumor and ocular metastasis is usually about six months but may be ten years or longer (Fig. 18.5).

Pseudotumor: With any tumefaction consideration must be given to inflammatory granulomas (syphilis, tuberculosis, sarcoidosis, foreign bodies, leukemia). Hemorrhagic proliferating retinopathy may simulate a tumor. Disciform macular degeneration (Kuhnt-Junius) includes hemorrhages and scar tissue, and pseudotumor formation. The lesions tend to be bilateral but are often asymmetric in appearance.

Differential diagnosis: In differentiating between choroidal detachment and choroidal melanoma it is important that with choroidal detachment hypotony is marked. The melanoma fails to transilluminate while a choroidal detachment transilluminates well. On transillumination a tumor appears as a dark area in the bright red glow of the surrounding posterior pole. Large subretinal hemorrhages can cast a similar shadow. Transillumination is normal with retinal detachment, subretinal fluid, choroidal detachment, pigment epithelial and ciliary body cysts, Coats' disease and serous retinal detachment. Infrared photography aids in the recognition of melanin-containing tumors.

Melanin-containing tumors are easily recognized by means of infrared photography.

Hemorrhages, especially beneath the pigment epithelium, reabsorb within weeks, often leaving a gray or darkly pigmented area behind.

Owing to their increased metabolic rate only malignant neoplasms concentrate radioactive material (P^{32}) to a greater extent than normal tissue. Using a Geiger-Müller counter, comparison of beta-ray emission is made between normal and involved portions of the eye. Properly performed (transscleral approach, probe placement, fresh P^{32}, etc.), the test is of a certain value (Lommatzsch and Guntermann 1967; Meyerratken 1963; Vogel and Strötges 1971). The concentration of tetracycline by melanomas and its visibility by fluorescence (Barkhoff 1968) is not yet a practical test.

Ultrasound can differentiate a solid tumor from subretinal fluid (Coleman 1972). Fluorescein angiography differentiates choroidal lesions: choroidal hemangiomas show diffuse spongelike staining in the early arterial phase. Choroidal nevi have fine fluorescing points. Malignant melanomas characteristically show fine granular spots made up of bright fluorescent points near the border. Metastatic tumors tend to have diffuse late staining. Subretinal hemorrhages block choroidal fluorescence and appear as dark shadows (Tenner and Honegger 1972).

References

Aicardi, J., J. Lefebre, A. Lerique: Spasm in flexion, callosal agenesis, ocular abnormalities: a new syndrome. Electroenceph. clin. Neurophys. 19 (1969) 609

Asbury, T.: The status of presumed ocular histoplasmosis: Including a report of a survey. Amer. Trans. ophthal. Soc. 64 (1966) 371–400

Barkhoff, E. R.: Diagnostik intraocularer Tumoren mittels Tetrazyklin-Fluorescenz. Klin. Mbl. Augenheilk. 153 (1968) 80–84

Blagojević, M., M. Arambrašić: Les affections des nerfs optiques dans les méningites tuberculeuses. Bull. Soc. Ophtal. Fr. 69 (1956) 315–327

Böke, W.: Neuritische Sehnervenveränderungen bei der Meningitis tuberculosa. Klin. Mbl. Augenheilk. 126 (1955) 678–684

Chisholm, I. H., R. K. Blach: Choroidal haemangioma, a diagnostic and therapeutic problem. Trans. Ophthal. Soc. UK 93 (1973) 161–169

Coleman, D. J.: Reliability of ocular and orbital diagnosis with B-Scan ultrasound. Am. J. Ophthalm. 73 (1972) 501–516

Cramer, F. E. K.: El examen del fondo del ojo como elemento de inicio diagnostico, pronostico en la meningitis tuberculosa. Arch. argent. Pediat. 38 (1952) 107–116

Custodis, E., K. Heinemann: Durch Streptomycin ermöglichte, länger dauernde Beobachtungen von Fundusveränderungen bei Meningitis-Tuberkulose und Miliar-Tuberkulose. Klin. Mbl. Augenheilk. 114 (1949) 356–363

Domke, H., M. Tost: Zur Histologie der Angioid streaks. Klin. Mbl. Augenheilk. 145 (1964) 18–29

Franceschetti, A.: A curious affection of the fundus oculi. Helicoid peripapillar chorioretinal degeneration. Docum. ophthal. 16 (1962) 81–110

Franceschetti, A., J. François, J. Babel: Chorioretinal heredodegenerationes. Charles C. Thomas, Springfield, Ill. 1974

François, J.: Toxoplasmose oculaire. Bull. Acad. roy Méd. Belg. Sér. 6, 19 (1954) 84–108

Gamringer, H., E. Schreck, J. Wollensak: Zur Pathogenese und Therapie der Cyclitis anularis exsudativa pseudotumorosa. Klin. Mbl. Augenheilk. 135 (1959) 638–646

Hamilton, A., A. Bird: Geographical chorioidopathy. Brit. J. Ophthal. 58 (1974) 784

Heinemann, K.: Augenhintergrundveränderungen bei Tbc-Meningitis unter Streptomycinbehandlung. Klin. Mbl. Augenheilk. 115 (1949) 171

Heinsius, E.: Metastatische Ophthalmie durch Blastomyzeten. Klin. Mbl. Augenheilk. 117 (1950) 136–141

Hogan, M. J.: Ocular toxoplasmosis. Trans. Amer. Acad. Ophthal. Otolaryng. 62 (1958) 7–37

Janku, J.: Pathogenese und pathologische Anatomie eines sogenannten angeborenen Maculakoloboms in einem normal großen Auge und in einem Mikrophthalmus mit Parasiten in beiden Netzhäuten. Cas. Lék. ces. 62, No. 39, 1021–1027; No. 40, 1054–1059; No. 41,1081–1085; No. 42, 1111–1115; No. 43, 1138–1144, 1923

Kalina, R. E.: Facial angiomatosis with angioid streaks. Am. Arch. Ophthalm. 84 (1970) 528

Kraffel, G.: Beitrag zur Chorioiditis striata. Klin. Mbl. Augenheilk. 127 (1955) 664–669

Krill, A. E.: Hereditary retinal and chorioidal diseases. Harper and Row, Hagerstown, Maryland, New York, Evanston, London 1972

Lommatzsch, P., S. Guntermann: Welche diagnostische Sicherheit bietet der Radiophosphortest bei Verdacht auf Aderhautmelanoblastom. Klin. Mbl. Augenheilk. 151 (1967) 514–518

Meyerratken, E.: Über die Brauchbarkeit des Radiophosphortests bei der Diagnose intraocularer Tumoren. Klin. Mbl. Augenheilk. 142 (1963) 874–892

Müller, F.: Toxoplasmose unter besonderer Berücksichtigung der Augenerkrankungen. Marholt, Halle 1954

Neumann, E., A. E. Gunders: Ocular lesions of onchocerciasis in Liberia. Amer. J. Ophthal. 56 (1963) 573–588

Nover, A.: Beiderseitige metastatische Ophthalmie durch Pilzembolien. Klin. Mbl. Augenheilk. 117 (1950) 127–135

Oksala, A.: Observations on chorioidal detachment by means of ultrasound. Acta ophthal. 36 (1958) 651–657

Pameyer, J. K., P. J. Waardenburg, H. E. Henkes: Choroideremia. Brit. J. Ophthal. 44 (1960) 724–738

Pau, H.: Über die Amotio chorioideae (Spongiosis chorioideae). Klin. Mbl. Augenheilk. 130 (1957) 347–371

Pau, H.: Chorioretinitis exsudativa centralis (haemorrhagica). Klin. Mbl. Augenheilk. 152 (1968) 348–357

Pau, H.: Der Zeitfaktor bei der expulsiven Blutung. Klin. Mbl. Augenheilk. 132 (1958) 865

Perkins, E. S.: Ocular toxoplasmosis. Brit. J. Ophthal. 57 (1973) 1–17

Redslob, E.: A la recherche de la pathogénie de l'ophthalmie sympathique. Ann. Oculist. (Paris) 189 (1956) 53–64

Remky, H.: Toxoplasmosis. Argumenta et documenta ophthalmologica. Lehmanns, München 1962

Remky, H.: Vergleichende Untersuchungen von Kammerwasser und Serum mittels des Dye-Tests. Klin. Mbl. Augenheilk. 153 (1968) 617–623

Rieger, H.: Zur Klinik der im Erwachsenenalter erworbenen Toxoplasmose. Klin. Mbl. Augenheilk. 119 (1951) 459–476

Rougier, J., J. P. Garin: La toxoplasmose oculaire. Ann. Oculist. (Paris) 188 (1955) 493–534

Ryan, S. J., R. E. Smith: The eye in systemic disease. Grune and Stratton, New York, London 1974

Schildberg, P., A. Wessing: Die fokale hämorrhagische Chorioiditis. Klin. Mbl. Augenheilk. 166 (1975) 651–659

Schlaegel, T. F.: Ocular Histoplasmosis. International Ophthalmology Clinics, Vol. 15, Little, Brown & Co., Boston, 1975

Sorsby, A., J. B. Davey: Generalized choroidal sclerosis. Brit. J. Ophthal. 39 (1955) 257–275

Sorsby, A., A. Franceschetti, R. Joseph, J. B. Davey: Choroideremia. Brit. J. Ophthal. 36 (1952) 547–581

Straub, W.: Toxoplasmose des Auges. Karger, Basel 1955

Straub, W.: Unsere heutige Ansicht über die Toxoplasmose des Auges. Docum, ophthal. 14 (1960) 308–329

Symposium sur les parasitoses endo-oculaires. L'onchocercose. Bull. et mém. soc. Franç. d'ophtal 71 (1958) 239–293

Tenner, A., H. Honegger: Ciba-Bericht 1972

Thiel, R., J. Otto, L. Toppel: Statistische Untersuchungen über das intraoculare Melanoblastom und Retinoblastom. Klin. Mbl. Augenheilk. 138 (1961) 682–704

Tillmann, W., H. v. Bernuth: Das Aicardi-Syndrom. Klin. Mbl. Augenheilk. 167 (1975) 496–499

Vogel, M. H., M. W. Strötges: Der Wert des 32 P-Tests bei der Diagnose intraokularer Aderhautmelanome. Klin. Mbl. Augenheilk. 159 (1971) 375–382

Wahle, H.: Die erworbene Toxoplasmose. Fortschr. Neurol. Psychiat. 26 (1958) 6–48

Waubke, Th.: Ein Beitrag zur Pathogenese der Chorioretinitis Jensen und die Möglichkeit einer therapeutischen Beeinflussung. Klin. Mbl. Augenheilk. 134 (1959) 627–643

Wollensak, J.: Weiteres zur Klinik und Differentialdiagnose der Cyclitis anularis exsudativa pseudotumorosa. Klin. Mbl. Augenheilk. 141 (1962) 559–568

19 Intraocular Pressure

Physiologic Intraocular Pressure

Intraocular pressure depends on the aqueous level, hydration of the vitreous, intraocular blood volume and rigidity of the ocular coats. The normal intraocular pressure ranges from 10 to 20 mm Hg, the average being around 16 mm Hg. Pressures above 23 are considered suspect for glaucoma.

There is a pulsatile fluctuation of intraocular pressure with blood pressure, as well as diurnal variations (usually highest on awakening, e.g., 5 to 7 A.M.). Intraocular pressure changes with illumination (bright = lower pressure, dark = higher pressure), posture (vertical = lower, horizontal = higher). In normal eyes these pressure variations are no greater than 2 to 3 mm Hg.

In terms of absolute values, the intraocular tension and blood pressure are unrelated. Fluctuations of the blood pressure are reflected by appropriate changes in intraocular tension.

Aqueous secretion is governed by the ciliary body epithelium and flows from the posterior chamber through the pupil into the anterior chamber, the chamber angle, Schlemm's canal and via aqueous veins into episcleral veins.

Aqueous volume is between 0.12 and 0.3 cm^3 with a normal protein content of about 20 mg percent. Aqueous outflow is continuous through aqueous veins at a rate of about 2 mm^3 per minute.

Formerly intraocular tension was investigated with indentation tonometers; today, however, mostly applanation tonometers are used. Tonography may be helpful when the recorded pressures are nondiagnostic. Diurnal curves and provocative testing may also be of value (water loading, dark room, mydriatics, Priscoline test of Leydhecker).

Intraocular Pressure Elevation; Glaucoma

Primary Glaucoma

Acute glaucomatous attack – Chronic-congestive glaucoma – Glaucoma simplex – Absolute glaucoma – Congenital, i.e., infantile glaucoma (buphthalmos, hydrophthalmos).

Narrow angle or *closed angle glaucoma* may be acute or chronic (includes malignant glaucoma). *Open angle glaucoma* is known as glaucoma simplex.

An **acute angle closure attack** (Fig. 19.1) is alarming. There is almost unbearable pain in the eye, brow and head along with vomiting. Vision declines rapidly. At first, rainbow colors are seen, then cloudy vision and finally marked vision loss occur. There is rapid concentric constriction of the visual field. Corneal sensitivity is decreased. The stroma and epithelium are edematous. Besides marked ciliary injection, conjunctival hyperemia and chemosis may occur. The anterior chamber is shallow

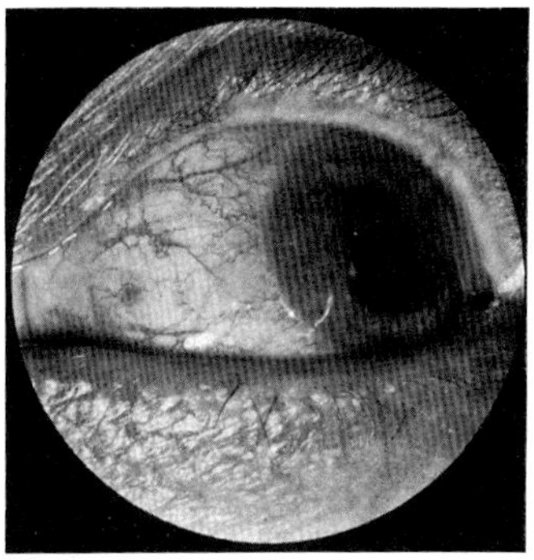

Fig. 19.1 Acute glaucoma attack: Corneal edema, flat anterior chamber, ciliary injection

and the chamber angle is closed. The pupil is mid-dilated while iris details appear blurred. The retinal artery may pulsate spontaneously at the optic disc.

The eye feels "rock hard" with pressures up to 80 to 100 mm Hg, or more. Glaucomatous cataracts (see page 250) may remain on the lens after an acute glaucoma attack. When there is a predisposition to angle closure, precipitating factors include: fright, fear, pain, etc. (epinephrine outpouring).

The *differential diagnosis* from acute iritis is important: with acute glaucoma the pupil is mid-dilated; it is constricted in iritis.

Chronic angle closure glaucoma implies a series of minor attacks of pressure elevation. The pressure rises to 40, 50, or 60 mm Hg with clouding of vision and rainbows or halos appearing around lights. A headache is usually present. Pupillary dilatation, epithelial edema and mild ciliary injection (Plate XVI, Fig. 5, page 192 h) are present during the pressure rise. There may be optic disc cupping and nasal shift of vessels. Optic atrophy results from repeated or longstanding attacks along with Bjerrum scotomata, nasal steps and other forms of glaucomatous visual field loss (see glaucoma simplex).

Glaucoma simplex (chronic open angle glaucoma) has no subjective symptoms. The chamber angle is open. Over a period of time the following appear: excavation of the optic disc (Plate XVI, Fig. 6, page 192 h), nasal shift of vessels with a bayonet-like angulation on crossing the disc margin, optic atrophy, and a glaucomatous circumpapillary halo. The disease is bilateral but usually asymmetric in the degree of involvement. Central vision loss may not be noticed until the less affected eye is accidentally covered. Nerve fiber bundle defects appear in the visual fields (Figs. 3.7 to 3.9, 19.2, 19.3). These are Bjerrum scotomata arching from the blind spot around the visual center, and nasal steps and nasal quadrant defects which infrequently extend temporally. The intraocular pressure is variably elevated, often to around 30 to 40 mm Hg. About two percent of the population past age 40 have chronic open angle glaucoma (glaucoma simplex).

Chronic corticosteroid therapy can cause increased resistance to aqueous outflow with pressure elevation, especially when a predisposition for glaucoma exists. Remission is usually spontaneous once the medication is stopped (Armaly 1963; Becker and Mills 1963).

Thyroid ophthalmopathy usually has an

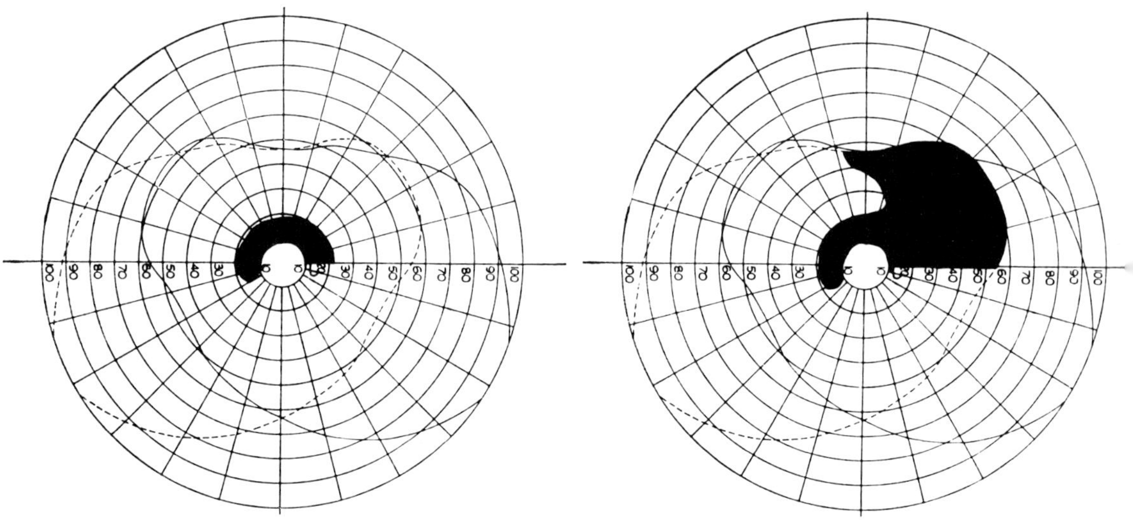

Figs. 19.2 and 19.3 Glaucomatous visual field loss in the left eye: 19.2 = Bjerrum scotoma; 19.3 = nasal step

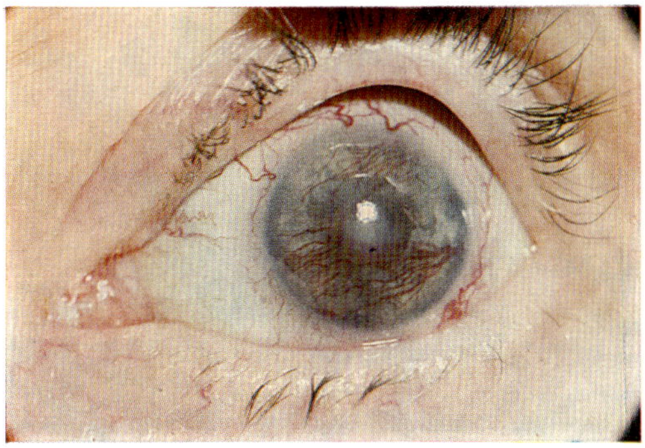

Fig. 1 Absolute glaucoma. Deep corneal vascularization, iris atrophy, cataract (see page 225)

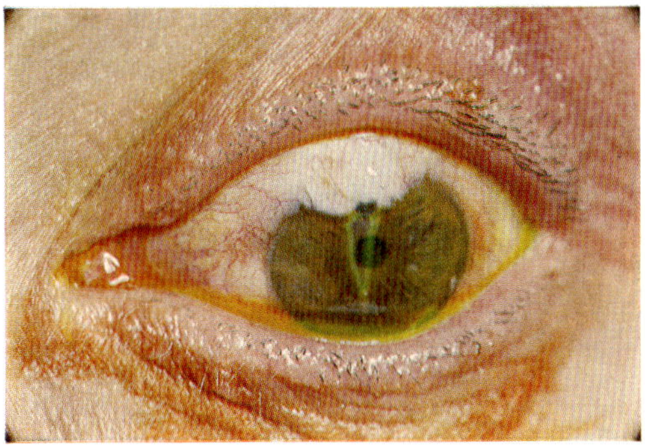

Fig. 4 Fistulizing scar after Elliot trephination. Seidel test + + = stream of fluorescein (♂ 38 yrs.) (see page 228)

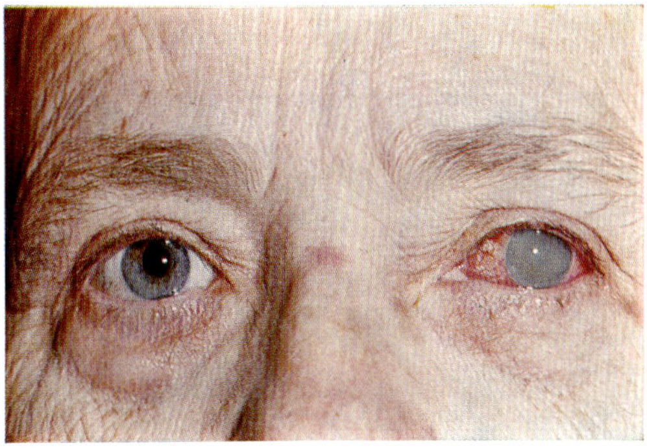

Fig. 2 Hypermature cataract with a gray-yellow protein-rich aqueous and secondary glaucoma in the left eye (♂ 70 yrs.) (see page 227)

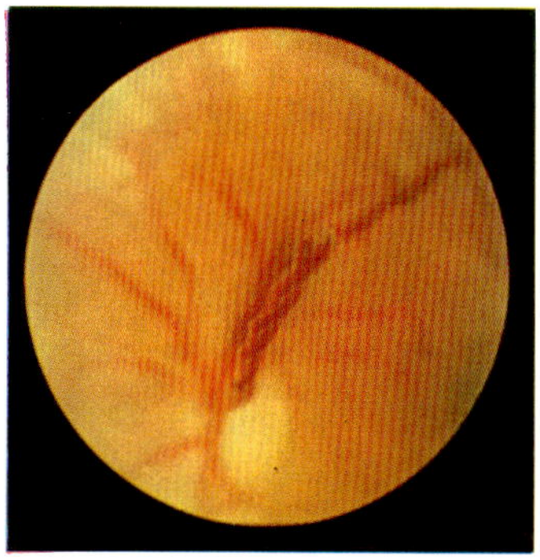

Fig. 5 Blood carrying a persistent hyaloid artery = two vessels twisted about each other (see pages 234, 306)

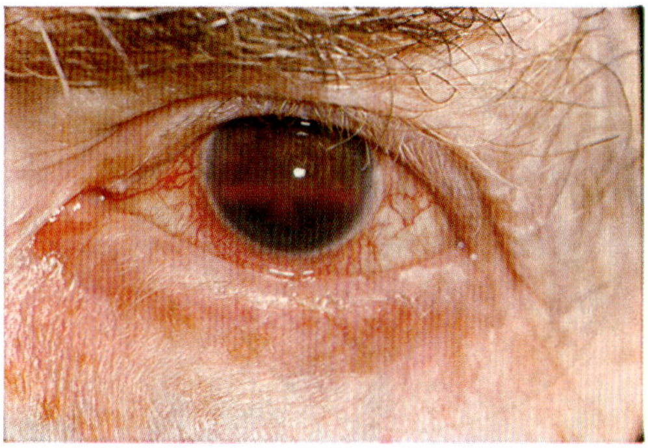

Fig. 3 Anterior chamber hemorrhage with hyphema in long-standing diabetes (♂ 86 yrs.) (see page 228)

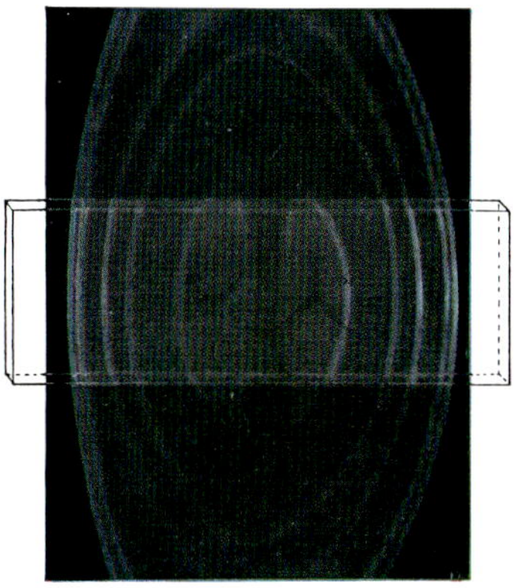

Fig. 6 Discontinuity zones of the lens. A narrow sagittal optical section of an adult lens reveals the following zones of discontinuity: Anterior-posterior capsule; anterior and posterior bands of dysjunction; anterior and posterior bands of the adult nucleus; anterior and posterior outer embryonic nuclear zone; anterior and posterior inner embryonic nuclear zone; central interval (from: R. Thiel, Atlas of Diseases of the Eye, 6th ed., Thieme, Stuttgart, 1963) (see page 238)

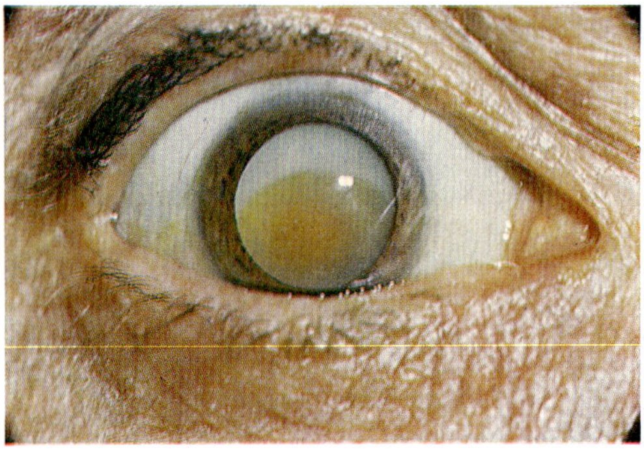

Fig. 1 Morgagnian cataract (the brunescent nucleus has settled downwards in the liquefied cortex) (♂ 75 yrs.) (see page 239)

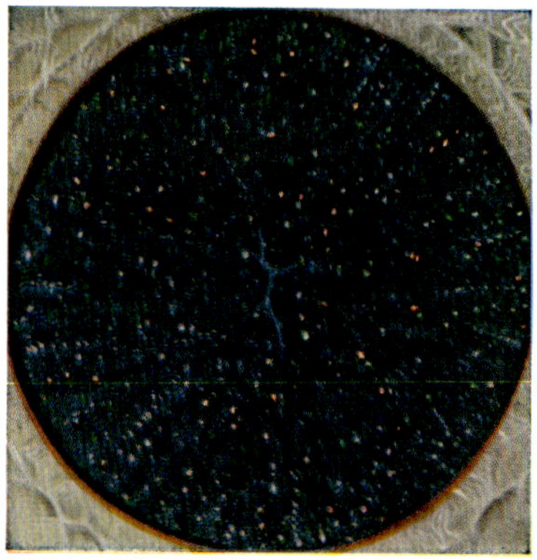

Fig. 4 Myotonic cataract (see page 241)

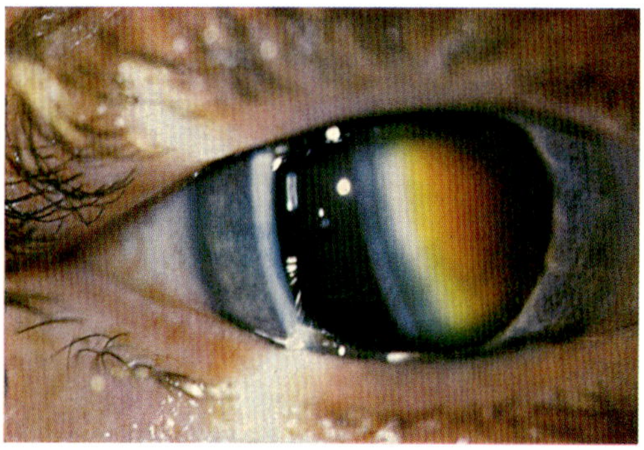

Fig. 2 Brunescent nuclear cataract (♀ 63 yrs.) (see pages 239, 248)

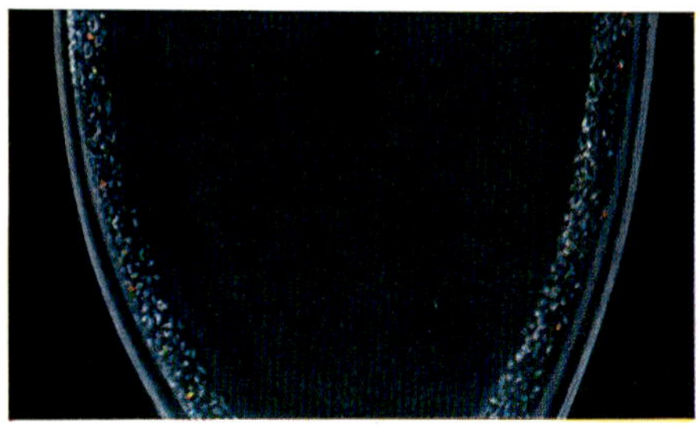

Fig. 5 Myotonic cataract (see page 241)

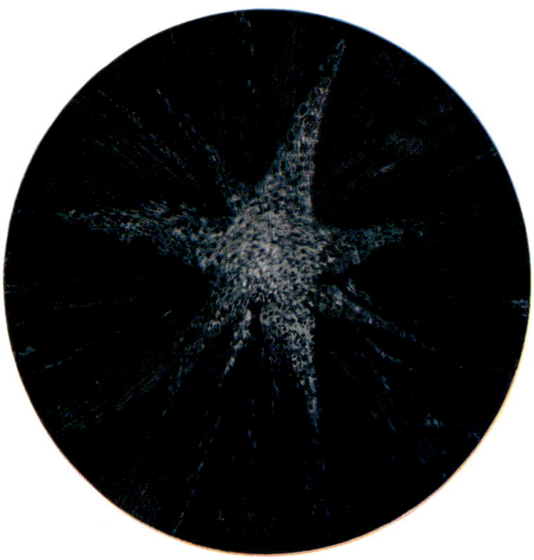

Fig. 3 Myotonic cataract (Figs. 3–6 from R. Thiel, Atlas of Diseases of the Eye, 6th ed., Thieme, Stuttgart, 1963) (see page 241)

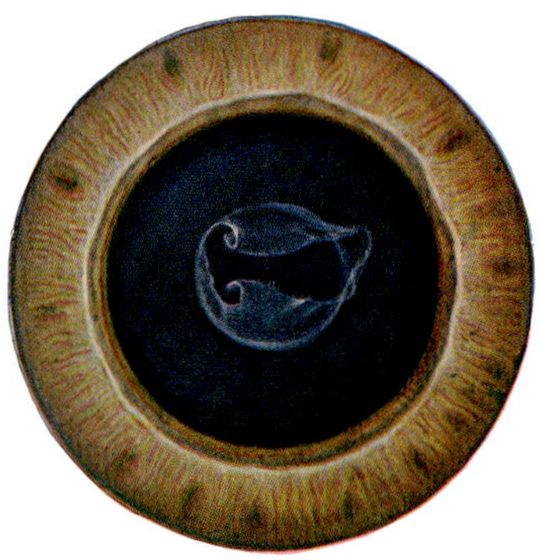

Fig. 6 Exfoliation of the superficial lamella of the lens capsule (glassblowers' cataract) (see page 242)

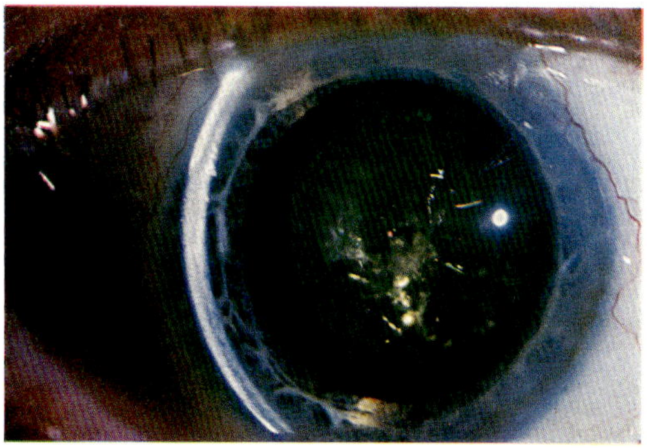

Fig. 1 Cholesterol crystals in the lens (♀ 69 yrs.) (see pages 243, 249)

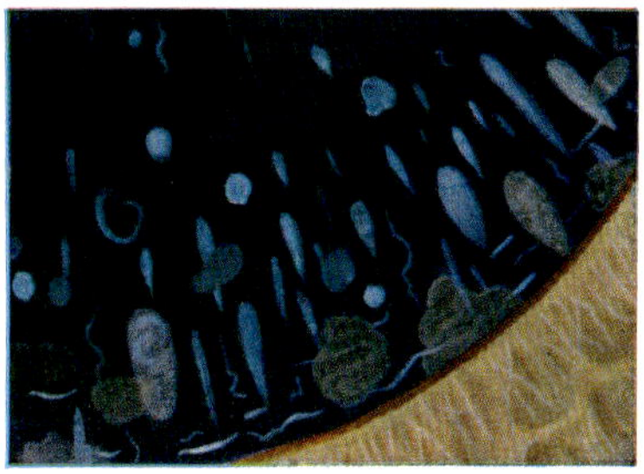

Fig. 2 Coronary, cerulean cataract (Figs. 2–5 from: R. Thiel, Atlas of Diseases of the Eye, 6 th ed., Thieme, Stuttgart, 1963) (see page 243)

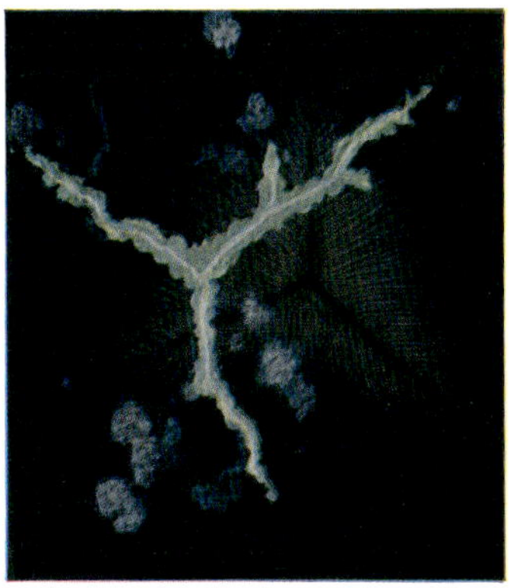

Fig. 3 Anterior embryonal sutural cataract (see page 248)

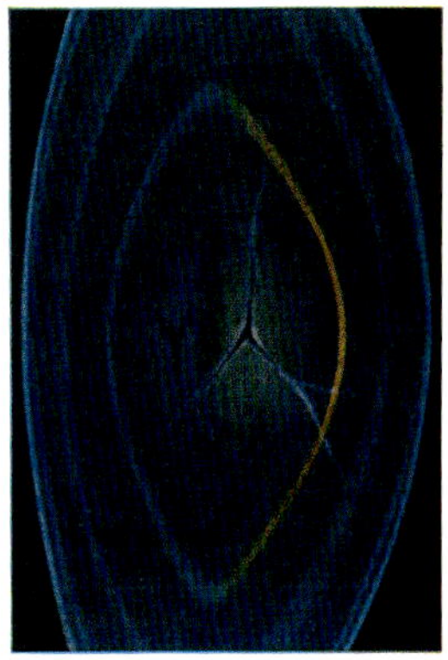

Fig. 4 Posterior brunescent bowl-shaped lens opacity (see page 247)

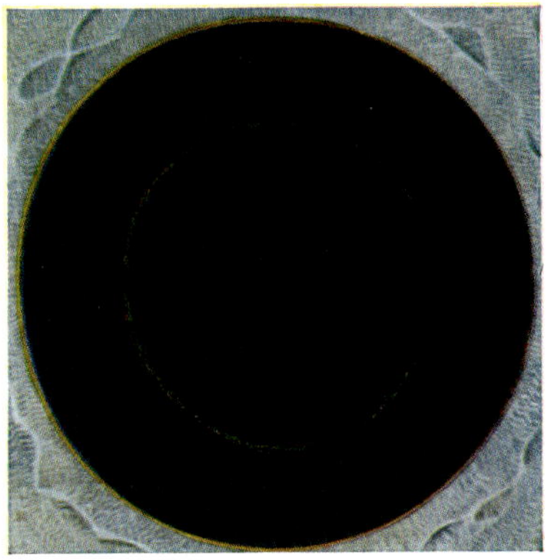

Fig. 5 Vossius' ring following a contusion injury. The transmitted pressure presses the iris against the anterior lens capsule leaving an imprint of iris pigment. In rare cases two rings may be seen. Traumatic cataract formation may appear later, independent of the Vossius' ring which is transient (see page 249)

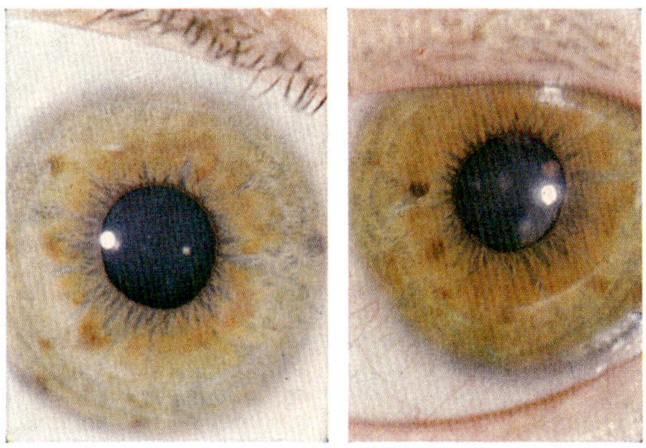

Fig. 6 Siderosis of the right lens and iris. Left-normal control (♂ 20 yrs.) (see pages 249, 250, 360)

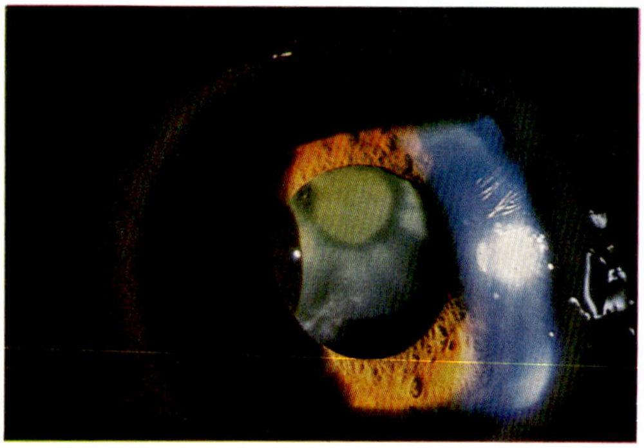

Fig. 1 Chalcosis lentis with a blue sunflower cataract. The lens is subluxated (♂ 45 yrs.) (see pages 249, 250, 360)

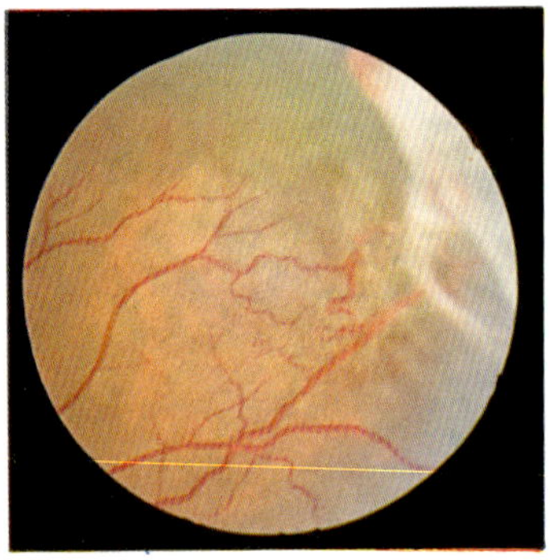

Fig. 4 Sickle cell anemia. Arteriovenous anastomoses, vitreous hemorrhages and exudates (♂ 23-year-old African) (see page 258)

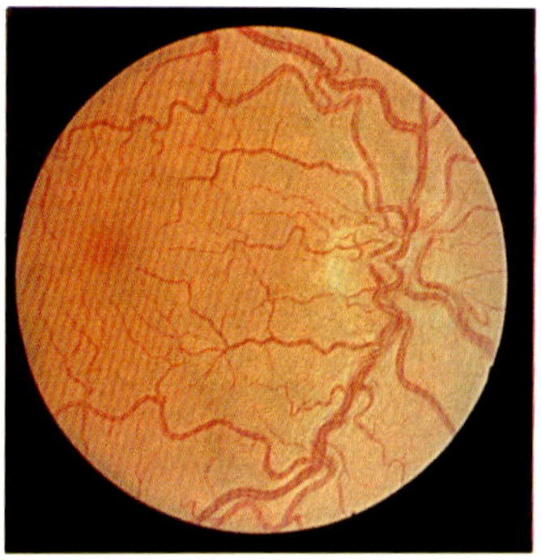

Fig. 2 Vascular tortuosity, pseudoneuritis (♂ 12 yrs.) (see pages 256, 306)

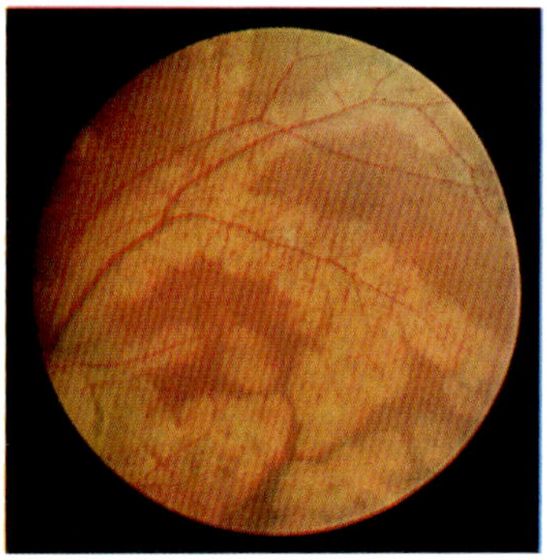

Fig. 5 Perivenous retinal-choroidal scarring in lymphogranulomatosis (♀ 46 yrs.) (see pages 258, 259)

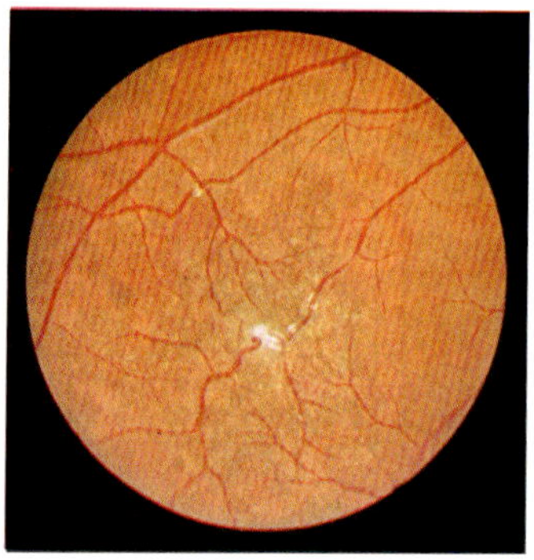

Fig. 3 Leber's miliary retinal aneurysms (♂ 33 yrs.) (see page 257)

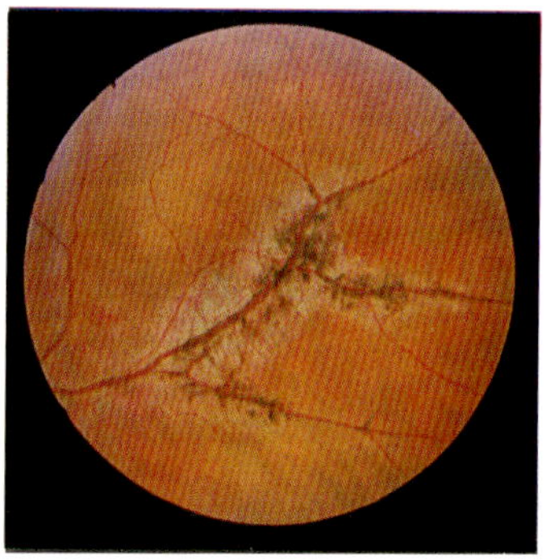

Fig. 6 Perivenous pigmentation–depigmentation in malignant hypertension (♂ 35 yrs.) (see pages 258)

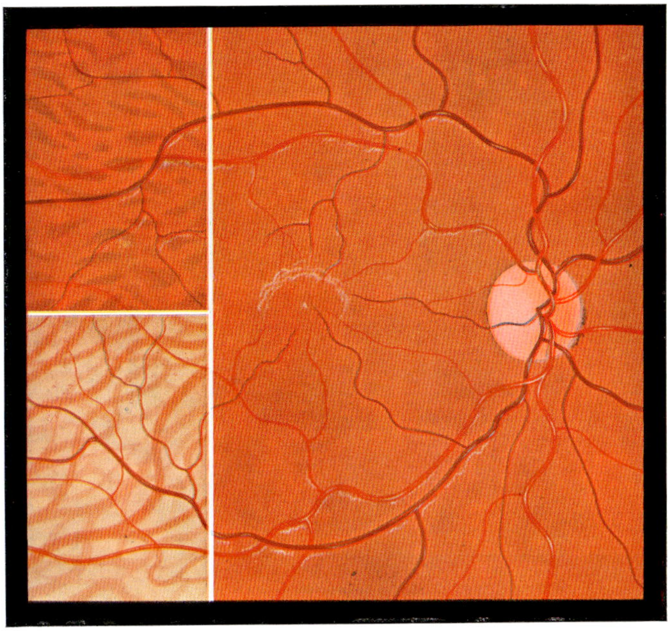

Fig. 1 Normal fundus (partially schematic)
Right: Homogeneous fundus pigmentation; choroidal vessels not visible.
Left top: Strongly pigmented (tessellated) background; pigment is located between choroidal vessels; choroidal vessels appear red on a dark brown background
Left bottom: Depigmented (albino) fundus; choroidal vessels appear red on a yellow-white background (from: R. Thiel: Atlas of Diseases of the Eye. 6th ed. Thieme, Stuttgart, 1963, p. 289), (see page 259).

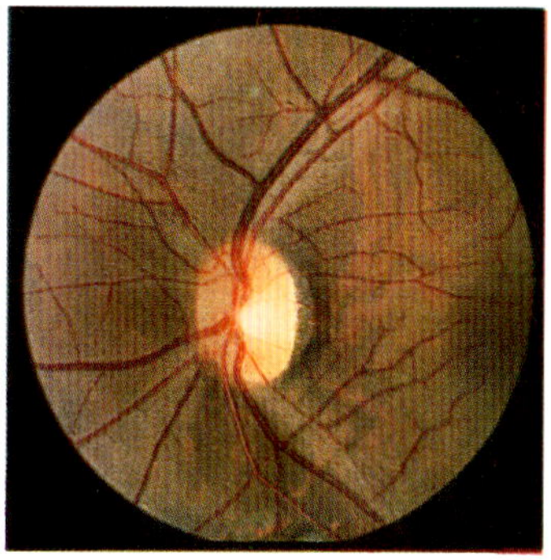

Fig. 2 Dark fundus (♂ 24 yrs.) of a Negro (see page 259)

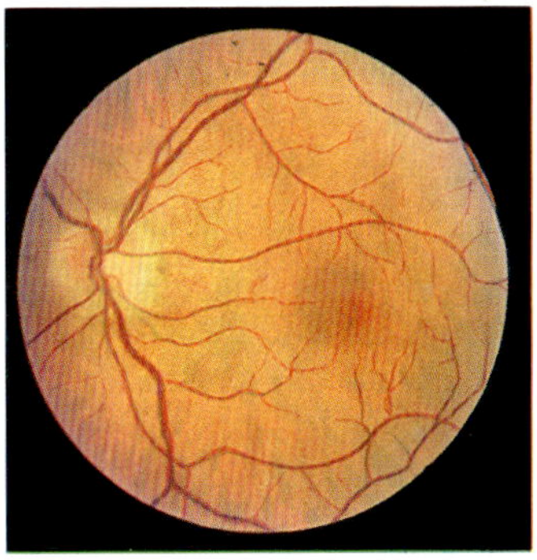

Fig. 4 Tessellated fundus (♂ 54 yrs.) (see page 259)

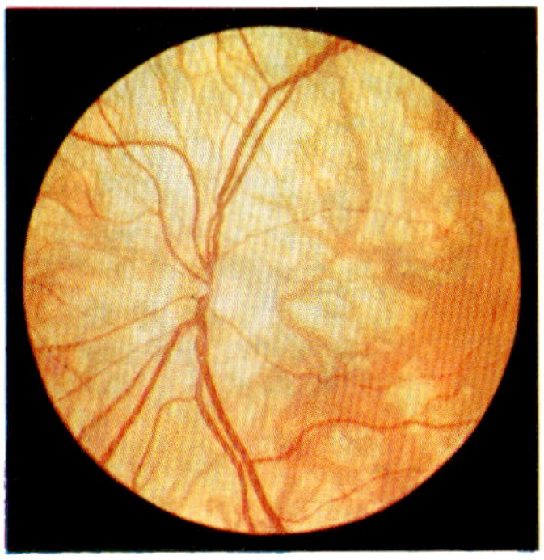

Fig. 3 Albinotic fundus (♂ 14 yrs.) (see pages 214, 259)

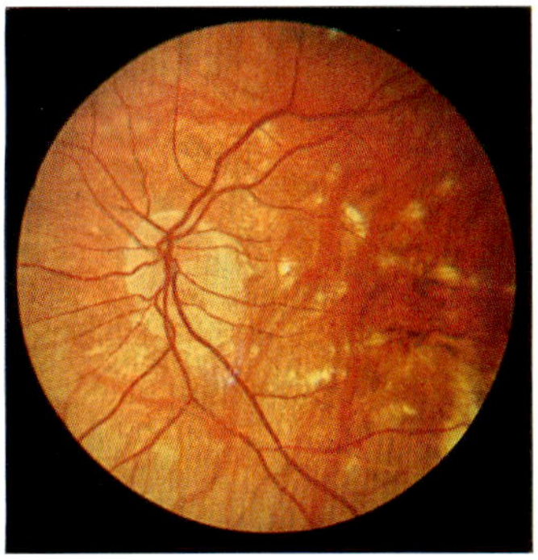

Fig. 5 Grade III myopia. Blond fundus, temporal myopic conus, stretched vessels, "lacquer cracks" in Bruch's membrane (♀ 32 yrs.) (see pages 214, 260, 282)

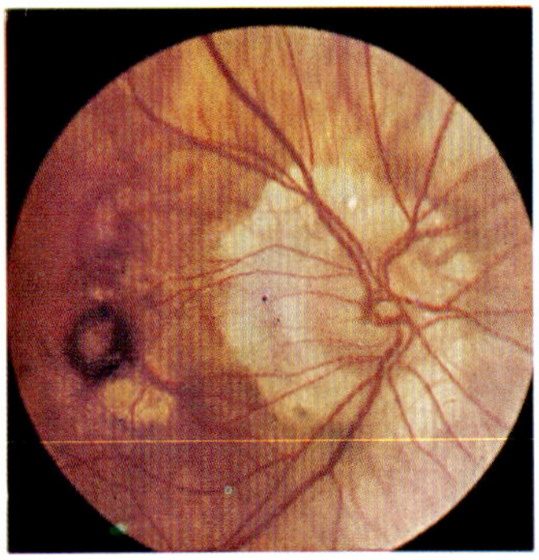

Fig. 1 Grade III myopia. Peripapillary myopic conus, stretch lesions and Fuchs' black spot in the macula (♂ 56 yrs.) (see pages 214, 260, 282)

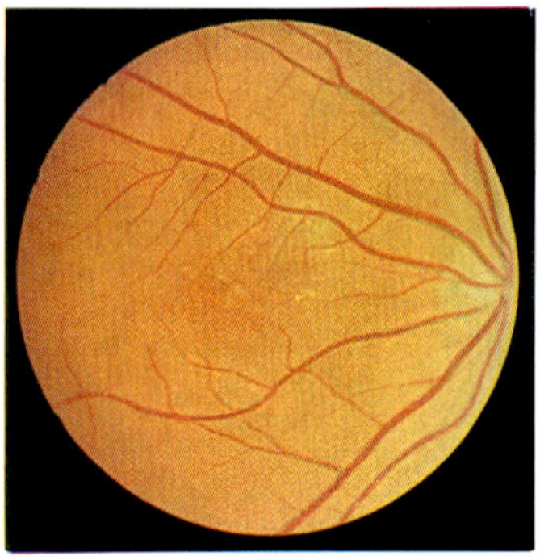

Fig. 2 Hypercholesterolemia with circinate yellow-white retinal deposits (♀ 54 yrs.) (see page 260)

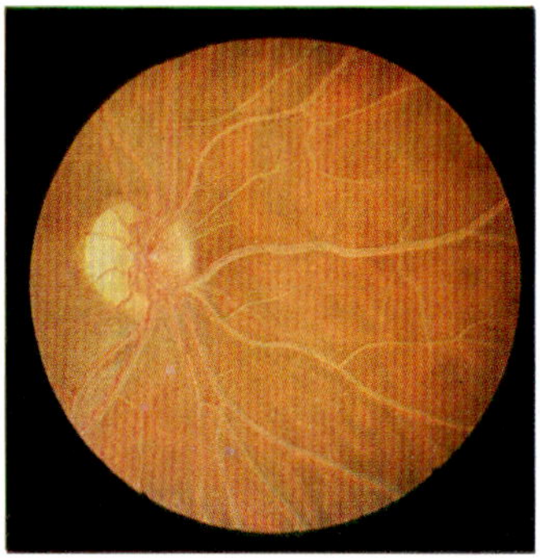

Fig. 3 Diabetes mellitus (blood sugar 400 mg per 100 ml) with symptomatic hyperlipemia (triglycerides over 5000 mg/100 ml) (♂ 35 yrs.) (see page 260)

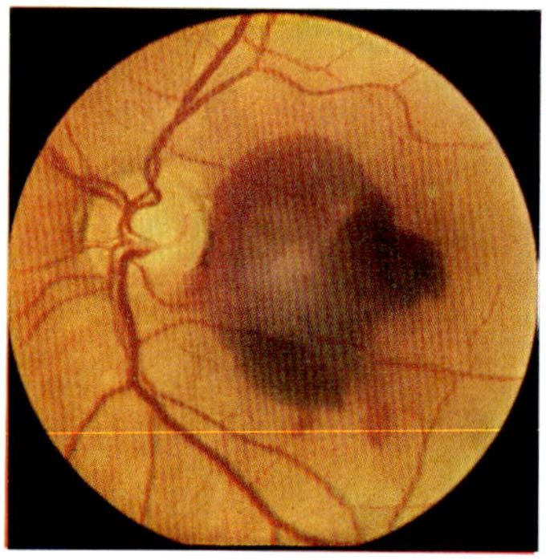

Fig. 4 Preretinal hemorrhage (♀ 71 yrs.) (see page 261)

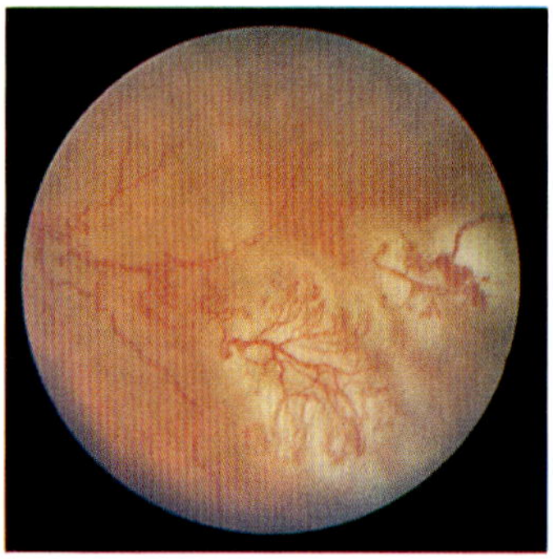

Fig. 5 Retinal periphlebitis. Rete mirabile photocoagulated (♂ 27 yrs.) (see page 261)

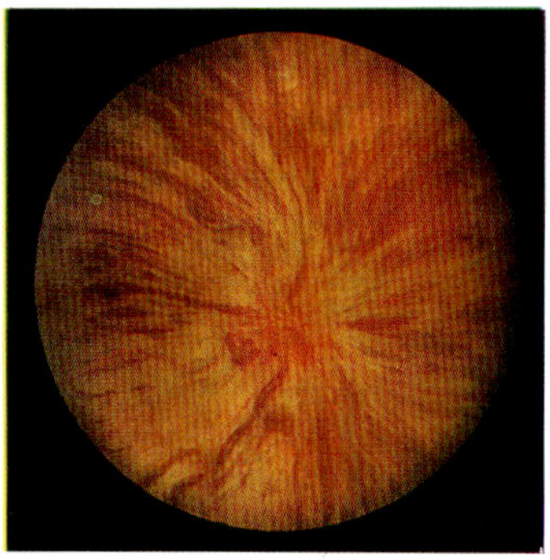

Fig. 6 Central vein thrombosis (♂ 57 yrs.) (see page 261)

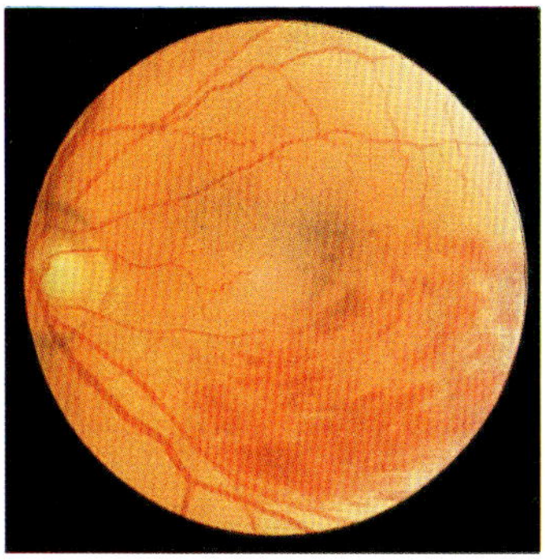

Fig. 1 Branch vein thrombosis (♀ 62 yrs.) (see page 262)

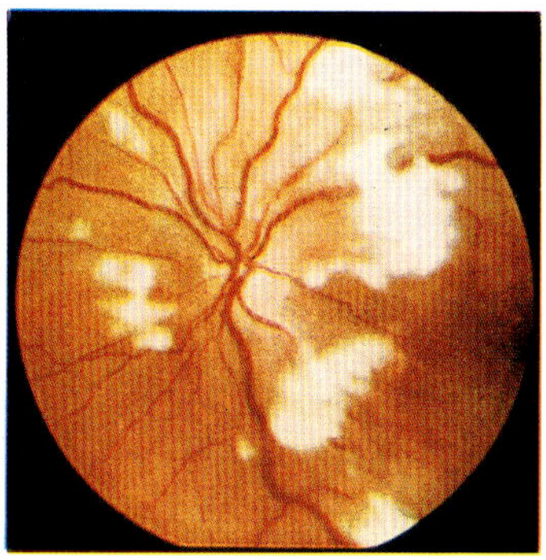

Fig. 2 Acute grade IV hypertensive retinopathy with cotton-wool spots (♀ 28 yrs.) (see pages 264, 268)

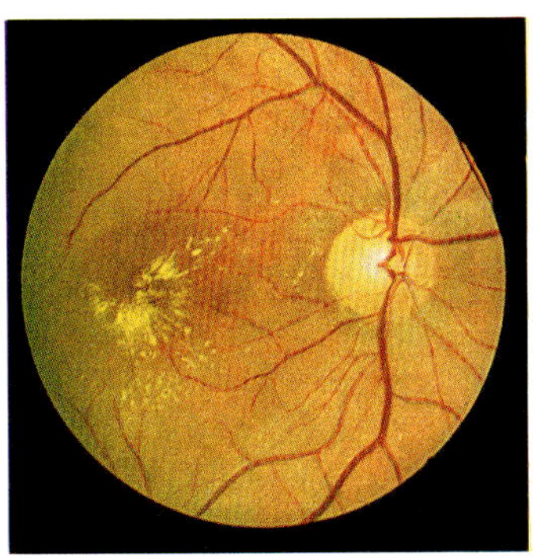

Fig. 3 Long-standing grade IV hypertensive retinopathy after bilateral nephrectomy. Narrow arteries, central-paracentral yellow star figure (♀ 36 yrs.) (see page 264)

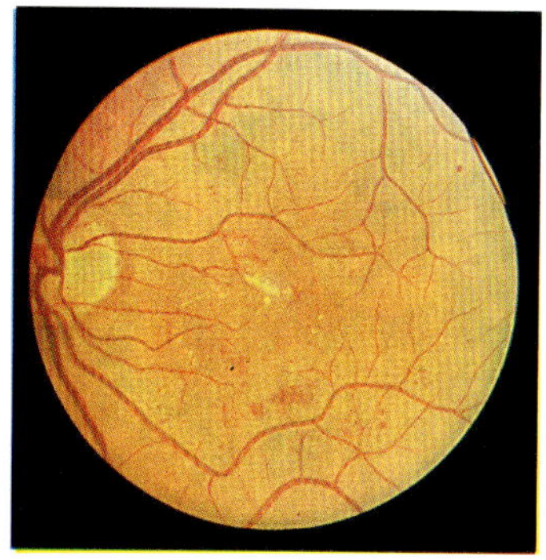

Fig. 4 Stage II diabetic retinopathy with flame-shaped hemorrhages and exudates (♀ 51 yrs.) (see page 266)

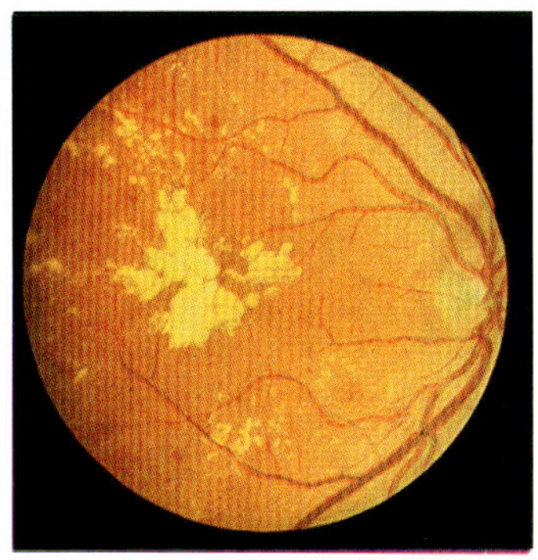

Fig. 5 Diabetic stage III retinopathy with punctate-macular exudates and hemorrhages (♀ 63 yrs.) (see page 266)

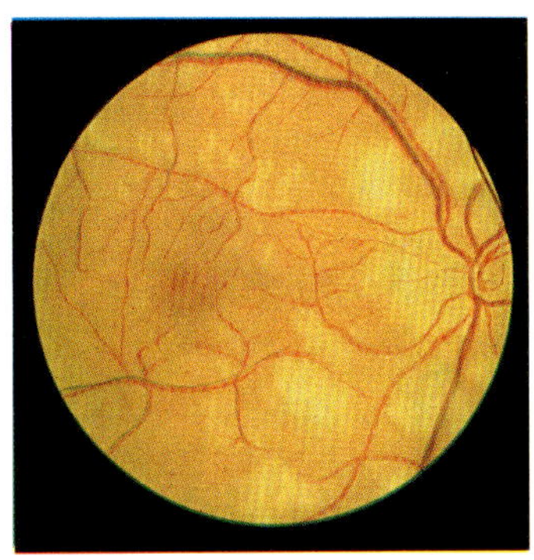

Fig. 6 Fundus in leukemia with yellow, soft, retina infiltrates (♀ 72 yrs.) (see page 267)

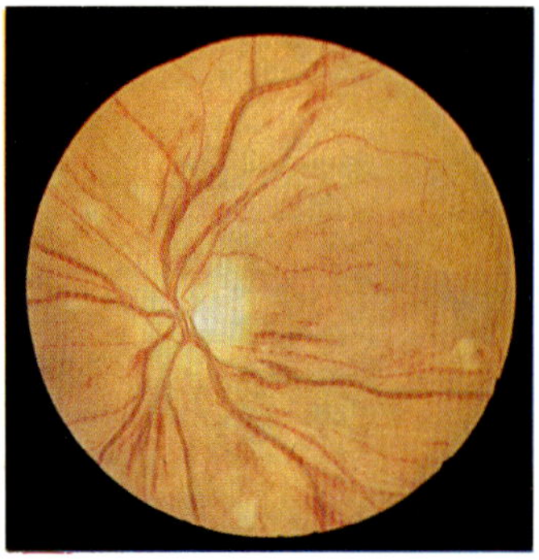

Fig. 1 Waldenström's paraproteinemia with hemorrhages, exudates, dilated retinal veins (♀ 46 yrs.) (see page 267)

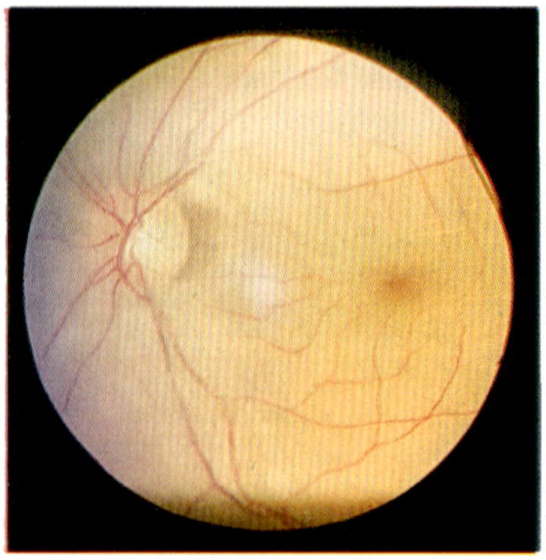

Fig. 4 Central retinal artery embolus with gray retinal edema and a cherry red spot (♀ 52 yrs.) (see pages 260, 270)

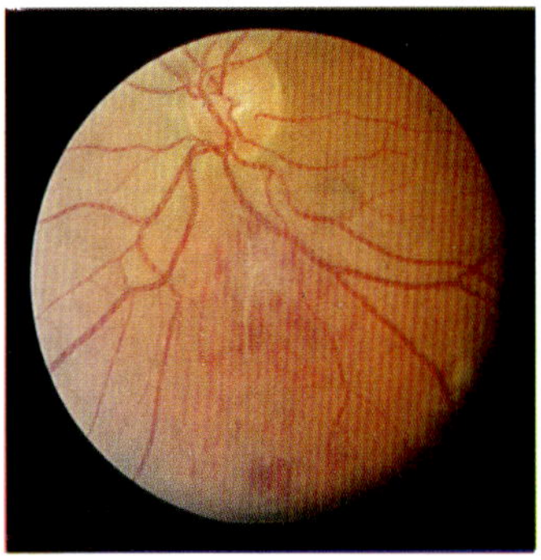

Fig. 2 Behçet's disease (recurrent hypopion iritis) with hemorrhages and vascular occlusions which are fleeting, changing daily (♂ 38 yrs.) (see page 203)

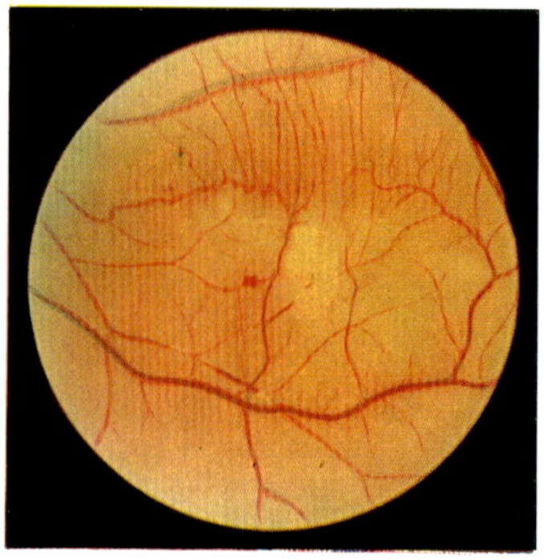

Fig. 5 Branch artery "embolus" in endarteritis obliterans (♂ 72 yrs.) (see page 271)

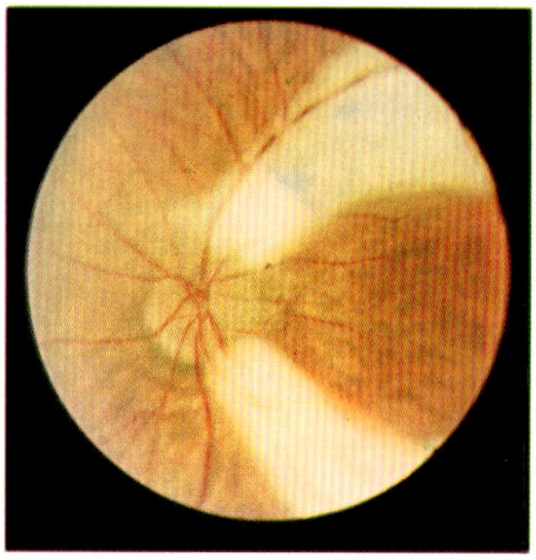

Fig. 3 Medullated nerve fibers (♀ 44 yrs.) (see page 269)

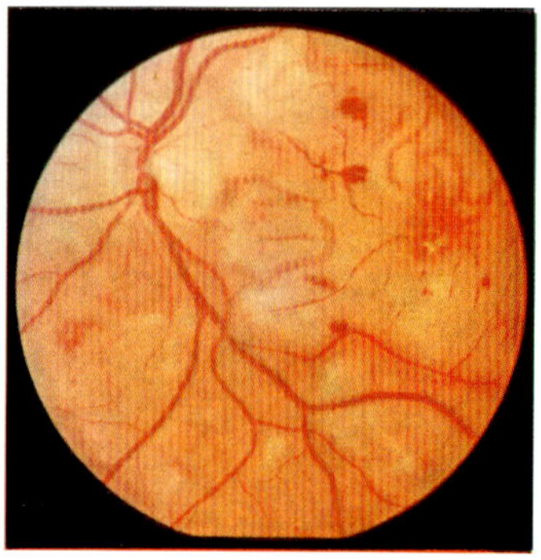

Fig. 6 Purtscher's traumatic angiopathy with small flame-shaped and larger blot hemorrhages and exudates, usually near vessels (♂ 22 yrs.) (see pages 272, 285)

elevated pressure which is only partly explained by the increased muscle tone on upgaze (Braley's sign).

Tonometry, perimetry and possibly tonography are necessary for an early diagnosis. In questionable cases stress testing may be helpful, e.g., water loading, caffein, etc.

Of *diagnostic importance* is the fact that glaucomatous cupping extends to the optic disc margin whereas with physiologic cupping a normal rim of tissue, which may be very narrow, remains even temporally.

With high myopia even longstanding pressure elevation may fail to cause glaucomatous cupping. Instead there is a posterior staphyloma. Optic atrophy and glaucomatous visual field loss, however, do occur.

Absolute glaucoma is any glaucoma leading to blindness. In the long run such blind eyes develop episcleral and conjunctival venous stasis, potentially with caput medusae, bullous keratopathy, band keratopathy, deep corneal vascularization (Plate XVII, Fig. 1, page 224 a), cataract formation and pain. There is always the suspicion of an intraocular neoplasm in such eyes.

Buphthalmos or hydrophthalmos: Infantile glaucoma causes hydrophthalmos or *buphthalmos* when it appears before birth or in the first years of life. Because of the distensibility of the ocular coats at this age the eye enlarges (Fig. 19.4) and appears prominent. The normal corneal diameter of 9 to 10 mm increases to 14 or even 16 mm. Because of the elevated pressure (40 to 50 mm Hg), the cornea appears gray-hazy and stippled in untreated cases. Descemet tears develop and remain permanently as double contoured lines (Haab's striae) (Fig. 19.5). These children are usually photophobic. The iris appears atrophic in the deepened anterior chamber. The enlarging globe stretches the zonular fibers which may tear, resulting in subluxation of the normally sized lens. The optic disc may be normal at first. If the intraocular pressure remains elevated, optic cupping and atrophy develop along with a glaucomatous field loss leading to blindness.

Congenital hydrophthalmos — Acquired hydrophthalmos — Differential diagnosis.

Congenital glaucoma is a developmental anomaly. Schlemm's canal is often poorly developed, missing or appears displaced. The chamber angle may be occluded by undifferentiated mesodermal tissue. In two thirds of cases signs of buphthalmos are already present at birth (Löhlein 1938).

Baillard (1947) found 23 percent of children in Paris schools for the blind to have hydrophthalmos. Jaeger (1968) confirms this figure. Buphthalmos is unilateral in 20 percent of cases (van der Helm 1963). In 359 patients evaluated by van der Helm, symptoms first appeared at birth in 29 percent, at one to three months of age in 17 percent, at three to six months in 32 percent and after six months in 22 percent.

Lacrimation and photophobia are often the first signs of congenital glaucoma.

On gonioscopy one sees atrophy of the peripheral iris root with radially coursing iris vessels. A translucent white tissue, Barkan's membrane (Worst 1964), or iris processes may be seen in the chamber

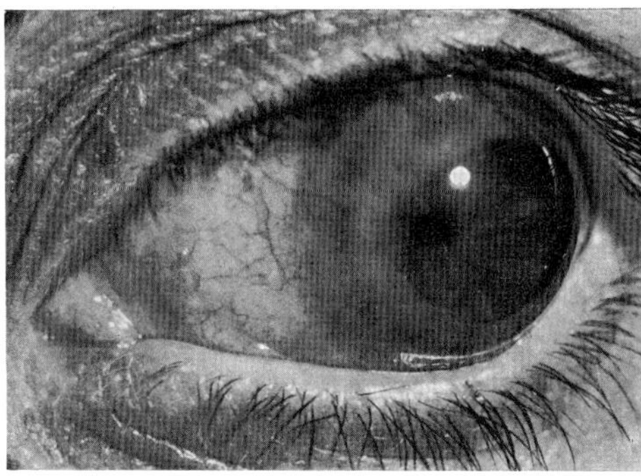

Fig. 19.4 Buphthalmos with ectasia and gray discoloration of the corneal periphery (♀ 23 yrs.)

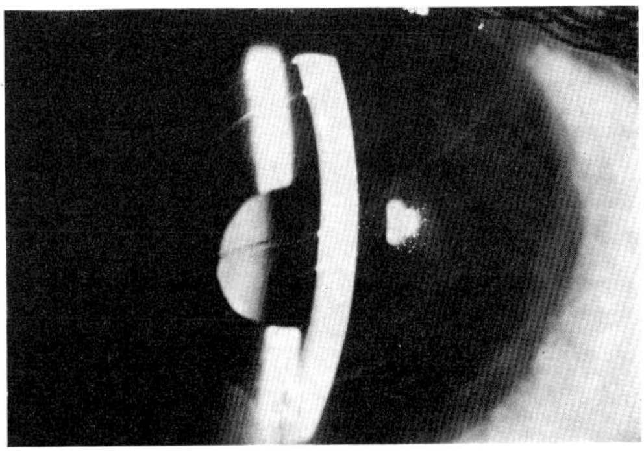

Fig. 19.5 Double contoured lines (Haab's striae) from Descemet tears in buphthalmos (♀ 27 yrs.)

angle extending between the iris root and trabeculum.

Hereditary congenital glaucoma is recessive in 80 percent and dominant in 20 percent (François et al. 1951). It is much more common than infantile glaucoma and secondary only to intraocular disease (birth trauma, perforating injury, iritis with pupillary occlusion, retinal glioma, etc.). Such acquired *hydrophthalmos* usually appears one or more years after birth.

Congenital or infantile glaucoma may appear in combination with other ocular anomalies or systemic diseases (Leydhecker 1973; Roy 1972; Kolker and Hetherington 1970).

Ocular anomalies associated with glaucoma include: megalophthalmos, megalocornea, microphthalmos, microcornea, posterior embryotoxon, microphakia, spherophakia, ectopia lentis, luxation-subluxation of the lens, iridocyclitis, essential iris atrophy, partial or total aniridia, mesodermal dysgenesis, Fuchs' heterochromia, Peters' anomaly (see page 145), iris coloboma, polycoria, tapetoretinal degeneration, retinoblastomas, persistent hyaloid artery, persistent primary hyperplastic vitreous, retrolental fibroplasia, choroidal hemangioma, and trauma, especially birth trauma.

The most important *systemic disorders* associated with hereditary glaucoma include: Marfan's syndrome (arachnodactyly, see page 251), Marchesani's syndrome (brachydactyly, see page 251), homocystinuria (see page 251), Hurler's syndrome (gargoylism, see page 171), Lowe's syndrome (oculocerebrorenal dystrophy, see page 246), Hallermann-Streiff syndrome (see page 332), oculo-dento-digital syndrome (see page 434), Ullrich's syndrome, and dyscraniopygophalangia (Ullrich-Feichtiger syndrome) (see page 333). Congenital glaucoma may occur with myopia or bilateral retinal detachments. It also occurs in the Pierre Robin syndrome, which includes micrognathia and cleft palate.

A variety of *embryopathies* (see page 244) are associated with glaucoma. The same is true of some *chromosomal disorders* (see page 329), for example, trisomy 13–15, trisomy 16–18, trisomy 21 (Down's syndrome, mongolism), Ullrich-Turner syndrome (see page 330).

Phakomatoses (see page 296) are often associated with glaucoma: von Recklinghausen's neurofibromatosis, tuberous sclerosis, von Hippel-Lindau disease (retinal angiomatosis), the Sturge-Weber syndrome, and the Klippel-Trenaunay syndrome (congenital dysplastic angiectasia).

The *Sturge-Weber syndrome* is one of the phakomatoses. It includes nevus flammeus of the face with *ipsilateral glaucoma* (Plate III, Fig. 6, page 128 c), epilepsy, potential hemiparesis and mental retardation. These changes can appear within a few months of birth (Bergstrand et al. 1936).

Nevus flammeus involves the area of distribution of the trigeminal nerve including lids, conjunctiva and sclera (Olesen 1950; Joy 1950; Djacos and Joannidès 1951; Binkhorst 1949 and others). Choroidal involvement leads to glaucoma and presents the greatest danger to the eye (Koch 1949; Berliner and Breinin 1951; Givner et al. 1957). Unilateral glaucoma with nevus flammeus can be divided into three groups (Kreibig 1941):

a) Port-wine stain with congenital or infantile glaucoma causing buphthalmos.

b) Port-wine stain without buphthalmos, but with late onset glaucoma.

c) Glaucoma caused by choroidal hemangiomas.

The *Klippel-Trenaunay syndrome* is associated with extensive angiectasias of an entire extremity or one-half of the body. Superficial and deep veins are dilated, and bony or even muscular hemihypertrophy occurs. This is an extreme variation of Sturge-Weber syndrome.

Differential diagnosis: Megalocornea, where only the cornea is enlarged, simulates buphthalmos. With megalophthalmos (megaloglobus) the entire eye is abnormally large without glaucoma or other disease.

Secondary Glaucoma

Secondary glaucomas can also be divided into those with *open* and those with *closed* chamber angles.

Secondary glaucoma with open chamber angle — Secondary glaucoma with angle closure — Ocular inflammation — Rubeosis iridis — Chemical and thermal burns — Lens-induced glaucoma — Malignant glaucoma — Postoperative — Malformations — Hyphemia — Tumors — Intraocular foreign body — Drug-induced glaucoma — Glaucomatous cyclitic crisis.

Secondary glaucoma with open chamber angles includes *pigmentary glaucoma* with pigment deposition in the chamber angle (Sautter 1971). Pigment generally deposits on the trabecula and posterior cornea, around Schlemm's canal, and forms a pigment ring at Schwalbe's line. A Krukenberg spindle may be present.

Pseudoexfoliation (see page 251) is associated with glaucoma owing to obstruction of the trabecula by an amorphous floccular material which is deposited throughout the anterior chamber.

Glaucoma from trabecular obstruction by cells (blood, macrophages, inflammatory exudate).

Glaucoma after blunt trauma.

Glaucoma caused by tumor cell obstruction.

Glaucoma in Fuchs' endothelial dystrophy.

Glaucoma with endocrine exophthalmos, pressure elevation in the orbit (tumor, hemorrhage, infection), and *pulsating exophthalmos* should be kept in mind.

Secondary angle closure glaucoma occurs with anterior synechiae formation in inflammation (postsurgical, flat chamber, hemorrhagic glaucoma, iridocyclitis, etc.).

Pupillary blockage with iris bombé (Fig. 19.6) results in secondary obstruction of the chamber angle.

Most severe ocular inflammations lead to an elevation of intraocular pressure. Since a predilection for glaucoma (primary) is common, the normal eye must also be checked.

Longstanding secondary glaucoma causes subjective (vision loss, cloudy vision, headaches, ocular pain) and objective (ciliary injection, corneal edema, hyperemia of the iris, glaucomatous cupping) symptoms.

Iridocyclitis should raise the suspicion of secondary glaucoma. Iritis caused by ophthalmic *zoster* is frequently associated with glaucoma. The greater the *anterior* or *posterior synechiae* formation, the more likely it is that glaucoma will develop. Scleritis often causes glaucoma; keratitis, retinitis, choroiditis rarely do so. Glaucoma occurs in one-fifth of patients with heterochromia complicata (Fuchs).

Rubeosis of the iris (see page 204) is caused by vascular dilatation and new vessel formation occurring mainly at the pupillary border and periphery of the iris (Plate XIV, Fig. 3, page 192 f). Hemorrhagic glaucoma almost invariably results. The most common cause is central retinal vein thrombosis or diabetic retinopathy.

Injury and *burns* cause glaucoma either directly by scar formation or indirectly from iridocyclitis. A traumatic increase in anterior chamber protein or hemorrhage is often associated with glaucoma.

A swollen lens *(intumescent cataract)* can cause angle closure glaucoma. Injury to the lens (perforation, discission) may release lens protein which obstructs the chamber angle. Loss of lens protein (hypermature cataract, Plate XVII, Fig. 2, page 224 a) causes *phacolytic glaucoma* despite an intact capsule. *Anterior luxation* of the lens almost always results in an acute pressure rise. *Posterior luxation* causes

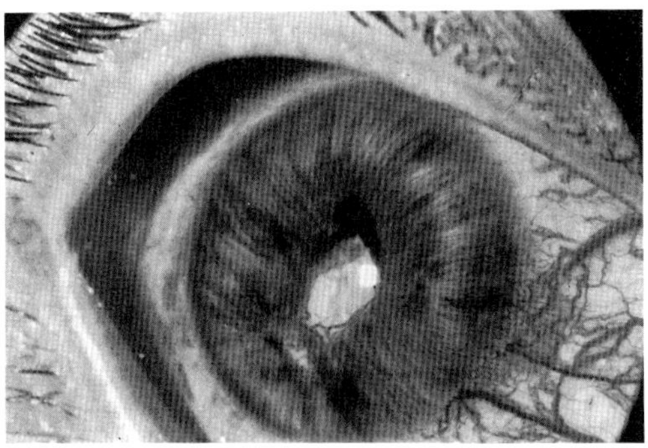

Fig. 19.6 Pupillary occlusion with iris bombé and cataract (♀ 20 yrs.)

glaucoma less often. If glaucoma does occur it is usually delayed.

Antigenicity to lens protein and other factors causes phacoanaphylactic glaucoma (Müller 1952) (see page 200).

In *malignant glaucoma* the lens and iris diaphragm are displaced forward creating a shallow chamber and angle closure with all the signs and symptoms of acute angle closure. It is caused by aqueous humor trapped behind the vitreous rather than flowing freely through the pupil into the anterior chamber. If the pressure is not relieved by mydriatics, the lens may need to be removed. Malignant glaucoma is seen most commonly after surgery (Elliot trephination, iridencleisis, etc.).

Prolonged loss of the *anterior chamber* after surgery (cataract, fistulizing glaucoma surgery) may lead to synechiae formation and secondary glaucoma.

The use of alpha chymotrypsin at cataract surgery may result in a transient postoperative pressure rise. Postoperative hemorrhage is a common cause of pressure elevation. Intraocular pressure needs to be watched after retinal detachment surgery. Epithelial downgrowth is invariably associated with a therapeutically unresponsive glaucoma.

Congenital anomalies (aniridia, mesodermal dysgenesis, microphthalmos, Sturge-Weber syndrome, etc.) are often associated with glaucoma.

Anterior chamber hemorrhages (Plate XVII, Fig. 3, page 224 a), and rarely vitreous hemorrhages of long standing, may lead to pressure elevation. Because of their slow growth, glaucoma is a late manifestation of intraocular neoplasms.

With any intraocular foreign body (including lens implants, silicone) glaucoma is a constant danger.

Drug-induced glaucoma: Topical (to the eyes) or systemic corticosteroid use can result in glaucoma which usually regresses once the medication is stopped. *Psychoanaleptic agents* may cause similar pressure elevation (Appelmans et al. 1963).

Sanguinarine leads to "Bengal glaucoma" through a severe generalized vasodilatation (Heidenreich 1966).

Glaucomatocyclitic crisis (Posner and Schlossman 1948) is a unilateral recurrent pressure elevation (40 to 70 mm Hg) in a white eye; vision is usually maintained. The chamber angle is open. Corneal precipitates are present but disappear after one to two weeks. The pressure then returns to normal (Merté 1959; Simpson 1960) (see page 211).

Decreased Intraocular Pressure

Marked hypotony occurs with phthisis, severe dehydration (cholera, dysentery, diabetic coma); choroidal detachment (Plate XVI, Fig. 2, page 192 h), severe hypotension (circulatory collapse, medications), and with carotid artery thrombosis (see page 315). It also occurs with poisoning by formaldehyde or formalin (either as a gas or liquid) which causes conjunctivitis and keratitis, and potential corneal ulcerations, iritis and ocular hypotony. Carbon disulfide poisoning causes neuritis, hypotony and ophthalmoplegia (Jaensch 1963).

Severe hypotony may occur after surgery, especially with filtering procedures (Plate XVII, Fig. 4, page 224 a). Intraocular pressure is lowered by topical miotics (mintacol, pilocarpine, prostigmine, etc.) and sympathomimetics (epinephrine etc.), as well as by orally or parenterally administered hyperosmotic agents (urea, glycerine, mannitol).

References

Appelmans, M., J. Michiels, M. Verdonck: Troubles neuro-végétatifs de l'appareil visuel au cours des traitments par les psychotropes. Bull. Soc. belge Ophtal. 135 (1963) 399–412

Armaly, M. F.: Effect of corticosteroids on intraocular pressure and fluid dynamics. Arch. Ophthal. 70 (1963) 482–499

Baillart, P.: Le glaucome infantile à l'institution nationale des jeunes avaugles. Ann. Oculist. (Paris) 180 (1947) 257–262

Barkan, Otto: Pathogenesis of congenital glaucoma. Gonioscopic and anatomic observation of the angle of the anterior chamber in the normal eye and in congenital glaucoma. Amer. J. Ophthal. 40 (1955) 1–11

Becker, B., D. W. Mills: Corticosteroids and intraocular pressure. Arch. Ophthal. 70 (1963) 500–507

Bergstrand, H., H. Olivecrone, W. Tönnis: Gefäßmißbildungen und Gefäßgeschwülste. Thieme, Leipzig 1936

Berliner, M., G. M. Breinin: Angioma of the choroid. A clinico-pathologic report of two cases of partial and complete encephalotrigeminal angiomatosis. Arch. Ophthal. 46 (1951) 39–48

Binkhorst, C. D.: Naevus flammeus faciei with homochoroideremia and secondary pigmentary degeneration of the retina. Ophthalmologica (Basel) 117 (1949) 360–361

Djacos, C., Th. Joannidès: La maladie de Sturge-Weber-Krabbe. Ann. Oculist. (Paris) 184 (1951) 994–1014

Duke-Elder, S.: Diseases of the lens and vitreous, glaucoma and hypotony. System of ophthalmology XI. Kimpton, London 1969

François, J., J. P. Deweer, J. van den Berghe: Glaucome chronique simple à hérédité dominante. Ann. Oculist. (Paris) 184 (1951) 404–422

Givner, I., L. Roizin, H. H. Berman, G. Gold: Sturge-Weber-Dimitri syndrome. Trans. Amer. Acad. Ophthal. Otolaryng. 61 (1957) 475–481

Heidenreich, A.: Chemisch-toxische Schäden des Auges (Vergiftungen, Berufskrankheiten). Klin. Mbl. Augenheilk. 149 (1966) 145–165

Helm, van der, F. G.: Hydrophthalmia and its treatment. A general study based on 630 cases in the Netherlands. Bibl. ophthal. (Basel) 61 (1963)

Jaeger, W.: Die Erblindungsursachen im Laufe der letzten 80 Jahre demonstriert an den Zöglingen der Blindenschule Ilvesheim. Klin. Mbl. Augenheilk. 152 (1968) 102–103

Jaensch, P. A.: Verletzungen, physikalische Schädigungen und Giftwirkungen. In: Der Augenarzt. Vol. V, ed. by K. Velhagen. Thieme, Leipzig 1963 (pp. 837–946)

Joy, H. H.: Naevus flammeus associated with glaucoma. Amer. J. Ophthal. 33 (1950) 1401–1408

Koch, G.: Sturge-Webersche Krankheit. Ärztl. Forsch. 3 (1949) 551–557

Kolker, A. E., J. Hetherington: Becker and Shaffer's Diagnosis and therapy of the glaucomas. Mosby, St. Louis 1970

Kreibig, W.: Zur klinischen Diagnose des Aderhautangioms. Klin. Mbl. Augenheilk. 107 (1941) 597–621

Kreibig, W.: Feuermal des Gesichtes, Glaukom und Skelettveränderungen. Klin. Mbl. Augenheilk. 110 (1944) 208–216

Leydhecker, W.: Glaukom. Ein Handbuch. Springer, Heidelberg 1973

Löhlein, W.: Glaukom als Erbleiden. In: Handbuch der Erbkrankheiten, Vol. V, ed. by A. Gütt. Thieme, Leipzig 1938 (pp. 35–64)

Merté, H. J.: Über glaukomatozyklitische Krisen. Klin. Mbl. Augenheilk. 135 (1959) 434–435

Müller, H.: Tierexperimentelle Untersuchungen zur Ophthalmia pathogenetica. Albrecht v. Graefes Arch. klin. exp. Ophthal. 153 (1952) 1–35

Olesen, O. S.: A case of angioma cavernosum of the choroid associated with facial naevus flammeus. Acta ophthal. (Kbh.) 28 (1950) 103–111

Pietruschka, G.: Zur Symptomatik der Syndrome nach Sturge-Weber und Kippel-Trénaunay. Klin. Mbl. Augenheilk. 137 (1960) 545–557

Posner, A., A. Schlossman: Syndrome of unilateral recurrent attacks of glaucoma with cyclitic symptoms. Amer. Arch. Ophthal. 39 (1948) 517–535

Roy, F. H.: Ocular differentialdiagnosis. Lea and Febiger, Philadelphia 1972

Sautter, H.: Zur klinischen Morphologie des Kammerwinkels. Glaukom-Probleme, Bücherei des Augenarztes, 56. Enke, Stuttgart 1971 (pp. 55–74)

Simpson, D. G.: Glaucomatocyclitic crises. Amer. J. Ophthal. 50 (1960) 163–165

Worst, J. G. F.: The cause and treatment of congenital glaucoma. Trans. Amer. Acad. Ophthal. Otolaryng. 68 (1964) 766–788

20 Vitreous Body

Important to the various changes seen in the vitreous (and peripheral retina) is the fact that structure and topography of the vitreous are determined by the former (now obliterated) embryonic hyaloid vessels (Pau 1969).

Vitreous Opacities

Muscae volitantes ("flies") — Hemorrhage — Cellular opacities — Parasites — Pigment — Asteroid bodies — Synchysis scintillans — Siderosis

Muscae Volitantes

Any vitreous opacity obstructs reflected light and is seen entoptically as dots, points or lines. These are best appreciated when viewing a bright, light homogeneous background (sky, snow, ceiling). They may be caused by normal vitreous structures, such as folded membranes, Cloquet's canal, etc. which become torn and mobile, or by vitreous synchysis and syneresis and posterior vitreous detachment. Their number and mobility increase with age and in myopia. On ocular movement entopsias move rapidly, opposite to the direction of gaze, and then return slowly to the direction of gaze. Any acquired vitreous opacity (see page 231) causes a similar picture.

The normal vitreous *fibrillar structure* is visible with the slit lamp on *direct illumination*, more so in younger than in older eyes.

Hemorrhages

Fresh *hemorrhages* appear as *red threads* or veils. Like any vitreous exudate, they leave behind gray-white, torn structures or veils after a few weeks. In transmitted light all vitreous opacities (vitreous structure, blood, exudate, etc.) appear as dark points, lines or floccules which move with the eye and sink towards the bottom when the eye is at rest.

The etiology of *vitreous hemorrhages* includes (Pietruschka 1964; Brini et al. 1968):

Trauma — Inflammation — Vascular disease — Hematologic disorders — Subarachnoid hemorrhages — Retinal detachment — Retrolental fibroplasia — Parasites — Endocrine disorders — Tumors — Takayasu's disease — Posterior vitreous detachment.

Trauma: Perforating and blunt trauma, surgery, birth, posttraumatic shock.

Inflammation: Periphlebitis, chorioretinitis with toxoplasmosis, listeriosis, viral infections, syphilis, tuberculosis, focal disease, intraocular parasites.

Vascular disease: Hypertension, arteriosclerosis, prediabetes, diabetes, central retinal vein occlusion, thromboangiitis obliterans (Buerger's disease) and congenital vascular anomalies.

Hematologic disorders: Hemorrhagic diathesis with coagulopathies, thrombosis, capillary fragility, anemia, leukemia, dysparaproteinemia, polycythemia and sickle cell hemoglobinopathy. Nine percent of American Negroes have SA, SS or SC hemoglobin (Isbey et al. 1958).

Subarachnoid hemorrhages: Ruptured aneurysm, hemorrhage from a hemangioma, brain tumor, arteriosclerosis, syphilis, trauma, hypertension. About one-fifth of patients with subarachnoid hemorrhage have an intraocular hemorrhage. About one-sixth have papilledema (Manschot 1954):

with the onset of *retinal detachment;*

from *retrolental fibroplasia;*

with *parasites* (tapeworms, ascarides);

with *endocrine disorders,* especially menstrual;

with *vicarious menstruation;*

with *posterior vitreous detachment;*
with *tumors* (retinal angiomatosis).
Vitreous hemorrhages may occur in Takayasu's disease, i.e., pulseless disease (see page 258, 315).
Vitreous hemorrhages occur most often with diabetic retinopathy and retinal periphlebitis (recurrent, juvenile vitreous hemorrhage). With any vitreous hemorrhage a detailed search must be made for a retinal tear which could lead to retinal detachment.

Cellular Opacities

Cells appear as gray-white punctate or linear opacities often forming a gray veil. These are seen in the various forms of cyclitis (usually with iritis) as well as with vitreous abscess, endophthalmitis, panophthalmitis, after perforating injury or metastatic ophthalmia (furunculosis, septicemia, etc.).
Tumor cells, especially retinoblastoma, may appear as small multiple tumor seeds in the vitreous (even anterior chamber).
Fungi occur in the eye after perforation of a fungal corneal ulcer, injury, postsurgically, as emboli from intravenous cannulae, and from unknown causes (François et al. 1962).

Parasites

Parasites rarely enter the vitreous, where they evoke an exudative reaction (*Cysticercus, Echinococcus*, ophthalmomyiasis).

Pigment

Pigment is frequently seen within the vitreous. With the slit lamp it appears as small yellow or brown punctate deposits.
The etiology includes: retinal detachment, cyclitis, retinitis, injury, siderosis, choroidal melanoma, etc.

Asteroid Bodies

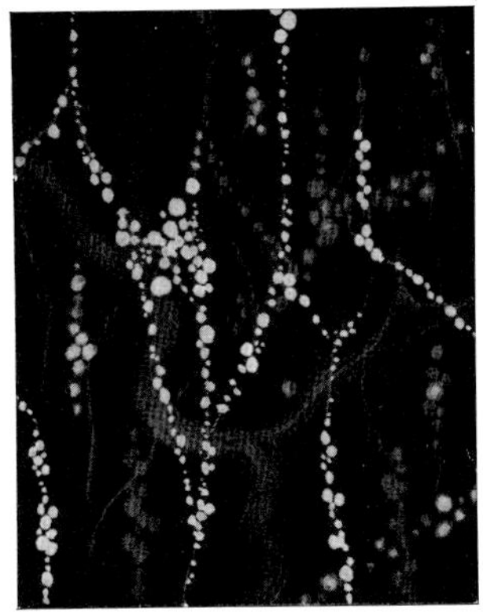

Fig. 20.1 Asteroid bodies (from: R. Thiel, Atlas of Diseases of the Eye, 6th Ed., Thieme, Stuttgart, 1963)

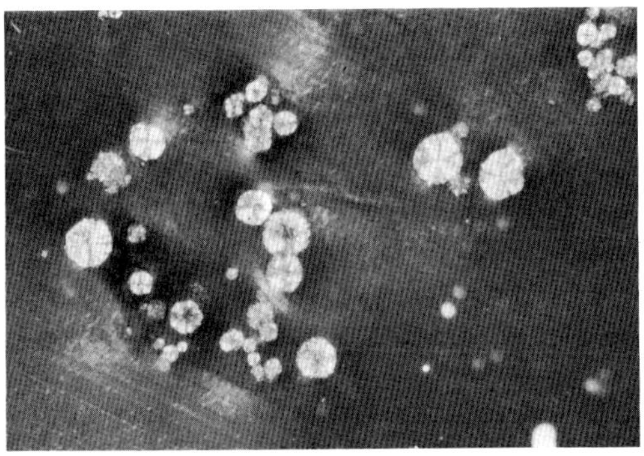

Fig. 20.2 Asteroid bodies (birefringence in polarized light)

Asteroid bodies are round white or yellow pearls (Fig. 20.1) attached to the vitreous fibrils. They are highly birefringent in polarized light (Fig. 20.2). Contrary to previous opinion they do not appear to be associated with diabetes or any known disease. They are overwhelmingly unilateral and appear to be formed by pigment epithelial cells which wander into the vitreous (Pau 1957). These are seen in the vitreous on slit lamp examination adjacent to the asteroid bodies (Pau 1957). They have been reported in association with choroidal melanomas.

Synchysis Scintillans

This consists of glistening yellow-white cholesterol crystals which appear in the vitreous after hermorrhage.

Siderosis, Chalcosis

Intraocular foreign bodies containing iron

cause siderosis of the vitreous. Hyaluronic acid is depolymerized with vitreous syneresis and brown-yellow pigment deposits. Copper-containing intraocular foreign bodies (brass) cause *chalcosis* with a blue-green-gray discoloration of vitreous strands.

Retinitis Proliferans

Connective tissue ingrowth into the vitreous (retinitis proliferans) occurs in periphlebitis, diabetic retinopathy, perforating injury, *retrolental fibroplasia* or congenitally with persistent hyperplastic primary vitreous. Gray retrolental connective tissue also occurs in Norrie's disease (see page 329).

Liquefaction (Syneresis) of the Vitreous

Vitreous *syneresis* occurs with axial myopia, age, longstanding uveitis and intraocular metal foreign bodies (iron, copper). With the slit lamp the liquefied lacunae appear as optically empty spaces. The vitreous fibrillae are disrupted and thickened, moving freely within the eye. This is observed entoptically and by ophthalmoscopy. Uveitis, endophthalmitis, hemorrhages, intraocular metal foreign bodies, retinal detachment, intraocular tumors, tapetoretinal degeneration, and hyaloid bodies demonstrate vitreous syneresis as well as cellular, corpuscular or metallic deposits. Perforating retinal injury results in thick strands of vitreous attaching to the perforation site.

Anterior Vitreous Detachment

Once liquefaction occurs the vitreous may detach from the underlying structure. Anterior (prebasal) vitreous detachment is primarily of theoretical interest. With the slit lamp a separation of the anterior vitreous face from the posterior lens surface can be discerned. Possible causes include: an old perforating injury, contusion, uveitis, retinal detachment, intraocular hemorrhage.

Posterior Vitreous Detachment

The vitreous detaches from the retina and optic disc. The detachment may be partial, usually beginning superiorly with collapse of the formed elements. Rarely, partial posterior vitreous detachment begins at other locations. A partial vitreous detachment usually evolves into total vitreous detachment and collapse.

The most common causes are age, axial myopia and retinal detachment. The posterior vitreous face in posterior vitreous detachment is often intermittently thickened and hazy with small, round droplet plaques or with circular, spindle-shaped, or polymorphous opacifications. These are noticed entoptically.

Posterior vitreous detachment is generally "acute." Photopsias appear suddenly, especially temporally. Entopsias, as previously described, become more numerous and mobile. Small, at times massive peripapillary and equatorial retinal hemorrhages appear, especially near vessels. These last for a few weeks and mark the detachment site. A retinal tear, which could potentially develop into retinal detachment, must be sought for in any acute posterior vitreous detachment.

A diagnosis of photopsias, entopsias, vitreous or retinal hemorrhages from posterior vitreous detachment may only be made if a meticulous search of the fundus fails to reveal any retinal tears.

Vitreous Loss and Macular Damage

The *Irvine-Gass syndrome* (see page 282) is the development of retinal edema and cystic maculopathy after cataract extraction. Presumably this is caused by incarceration of vitreous in the wound with tugging at the macula by vitreous strands. The eye may be irritated for months to years.

Vitreoretinal Degeneration

This is differentiated into (Ricci 1960; Hauschild et al. 1970 [see page 273]):

1. Sex-linked congenital retinal detachment (Norrie's disease)
2. Sex-linked juvenile retinoschisis
3. Autosomal, dominantly inherited, vitreoretinal degeneration (Wagner's degeneration)
4. Autosomal, recessively inherited, vitreotapetoretinal degeneration (Favre-Goldmann)
5 Macrofibrillar vitreoretinal degeneration (Favre).

In sex-linked, recessive, hereditary retinal detachment (Norrie's disease [see page 329]) vascularized retrolental membranes, which may

Table 20.1 Vitreoretinal Degenerations (after Blach)

Characteristics	Juvenile Idiopathic Retinoschisis	Hyaloideotapetoretinal Degeneration (Favre-Goldmann)	Hyaloideoretinal Degeneration (Wagner)	Macrofibrillary Hyaloideoretinal Degeneration (Favre)
Heredity	X-linked recessive	Autosomal recessive	Autosomal dominant	Autosomal dominant
Vision	Normal	Defective	Normal	Normal
Fields	Defective	Defective	Central scotomata	Normal
Macula	Rarely, cystic change	Cystic change	Normal	Normal
Retina	Schisis	Schisis Retinitis pigmentosa	Peripheral schisis Pigment clumps	Detachment
Vitreous	Membranes Cords Detachment	Degeneration Strands	Destruction Glial membranes	Macrofibrillary degeneration Myopic degeneration
Lens	Clear	Complicated cataract	Presenile cataract	Lens opacities
Refraction	Hypermetropia	Hypermetropia, Myopic astigmatism	Myopia	High myopia but may be emmetropic
ERG	Reduced	Absent	— — —	— — —
Night vision	Normal	Absent	Reduced	— — —

appear within the first week of life, develop. Months to years later, cataracts, corneal clouding and, finally, phthisis develop. Deafness and mental retardation may be present.

Idiopathic sex-linked juvenile retinoschisis has a recessive sex-linked heredity. The disorder appears in non-myopes, usually young hyperopes. Retinoschisis is greatest *inferior temporally* with bilateral, translucent veil-like schisis membranes. Tears in the inner retinal layer result in large bow-shaped lacunae. These may simulate ora tears. Vascularized sails or membranes do not form in the vitreous. Perivascular gliosis, pigment clumping and dispersion, as well as peripheral vascular tortuosity, are present. Cystic macular edema, pigment dispersion and linear radial reflexes appear in the macula causing vision loss. In 50 percent of cases the macular changes are the only symptoms (Jager 1959; Lisch 1968; Ricci 1960). Optic atrophy and retinal detachment may develop.

Peripheral retinoschisis, with preretinal membranes and vitreous syneresis, is seen in the autosomal recessive *hyaloideotapetoretinal degeneration (Favre-Goldmann)* (see page 274). The vitreous membranes and retinoschisis are not limited to the lower retinal half. Of greatest importance is the simultaneous tapetoretinal degeneration (retinitis pigmentosa) with loss of the electroretinogram. Cystic macular degeneration also occurs.

Wagner's hyaloideoretinal degeneration is an autosomal dominant disorder. There is a fibrillar degeneration of the vitreous with formation of avascular, transparent preretinal membranes near the equator. These are discontinuous and riddled with holes. They attach to the inner layer of the retina. Retinoschisis is normally not present. Peripheral retinal vessels are white from segmental sheathing. The vitreous is liquefied. Pigmentary disruption simulating retinitis pigmentosa slowly develops. The ERG may be subnormal but dark adaptation remains unaffected. Presenile cataracts, glaucoma and retinal detachment are common. Most patients are myopic (Böhringer et al. 1960).

Macrofibriallary hyaloideo-retinal-degeneration (Favre 1958) demonstrates early vitreous syneresis with development of macrofibrils, hyaloideoretinal adhesions and sclerotic degenerative retinal areoles. Inheritance is dominant and retinal detachment is common.

Pseudoglioma

A pseudoglioma (see page 295) is any gray-white vitreous opacity. This causes a gray-white pupillary reflex (amaurotic cat's eye pupil) and blindness. The primary causes of pseudoglioma are:

Congenital anomalies (persistent hyaloid artery; persistent hyperplastic primary vitreous; retinal dysplasia, congenital encephalo-ophthalmic dysplasia [Krause syndrome]; Norrie's disease; D-Trisomy [13–15]; incontinentia pigmenti; congenital falciform retinal folds [see page 295]) — Retrolental fibroplasia — Vitreous abscess — Intravitreal parasites — Old vitreous hemorrhage — Differential diagnosis of pseudoglioma.

Congenital anomalies: persistent hyaloid artery, persistent hyperplastic primary vitreous (PHPV).

A *persistent hyaloid artery* can present different clinical pictures. The entire artery may persist from the optic disc to the lens or extend only partly into the vitreous (Plate XVII, Fig. 5, *page 224 a*). It may be accompanied entirely or in part by varying amounts of connective tissue or only segments of connective tissue may remain. These may reach to the ciliary body or equatorial retina.

Persistent hyperplastic primary vitreous (Reese 1955) is overwhelmingly unilateral, occuring in infants born at term. The eye is normally microphthalmic with a white, vascularized fibrous membrane present behind the lens. The lens is flatter than normal with dehiscence and opacification of the posterior capsule. On mydriasis one can see that the ciliary processes are pulled towards the connective tissue mass. Vitreous hemorrhages, corneal opacification, posterior synechiae and secondary glaucoma may develop.

In *retinal dysplasia* (Reese and Blodi 1950) clinical findings are bilateral microphthalmos, persistent pupillary membranes, cataracts, persistent primary vitreous and retinal folds with rosettes. Central nervous system anomalies are common: mental retardation, cortical hypoplasia, hydrocephalus, etc. Other organs may also be malformed. Congenital encephalo-ophthalmic dysplasia (Krause 1946) is probably the same disorder.

In *congenital encephalo-ophthalmic dysplasia* (Krause 1946) or retinal dysplasia, bilateral microphthalmos is present at birth. The retina is detached, lying in a mass of retrolental connective tissue in association with a persistent tunica vasculosa and hyaloid artery. Hemorrhages, gliosis, as well as cataracts and glaucoma, develop.

Additional malformations: hydrocephalus, encephalocele, microcephaly.

Congenital progressive oculoacousticocerebral degeneration (Norrie's disease) has a sex-linked recessive heredity and congenital retinal detachment (see page 193, 329). At birth or shortly thereafter pseudoglioma, vitreous opacification, retinal detachment and preretinal membrane proliferation develop. During childhood cataracts form and the eyes become phthisical. Histologically the retina is aplastic. Mental retardation is the rule (Warburg 1965).

Patau syndrome is *trisomy D or 13–15*. This disorder seems more frequent as maternal age increases. Most children die by age six months (82.6 percent) and nearly all by the age of two or three years. Ophthalmologic findings include: microphthalmos, uveal colobomas, cataracts, persistent hyperplastic primary vitreous and retinal dysplasia, anophthalmos and hypoplasia or atrophy of the optic nerve (François and Hanssens 1970).

Pseudoglioma also occurs in incontinentia pigmenti (Bloch-Sulzberger syndrome) (Wollensak 1959 [see page 293]).

Retrolental fibroplasia (Terry's syndrome) (see page 235, 277) occurs in prematurely born infants, usually with a birth weight less than 1,900 grams, who received oxygen in the incubator (Foos 1975, Flynn 1975). Retrolental fibroplasia has been observed in children with a normal birth weight and without additional oxygen (Brockhurst and Chishti 1975).

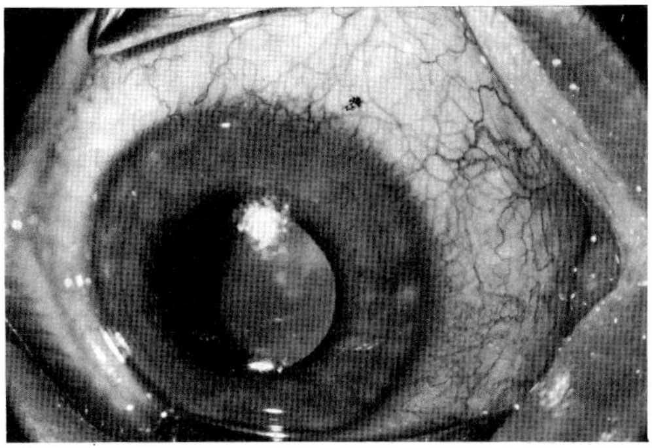

Fig. 20.3 Retrolental fibroplasia, gray retrolental mass (♀ 8 months)

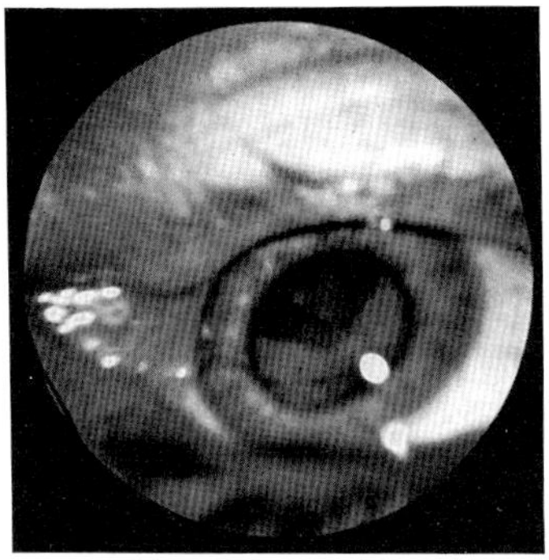

Fig. 20.4 Large vitreous cyst (dark mass in the upper-half of the pupil) (♀ 45 yrs.)

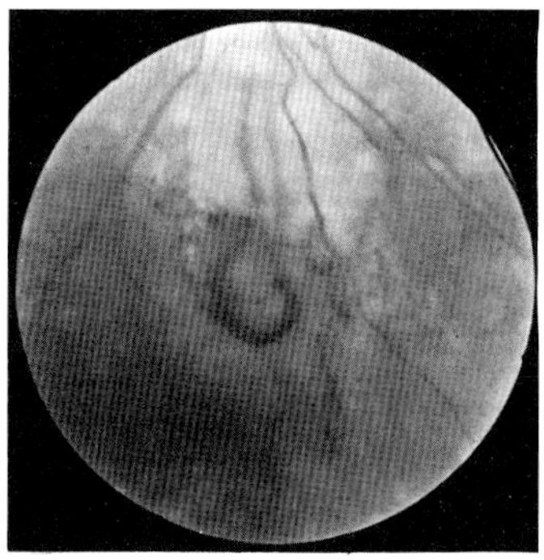

Fig. 20.5 Congenital, free-floating vitreous cyst (♂ 41 yrs.)

At first there is dilatation and tortuosity of peripheral retinal vessels followed by hemorrhages and tufts of new vessel ingrowth into the vitreous.

The vitreous becomes filled by a gliotic fibrous mass (Fig. 20.3). Flat traction detachment of the retina follows. Iris atrophy, cataracts, glaucoma, even phthisis bulbi, are not uncommon (Brown and Corner 1952; Kinsey and Hemphill 1955).

Although peripheral retinal changes begin soon after the incubator oxygen levels are lowered or withdrawn, the full-blown picture of retrolental fibroplasia appears about one to three months after birth. Levels greater than 40 percent oxygen should not be used, but lower levels are no guarantee against the appearance of retrolental fibroplasia or its forme fruste.

Four to ten percent of prematurely born infants have evidence of mental retardation. According to various authors, if retrolental fibroplasia is also present the incidence of mental retardation rises to between 10 and 40 percent with an average of 30 percent (Williams 1958).

Vascular anomalies similar to those occurring in the retina may appear in the brain (Szewszyk 1951): reactive proliferation follows vasoconstriction. Among a large number of patients with retrolental fibroplasia, Krause (1955) found many with below average intelligence and severe physical and neurological deficits.

A relationship between retrolental fibroplasia and falciform retinal detachment has frequently been suggested (Tasmar 1975) (see page 278).

Vitreous abscess: Inflammation (endophthalmitis, glaucoma, or phthisis) results in a yellow reflex and synechiae.

Pseudoglioma from metastatic vitreous abscess can occur in children with meningococcal septicemia or toxoplasmosis.

Parasites, such as filariae, echinococci, or fly larvae (ophthalmomyiasis), are rarely found in the vitreous but will cause massive vitreous exudates and retinal detachment as well as vitreous cysts (Fig. 20.4). The latter also occur as a congenital anomaly (Fig. 20.5).

Toxocara canis larvae are a not uncommon cause of pseudoglioma in children (Remky and Kraft 1964).

Nematode endophthalmitis from toxocarae can have a chronic, almost asymptomatic, course (Wilder 1950).

Every old *vitreous hemorrhage* appears as a depigmented gray-white pseudoglioma (see page 295).

Differential diagnosis: Retinoblastoma as opposed to congenital anomalies – especially persistent hyperplastic primary vitreous – is not associated with microphthalmos. Furthermore, while the fleshy red-white tumor may fill the vitreous, it is not attached to the lens and a cataract is not present. There is no elongation of the ciliary processes. Echography is a helpful diagnostic procedure to differentiate from tumors/pseudotumors (Oksala 1960). Congenital cataracts are usually bilateral and microphthalmos is rare. The lenticular opacities are generally not in the posterior part of the lens. Retrolental fibroplasia is a predominantly bilateral disease found in prematurely born infants of less than 1,900 g birth weight who received oxygen. Cataracts are rare. With other congenital anomalies the systemic findings stand out. Congenital vitreous cysts reach 1 to 5 mm in size. These are stationary and benign compared to the increasing vitreous opacification, retinal detachment and glaucoma which typify parasitic cysts (cysticercus). Vitreous hemorrhages and abscesses usually do not present a diagnostic problem.

References

Blach, R. K.: The hereditary hyalo-retinopathies. Brit. J. Ophthal. 53 (1969) 136–137

Böhringer, H. R., P. Dieterle, E. Londolt: Zur Klinik und Pathologie der degeneratio hyaloideo-retinalis hereditaria (Wagner). Ophthalmologica 139 (1960) 330–338

Brini, A., A. Bronner, J. P. Gerhard, J. Nordmann: Biologie et chirurgie du corps vitré. Masson, Paris 1968

Brockhurst, R. J., M. Chischti: Cicatricial retrolental fibroplasia. Its occurrence without oxygen administration and full term infants. Albrecht v. Graefes Arch. Klin. exp. Ophthal. 195 (1975) 113–128

Brown, C. A., B. Corner: Retrolental fibroplasia. Brit. J. Ophthal. 36 (1952) 281–302

Duke-Elder, S.: Diseases of the lens and vitreous, glaucoma and hypotony. System of ophthalmology XI. Kimpton, London 1969

Favre, M.: A propos de deux cas de dégénérescence hyaloideo-retinienne. Ophthalmologica 135 (1958) 604–609

Flynn, J. T.: Acute proliferative retrolental fibroplasia. Evolution of the lesion. Albrecht v. Graefes Arch. Klin. exp. Ophthal. 195 (1975) 101–111

Foos, R. Y.: Acute retrolental fibroplasia. Albrecht v. Graefes Arch. Klin. exp. Ophthal. 195 (1975) 87–100

François, J., E. de Vos, M. Hanssens, M. Elewaut-Rijsselaere: Mycoses intra-oculaires. Ann. Oculist. (Paris) 195 (1962) 97–119

François, J., M. Hanssens: Les manifestations oculaires de la trisomie D 1. Etude clinique et histo-pathologique. Ann. Oculist. (Paris) 203 (1970) 873–914

Hauschild, E., H. Hiller, A. Heydenreich: Beitrag zum Krankheitsbild der vitreo-retinalen Degeneration. Klin. Mbl. Augenheilk. 156 (1970) 628–643

Irvine, S. R.: A newly vitreous syndrome following cataract surgery. Amer. J. Ophthal. 36 (1953) 599–619

Isbey, E. K., G. O. Clifford, K. R. Tanaka: Vitreous haemorrhage. Amer. J. Ophthal. 45 (1958) 870–879

Jager, G. M.: A hereditary retinal disease. Trans. ophthal. Soc. U. K. 73 (1959) 617

Kinsey, V. E., F. M. Hemphill: Etiology of retrolental fibroplasia and preliminary report of cooperative study of retrolental fibroplasia. Trans. Amer Acad Ophthal. Otolaryng. 59 (1955) 15–24

Krause, A. C.: Congenital encephalo-ophthalmic dysplasia. Arch. Ophthal. 36 (1946) 387

Krause, A. C.: Effect of retrolental fibroplasia in children. Arch. Ophthal. 53 (1955) 522–529

Lisch, K.: Idiopathische hereditäre Retinochisis. Klin. Mbl. Augenheilk. 153 (1968) 204

Manschot, W. A.: Subarachnoid haemorrhage. Amer. J. Ophthal. 38 (1954) 501–505

Norrie, G.: Causes of blindness in children. Acta ophthal. (Kbh.) 5 (1927) 357

Oksala, A.: Das Echogramm in der Diagnostik von Augenkrankheiten. Klin. Mbl. Augenheilk. 137 (1960) 72–87

Pau, H.: Die Scintillatio nivea corporis vitrei. Klin. Mbl. Augenheilk. 137 (1957) 610–615

Pau, H.: Die Strukturen des Glaskörpers in Beziehung zu embryonalen Blutgefäßen und Glaskörperrindenzellen. Albrecht v. Graefes Arch. 177 (1969) 261–270

Pietruschka, G.: Zur Ätiologie und Therapie von Glaskörpereinblutungen. Klin. Mlb. Augenheilk. 144 (1964) 641–670

Reese, A. B., F. C. Blodi: Retinal dysplasia. Amer. J. Ophthal. 33 (1950) 23–32

Reese, A. B.: Persistent hyperplastic primary vitreous. Trans. Amer. Acad. Ophthal. Otolaryng. 59 (1955) 271–296

Remky, H., H. Kraft: Intraoculare Toxocara-canis-Infestation. Klin. Mbl. Augenheilk. 147 (1964) 692–702

Ricci, A.: Clinique et transmission génétique des différents formes de dégénérescences vitréo-retiennes. Ophthalmologica 139 (1960) 338–343

Szewczyk, Th. S.: Retrolental fibroplasia etiology and prophylaxis. Amer. J. Ophthal. 34 (1951) 1649–1650

Tasman, W.: Retinal detachment in retrolental fibroplasia. Albrecht v. Graefes Arch. Klin. exp. Ophthal. 195 (1975) 129–139

Warburg, M.: Norrie's disease. Trans. ophthal. Soc. U. K. 85 (1965) 391–408

Wilder, H. C.: Nematode Endophthalmitis. Trans. Amer. Acad. Ophthal. Otolaryng. 55 (1950) 99–109

Williams, C. E.: Retrolental fibroplasia in association with mental defect. Brit. J. Ophthal. 42 (1958) 549–557

Wollensak, K. J.: Charakteristische Augenbefunde beim Bloch-Sulzberger-Syndrom (Incontinentia pigmenti). Klin. Mbl. Augenheilk. 134 (1959) 692–704

21 Lens

Cataract, Zones of Discontinuity, Location of Opacities

Any opacification of the lens is called a *cataract*. True lens opacities should not be confused with the zones of discontinuity visible with the slit lamp (Plate XVII, Fig. 6, page 224 a).

The ectodermal lens is surrounded by a lens capsule over which lies the zonula lamellae (the embryonic tunica vasculosa lentis) into which the ciliary zonules of Zinn merge. Under the anterior capsule there is a single epithelial cell layer which at the equator forms the lens fibers. Here they still retain their cell nuclei. The newly formed fibers layer themselves over previously formed lens parenchyma. Protein comprises 35 percent of the lens. The refractive index varies abruptly with the varying zones of discontinuity from the anterior zone of disjunction to the adult, the peripheral fetal and the central embryonic nuclei. The age of a circumscribed opacity is reflected in its relationship to the zones of discontinuity. With the slit lamp the discontinuous layers are seen as alternating light and dark bands. The water content of the older parts of the lens continuously decreases with age and previously soluble protein becomes insoluble.

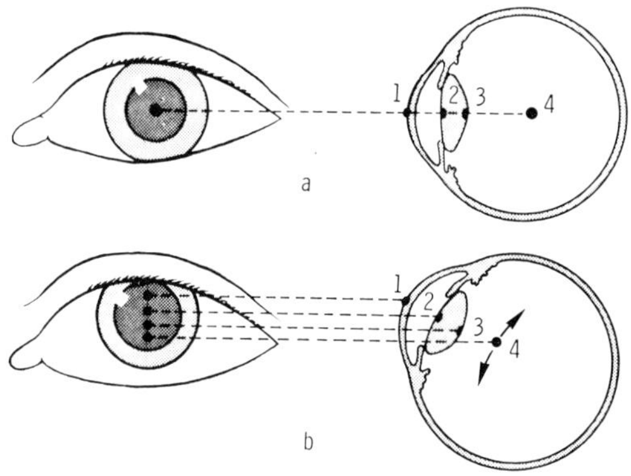

Fig. 21.1 Schematic representation of parallactic shift of opacities in the optical mediae
a) gaze straight ahead: opacities 1, 2, 3, and 4 cover one another;
b) gaze to the side: corneal opacity (1) anterior to the pupillary plane moves in the direction of gaze while opacity (3) at the posterior pole of the lens moves in the opposite direction. Opacity (2) which is in the pupillary plane stands still. Opacity (4) in the vitreous has an undulating motion.

Even without a slit lamp the *location of ocular opacities* can be determined by parallax (Fig. 21.1). Opacities anterior to the pupillary plane move in the same direction, those posterior to the pupillary plane opposite to the direction of movement of the eye. Vitreous opacities also have an independent floating movement.
Lens opacities appear gray with oblique illumination and black in light reflected from the fundus.

Pathogenesis of Cataracts

Differentiation of cataract types allows a correlation to their *pathogenesis* (Pau and Graeber 1969):

1. *New formations*, specifically malformation, of lens fibers-epithelium: membranous cataract, capsular cataracts, white riders in zonular cataract, new tissue formation in siderosis lentis

2. *Aging* of lens protein: primarily gray or brown nuclear sclerosis

3. Age related, *mechanical* disruption of structures (between cortex and nucleus) results in water clefts: typical gray cataract of age

4. Opacification through *increased water entering from the outside*
a) generalized *damage of the cation pump:* subcapsular cataracts, permeability cataracts, cataracta complicata, intumescent cataracts, secondary gray nuclear cataracts
b) *temporary* generalized *disruption of the cation* pump: congenital cataracts of the fetal nucleus, lamellar cataracts, traumatic rosettes
c) *Disruption of the cation pump* limited in time and area: Glaucomflecken, post-traumatic late

rosettes, coronal cataracts, circumscribed congenital cataracts
5. *Deposition* in the lens: connective and fatty tissue (after injury to the capsule), cholesterol, calcium, copper (chalcosis), gold (chrysosis), mercury, silver (argyrosis), iron (siderosis), phenothiazine.

Subjective Symptoms with Cataracts

Subjective symptoms of cataracts are primarily blurred or unclear vision. Monocular diplopia or multiple images may be seen. Photophobia and dazzling are present. In twilight the patient may see better because pupillary dilatation allows him to see around the opacity.

Acquired Cataracts

Stages of opacification — Nuclear cataract — Senile cataract — Metabolic cataract — Cataracta complicata — Transient refractive errors — Intumescent cataract — Cholesterol crystals in the lens — Coronary cataract — Phenothiazine deposition.

Stages of Opacification

Incipient cataract is a simple clouding of the lens; in premature cataract a red fundus reflex can be seen; in mature cataracts the opaque lens no longer allows the red fundus reflex to be seen; in hypermature cataract the brown nucleus sinks in the liquefied cortex (Morgagnian cataract) (Plate XVIII, Fig. 1, page 224 b); in intumescent cataract the lens is swollen with the appearance of mother of pearl.

Frequency of various types of senile cataract

Percentage of occurrence in 1,000 senile cataracts: typical gray senile opacity (supranuclear cataract) 23 percent, permeability cataract (subcapsular cataract) 36 percent, gray nuclear cataract 37 percent, brown nuclear cataract 5 percent, mature cataract 4 percent, hypermature cataract 1 percent, intumescent cataract 11 percent. These types of cataract were seen in various combinations.

A frequent combination is a dense permeability cataract (supcapsular cataract) with a dense gray nuclear opacity. The typical gray senile cataract (supranuclear cataract) is usually associated with a clear nucleus. In contrast a brown-black nuclear opacity (cat. brunescence-negra) is usually associated with a clear cortex (Pau 1976).

Nuclear Cataract

Brown and *gray nuclear cataracts* must be differentiated. A brown nucleus (cataracta brunescens, rubra, nigra) (Plate XVIII, Fig. 2, page 224 b) is an aging process. It occurs with old age, high myopia, chronic iridocyclitis, absolute glaucoma, etc. Brunescense of the lens develops slowly over many years. At first, vision loss may be minimal (biochemical changes, see Pau and Graeber 1969).

Primary gray nuclear cataracts must be differentiated from *secondary gray nuclei* owing to absorbtion of fluid by the lens. The secondary gray nuclear opacity develops within a few months. It develops rapidly and is almost always associated with a subcapsular or permeability cataract (see page 240, Fig. 21.5).

Primary gray nuclear cataract is particularly common in myopes, with old perforating injuries, early syneresis of the vitreous, retinal detachment etc. The opacity develops slowly over years. Early gray nuclear cataract leads to lenticular myopia (5 to 10 diopters) and sometimes monocular diplopia owing to two (even triplopia from three) focal points of the lens. A primary gray nuclear cataract may become brunescent.

Simple nuclear sclerosis which increases with age and progresses very slowly may be present without clouding.

Senile Supranuclear Cortical Cataract

The most common senile cataracts are the typical cortical opacities. These begin as water clefts and lamellar separation. They appear supranuclearly but not subcapsularly as do cataracta complicata or permeability cataracts. In time, the clear water clefts accumulate opaque material and become gray fissures (Fig. 21.2) while the lamellar disruptions become gray cuneiform opacities (Fig. 21.3). As the opacification increases to a mature cataract, its origin as a supranuclear or a subcapsular cortical cataract can no longer be determined (Fig. 21.4). The gray supranuclear cortical cataract is an age-dependent occurrence which may appear as early as age 45. It has not as yet been reproduced experimentally. Typically, progression is slow over many months to years. Its etiology may be a mechanical disruption with accumulation of fluid between the sclerotic hard nucleus and the softer cortex. The relationship of cations to each other is essentially that of the normal clear lens (Pau and Leithäuser 1964).

Cataracta Complicata – Permeability (Subcapsular Cortical) Cataract

Subcapsular (not supranuclear as with cortical cataracts) gray or white vacuoles, tufts, and linear opacities develop. At first these lie centrally beneath the posterior (Fig. 21.5) and then beneath the anterior capsule. Later they extend beneath the entire capsule and into deeper cortical layers. Often there is a simultaneous gray opacification of the nucleus (Fig. 21.5). Once the cataract is mature it is no longer possible to tell if it began in the deep cortex (typical cortical cataract) or subcapsularly (permeability-cataract).

All experimental cataracts and those caused by blunt trauma are permeability cataracts.

In these forms of cataract, the physiologic permeability of the lens (high K^+, low Na^+ intra-

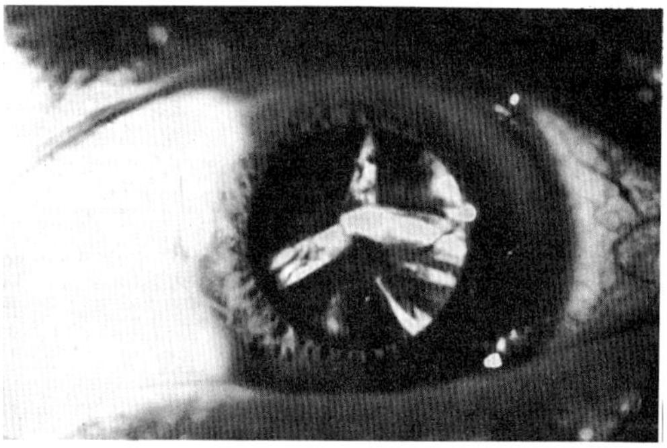

Fig. 21.2 Typical cortical opacities (supranuclear cataract) with gray fissures (♀ 60 yrs.)

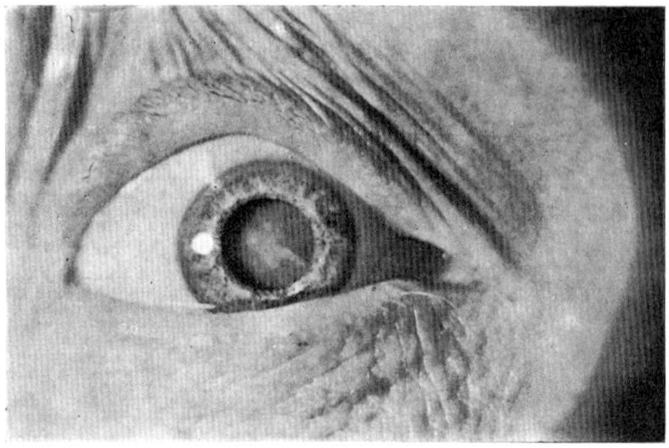

Fig. 21.4 Mature cataract with gray fissures

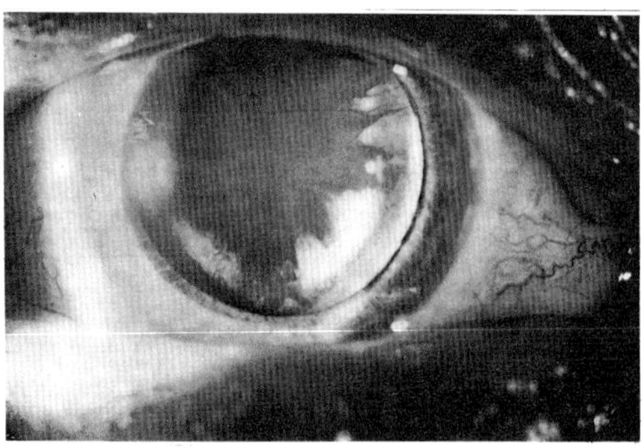

Fig. 21.3 Typical cortical cataract (supranuclear cataract) with cuneiform opacities (♀ 71 yrs.)

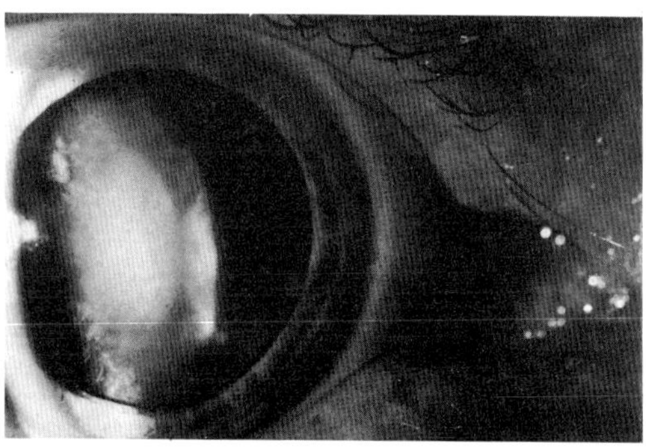

Fig. 21.5 Tufts of posterior and (minimal) anterior subcapsular opacities (permeability cataract and gray nuclear opacification) (♂ 63 yrs.)

lenticularly) is lost in the superficial layers of the lens. The electrolyte concentrations approximate those of the aqueous and vitreous, i.e., high Na^+, low K^+. The increased osmotic pressure (Gibbs-Donnan effect) results in increased fluid content and subcapsular opacities (Pau 1974; Pau and Graeber 1969; Pau et al. 1973).

Important causes of *permeability cataracts:*

Diabetes — Tetany, myotonia — Syndermatotic cataracts — Poisoning — Ocular diseases — Metabolic damage — Radiation damage — Heat, glassblower's cataract.

Diabetes: The incidence of cataract with diabetes mellitus varies in different reports between 1 and 10 percent (Heinsius and Arndt 1950). Diabetic cataracts have been seen as early as age 11 months (Fig. 21.6). As long as the fluid accumulation in a permeability cataract (for example with diabetes mellitus) is purely subcapsular, without molecular disruption, the opacity is reversible. Rapid normalization of metabolism may restore the electrolyte balance in the lens, allowing a return to the normal water content. Once denaturation of proteins has occurred the opacification is no longer reversible.
Purely senile cataracts (typical cortical, brunescent) appear more frequently and at an earlier age in diabetics.

Tetany, especially hypoparathyroid: serum calcium levels are lowered, resulting in muscular hyperirritability. This is demonstrated by tapping the facial nerve (Chvostek's phenomenon) as well as by Erb's and Trousseau's sign. Besides a permeability cataract, the lens diameter in tetanus may be smaller than normal.

Myotonic Dystrophy or the Curschmann-Steinert Syndrome
Subcapsular permeability cataracts develop in myotonic dystrophy but not in myotonia congenita of Thomsen. They are often associated with numerous, small, colored, punctate cholesterol crystals in the lens cortex (Plate XVIII, Fig. 3–5, page 224 b).

Syndermatotic Cataracts (Kugelberg 1934) appear in the third to fourth decade in disseminated neurodermatitis (late exudative eczema, endogenous eczema), in the fourth to fifth decade with scleroderma and by age two to six in Rothmund's syndrome (Huerkamp 1948).

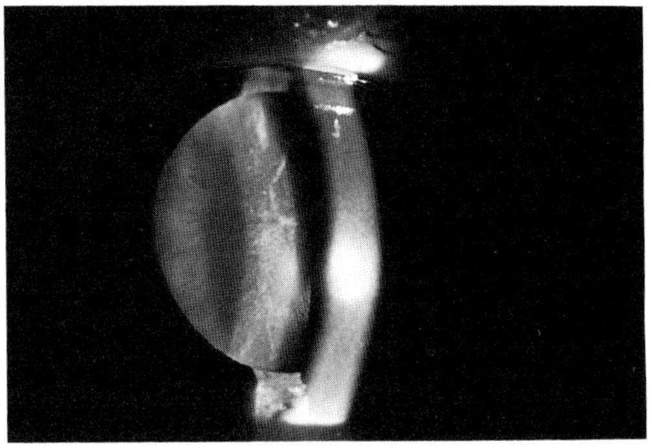

Fig. 21.6 Diabetic cataract: anterior and posterior subcapsular cataract (♂ 41 yrs.)

Werner's syndrome involves sclerodermatitis with loss of adipose tissue and muscle, de- or hyperpigmentation, endocrine dysfunctions and syndermatotic cataracts.
Rothmund's syndrome (poikiloderma atrophicans vasculare) (see page 247) includes bilateral cataracts and gonadal atrophy. Heredity is recessive (Rothmund 1968; Schnyder 1935; Siegrist 1928; Seefelder 1935; Vogt 1931) with consanguinity allegedly playing a special role. Endocrinologic findings are marked; they include brittle hair, sparse hair growth (Seefelder 1935; Siegrist 1928; Schnyder 1935), dwarfism, undescended testes, thyroid hypoplasia. The disease is rare and seen only in isolated, inbred (mountain) communities, There is no relationship to the poikiloderma of dermatomyositis.
With endogenous eczema, besides the typical posterior capsular cataracts, early central anterior capsular plaques may be seen.
Poisoning: With *ergotamine* poisoning, mature cataracts are alleged to develop within two to three months in children, and within eight to eleven months in adults. The validity of this claim is questionable.
Naphthaline and *thallium* cause cataracts in animals. *Dinitrophenol* and *dinitrocresol* (weight-reducing agents), as well as halogenated-hydrocarbons (chlorbenzol and dichlorbenzol) can cause cataracts. Concentrated acid instilled in the conjunctival sac, or bee or wasp venom injected into the eye may lead to cataract formation (Sautter 1960).

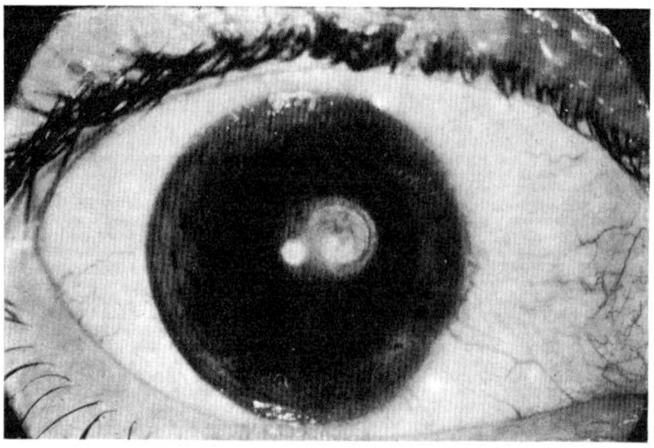

Fig. 21.7 Disciform posterior subcapsular opacity (radiation cataract) (♂ 29 yrs.)

Ocular Diseases: Subcapsular or permeability cataracts occur with iridocyclitis, retinitis pigmentosa, retinal detachment, and heterochromia complicata (Fuchs). Onchocercosis may also lead to cataracts. Cataracts can develop with varying rapidity in pulseless Takayasu's disease.

Of great importance are lens changes resulting from lowered pH (acidosis) (Pau and Augstein 1977).

Metabolic Damage: *Galactosemia* leads to cataract formation. Other findings in galactosemia include anemia, hepatosplenomegaly and mental retardation (Müller et al. 1967).

Bilateral cataracts are part of the *oculocerebrorenal syndrome* of Lowe, along with nystagmus, hydrophthalmos, strabismus, rickets, ketonuria, glycosuria, proteinuria and deficient ammonia excretion (see page 246).

Systemic corticosteroid therapy can cause posterior subcapsular plaques. High dosages must be given over some years (Crews 1963).

In animals, cataracts can be produced experimentally by *alloxan poisoning* (alloxan diabetes) and a *galactose* diet.

Radiation Cataracts: Cataracts may develop after irradiation of the eye. The latent period varies between two to ten months and eight years. The average time of onset is three years after radiation (Rohrschneider 1932). Minimal dosages claimed to produce cataracts range between 400 and 900 rads. Growing fetal and infant lenses are particularly susceptible. Among 520 Hiroshima survivors, 138 cases of radiation cataract were found, primarily among younger persons (Kandor 1956) (see page 354).

Radiation cataract begins with a round, gray posterior subcapsular cortical disk (Fig. 21.7) or an equivalent area of vacuoles (permeability cataract). The cortical opacification may then progress to involve the entire lens. Early radiation damage is less common but can result in a rapidly progressing cataract within a few days.

Glassblower's Cataract: Infrared radiation (heat) may cause a permeability cataract which is often associated with *exfoliation* of the *capsular lamellae* (Plate XVIII, Fig. 6, page 224 b) (not to be confused with *senile pseudoexfoliation* [see page 251]). *Electric-lightning* cataract should be mentioned here. High voltage or lightning injuries may result in cataracta electrica. These appear after two to eight months, rarely immediately or years after the injury.

Transient Refractive Errors

(see page 26)

Transient refractive errors are a precataractous sign and represent changes in the refractive power of the lens. These result from an increase in the refractive index of the lens (Granström 1933), changes in colloidal status (Braun 1937) and variations in the degree of hydration of the lens (Pau 1954). Lenticular hydration, owing to permeability changes at the lens surface from metabolic damage, increases the curvature of the lens causing myopia. The myopia is reversible if the metabolic upset is corrected. The most common cause of such transient myopia is poorly controlled diabetes, fluid and electrolyte imbalance with diarrhea, influenza, typhus and similar disorders, as well as sulfonamide, salicylate and arsphenamine (Salvarsan) therapy. Insulin administration may cause the converse picture of a transient hyperopia.

Intumescent Cataract

The entire lens (Fig. 21.8) is opaque and swollen with the blue-white appearance of mother of pearl. This is caused by a relatively rapid collapse of the normal permeability of the lens with ingress of water. It can occur within

hours and represents the most severe form of permeability cataract.
Intumescence is part of any rapidly appearing permeability cataract (see page 240) or lens perforation. Sudden appearance of an intumescent cataract has been reported after renal dialysis (Straub and Freund 1970).

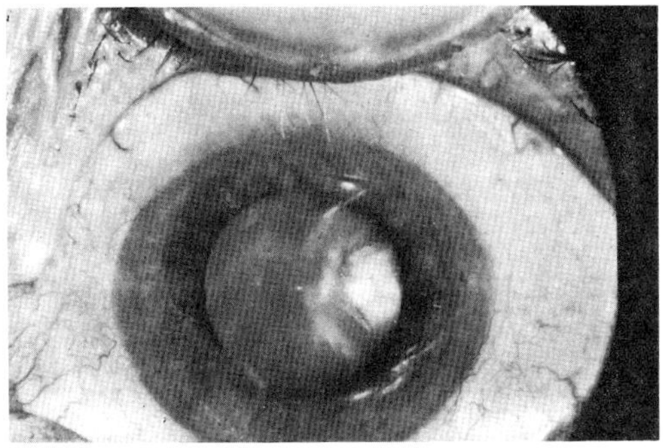

Fig. 21.8 Intumescent cataract (♀ 75 yrs.)

Cholesterol Crystals

Small yellow-red-green-blue *shimmering* crystals (usually cholesterol) which glisten like "Christmas tree ornaments" (Plate XIX, Fig. 1, page 224 c) are sometimes found in the senile lens.

Coronary Cataract

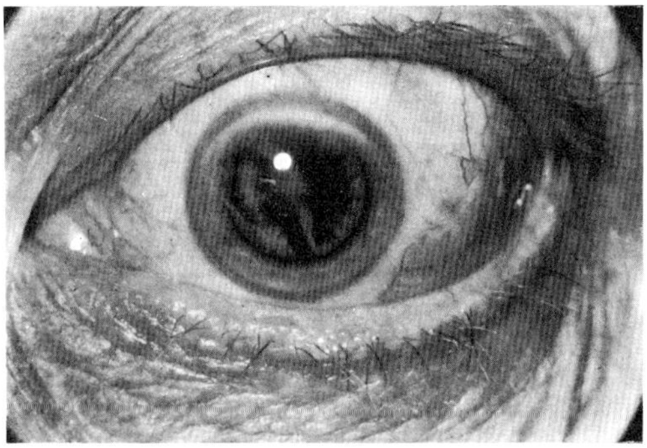

Fig. 21.9 Cataracta coronaria with numerous clublike equatorial opacities (in addition typical gray senile cataract with spoke-shaped opacities)

Coronary cataracts appear at or after puberty in some 20 to 25 percent of the population. Club shaped opacities are arranged like a crown in the peripheral inner and outer cortical layers where they bend around the equator (Fig. 21.9, Plate XIX, Fig. 2, page 224 c). Since they are peripheral they do not obstruct vision and can only be seen after pupillary dilatation. With age these can extend into the cortex as water clefts. Coronary opacities are thought to be caused by transient damage to the lens surface (with entry of fluid) by the tug of zonules at their insertions to the lens (Pau 1961).

Phenothiazine Deposition

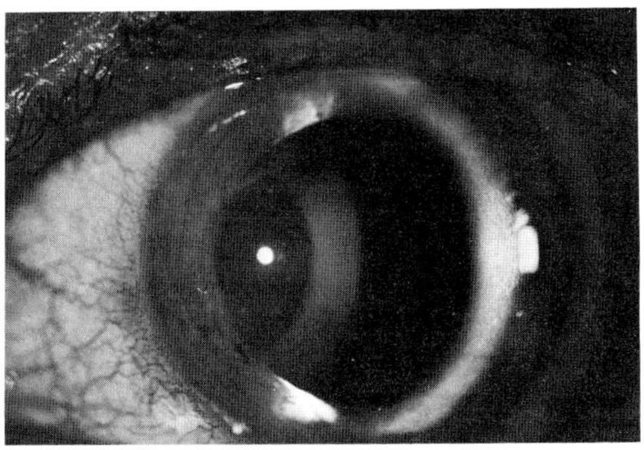

Fig. 21.10 Dense subcapsular and capsular discoloration following Valium use (♀ 53 yrs.) (Klin. Mbl. Augenheilk. 164, [1974] 447.)

After *phenothiazine* administration some eight percent of patients develop brown pigmentation in the interpalpebral conjunctiva. Brown, yellow and white dots appear in the corneal stroma and endothelial layer, particularly in the interpalpebral fissure area. Yellow-brown granules appear superficially (capsule, subcapsular) in the center of the lens in a star-shaped or disklike pattern. (Pau 1976). (Fig. 21.10). Retinal pigmentation appears in the form of pseudoretinitis pigmentosa (Mathalone 1967) (see page 291).

Congenital Cataracts

Congenital cataracts are usually *zonular* (lamellar). The *white zonular* cataract lies beneath a layer of clear cortex (Fig. 21.11). It takes the form of a central nuclear opacity or concentric sheet often surrounded by white bands called riders (Fig. 21.12). These riders probably represent newly formed lens fibers (Pau 1964). A *pulverulent cataract* is a variant of zonular (lamellar) cataracts.

Variants of congenital cataracts include incomplete lamellar cataracts, punctate cataracts, thin irregular sheets (dilacerated cataract) and crystal deposits. The variable clinical appearance of congenital cataracts is reflected in their many names (Vogt 1931): laurel-branchlike (Fig. 21.13) flowerlike (cat. floriformis) (Fig. 21.14) fishlike (cat. pisciformis) (Fig. 21.10), ring-shaped, fleck, spearlike, spiraliform, threadlike, flat-ragged-fenestrated (cat. dilacerata). The opacities are limited to the lens nucleus (embryonal or senile) and may be multicolored, ranging from blue to blue-green to gray.

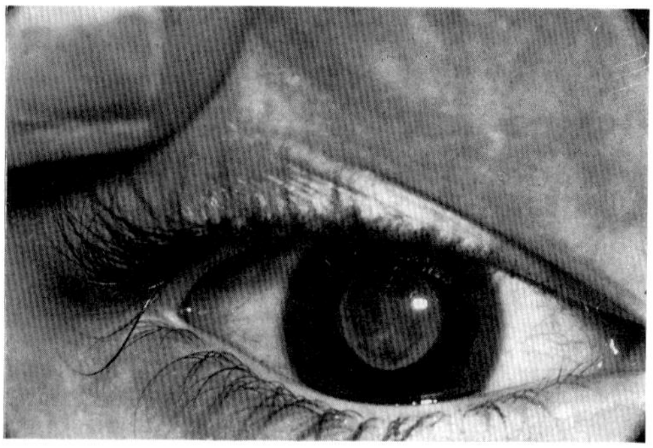

Fig. 21.11 Zonular (lamellar) cataract (♂ 5 yrs.)

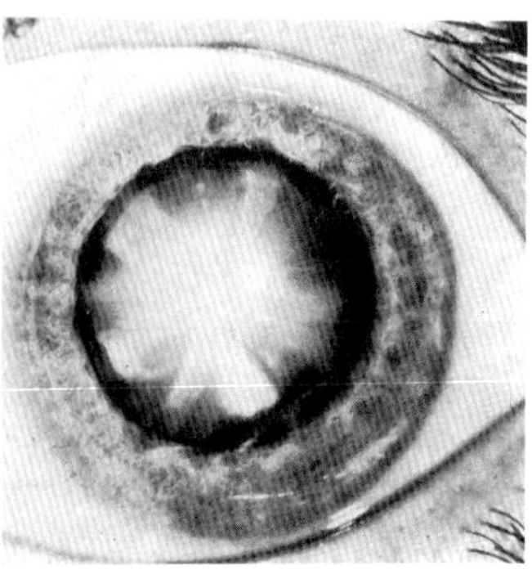

Fig. 21.12 Lamellar cataract with "riders" (♀ 19 yrs.)

Congenital zonular cataracts are usually associated with varying degrees of amblyopia. Many lamellar cataracts can be considered a form of permeability cataract. Damage during embryonic development caused lens opacities which were later surrounded by clear, newly formed lens fibers. With time, the original opacities end up deep within the lens. The precise, often hereditary, metabolic disturbance that is present at a specific time in embryonic development cannot usually be ascertained.

Heredity — Embryopathies — Galactose cataract — Congenital cataracts in various syndromes — Chromosomal aberrations — Congenital syndermatotic cataracts — Congenital brunescent lamellar sheets — Membranous cataracts — Pseudophakia, vascular, fibrous, adipose calcification, bone formation — Cerulean cataract — Sutural (stellate) cataract — Capsular cataract — Polar cataract.

Heredity

The most common etiology of zonular cataracts is genetic. Central concentric sheets of opacities with overlying bands or "riders" were observed by Marner (1949) over eight successive generations. It is generally difficult to determine if the lamellar cataract is congenital or caused by exogenous noxious agents (Meesmann 1942).

Congenital cataracts may be associated with polydactyly, syndactyly or tapetoretinal degeneration. Oxycephaly has an associated cataract besides the optic atrophy and exophthalmos.

Embryopathies

The etiology of cataracts is more obvious in the embryopathies (see page 54). There is a phase-specific reaction to a variety of noxious stimuli depending on the gestational stage. Blastopathies occur in the first 14 days. After differentiating into embryoblasts and trophoblasts, embryopathies occur. Fetopathies develop after the third month of gestation. Besides hereditary factors there are exogenous noxious agents: mechanical-physical and chemical, metabolite deficiencies, serologic incompatibility and infectious organisms (Goerttler 1964).

Virus infections — Syphilis — Toxoplasmosis — Diabetes — Hypocalcemia — Thalidomide — Radiation damage to the embryo.

Virus Infections: Virus infections of the mother which cause congenital cataracts in the infant usually occur within the first three months of pregnancy. Common viruses are *rubella* (40 to 60 percent), *mumps* (16 to 22 percent) and *Hepatitis* (16 percent). *Measles, poliomyelitis, epidemic encephalitis, herpes zoster, varicella, variola,* and *infectious mononucleosis* are less common (Froewis and Plattner 1956; François 1959).
Virus infections in the second half of the pregnancy apparently do not affect the lens.

Some 10 percent of human congenital malformations are probably related to viral embryopathies. During the second month of gestation, where susceptibly is high, the risk of malformation with a viral infection declines from 30 to 50 percent at the beginning, to 10 to 15 percent at the end of the month. The peak risk (occurrence) of malformation (including the eye) is from the third to eighth week (Goerttler 1964).
With congenital *rubella* the significant findings are (François 1959, 1963; Lindström 1962; Velaszquez 1963): cataracts (40 to 60 percent), *microphthalmos* (unilateral), *pseudoretinitis pigmentosa* (Franceschetti and Bourquin 1946), *inner ear deafness* (50 percent), *congenital heart defects* (50 percent), *brachymicrocephaly* (rare), *dental malformations, spina bifida, gastrointestinal occlusion,* and *mental retardation* (Nick 1953; Emerson 1958; Töndury 1952; Agarwal and Raizada 1954; Budolfsen 1956). Ophthalmic findings also include glaucoma, posterior synechiae, iris atrophy, anophthalmos, corneal clouding, nystagmus and strabismus (Alfano 1966).

Congenital Syphilis: This may cause a typical brown, supranuclear cortical cataract affecting the surface layer of the fetal nucleus (see page 249).
Congenital Toxoplasmosis: Of the parasitic infestations the one most commonly causing congenital cataracts is toxoplasmosis. These eyes are usually microphthalmic with persistent pupillary membranes.
Diabetes, Hypocalcemia: Congenital cataracts can occur when the mother has diabetes during pregnancy. Congenital cataracts may also occur when the *mother* is markedly *hypocalcemic (hypophosphatasia, hypoparathyroidism).*
Thalidomide: *Thalidomide ingestion* 28 to 40 days after conception causes widespread malformations only rarely including cataracts (Wiedemann 1961; Lena and Knapp 1962; Cullen 1967). Papst (1964) found *motility problems* when ingestions was on days 35 to 39 whereas days 40 to 42 were associated with *microphthalmos* and *anophthalmos* usually accompanied by phocomelia. The motility problems included *abducens paresis,* rarely *oculomotor nerve paresis* (with facial nerve paresis), *horizontal gaze paresis* and *Duane's syndrome.* Abducens nerve paresis (potentially with facial nerve paresis) was usually present whenever the ears were malformed (Papst 1964; Miehlke and Partsch 1963; J.G.H. Schmidt 1964). *Retinal and choroidal colobomas* have been observed in thalidomide embryopathy (Honegger and Pape 1964).

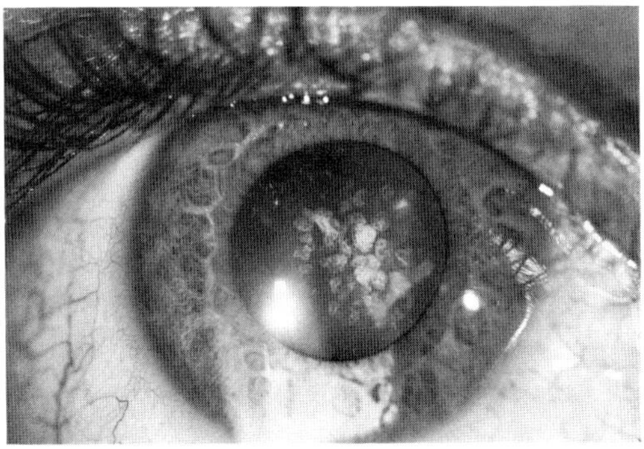

Fig. 21.13 Congenital blue nuclear and coronary opacity resembling a laurel wreath. (♀ 67 yrs.)

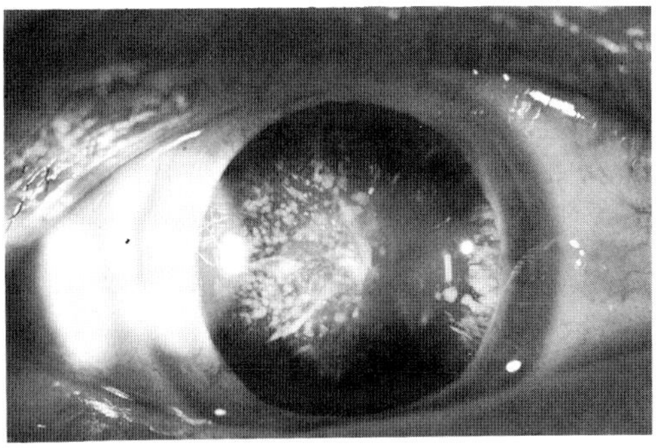

Fig. 21.14 Floriform cataract. Congenital nuclear opacity resembling flowers. (♀ 17 yrs.)

Radiation of the Embryo: Direct radiation of the embryo (over 500 rad) within the first few months of gestation results in severe congenital malformations of the nervous system, eye, skeleton, and urogenital system. The most dangerous period is during the third to tenth week of gestation. Ocular malformations include: microphthalmos, congenital cataracts and a picture similar to retinitis pigmentosa (François et al. 1962). After the third month, malformations caused by radiation are less common and less severe.

Galactose Cataract

Glactosemia (Galactosuria) is a hereditary metabolic disorder which causes cataracts (lack of galactose-l-phosphate-uridyl-transferase).

These are not truly congenital cataracts but are acquired early as cortical vacuoles, lamellar opacities and, finally, total white-gray clouding. This may appear within the first few days to weeks of life. Galactose cataracts appeared before age three months in 60 percent and during the first month in 36 percent of cases. Other findings include hepatomegaly, cirrhosis, icterus, galactosuria, albuminuria, digestive disorders, dwarfism, mental retardation, and recessive inheritance (Johnson 1953; Patz 1953). Galactose cataracts can also result from **galactokinase deficiency** without systemic findings.

Congenital Cataracts in Various Syndromes

Lowe's syndrome — Congenital hemolytic icterus — Mandibulo-oculo-facial dysmorphia (Hallermann-Streiff) — Craniofacial dysostosis (Crouzon) — Sjögren's syndrome — Marinesco-Sjögren syndrome — Sjögren-Larsson syndrome — Ehlers-Danlos syndrome — Osteogenesis imperfecta (Lobstein syndrome) — Congenital stippled epiphyses (Conradi-Hühnermann syndrome) — Alport syndrome — Osteodystrophic fibrosis (Albright's syndrome).

Lowe's Syndrome: The oculocerebrorenal syndrome includes *congenital cataract, congenital glaucoma,* nystagmus, buphthalmos and iris atrophy. There is hyperaminoaciduria and glycosuria, albuminuria, osteomalacia and generalized debility. The renal tubules and glomeruli are affected causing renal rickets, muscular atrophy-hypotony and growth retardation. Heredity is sex-linked recessive (Trautmann 1964; Jacoby and Tympner 1966; Haut and Joanides 1966).

Congenital hemolytic icterus includes icterus, splenomegaly and anemia with congenital cataracts, and rarely microphthalmos and heterochromia of the iris.

Hallermann-Streiff Syndrome, also called bird facies or mandibulo-oculo-facial dysmorphia (see page 332), includes dyscephaly, anomalous dentition, atrophy of the skin, microphthalmos and congenital cataracts.

Craniofacial dysostosis (Crouzon) (see page 334) may develop cataracts.

Sjögren's Syndrome: oligophrenia with congenital cataracts (lamellar, total or posterior pole), ectopia lentis, nystagmus; potentially microphthalmos, keratoconus, megalocornea and strabismus. Heredity is autosomal recessive.

Marinesco-Sjögren's Syndrome: In addition to Sjögren's syndrome there is mental retardation, cataracts, spinocerebellar ataxia and potentially skeletal anomalies.

Sjögren-Larssen Syndrome includes congenital cataract, mental deficiency, spastic ataxia and ichthyosis.

Ehlers-Danlos Syndrome: Cutis laxa, hyperelastosis of the skin (Indian rubber man syndrome): elastic, excess skin folds on the lids, epicanthus, subluxated lenses, cataract.

Lobstein's Syndrome (osteogenesis imperfecta tarda): Fragility of the bones, blue sclera, otosclerosis, hyperextensible joints, occasional cataract; dominant heredity.

Congenital Stippled Epiphyses (Conradi-Hühnermann syndrome, *fetal calcinosis, chondrodystrophia calcificans congenita punctata)* is a hereditary disorder with generalized debility, and retarded growth of long bones owing to punctate calcific epiphyseal deposits that are visible rachographically. Cataracts are found in 50 percent of cases. Heredity is recessive or dominant. Death usually occurs before age two.

Alport syndrome is a familial nephritis of variable inheritance. Ocular findings include cataracts and anterior lenticonus. Hematuria, pyelonephritis and deafness are further findings.

Albright's syndrome *(fibrous osteodystrophy)* may include cerulean cataracts, exophthalmos and optic atrophy.

Chromosomal Aberrations

(see page 329)

Mongoloid idiocy (Down's syndrome, Trisomy-21) is associated with a variety of different lens opacities.
Trisomy 13–15 (Patau syndrome): These children usually survive for only a few weeks; ocular findings include: microphthalmos, cataract, retinal dysplasia, iris-ciliary body colobomata (Heinemann 1963). Trisomy 16–18 (Edward's syndrome) (see page 329) may include cataracts, optic atrophy and secondary glaucoma.
Turner's syndrome with pterygium colli (webbed neck): Congenital cataracts may be present. Other findings are: hyperelasticity of the skin (cutis laxa), lymphangiectatic edema, mental retardation, paralytic strabismus and facial paresis. The genotype is XO chromatin negative (see page 330).

Congenital Syndermatotic Cataracts

Syndermatotic congenital cataracts include (François 1959):
infantile poikiloderma (Zinsser-Thomson) or Rothmund's syndrome,
congenital dyskeratosis (Schäfer's syndrome),
congenital ichthyosis,
congenital ectodermal dysplasia (Siemen's syndrome), and incontinentia pigmenti.

Infantile poikiloderma, Rothmund's syndrome — Palmoplantar keratosis, Schäfer's syndrome — Congenital ichthyosis — Siemens' syndrome — Incontinentia pigmenti.

Infantile poikiloderma, Rothmund's syndrome: Werner's syndrome begins after puberty but *Rothmund's syndrome* (page 241) becomes manifest between the third and sixth months of age with skin eruptions leading to sclerosis and scarring, pigment dispersion and telangiectasias. Cataracts develop over a few weeks or months during the second to fourth year of life. Hypogonadism is present.

Palmoplantar keratosis: *Schäfer's syndrome* is a combination of congenital cataracts and dyskeratosis: There is palmoplantar keratosis along with disseminated follicular hyperkeratosis of the skin, hyperhidrosis, pachyonychia, and developmental retardation. Heredity is autosomal dominant.
Congenital Ichthyosis: Congenital ichthyosis or congenital ichthyform erythrodermia of Bocq demonstrates diffuse erythema and hyperkeratosis, especially around joints, palms and soles of the feet. Congenital cataracts are common.
Siemens' Syndrome: Findings are congenital cataracts with dermal hypoplasia. Recessive heredity.
Incontinentia Pigmenti (Bloch-Sulzberger, see page 293): Pigmented spots and stripes appear on the skin either congenitally, within the first few weeks of life or, rarely, at a later date. One-fourth of patients develop pseudogliomas with optic atrophy and strabismus; congenital cataracts are more common. One-fourth of patients have dental anomalies and another fourth develop alopecia. Heredity is X-linked and lethal to male embryos so that only females are affected. Female carriers may show retinal vascular anomalies.
Congenital brunescent lamellar cataracts are supranuclear after chorioretinitis which occurs in utero or within the first years of life (Remler 1952; Dubler 1960). When the cataract occurs only posteriorly (Plate XIX, Fig. 4, page 224 c), congenital lues is particularly suspect.

Membranous Cataract

A membranous cataract is a more or less thin membranous capsular lens remaining after aspiration of the lens mass, absorption of cortex, following rupture of the capsule, after intraocular inflammation or with persistent hyperplastic primary vitreous (see page 234).

Pseudophakia, Calcification, Ossification

Following a tear in the lens capsule, vascularized connective tissue ingrowth (may be congenital) leads to a *vascular cataract*. Rarely the lens will *calcify*, even *ossify*.

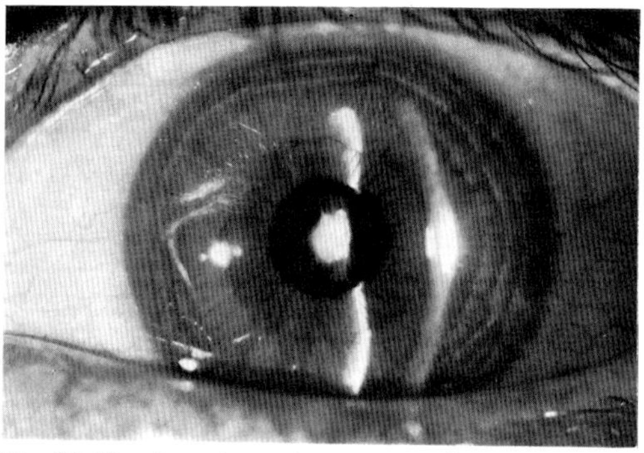

Fig. 21.15 Anterior polar cataract (♂ 25 yrs.)

Pseudophakia with the lens replaced by *fibrous* or *adipose* tissue occurs as a congenital malformation. Such fibrous or lipomatous pseudophakia always appears in conjunction with a persistent hyaloid membrane (Rintelen and Staufenegger 1957). Usually there is persistence of hyperplastic primary vitreous (see page 234). The term is also used for patients with an intraocular lens implant after cataract surgery.

Cerulean Cataract

Cerulean cataracts consists of thin blue or blue-green rings or sheets which, unlike coronary cataract, are not in the peripheral cortex but in the adult nucleus. Cerulean cataracts are often associated with coronary cataracts beginning at puberty. Cerulean cataracts and stellate (sutural) cataracts are often found in Down's syndrome.

Sutural Cataracts

Congenital sutural cataracts (anterior, axial embryonic cataracts or stellate cataracts) are common and usually do not affect vision (Plate XIX, Fig. 3, page 224 c).

Capsular Cataract

Capsular cataract — Anterior polar cataract — Posterior polar cataract.

Capsular Cataract: These are small, white, slightly prominent opacities at the anterior capsule. Capsular cataracts are congenital and are caused by adhesion of the pupillary membrane. They may also follow embryonal intraocular inflammation. They may be acquired as slowly developing permeability cataracts (for example syndermatotic cataracts), with age, perforating injuries or hypermature cataract.

Polar Cataracts: *Anterior polar* cataracts (Fig. 21.15) are small, white, anteriorly located prominences. In essence they are a form of capsular cataract. Histologically capsular cataracts consist of connective tissue metaplasia and reactive hyperplasia of the lens epithelium (Pau and Caesar 1967). In polarizing microscopy the newly formed tissue is birefringent.

Posterior polar cataracts are far more rare than anterior ones. There may be an association with the insertion of the fetal or persistent hyaloid artery.

Color Changes

During youth the lens is colorless and transparent. With increasing age it becomes yellow-brown, accounting in part for the age-dependent loss of sensitivity for blue.

Increasing brown coloration leads to *brunescent cataracts* (see page 239; Plate XVIII, Fig. 2, page 224 b).

The rapidly developing intumescent cataract (see page 242) is swollen and has a mother of pearl (Fig. 21.8) blue-white color.

Early in the development of *cataracta complicata*, specifically *permeability cataract*, the shagreen of the posterior lens capsule becomes more prominent and develops a multicolored sheen (reflection from thin plaques). These progress to typical posterior plaques.

Calcium deposition can cause the lens to be pure white (Fig. 21.16).

Myotonic cataracts (see page 241) can have multiple, small, red-green-blue *cholesterol crystals* in the lens cortex.

Colorful glistening cholesterol crystals reminiscent of Christmas tree ornaments (see page 243) may deposit in the lens nucleus of older patients. These are usually but not necessarily associated with other senile opacities.

Congenital *cerulean cataract* (see page 248) has thin blue or green rings or sheets in the region of the adult nucleus; in addition coronary cataracts commonly occur later.

The congenital *stellate cataract* often *looks blue* but is usually more white-gray.

The congenital or early acquired brown zonular cataract is usually located in the peripheral zone of the embryonic nucleus. Congenital syphilis is likely when the opacity is limited to the posterior part of the lens. Chorioretinitis of different etiology should be considered when the brunescent zonular cataract occurs both at the anterior and posterior borders of the embryonal nucleus (see page 247).

Sunflower cataracts are blue-green and are just subcapsular (Plate XX, Fig. 1, page 224 d). Their etiology is either an intraocular foreign body containing copper or Wilson's disease. A Kayser-Fleischer ring may be present in either case. *A yellow sunflower cataract* is seen with intraocular gold deposition (chrysiasis) (see page 250). Brown subcapsular spots associated with increasing subcapsular plaques, brown discoloration of the iris, and retinal damage occur in siderosis (Plate XIX, Fig. 6, page 224 c) resulting from intraocular foreign bodies containing iron (see page 250).

Prolonged *phenothiazine therapy* can cause *yellow-brown granular subcapsular* deposits, as well as corneal and conjunctival pigment deposition and pseudoretinitis pigmentosa (see page 243). The lenticular pigment granules are subcapsular in the pupillary zone. The deposits may be ring-shaped or concentrated along suture lines. They appear to be reversible (Heermans 1972). *Contusion injury* to the eye can result in a ring of iris pigment impressed onto the anterior lens capsule (Vossius' ring, see below). Vascular ingrowth after rupture of the capsule (*vascular cataract* see page 247) appears *gray-red*. A hypermature cataract may contain numerous mobile cholesterol crystals. Colored gold cholesterol crystals resembling "Christmas tree" decorations (Plate XIX, Fig. 1, page 224 c) may appear in a senile lens. A congenital *lipoid pseudolens* (see page 248) has a *yellow-white* appearance.

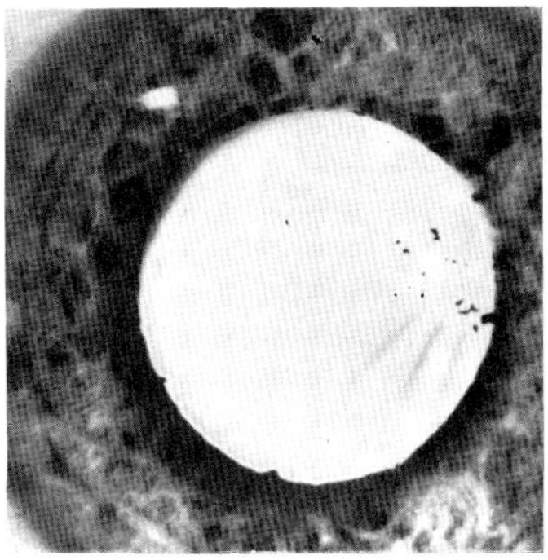

Fig. 21.16 Calcification of the lens (♂ 14 yrs.)

Traumatic Cataracts

Vossius' ring — Posttraumatic late rosettes — Perforation rosette, phacogenic ophthalmia — Glaucomflecken — Siderosis lentis — Sunflower cataract — Aftercataract.

Vossius' Ring

This is nothing more than the imprint of iris pigment epithelium on the lens after blunt trauma (Plate XIX, Fig. 5, page 224 c). The size of the ring depends on the width of the pupil at the time of injury. The ring disappears within a few days.

Capsular tears are rare with blunt trauma.

Posttraumatic Late Rosette, Contusion Rosette

This appears under the anterior and, rarely, also beneath the posterior lens capsule after severe blunt trauma to the eye. Usually only part of a rosette forms. The gray areas lie *between the lens sutures* (Fig. 21.17) and after a few weeks to months turn a sharply demarcated white. With time, as new clear lens fibers are deposited over the opacity, it recedes into the lens but remains sharply defined. Visual loss is usually minimal. Histologically, these opacities consist of tubules and vacuoles filled with a homogeneous substance (Pau 1974).

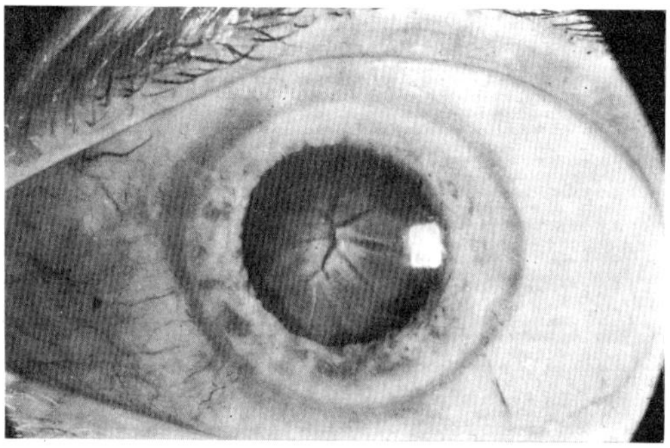

Fig. 21.17 Posttraumatic late rosette (♂ 60 yrs.)

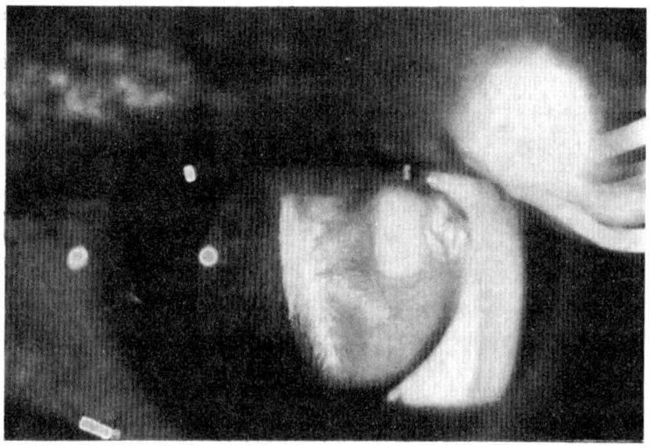

Fig. 21.18 Perforation rosette of the lens; feathery opacities along suture lines beneath the posterior capsule

Perforation Rosette

These are feathery opacities corresponding to lens sutures beneath the posterior lens capsule independent of the lens perforation site (Fig. 21.18). The rosettes are composed of small fluid-filled vacuoles and disappear within a few weeks if a small perforation site manages to close itself. If lens protein has been released, usually after injury, and additional noxious agents (foreign protein adjuvants, infection, etc.) are superimposed, a chronic inflammation (phakogenic reaction, phakogenetic ophthalmia) occurs (Irvine and Irvine 1952; H. Müller 1953/54) (see page 200).

Glaucomflecken

Glaucomflecken (cataracta glaucomatosa disseminata subepithelialis acuta, Vogt) appear after an acute glaucoma attack. They are small, round or oval, amoeboid, gray-white spots under the anterior capsule. Ultimately these are displaced deeper into the lens as new, clear lens fibers are superimposed.

Siderosis of the Lens

Perforation and intraocular retention of foreign body containing iron results in siderosis lentis (foreign bodies containing copper cause *chalcosis lentis).*

Siderosis lentis leads to circumscribed, brown, subcapsular spots (Figs. 21.19, 21.20, Plate XIX, Fig. 6, page 224 c) and increasing subcapsular (permeability) cataracts. Histologically, iron-containing connective tissue is present in the area of the brown spots (capsular cataract) (Pau 1976). Siderosis of the iris (see page 193) and retina also occur. Retinal siderosis may simulate retinitis pigmentosa.

Sunflower Cataract

Chalcosis of the lens leads to a bluish *sunflower cataract* (Plate XX, Fig. 1, page 224 d). Copper is deposited particularly where the iris rests against the lens. Chalcosis lentis can regress without sequelae (no permeability cataract) once the copper foreign body is removed from the eye.

The same sort of sunflower cataract can be seen in Wilson's disease, along with a Kayser-Fleischer corneal ring (Rix 1965).

Intraocular *gold (chrysiasis), mercury* (Abrams 1964; Rosen 1950 b) and *silver* (argyrosis) (Rosen 1950 a) can produce similar sunflower cataracts.

Aftercataract

Aftercataracts of varying thickness may remain following lens injury, extracapsular cataract extraction, or spontaneous reabsorption of the lens. Regenerating lens fiber remnants can cause Soemmering rings.

Senile Pseudoexfoliation

In *senile pseudoexfoliation* a gray-white material lies in powdery granules, flakes or shredded sheets on the lens capsule, especially in the pupillary region and lens periphery (Fig. 21.19). Similar dandrufflike material collects on the iris margin, iris stroma and chamber angle. Glaucoma is frequently present, presumably caused by blockage of outflow channels by the exfoliated material. Bertelsen et al. (1964) call the condition "fibrillopathia epithelio capsularis" because lens epithelium fibrils seemingly extend through the lens capsule into the anterior cortex. Benedikt (1973) believes the exfoliated material is produced directly at its location.

Pseudoexfoliation of the lens is not to be confused with true exfoliation of the zonular lamella from the anterior lens capsule (see page 242) (glassblowers' cataract). True exfoliation resembles a glassy membrane peeling from the anterior capsule.

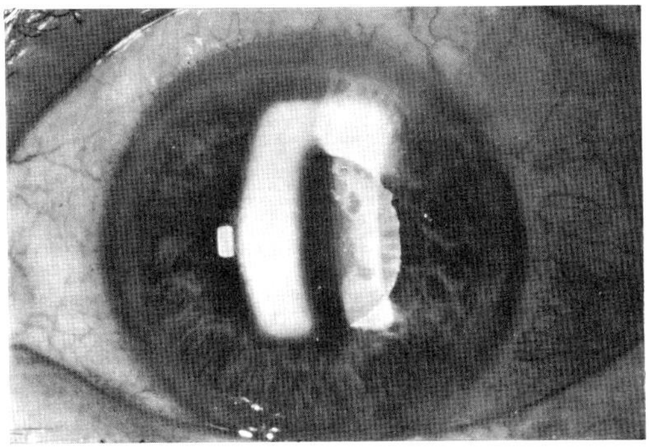

Fig. 21.19 Pseudoexfoliation of the anterior lens capsule

Changes in Shape or Location of the Lens

Spherophakia, microphakia — Subluxation, ectopia lentis — Posterior luxation — Anterior luxation — Lenticonus, coloboma of the lens — Aphakia.

Spherophakia, Microphakia

Spherophakia, or microphakia resulting from partial absence, weakness or elongation of the zonules produces a refractive myopia. Congenital subluxation (i.e., ectopia, Fig. 21.20) of the small lens is usually present. Frequently the lens is flattened, even colobomatous in the area of the missing zonules. *Ectopia lentis* rarely appears without spherophakia. It is a frequent finding in dystrophia ectodermalis congenita hypoplastica (arachnodactyly: Marfan's syndrome) and in the less common Marchesani's syndrome (dystrophia mesodermalis congenita hyperplastica, brachymorphia with spherophakia). The small lenses are frequently eccentric (ectopia lentis), often luxating into the vitreous, potentially causing glaucoma and retinal detachment. The luxation may follow trauma.

In addition to their above average height and long, delicate bones, *Marfan* patients have a paucity of subcutaneous fat and a poorly developed musculature. There is dolichocephaly with long, narrow, masklike facies. The spinal column and narrow breast cage are often deformed. Cardiac defects are common. The pupils may be miotic and difficult to dilate. The lenses in Marfan's syndrome are bilaterally dislocated upwards.

Besides dislocated lenses, arachnodactyly is an important finding in Marfan's syndrome (Weve 1931). The disorder has been described in monozygotic twins (Becker 1935; Schwarzweller 1937) and Negroes (Gilston 1955). Heredity is dominant or occasionally recessive.

Homocystinuria (see page 364) has to be con-

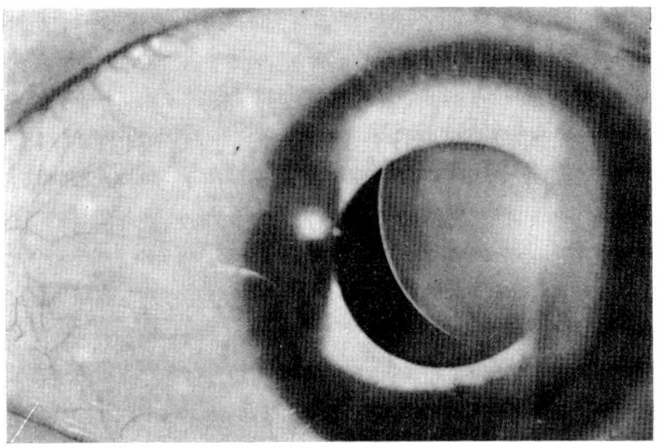

Fig. 21.20 Microphakia, spherophakia, ectopia lentis in Marfan's syndrome (♀ 17 yrs.)

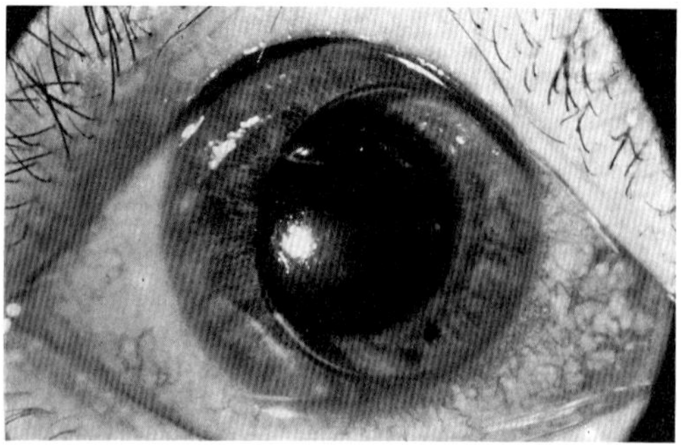

Fig. 21.21 Anterior luxation of the lens (♀ 49 yrs.)

sidered in a patient with ectopia lentis, microspherophakia and the Marfan's symptom complex (Henkind and Ashton 1966; Spaeth and Barber 1965; Ramsey, Yanoff and Fine 1972). Homocystinuria leads to a degeneration of the nonpigmented ciliary body epithelium, which develops an overlying hyaline connective tissue layer along with degeneration of the zonules and luxation of the lens.

Spherophakia alone occurs as a recessively inherited congenital anomaly (Fleischer 1916; Franceschetti 1946). It is seen most commonly, however, as part of Marfan's or Marchesani's syndromes (Marchesani 1939). In Marchesani's syndrome there is a generalized brachymorphia along with fat, stubby fingers (brachydactyly). The hereditary pattern of Marchesani's syndrome is not defined. Family studies were reported by Meyer (1954), Probert (1953), Kloepper and Rosenthal (1955) among others.

Ectopia lentis can occur in *Ehlers-Danlos syndrome*. Other possible ocular findings are epicanthus, microcornea, keratoconus, blue sclera, retinal hemorrhages and vascular proliferation. These "Indian rubber men" have "cutis laxa" hyperextensibility of joints which often luxate, kyphoscoliosis, aneurysms, etc.

Besides the hereditary nephropathy, hematuria, and deafness, that occur in *Alport's syndrome*, there may be spherophakia, anterior lenticonus and tapetoretinal degeneration.

Lowe's syndrome (see page 246) can be associated with spherophakia.

Subluxation, Ectopia Lentis

The anterior chamber depth is irregular when the lens is *subluxated*. The iris and lens have trembling movements. The vitreous may herniate. Congenital subluxation of the lens is called *ectopia lentis*.

Posterior Luxation of the Lens

The eye appears aphakic with iridodonesis, a deep anterior chamber, and vitreous herniating through the pupil. The lens usually lies inferiorly (position dependent) and floats freely in the liquefied vitreous. Danger: retinal detachment, secondary glaucoma.

Anterior Luxation of the Lens

The lens resembles an oil drop in the anterior chamber (Fig. 21.21).

Glaucoma occurs almost immediately with severe head-eye pain, corneal edema, ciliary injection and vision loss. Often the lens was dislocated by trauma, in which case sphincter tears, iridodialysis and hyphema may be present. If the sclera has ruptured, iris and lens may be displaced beneath the conjunctiva or even completely expulsed from the eye. Scleral ruptures almost always occur contralateral to the impact site. The lens may luxate spontaneously whenever zonules are easily torn. Thus, luxation may occur with age, shrunken cataracts, chronic cyclitis, old intraocular hemorrhage and absolute secondary glaucoma. Luxation of the lens, when familial, tends to occur between ages 20 to 65.

Lenticonus and Lens Colobomata

Anterior and posterior lenticonus are rare. They consist of an anterior or posterior central bulging of the lens. Anterior lenticonus may be associated with pseudoneuritis, optic disk drusen, or more frequently *Alport's syndrome*. The latter includes familial nephropathy and deafness (Friedburg 1968).

Zonular fibers are frequently missing in the region of a congenital iris coloboma. There is a notch in the edge of the lens at this point *(lens coloboma)*.

Aphakia

Aphakia is also known as deep anterior chamber, dark pupil, or iridodonesis (Fig. 21.22). Primary congenital aphakia occurs in D-trisomy (Manschot 1969) and may be associated with microphthalmos, colobomata, cataracts and retinal dysplasia.

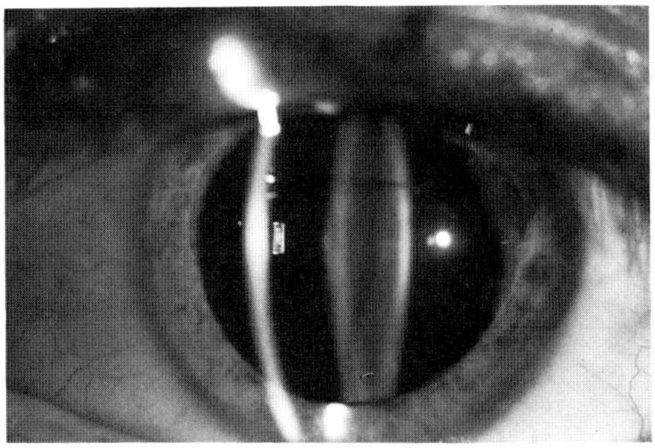

Fig. 21.22 Anterior lenticonus (central protrusion of the lens capsule) in Alport's syndrome (♀ 25 yrs.) ▶

References

Abrams, J. D.: Jatrogenic mercurialentis. Trans. ophthal. Soc. U. K. 83 (1964) 263–269

Agarwal, L. P., J. N. Raizada: Congenital membranous cataract, dentigerous cyst, and multiple fibrolipomata. Brit. J. Ophthal. 38 (1954) 383–384

Alfano, J. E.: Ocular aspects of the maternal rubella syndrome. Trans. Amer. Acad. Ophthal. Otolaryng. 70 (1966) 235–266

Becker, F.: Linsenektopie in der I., II. und III. Generation. Klin. Mbl. Augenheilk. 94 (1935) 547–548

Benedikt, O.: Morphologische Veränderungen beim sog. Exfoliationssyndrom. Klin. Mbl. Augenheilk. 162 (1973) 465–472.

Bertelsen, T. I.: Fibrillopathia epithelio-capsularis. The so-called senile exfoliation or pseudo-exfoliation of the anterior lens capsule. Acta ophthal. 44 (1966) 737–750

Bertelsen, T. I., .P A. Drablös, P. R. Flood: The so-called senile exfoliation (pseudo-exfoliation) of the anterior lens capsule, a product of the lens epithelium. Fibrillopathia epithelio-capsularis. Acta ophthal. 42 (1964) 1096–1113

Braun, R.: Retinitis diabetica. Albrecht v. Graefes Arch. klin. exp. Ophthal. 136 (1937) 256–302

Budolfsen, Sv. E.: Mißbildungen nach Rubeola während der Gravidität. Ugeskr. Laeg., 1956, 859–863

Crews, S. J.: Toxic effects on the eye and visual apparatus resulting from the systemic absorption of recently introduced chemical agents. Trans. ophthalm. Soc. U. K. 82 (1963) 387–406

Cullen, J. F.: Teratogenic agents and thalidomide. Trans. ophthal. Soc. U. K. 86 (1967) 101–117

Dubler, H.: La cataracte brune en soucoupe postérieure du cristallin. Premier examen histologique. Arch. Ophtal. (Paris) 20 (1960) 389–401

Duke-Elder, S.: Diseases of the lens and vitreous, glaucoma and hypotony. System of ophthalmology XI. Kimpton, London 1969

Emerson, E.: Retinitis: pigmentosa or rubella? Amer. J. Ophthal. 45 (1958) 93–101

Fleischer, B.: Abnorme Kleinheit und abnorme Kugelgestalt der Linse bei zwei Geschwisterpaaren. Klin. Mbl. Augenheilk. 80 (1916) 248–258

Franceschetti, A., J. J. B. Bourquin: Rubéole pendant la grossese et malformations congénitales de l'enfant. Ann. Oculist (Paris) 179 (1946) 623–626

François, J.: Les cataractes congénitales. Masson, Paris 1959 (p. 313)

François, J.: Syndromes with congenital cataract. Amer. J. Ophthal. 52 (1961) 207–238

François, J.: Ätiologie der kongenitalen Katarakte, Entwicklung und Fortschritt in der Augenheilkunde. Enke, Stuttgart 1963 (pp. 419–434)

François, J., G. Hooft, R. de Blond, F. Loore: Amblyopathie par radiations ionisantes. Ophthalmologica (Basel) 143 (1962) 163–186

Friedburg, D.: Pseudoneuritis und Drusenpapille beim Alport-Syndrom. Klin. Mbl. Augenheilk. 152 (1968) 379–383

Froewis, J., W. Plattner: Viruserkrankungen in der Schwangerschaft und Embryopathien. Wien. klin. Wschr. 68 (1956) 645–647

Gilston, R. J.: Marfan's syndrome. Med. Ann. D. C. 24 (1955) 127–129, 158

Goerttler, K.: Ätiopathogenese der Entwicklungsstörungen. Ber. dtsch. ophthal. Ges. 65 (1964) 136–160

Granström, K. O.: Refraktionsveränderungen bei Diabetes mellitus. Acta ophthal. (Kbh.) 11 (1933) 1–160

Gregg, N.: Congenital anomalies due to maternal infections especially in the early months of pregnancy. Trans. Amer. Acad. Ophthal. Otolaryng. 60 (1956) 199–205

Haut, J., Z. Joannides: A propos de 55 cas de syndrome de lowe. Arch. Ophtal. (Paris) 26 (1966) 21–28

Heimann, K.: Mikrophthalmussyndrome und 13 bis 15 Trisomie. Ber. dtsch. ophthal. Ges. 65 (1963) 32–38

Heinsius, E., G. Arndt: Über Häufigkeit des Vorkommens, Form und Genese der echten diabetischen Katarakt und Katarakt bei Diabetes. Albrecht v. Graefes Arch. klin. exp. Ophthal. 150 (1950) 555–571

Henkind, P., N. Ashton: Ocular pathology in homocystinuria. Trans. ophthal. Soc. U. K. 85 (1966) 21–38

Hermans, G.: Les phenothiazines. Bull. Soc. Belge d'Ophtalm. 160 (1972) 51–69

Honegger, H., R. Pape: Thalidomid und angeborene Fehlbildungen der Augen. Ber. dtsch. ophthal. Ges. 65 (1964) 222–223

Huerkamp, B.: Grundsätzlich verschiedene Arten der als „Caracta syndermatotica" zusammengefaßten Starformen. Klin. Mbl. Augenheilk. 113 (1948) 318–328

Irvine, S. R., A. R. Irvine: Lens-induced uveitis and glaucoma. Amer. J. Ophthal. 35 (1952) 177–186; 370–375

Jacobi, K. W., K. D. Tympner: Das okulo-cerebro-renale Syndrom (Lowe) aus ophthalmologischer Sicht. Klin. Mbl. Augenheilk. 149 (1966) 867–871

Johnson, J.: Cataracts in galactosemia. Amer. J. Ophthal. 36 (1953) 1380–1386

Kandori, F.: Studies on radiation cataract. I. Decomination of the threshold dose level of radiation cataract. Amer. J. Ophthal. 41 (1956 a) 627–632

Kandori, F.: Studies upon the radiation cataract. II. Commentary on the radiation cataract. Amer. J. Ophthal. 41 (1956 b) 1006–1019

Kloepfer, H. W., J. W. Rosenthal: Possible genetic carriers in the spherophakia-brachymorphie-syndrome. Amer. J. hum. Genet. 7 (1955) 398–425

Kugelberg, J.: Juvenile Katarakt bei Dermatosen. Cataracta syndermatotica. Klin. Mbl. Augenheilk. 92 (1934) 484–508

Lenz, W., K. Knapp: Die Thalidomid-Embryopathie. Dtsch. med. Wschr. 87 (1962) 1232–1242

Lundström, R.: Rubella during pregnancy. Acta paediat. (Stockholm) 51, suppl. 133 (1962) 9–110

Manschot, W. A.: Die kongenitale primäre Aphakie in genetischer Sicht. Klin. Mbl. Augenlheilk. 154 (1969) 1–11

Marchesani, O.: Brachydaktylie und angeborene Kugellinse als Systemerkrankung. Klin. Mbl. Augenheilk. 103 (1939) 392–406

Marinesco, G., S. Draganesco, D. Vasiliu: Nouvelle maladie familiale charactérisée par une cataracte congénitale et un arrêt du développement somato-neuropsychique. Encéphale 26 (1931) 107–109

Marner, E.: A family with eight generations of hereditary cataract. Acta Ophthal. (Kbh.) 27 (1949) 537–551

Mathalone, M. B. R.: Ocular complications of phenothiazines. Trans. ophthal. Soc. U. K. 86 (1967) 77–88

Meesmann, A.: Über die Ursache des Schichtstars, mit Bericht über Schichtstar bei eineiigen Zwillingen. Albrecht v. Graefes Arch. klin. exp. Ophthal. 144 (1942) 216–226

Meyer, E. T.: Familial ectopia lentis and its complications. Brit. J. Ophthal. 38 (1954) 163–172

Miehlke, A., C. J. Partsch: Ohrmißbildung, Facialis- und Abducenslähmung als Syndrom der Thalidomidschädigung. Arch. Ohr-, Nas.-, u. Kehlk.-Heilk. 181 (1963) 154–174

Müller, H.: Die Morphologie der phakogenetischen Reaktion im Menschenauge. Albrecht v. Graefes Arch. klin. exp. Ophthal. 154 (1953/54) 224–243

Müller, Ch., G. Pietruschka, H. Kirchmair: Klinischer Beitrag zum okulo-cerebro-renalen Syndrom (Lowe-Syndrom) mit ätiologischen, genetischen und differentialdiagnostischen Erwägungen. Klin. Mbl. Augenheilk. 151 (1967) 648–662

Nick, J.: Über die Untersuchung von Herzen menschlicher Keimlinge mit den Zeichen einer Embryopathia rubeolica. Schweiz. Z. allg. Path. 16 (1953) 653–665

Papst, W.: Thalidomid und kongenitale Anomalien der Augen. Ber. dtsch. ophthal. Ges. 65 (1964) 209–215

Patz, A.: Cataracts in galactosemia. Amer. J. Ophthal. 36 (1953) 453–462

Pau, H.: Braune Einlagerung in die Linse nach Diazepam-(Valium-)Gabe. Klin. Mbl. f. Augenheilk. 164 (1974) 446–448

Pau, H.: The pathogenesis of subcapsular opacities of the lens (permeability cataract). Docum. ophthal. (The Hague) 37.1 (1974) 47–57

Pau, H.: Die Permeabilitätskatarakt. Stuttgart, Enke 1954

Pau, H.: Die Cataracta coronaria. Klin. Mbl. Augenheilk. 138 (1961) 345–359

Pau, H., R. Caesar: Elektronenmikroskopische Studien zur Herkunft der Kollagenfasern im Kapselstar. Albrecht v. Graefes Arch. klin. exp. Ophthal. 171 (1967) 327–336

Pau, H.: Zur Entstehung der "Reiterchen" beim Schichtstar (Kat. zonularis). Graefes Arch. 166 (1964) 545–555

Pau, H.: Histologie der posttraumatischen Spätrosette (Kontusionsrosette). Albrecht v. Graefes Arch. klin. exp. Ophthal. 189 (1974) 99–104

Pau, H.: Siderosis lentis. Klin. Mbl. f. Augenheilk. 168 (1976) 478–482

Pau, H.: Die Häufigkeit der verschiedenen Formen der Alterskatarakt. Klin. Mbl. Augenheilk. 169 (1976) 158–164

Pau, H., E. M. Augstein: Durch Acidose (Senkung des PH) bedingte Linsenveränderungen. Albr. v. Graefes Arch. klin. u. experiment. Ophthalm. 202 (1977) 223–229

Pau, H., U. Leithäuser: Die „Kationenpumpe" in ihrer Bedeutung für die verschiedenen erworbenen Katarakte. Graefes Arch. 166 (1964) 440–450

Pau, H., W. Graeber: Physiologische Chemie. Der Augenarzt. Thieme, Leipzig, ed. by K. Velhagen, Vol. 1, 2nd Ed. (1969) pp. 290–357

Pau, H., R. Kuhlmann, I. Schröter: Die Kationenpumpe in ihrer Bedeutung für die Flüssigkeitsverschiebung in der Linse und die Permeabilitätskatarakt. Graefes Arch. 186 (1973) 165–174

Probert, L. A.: Spherophakia with Brachydactyly. Amer. J. Ophthal. 36 (1953) 1571–1574

Ramsey, M. S., M. Yanoff, B. S. Fine: The ocular histopathology of homocystinuria. Amer. J. Ophthal. 74 (1972) 377–385

Remler, O.: Über die sogenannte braune, schalenförmige Linsentrübung. Klin. Mbl. Augenheilk. 121 (1952) 647–653

Rintelen, F., U. Stauffenegger: Die Pathogenese der Pseudophakia fibrosa. Albrecht v. Graefes Arch. klin. exp. Ophthal. 159 (1957) 411–419

Rix, J.: Verlaufskontrollen bei familiär auftretender Wilsonscher Krankheit (Kayser-Fleischer-Ring, Sonnenblumenkatarakt, Glaskörperpigmentierung). Klin. Mbl. Augenheilk. 146 (1965) 695–708

Rohrschneider, W.: Untersuchungen über die Morphologie und Entstehung der Röntgenstrahlenkatarakt bei Menschen. Arch. Augenheilk. 106 (1932) 221–254

Rosen, E.: Argyrolentis. Amer. J. Ophthal. 33 (1950 a) 797–800

Rosen, E.: Mercurialentis. Amer. J. Ophthal. 33 (1950 b) 1287–1288

Rothmund, A.: Über Cataracte in Verbindung mit einer eigentümlichen Hautdegeneration. Albrecht v. Graefes Arch. klin. exp. Ophthal. 14 (1868) 159–182

Sautter, H.: Erkrankungen der Linse. In: Der Augenarzt, Vol. III, ed. by K. Velhagen. Thieme, Stuttgart 1960 (pp. 539–652)

Schäfer, E.: Zur Lehre von den kongenitalen Dyskeratosen. Arch. Dermat. Syph. 148 (1925) 425

Schmidt, J. G. H.: Augenmuskelparesen bei Thalidomid-Embryopathie. Ber. dtsch. ophthal. Ges. 65 (1964) 215–220

Schnyder, W. F.: Über Katarakt im Kindesalter bei gleichzeitigem Vorkommen von Poikilodermia atrophicans. Familiäres Vorkommen in der Schweiz (Rothmundsche Krankheit). Schweiz. med. Wschr. 65 (1935) II, 719–721

Schwarzweller, F.: Die konstitutionelle Bedingtheit der sogenannten Arachnodaktylie. Erbarzt 4 (1937) 96–101 (Sonderbeil. z. Dtsch. Ärztebl. 1937, 31)

Seefelder, R.: Über familiäres Auftreten von Katarakt und Poikilodermie. Z. Augenheilk. 86 (1935) 81–97

Siegrist, A.: Der graue Altersstar, seine Ursachen und seine nichtoperative Behandlung. Urban & Schwarzenberg, Berlin 1928

Siemens, H. W.: Studien über Vererbung von Hautkrankheiten. XI. Ichthyosis congenita. Arch. Dermat. Syph. 158 (1928) 111

Sjögren, T.: Klinische und Vererbungsmedizinische Untersuchungen über Oligophrenie mit kongenitaler Katarakt. Z. ges. Neurol. Psychiat. 152 (1935) 263–292

Spaeth, G. L., G. W. Barber: Homocystinuria. Trans. Amer. Ophthal. Otolaryng. 69 (1965) 912–930

Straub, W., J. Freund: Katarakt nach extrakorporaler Dialysebehandlung. Klin. Mbl. Augenheilk. 157 (1970) 50–52

Töndury, G.: Zur Wirkung des Erregers der Rubeolen auf den menschlichen Keimling. Helv. paediat. Acta Ser. D, 7 (1952) 105–135

Trautmann, J.: Das Lowe-Syndrom. Klin. Mbl. Augenheilk. 145 (1964) 60–66

Velasquez, O.: Congenital ocular malformations as a result of rubella in the pregnant mother. Ophthal. ib.-amer. 23 (1962) 121–146; ref. in: Zbl. ges. Ophthal. 88 (1963) 131

Vogt, A.: Lehrbuch und Atlas der Spaltlampenmikroskopie des lebenden Auges, Vol. II. Springer, Berlin 1931

Weve, H.: Über Arachnodaktylie (Dystrophia mesodermalis congenita, Typus Marfan). Arch. Augenheilk. 104 (1931) 1–46

Wiedemann, H. R.: Hinweise auf eine derzeitige Häufung hypo- und aplastischer Fehlbildungen der Gliedmaßen. Med. Welt 37 (1961) 1863

22 Retina

Retinal Vessels

The ratio of retinal vessel caliber is 2 : 3 (artery : vein). The central retinal artery has the caliber of an arteriole. Retinal vessels, like cerebral vessels, are end arteries. They supply only the inner retinal layers up to the bipolar cells. The outer retinal layers are nourished by diffusion from the choroid.

Outer retina: the sensory epithelium includes rods (75 to 100 million) and cones (3 to 7 million); then the first neuron or bipolar cells.
Inner retina: second neuron or ganglion cells whose axons form the optic nerve; partial decussation at the chiasm, then optic tract to the lateral geniculate body; from here the third neuron proceeds via Gratiolet's optic radiation to the calcarine fissure.
Developmentally the retina is part of the brain, the optic nerve a cerebral commissure. In a sense, vitreous and choroid represent meninges.

Vascular Tortuosity

Severe, often bizarre tortuosity of retinal vessels (Plate XX, Fig. 2, page 224 d) can be purely congenital (Cagianut and Werner 1968).
Macular hemorrhages may occur with hereditary tortuosity of small retinal vessels. Frequently, vascular tortuosity is associated with hyperopia. However, marked tortuosity of macular venules can result from cardiac insufficiency with venous stasis (superior vena cava syndrome). Children with severe congenital heart defects (blue babies) have particularly tortuous vessels filled with dark red blood. Tortuosity is also seen in congenital aortic stenosis (Bonnet 1954).
Hereditary hemorrhagic telangiectasia (Rendu-Osler-Weber), sickle cell anemia, and polycythemia can all be associated with tortuous vessels.
Cystic fibrosis (mucoviscidosis) includes venous stasis, vascular tortuosity, retinal hemorrhages, papilledema, and cystic maculopathy. There is an increase in the NaCl concentration and viscosity of mucous secretions (hence the name mucoviscidosis), as well as increased trypsin concentration in the duodenum. The tear, pancreas, salivary, sweat, mucous, and many endocrine glands are affected. These children develop malabsorption steatorrhea, emphysema and bronchopneumonia.

Crossing Phenomena

Crossing phenomena such as Gunn's sign (venous narrowing at A-V crossings) and Salus' sign (disappearance of the vein under an artery) were formerly thought to have diagnostic implications in various forms of hypertension. Since the work of Seitz (1961), these crossing phenomena are no longer considered to be exclusive for hypertension. Actually, they are optic phenomena caused by a lack of transparency in perivascular connective tissue.

Aneurysms

Endangiitis obliterans — Vascular disease — Ataxia telangiectasia (Louis-Bar) — Neuro-oculofacial arteriovenous aneurysm — Retinal angiomatosis (von Hippel) — Arteriovenous aneurysms (anastomoses) — Angiokeratoma corporis (Fabry) — Cilioretinal arteries — Caput medusae — Leber's miliary aneurysms with retinal degeneration — External exudative retinitis (Coats) — Pulseless disease (Takayasu) — Sickle cell anemia.

Endangiitis obliterans: Aneurysms or tiny loops are found on small venules in the retinal periphery. Conjunctival and episcleral vessels also show aneurysms and rete mirabile. The latter can also be a normal finding (Haimböck 1960).

Vascular diseases: Newly formed retinal aneurysms are seen in a variety of vascular diseases: periphlebitis, diabetic retinopathy, central vein thrombosis, arteriosclerotic retinopathy.
Hereditary hemorrhagic telagiectasia (Rendu-Osler-Weber syndrome) can include: intermittent exophthalmos, telangiectasias, vascular tortuosity potentially with hemorrhages, numerous angiomas and hemorrhages. The disorder has a dominant inheritance.

Ataxia telangiectasia (Louis-Bar syndrome): Ocular findings in ataxia telangiectasia (Heimann et al. 1969) include telangiectasias of the bulbar conjunctiva, particularly in the peripheral interpalpebral fissure area, and of retinal veins. Lids or other exposed areas of skin may also have telangiectatic vessels.
The most striking symptom is a cerebellar ataxia. This usually has its onset in early youth and leads to a complete inability to walk. Extrapyramidal symptoms may occur. Ocular nystagmus, motility problems and partial ophthalmoplegia are possible. Heredity of the Louis-Bar syndrome is autosomal recessive. Death usually occurs during adolescence (see page 134).
Neuro-oculo-facial arteriovenous aneurysms: Here, extensive facial skin angiomas are associated with harmless retinal vascular loops (Fig. 22.1). The disorder is one of the phakomatoses (see page 296).
Angiomatosis retinae of von Hippel (see page 296): This is one of the phakomatoses (Plate XXIX, Fig. 2, page 288 e).
Arteriovenous anastomoses (aneurysms): A retinal arteriovenous aneurysm (anastomosis) may appear in the retinal circulation, between retina and choroid, or as a shunt between a vascular loop or precapillary net. This unilateral condition leads to vision loss because of hemorrhages, thrombosis, retrobulbar hemorrhages or secondary glaucoma. The classic finding is a convoluted dilated vessel usually over the optic disc. Vascularized nevi of the face and cerebral vascular malformations (angioma) are a common accompaniment (Cagianut 1962). *Racemose aneurysm* of Leber and direct arterio-venous shunts (Stucchi and Höpping 1966) are part of the differential diagnosis. Most direct arterio-venous shunts are secondary to an old central vein thrombosis.

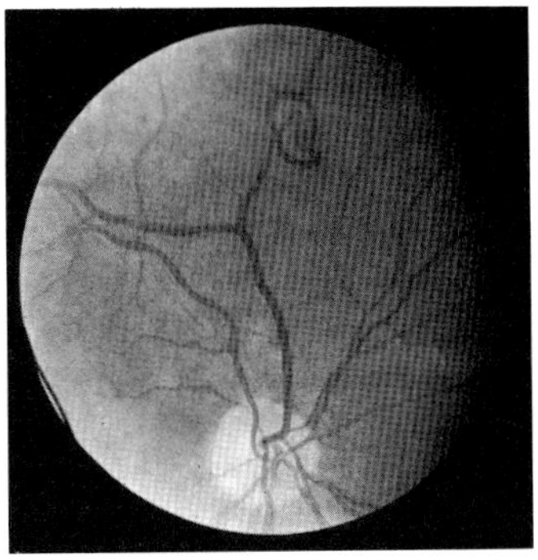

Fig. 22.1 Aneurysm of the superior temporal vein (♂ 59 yrs.)

Angiokeratoma corporis (Fabry): Beaded dilatation of retinal and conjunctival arteries and veins in combination with cornea verticillata (Fig. 22.2) (see page 167) is a combination exclusive to Fabry-Anderson's disease or angiokeratoma corporis. This is a glycolipid storage disease (see page 366).
Cilioretinal artery: Numerous cilioretinal arteries occur in Turner's syndrome, an aberration of the sex chromosomes (see page 330).
Caput medusae: Dilatation and proliferation of disc vessels can cause a form of caput medusae (Werncke 1940).
Leber's retinal degeneration: Leber's retinal degeneration has multiple miliary aneurysms of the peripheral retinal arteries (Plate XX, Fig. 3, page 224 d). The peripheral retina is opaque. Localized retinal detachments can occur.
Leber's miliary aneurysms appear primarily in young adult males (90 percent) (Paufique et al.

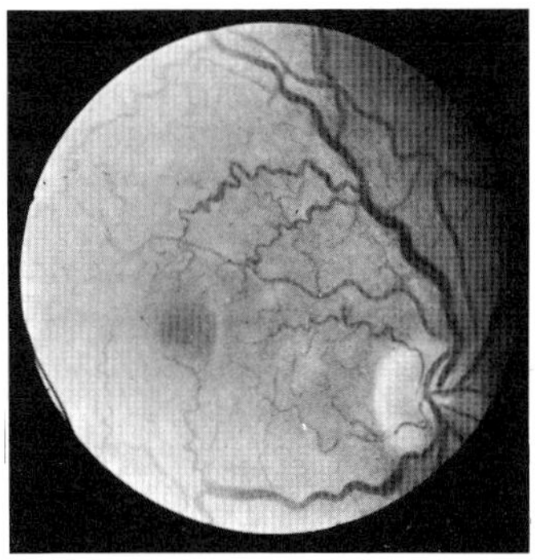

Fig. 22.2 Fabry's disease, beaded tortuous retinal vessels and aneurysms (♂ 37 yrs.)

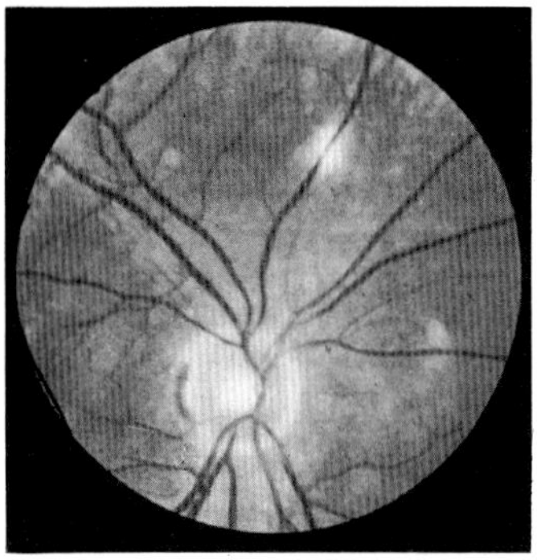

Fig. 22.3 Vascular sheathing in lupus erythematosus (♂ 30 yrs.)

1964). Involvement is almost invariably unilateral. Macular damage with vitreoretinal hemorrhages occurs. Small arterial branches (rarely veins) develop a variable number of exudative retinal lesions distributed like a garland or in a circinate pattern around the macula. Leber's miliary aneurysmal retinitis may be a special form of Coats' disease (Hiller 1971).

External exudative retinitis: In *Coats' disease* aneurysms appear like nits along blood vessels (Plate XXV, Fig. 4, page 288 a, Plate XXVIII, Fig. 5, page 288 d).

Pulseless disease (Takayasu): Takayasu's disease, pulseless disease, aortic arch disease = thrombosis at the aortic arch and the subclavian artery; presumably of allergic-immune etiology (Pillat 1955). Besides "boxcarring" of blood in the link-sausage-like dilated retinal veins, one finds arterio-venous shunts especially at the optic disc, vascular occlusion in the retinal periphery, trophic corneal ulcers, iris atrophy, ophthalmoplegia, and, as late complications: cataracts, optic atrophy (see page 315), vitreous hemorrhages, and retinal detachment.

Sickle cell anemia: This is a dominantly inherited (hemoglobin-S = AS, SS, SC) anemia in Negroes (Plate XX, Fig. 4, page 224 d). Ocular findings include: vascular tortuosity with dilatation of arterio-venous anastomoses, peripheral edema, vascular sheathing, microaneurysms, telangiectasias, neovascularization, hemorrhages, exudates, vascular occlusion, vitreous hemorrhages, and exudative retinal detachments (Lieb et al. 1960)

In C- + S-hemoglobinopathies, peripheral retinal changes often occur before the age of five; for example: glistening copper-colored deposits, preretinal hemorrhages, venous aneurysms, retinal pigmentation (Lewine and Kaplan 1965; Rummeld 1972; Cordon and Serjeant 1972).

Hemoglobin S occurs most commonly in Negroes of West African descent, rarely in Mediterranean races and along the Persian gulf and in India. Hemoglobin C is native to West Africa. Sickle cell anemia can resemble periphlebitis. Retinal detachment is due to traction in the latter, but is exudative in sickle disease. There are also similarities between sickling and Coats' disease in the form of aneurysms, anastomoses and vascular tortuosity. Sickle cell retinopathy is primarily peripheral, whereas Coats' disease affects the posterior pole (Munro and Walker 1960).

Reversible Vascular Sheathing

In *segmental reversible periarteritis* (Kyrieleis 1958; Filbry 1961), yellow or yellow-white rings, cuffs or punctate nodules develop along the arterial walls. These may remain for weeks, and are segmental and reversible. They occur with various uveitides, especially with solitary chorioretinal lesions (particularly juxtapapillary chorioretinitis) and cyclitits.

Reversible perivenous sheathing occurs in a variety of conditions: periphlebitis, endophthalmitis, cyclitis, diffuse chorioretinitis, sarcoidosis and multiple sclerosis. Inflammatory sheathing can scarify, as in lupus erythematosus (Fig. 22.3), the lymphogranulomatoses (Plate XX, Fig. 5, page 224 d) and in malignant hypertension (Plate XX, Fig. 6, page 224 d).

Sludged Blood Phenomenon

A picture similar to bilateral central vein thrombosis with dilatation and tortuosity of retinal veins to the point that they appear like sausage links occurs with dysproteinemia (multiple myeloma, Waldenström's macroglobulinemia, cryoglobulinemia and thalassemia (Berneaud-Kötz 1959). Boxcarring (sludging phenomenon) or segmental flow occurs in the veins. Hemorrhages, nodular retinal exudates, papilledema and exudative retinal detachments may be present. Crystals may deposit in the cornea (François and Rabaey 1960). The erythrocyte sedimentation rate is markedly elevated.

The sludged blood phenomenon is an aggregation of erythrocytes giving the appearance of discontinuous blood flow. The phenomenon is more noticeable in conjunctival than in retinal vessels and is due to an alteration of the erythrocyte surfaces, making them more adherent to each other. It is an accentuation of physiologic rouleaux formation.

Besides dys- and paraproteinemias, the sludged blood phenomenon occurs with trauma, heat or cold, vascular occlusion, infusion of colloidal substances (blood volume expanders), hyperlipemia, pregnancy and menstruation (Seitz 1961).

In Takayasu's disease *(pulseless disease,* aortic arch syndrome) (see page 315), there is hypotony cranially and hypertension caudally. Vision decreases with physical exertion. Boxcarring may be observed in retinal vessels. Potentially there is a granular appearance to the blood stream in the dilated link-sausage-like veins. The pupil may be dilated on the involved side with atrophy of the iris stroma. Late complications: cataract, retinal pigment dispersion, optic atrophy. In Takayasu's disease (Seitz 1961) there is occlusion of arteries originating from the aortic arch. Because of poor cerebral circulation, the patients tend to faint on standing. Trophic changes appear in the bony skull.

Fever, leukocytosis and an elevated erythrocyte sedimentation rate is common in pulseless (Takayasu-Onishi's) disease. Other etiologies include giant cell arteritis, arteriosclerosis with arteritis, endarteritis, thromboangiitis, and luetic vasculitis with obliteration of the large aortic arch branches. A differentiation between pulseless disease and bilateral carotid artery occlusion is possible with the help of ophthalmodynamography and ophthalmodynamometry (Hager 1963; Bettelheim 1968).

Paravenous, Para-Arterial Retinal-Choroidal Atrophy

Franceschetti (1962 a) described paravenous, granular, retinal pigmentary changes along large retinal veins and their branches as "pigmented paravenous retinal-choroidal atrophy." Such changes may *appear solely along arteries* (for example with Hodgkin's disease, Plate XX, Fig. 5, page 224 d) (Pau 1968).

Venous Dilatation

Venous dilatation (normal relationship, artery : vein = 2 : 3) occurs in blood dyscrasias (paraproteinemia, dysproteinemia, multiple myeloma, leukemia, polycythemia vera, sickle cell anemia), with congenital heart defects (venous stasis, superior vena cava syndrome, blue babies), with arterio-venous aneurysms of the internal carotid in the cavernous sinus, with congenital vascular tortuosity, Fabry's disease and retinal angiomatosis (von Hippel-Lindau), with central vein thrombosis, diabetic retinopathy, papilledema, and in the newborn. Polycythemia vera (Vaquez-Osler syndrome) leads to dilated, dark retinal veins potentially with retinal hemorrhages and generalized hemorrhages.

Color and Reflex

The color of the fundus depends on the pigment (chromatophores) and blood content of the choroid and the pigment content of the retinal pigment epithelium (Plate XXI, Fig. 1, page 224 e) (as well as the nature of the light source).

In a *homogeneous red fundus* the choroid is obscured by the even distribution of pigment in the pigment epithelium. The fundus is dark in pigmented races (Plate XXI, Fig. 2, page 224 e).

In a depigmented, *albinotic fundus* (Plate XXI, Fig. 3, page 224 e) the sclera gives a yellowish pale red background owing to paucity of pigment epithelial and choroidal pigmentation. The red choroidal vessels are clearly visible for the same reason.

In a pigmented *(tessellated)* fundus (Plate XXI, Fig. 4, page 224 e) the pigment epithelium is lightly pigmented and dark brown-black choroidal pigment is visible between red choroidal vessels.

In youthful fundi there is a strong variation of retinal and vascular reflexes, depending on the direction of illumination. The *foveal reflex* is particularly striking. There is a *paucity of reflexes* in the *senile fundus* and shallow excavation of the optic disc. Areoles of choroidal atrophy may be present. Senile pigmentation either as lines, fine dots or even bone spicules is common in the equatorial region (Pillat 1958).

Hyaline drusen on Bruch's membrane, formed by the pigment epithelium, are common degenerative changes in older people. These are small bright nodules often surrounded by a pigmented rim. They are preferentially located at the posterior pole or equator. Myopia causes stretching with thinning of all ocular coats (see page 26). As a result, a sparsely pigmented fundus is part of myopia. Retinal vessels, especially those serving the macula, appear stretched. In *excessive myopia*, central, paracentral and peripapillary (conus myopicus) stretch lesions occur (Plate XXII, Fig. 1, page 224 f). In the region of Bruch's membrane, circumscribed hemorrhages with connective tissue ingrowth and pigmentary deposits develop. Small subpigment epithelial hemorrhages are common in the region of the macula lutea in excessive myopia. These result in Fuchs' black spot (Plate XXII, Fig. 1, page 224 f) with severe vision loss.

Active hyperemia is rarely seen, for example with retinitis or chorioretinitis. The ever present question is whether a vitreous haze simulates hyperemia. A dark blue red color and dilated vessels occur with polycythemia.

Passive hyperemia (retinal cyanosis) results from venous stasis for any reason (cardiac insufficiency, retinal vein thrombosis, papilledema, tumors of the retina, choroid, optic nerve and orbit). A marked passive hyperemia is seen with cavernous sinus thrombosis, pulmonary venous obstruction as in cystic fibrosis, compression of the thorax (for example at birth), congenital heart defects, or polycythemia rubra.

The fundus is noticeably more *pale* in anemia when the color index of blood can be reduced by one half its normal value.

In Oguchi's disease, which is a form of congenital hemeralopia (see page 31), the fundus takes on a white-gray to brown color, especially in the macular and peripapillary region after exposure to light. After two to three hours of dark adaptation, the color of the fundus returns to normal (Mizuo's phenomenon).

Lipid storage disease develops a gray coloration of the fundus, potentially with a cherry red spot (Plate XXVII, Fig. 6, page 228 c). Tapetoretinal degeneration also occurs. Lipidoses (see page 289) include Tay-Sachs disease, Niemann-Pick disease, and Gaucher's disease. A cherry red spot is also seen with *retinal edema*. The nerve fiber layer, which becomes opaque with edema, is missing at the macula lutea, allowing the red choroid to be visible. This occurs after death, with central retinal artery embolus (Plate XXIV, Fig. 4, page 224 h) or with trauma (Berlin's edema), acute quinine poisoning, fresh chorioretinitis, etc.

Chronic primary or *secondary retinal ischemia* as occurs with absolute glaucoma, after extract of *Filicis maris*, quinine or optochinin poisoning, after old central retinal artery embolus and with tapetoretinal degeneration, retinal siderosis, grade IV hypertension, etc,, is recognized by the *narrowed retinal arteries* and *optic atrophy* but not by the color of the fundus, which is dependent on the choroid.

With *lipemia*, the *fundus* and retinal vessels appear creamy-yellow (Ericson 1955; Godde-Jolly 1961) (Plate XXII, Fig. 3, page 224 f).

Hyperlipemia occurs when the serum triglyceride level exceeds 2,500 mg/100 ml and reaches a maximum at 5,000 mg/100 ml (Vinger and Sachs 1970). Hyperlipemia can be differentiated into

a) secondary hyperlipemia, transport hyperlipemia (in diabetes mellitus, chronic alcoholism, deficiency disorders with starvation, dieting or anemia, poisoning with phosphor or chloroform, lipoid nephrosis, myxedema) and

b) retention hyperlipemia.

Hyperlipemia can cause (Dunphy 1950): retinal hyperlipemia, interstitial lipid keratitis, xanthomata on the eyelids (not to be confused with xanthelasma),

Circinate, yellow-white retinal exudates can be present in hypercholesterolemia (Plate XXII, Fig. 2, page 224 f).

Hemorrhages

Preretinal hemorrhages (Fig. 22.4, Plate XXII, Fig. 4, page 224 f) usually appear suddenly as round central or paracentral lakes of blood at the posterior pole of the eye. The hemorrhage lies in the potential space between retina and vitreous. A fluid level can occur as red blood cells settle out inferiorly. The lower cellular portion of the hemorrhage is darker than the serum-containing upper portion. The red color of the hemorrhage becomes (beginning 1–3 weeks later) increasingly gray.
Overwhelmingly one is dealing with younger patients, and a subarachnoid hemorrhage (hemorrhagic pachymeningitis) has to be considered. In infants with subarachnoid hemorrhages, preretinal hemorrhages and even a picture resembling central vein occlusion can occur (Schmidt and Trojan 1970). Of young children with subarachnoid hemorrhages (hemorrhagic pachymeningitis), 40 percent had retinal hemorrhages - mostly preretinal - and less commonly papilledema, optic atrophy or strabismus (Hentsch and Weissbach 1966).
Less common causes include all the retinal vascular disorders (arteriosclerosis, diabetes, periphlebitis, hematopoietic disorders, aneurysm, etc.), thrombosis of the retinal veins, vitreous detachment, blunt trauma, even vicarious menstruation.
Besides preretinal hemorrhages, subarachnoid hemorrhage will also cause intra- and subretinal hemorrhages as well as venous stasis and papilledema (Aust et al. 1968).
Complications (hemorrhage into the vitreous, retinitis proliferans, glaucoma) are rare. Usually vision returns on its own.

Eales' disease (Plate XXII, Fig. 5, page 224 f) was formerly know as recurrent juvenile vitreous hemorrhage. Young persons, especially males between ages 20 and 35, develop sudden severe vitreous hemorrhages and vision loss. After the hemorrhage reabsorbs, retinal hemorrhages and new vessel formation are visible around veins. The vitreous hemorrhages recur at irregular intervals and result in retinitis proliferans, which may lead secondarily to retinal traction detachments. On the average, the active vascular stage of the disease burns out after about three years. The cause is unknown. Possible etiologies include focal disease, tuberculosis, thromboangiitis proliferans, and hormonal disturbances (Doden 1963).
Intraretinal hemorrhages (see page 261 to 268), when superficial, have a feathery striate appearance corresponding to the nerve fiber layer. Therefore, they run radial to the disc. Hemorrhages in the deeper retinal layer have a more punctate or blotlike appearance.

Central vein thrombosis — Branch vein thrombosis — Trauma — Hemorrhages in newborns.

Central retinal vein thrombosis: With central retinal vein thrombosis there is a sudden decrease in visual acuity, which is less severe and therefore less alarming than the sudden blindness experienced with central retinal artery occlusion.
Retinal hemorrhages are the most impressive ophthalmoscopic finding. These are massive and may be radial in the nerve fiber layer (superficial) or blot-punctate (deeper) in the inner plexiform or even inner nuclear layer. Retinal edema is common. The veins are thickened, tortuous (Fig. 22.5) and filled with dark red blood. In certain areas they appear interrupted owing to opacity of the overlying edematous tissue. The optic disc is usually hemorrhagic and blurred (Plate XXII, Fig. 6, page 224 f); the picture may resemble severe papilledema. Generally, vision is severely decreased (hand motion 1/10). The lamina cri-

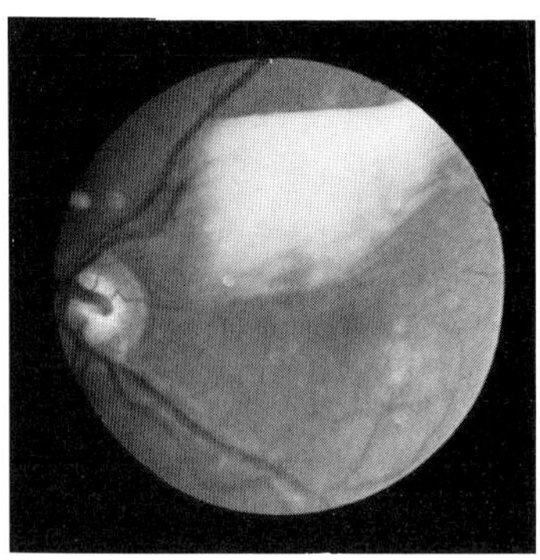

Fig. 22.4 Old preretinal hemorrhage, gray-white decoloration. (♂ 45 yrs.)

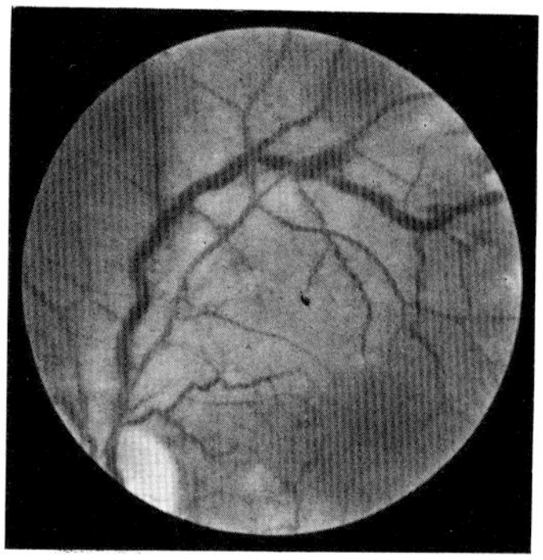

Fig. 22.5 Venous stasis and isolated retinal hemorrhages ("prethrombosis") (♂ 67 yrs.)

brosa and arterio-venous crossings are predisposed points for venous thrombosis.
White hard exudates form on the hemorrhagic disc with *long-standing venous thrombosis*. Circinate retinopathy can also develop. With time, hemorrhages ultimately resolve. Yellow-gray exudates can remain for some time along with circinate retinopathy. Neovascularization and arterio-venous anastomoses occur. Blood vessels may be interrupted or sheathe with irregular reflexes. The macula can become edematous or cystic, or develop holes or pigmentary changes.
Complications: The most common and unpleasant complication is therapy-resistant hemorrhagic glaucoma. This is usually accompanied by *rubeosis iridis*. Preretinal or vitreous hemorrhages are rare.
Etiologically, central vein thrombosis in children raises the question of syphilis, other infectious disorders, orbital tumor, or cystic fibrosis.
In older persons, central vein thrombosis is usually due to arteriosclerosis, hypertension, blood dyscrasias (leukemia, polycythemia vera, sickle cell anemia, emphysema with erythrocytosis, macroglobulinemia, hyperproteinemia, multiple myeloma, following renal dialysis), cardiac failure, aneurysms, carotid occlusion, diabetes, or poisoning. According to Altenberger, ophthalmoscopic changes with *polycythemia* occur only after the erythrocyte count exceeds 6.3 million. Besides retinal cyanosis, papilledema, central vein thrombosis and central artery occlusion may develop (Velhagen 1964).
Retinal vein thrombosis or pre-thrombosis has been observed with use of oral contraceptives (van Oye 1972). Histologically, actual thrombi are not found. Rather, venous stasis is brought about by endothelial swelling (Seitz 1961). The vessel walls can rupture.
With **branch vein thrombosis** (Plate XXIII, Fig. 1, page 224 g), the clinical picture of central retinal vein thrombosis is limited to a small area of the fundus. Complications are less frequent.

Trauma, Hemorrhages in the Newborn

Blunt or *sharp trauma – injury, birth trauma –* causes varying degrees of retinal hemorrhage.
Retinal hemorrhages are common in the *newborn* (Giles [1960] 40 percent; Krebs and Jäger [1966] 20 percent). Newborns of primiparous mothers have a higher incidence of hemorrhages than do those of a multipara. The incidence of hemorrhages increases with length of labor, birth weight, forceps, or vacuum delivery (Krebs and Jäger 1966). Asphyxiated children have the most hemorrhages (56 percent according to Lemmingson and Stark 1957).
Battered baby syndrome see page 268.

Hemorrhages and Exudates

A large number of systemic and retinal diseases cause *retinal hemorrhages* and *exudates*.

Arteriosclerosis of Retinal Vessels

Arteriosclerotic retinal vessels are of irregular caliber, appearing white in some parts, yellow in others (Fig. 22.6). The blood column looks narrowed in these areas. Punctate, or more rarely striate, hemorrhages and small gray-white exudates may appear in the retina.
Choroidal sclerosis (Fig. 22.25) is recognizable

only after loss of the overlying pigment epithelium. The *choroidal vessels* are then visible as *yellow-white bands* with narrow blood columns, or, when totally occluded, as white bands.

Hypertensive Retinopathy

Mild hypertensive retinopathy (grades I and II) elicits no or minimal (grade III) *symptoms*. Severe changes (grade IV) are associated with a variety of complaints (see page 264).

Objectively, the various causes and mechanisms for hypertension result in the same basic changes. The ophthalmoscopic picture depends on the duration, degree and evolution of the hypertension. There is a strong relationship between arterial changes and the diastolic blood pressure.

Young hypertensives usually demonstrate only an irregularity of the vessel reflex. Even months of elevated blood pressure in young patients causes only variations of vessel caliber.

In adults, long-standing *labile hypertension* leads to variations in vessel caliber and an irregular vessel reflex. Peripapillary capillary dilatation, best seen with red-free light, occurs in older persons.

Fixed hypertension, when acute, leads to disc and retinal damage, often with normal or minimally altered arteries. In contrast, chronic fixed hypertension can cause severe organic arteriolar changes with a minimum of retinal parenchymal injury.

Neubauer (1967) has a convenient classification of hypertensive fundus changes. Early changes, grades I and II, are called *hypertensive fundus*, while the more severe changes of grades III and IV are labeled *hypertensive retinopathy*. This classification is related to those of Keith, Wagener and Barker. A modification of the American classification was made by Renbi, Nowak and Witmer. Neubauer's classification makes similar divisions (Tables 22.1 and 22.2).

Hypertensive fundus I – Hypertensive fundus II – Hypertensive retinopathy III – Hypertensive retinopathy IV.

Hypertensive fundus grade I is characterized by minimal arteriolar constriction and venous dilatation. Venules (especially paracentrally) may be tortuous. Very exceptionally the arteries are packed, appearing as copper wire arteries as described by Thiel (1963).

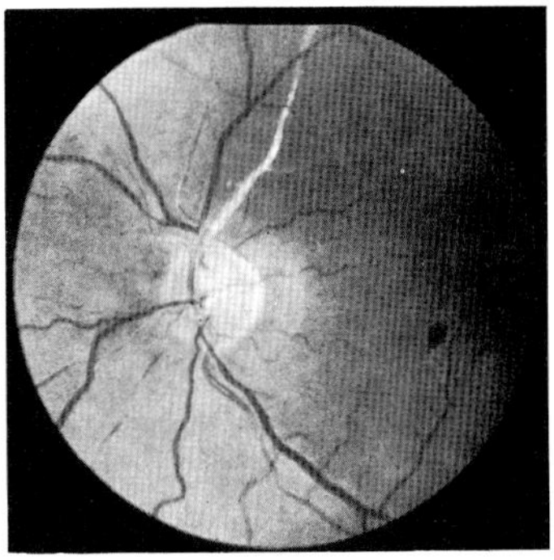

Fig. 22.6 Arteriosclerosis with a yellow-white obliterated vessel, round and striate hemorrhages (♂ 64 yrs.)

Hypertensive fundus grade II includes irregular caliber of arteries with an increased arterial reflex. The veins are slightly distended, and venules are increased and tortuous. Peripapillary capillary loops, isolated hemorrhages and gray exudates appear near vessels or at the posterior pole.

Grade III hypertensive retinopathy: The disc margins are slightly blurred, even elevated. Arteries are minimally to distinctly narrowed. The vessel walls are altered with an irregular light reflex and a beaded appearance due to segmental vascular constriction. The veins are minimally altered, perhaps slightly distended with increased tortuosity paracentrally.

Ectasia of peripapillary capillaries is increased. Besides isolated and grouped hemorrhages and gray exudates, an early star-shaped macular exudate may be present (grade III is equivalent to the early transition fundus).

Grade IV hypertensive retinopathy: The *subjective symptoms* vary enormously. These may be absent, or small positive scotomata corresponding to hemorrhages or exudates are noted. Large scotomata due to vascular occlusion, or varying degrees of vision loss from retinal edema or secondary detachment, cause more significant complaints.

Objective findings in grade IV hypertensive

Table 22.1 Classification of hypertensive retinopathy after Neubauer I (papilla, arterial vasculature, precapillaries)

Grade	Optic Disc	Major Branches	Arterioles
I	distinct, slightly hyperemic	normal, increased light reflex	**caliber** normal – low normal
II	distinct, slightly hyperemic	**caliber** is low normal, **reflexes** irregular and increased minimal changes in vessel walls over short distances	**caliber** low normal, intermittently constricted or completely constricted and irregular
III	usually blurred, flat or slightly prominent	**caliber** minimally distinctly constricted **reflexes** hard and irregular	**caliber** narrowed **vessel reflex hard** and irregular
IV	papilledema/optic disc swelling with peripapillary edema, occasional disappearance of vessels	irregular changes in the vessel walls similar to III or more pronounced	similar to III or more pronounced

retinopathy are: narrowing of retinal arteries, changes in retinal tissue, and papilledema.

Ophthalmoscopically, all *retinal arteries* (Plate XXIII, Fig. 3, page 224 g) are *narrowed* with thin blood columns and marked variations in their caliber. The vessel reflex may have the appearance of a narrow silver stripe (silver wire arteries). The partly obliterated vessels appear stretched. More commonly there is intermittent white sheathing of the vessels with partial obscuration of their terminal bifurcation (Thiel [1963] called this angiospastic retinopathy). The veins are moderately distended and basically normal except for their tortuosity. The capillaries are increasingly ectatic.

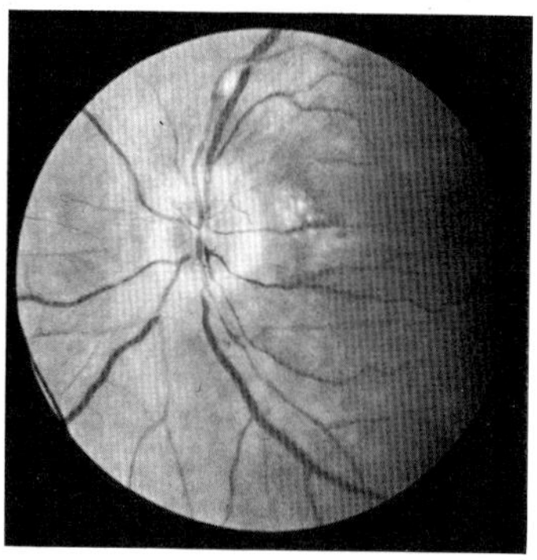

Fig. 22.7 Chronic grade IV hypertensive retinopathy with papilledema, narrowed arteries and linear exudates (♂ 40 yrs.)

Blurring of the *disc margin* can progress to frank *papilledema* (see page 308) (Fig. 22.7). This is usually also a sign of elevated intracranial pressure due to cerebral edema.

The retinal picture is primarily one of *hemorrhages, hard exudates* and *"cotton-wool spots"* (Plate XXIII, Fig. 2, page 224 g). The hemorrhages may be radial about the optic disc or of varying size elsewhere in the retina. This is also true of hard exudates. These appear as white lines on or near the optic disc and as small bright dots or spots positioned radially about the macula. Such a "macular star" is usually incomplete. Numerous soft exudates ("cotton-wool spots") are also present and are characteristic of grade IV hypertensive retinopathy.

Therapy is purely medical. If the blood pressure is brought under control, most fundus

Table 22.2 Classification of hypertensive retinopathy after Neubauer II (veins, capillaries, parenchyma)

Grade	Veins	Venules	Capillaries	Parenchyma
I	**filled** potentially slightly increased	**tortuous** potentially slightly increased	only visible on the disc	
II	**filled** potentially slightly increased	**tortuous** slight increase	isolated peripapillary capillary loops also visible	**hemorrhages,** usually isolated near arterio-venous crossings; isolated chronic ischemic **exudates** at the posterior pole; rarely acute "cotton-wool spots"
III	**filled** potentially slightly increased	**tortuous** slight increase	increasing **capillary ectasia**	**hemorrhages,** isolated and in groups generally in the vicinity of vessel crossings; potentially **prethrombosis/thrombosis** deep **capillary hemorrhages** chromic hypoxic lipid exudates (macular star figure)
IV	as in III or more pronounced	as in III or more pronounced	increasing **capillary ectasia**	overwhelmingly acute changes

changes, except for arterial narrowing, resolve.

Complications: Edematous exudate beneath the retina causes a flat retinal detachment. These areas appear more opaque and undulating. A sudden branch or central artery occlusion (embolic phenomenon), is a rare occurrence.

In view of the almost invariable presence of perimacular exudates, the generalized loss of central acuity is not surprising. With marked papilledema, the peripheral visual field may also be constricted.

Pathogenetically it is important that the same arterial narrowing observed in the eye occurs throughout the body. This gives the patients a pale pasty complexion (pale hypertension of Volhard). The systolic and particularly the diastolic retinal arterial pressure is elevated.

Histologically, edema develops in the area of a cotton-wool spot, which is a localized nerve fiber layer infarct. The infarcted nerve fibers develop terminal swellings of Cajal or "cytoid bodies" (Wolter 1961). Cotton-wool spots disappear after a few weeks, with resolution of the edema and degeneration of the nerve fiber endings. "Soft exudates" also result from swelling of nerve axons due to metabolic disturbances. In contrast, "hard exudates" are a true accumulation of fluid in the outer plexiform or even outer nuclear layer (Diezel-Willert 1961).

The prognosis of hypertensive retinopathy depends on the causes of the hypertension (and renal disease). The extent of resolution of retinal changes (less so of arterial narrowing) is often amazing, once the hypertension is controlled. The relationship be-

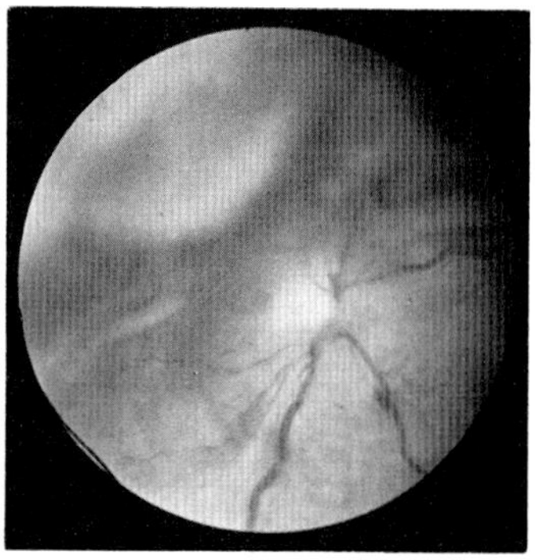

Fig. 22.8 Eclamptic retinopathy with very narrow arteries and exudative retinal detachment (♀ 22 yrs.)

tween retinal and renal findings is relatively good. Papilledema can be viewed as a sign of early renal insufficiency.

The question as to what extent hypertensive or arteriosclerotic fundus findings correlate with renal and cerebral changes is answered differently by various authors. Rintelen (1956) denies a close relationship. Lund (1960) finds an 80 percent correlation. Weigelin feels that if fundus findings are particularly marked or absent in hypertension, this is reflected in the cerebral arteries.

Differential diagnosis: Papilledema of other etiologies or central venous thrombosis, fresh chorioretinitis, primary retinal detachment and central retinal artery emboli must be considered. Constriction of the vein at arteriovenous crossings (A-V nicking), the increased angle of departure between an arteriole and its precapillary branch and arteriolar tortuosity cannot be considered signs of hypertension in adults (Kropp et al. 1970). Increased tortuosity of small veins and venules is more a sign of cardiac insufficiency than of hypertension.

Retinopathy of Pregnancy (Pre-Eclampsia)

Clinically the picture is one of grade III or IV retinopathy. Papilledema, hard exudates, cotton-wool spots and hemorrhages are present. At first, arterial changes are minimal (young patients). The nephropathy and hypertension result from a toxicity of pregnancy with hormonal and metabolic disturbances. Severe ocular changes, such as exudative retinal detachment (Fig. 22.8), extensive retinal edema or massive hemorrhages, may force therapeutic interruption of the pregnancy.

Diabetic Retinopathy

The appearance of diabetic retinopathy relates to the length and severity of the diabetes (Hill et al. 1973). Diabetic retinopathy can be expected after 5 to 8 years. After 15 years of diabetes, 60 percent of patients have retinopathy. Diabetic retinopathy may already appear in childhood (Heinsius 1956). At first, isolated punctate or striate retinal hemorrhages appear (stage I). Often these "dot" hemorrhages are microaneurysms. The optic disc and vessels remain normal. In stage II (Plate XXIII, Fig. 4, page 224 g) striate hemorrhages and white or yellow, sharply delineated, paracentral hard exudates are present. Circinate retinopathy is possible. The veins may develop nodular or spindle-shaped aneurysmal dilatations, especially in juvenile diabetics.

The exudation of protein across vessel walls is most readily seen by fluorescein angiography (Amalric 1971; Rosen 1969).

The hemorrhages become more massive and may be preretinal. Large preretinal hemorrhages lead to neovascularization (stage III, [Plate XXIII, Fig. 5, page 224 g]), with connective tissue organization, i.e. *retinitis proliferans*.

The most severe form of diabetic retinopathy (stage IV) involves large hemorrhages, often into the vitreous, with marked retinitis proliferans and traction detachment of the retina.

Long-standing diabetes, diabetic retinopathy and microaneurysms are usually associated with intercapillary glomerulosclerosis (Kimmelstiel-Wilson).

Secondary detachment with retinitis proliferans is the most common cause of blindness in long-standing diabetes. Recurrent, often non-reabsorbing, vitreous hemorrhages are also frequent. Hemorrhagic secondary glaucoma is one of the more common complications of severe diabetic retinopathy. This therapeutically recalcitrant glaucoma is nearly always associated with rubeosis of the iris.

Diabetic retinopathy is frequently combined with arteriosclerotic or hypertensive retinal changes but may appear independent of them.

Venous Stasis

Especially when chronic, these can lead to hard exudates, cotton-wool spots and macular star formations. *Etiology:* retinal vein thrombosis, papilledema, retrobulbar tumors, retrobulbar inflammation, cavernous sinus thrombosis – arteriovenous aneurysm, pulmonary stenosis, pulmonary emphysema.

Hematologic Disorders

Hemorrhages and gray-white exudates occur in nearly all *blood disorders,* white or red cell: anemia, leukemia, hemorrhagic diathesis, Henoch-Schönlein purpura, polycythemia (Gavey 1964). Sickle cell anemia, an inherited disorder common in Negroes, causes hemorrhages, tortuous vessels and microaneurysms.

Cachectic (malignancies, tuberculosis, etc.) *retinopathy* relates to the underlying anemia; it includes hemorrhages and cotton-wool spots. A similar picture occurs with *septic anemia* (subacute bacterial endocarditis, etc.).

Hemophilia and thrombocytopenic purpura *(Werlhof's disease)* can cause retinal hemorrhages, degeneration, or severe intraocular hemorrhages with resultant retinitis proliferans (Bruna 1949).

Pernicious anemia results in retinal hemorrhages when the hematocrit falls below 25 percent (Kearns 1956).

Large round white exudates with a red center (Plate XXIII, Fig. 6, page 224 g) occur in *leukemia* along with hemorrhages, white exudates, venous dilatation and vascular tortuosity.

Dys- and *paraproteinemia* (multiple myeloma, Waldenström's macroglobulinemia, cryoglobulinemia) and thalassemia (Mediterranean anemia) cause distention and tortuosity of retinal veins often with sausage-like dilatations, sludging phenomenon, hemorrhages, papilledema, and white exudates (Plate XXIV, Fig. 1, page 224 h).

The retinal changes in lymphogranulomatosis (Hodgkin) are those of anemia or the accompanying dysproteinemia. Malignant lymphogranulomatosis (Hodgkin) may result in tumorlike orbital nodules. Painless, slightly prominent, firm, gelatinous, reddish conjunctival nodules occur. Iritis has been observed in the end stages of Hodgkin's disease (Marquardt 1961).

Infectious Diseases, Intoxications, Occupational Diseases, Trichinosis

Infectious diseases: pyemia, sepsis (Fig. 22.10), malaria, recurrent fever, typhus, etc.

Intoxications: snakebite, carbon monoxide, nitrobenzene, lead, phosphorus, third degree burns. Rarely retinal hemorrhages and retrobulbar neuritis appear with streptomycin or sulfonamide therapy.

Occupational hazards causing retinal disease include (Merté 1969):

Arsenicals: pigment dispersion simulating retinitis pigmentosa.

Pentavalent arsenical combinations: retinal hemorrhages.

Benzene: retinal hemorrhages, neuroretinitis, conjunctival-corneal inflammation.

Nitro- and amino benzoles (methemoglobin formers): Nitronaphthalene: retinal hemorrhages, venous stasis, neuritis, severe corneal-conjunctival inflammation.

Lead: hemorrhages and exudates as in grade IV hypertensive retinopathy (angiospasm), narrowing of retinal arteries, optic neuritis.

Phosphorus: retinal hemorrhages, conjunctival icterus.

Chromium: narrowing of retinal arteries, optic atrophy.

Methanol: retinal hemorrhages, optic neuritis.

Carbon monoxide: retinal hemorrhages with venous dilatation and tortuosity, retinal edema, optic neuritis.

Trichinosis can cause retinal hemorrhages and edema (see page 198).

Collagen Disorders

The most important *collagen diseases – autoimmune disorders* include (Witmer 1970; see page 183):

Lupus erythematosus — Dermatomyositis — Scleroderma. Rheumatoid disorders: Primary chronic polyarthritis (see page 183); Ankylosing spondylitis (Marie-Strümpell-Bekhterev's disease), Still's disease, Felty's syndrome (see page 197); Sjögren's syndrome (see page 150) — Angiitides: Panarteritis, specifically panarteritis nodosa; hypersensitivity angiitis; Wegener's granulomatosis (see page 184); Goodpasture's syndrome – Behçet-Gilbert's disease (see page 203) – Reiter's syndrome (see page 128).

Disseminated lupus erythematosus (Kaposi-Libman-Sacks syndrome) (see page 93). This is a collagen disorder involving connective tissue and the vascular system. Ophthalmologically there is fleeting perivascular (Fig. 22.3) cuffing (exudates), gray cotton-wool spots (Clifton and Greer 1955; Hartmann and Massin 1956), exudative detachment, papilledema and episcleritis. Systemic findings include polyarthritis, lymphadenopathy, hepatitis, endocarditis, nephropathy and serum protein changes. Lupus erythematosus cells in the blood secure the diagnosis (Böke and Bäumer 1965).
Dermatomyositis: Cotton-wool exudates and striate retinal hemorrhages may appear.
Scleroderma: Scleroderma may be associated with cotton-wool spots, hard exudates, retinal hemorrhages and arterial occlusion. Progressive shrinkage of the lids is characteristic (Schreck 1960; Stucchi and Geiser 1967). Cataracts are not part of the clinical picture but are seen in pseudoscleroderma, such as Werner's syndrome.
Periarteritis nodosa: Most of the retinal changes of periarteritis nodosa are due to systemic hypertension. Primary vascular changes of the fundus may include (Pillat 1955): yellow-gray nodules along arteries, arterial occlusion, soft retinal exudates, gray choroidal nodules. External ocular findings include: myositis of extraocular muscles, nodules, scleritis with necrosis simulating scleromalacia perforans.
Mycosis fungoides may lead to exudation around the retinal arteries (Fig. 22.9).

Caisson Disease (The Bends)

Decompression disease: Retinal hemorrhages, papilledema, transient amaurosis, hemianopsia, fixed pupil, extraocular muscle palsy, edema and hemorrhage of the lid and conjunctiva. Air emboli develop in blood vessels (Kittel 1953).
The *battered baby syndrome* mostly includes bone fractures, subdural hematoma and in many cases also localized retinal or subretinal hemorrhages.

Gray, Circumscribed Retinal Lesions

Cotton-Wool Spots

Cotton-wool spots and retinal hemorrhages appear pathognomonically in grade IV *hypertensive retinopathy* (Plate XXIII, Fig. 2, page 224 g) and *eclampsia*. Similar changes are described (Hollwich 1963): with diabetes, lupus erythematosus, dermatomyositis, periarteritis nodosa, erythema multiforme, Hodgkin's disease, dysproteinemia, anemia, juxtapapillary chorioretinitis and internal carotid artery occlusion. Cotton-wool spots are fluffy, gray-white, poorly demarcated lesions over or under blood vessels. They disappear within a few weeks.
Hemorrhages, gray or white exudates, cotton-wool spots, and even papilledema occur with various blood disorders, such as pernicious anemia or secondary anemia: after severe hemorrhages, cachexia with neoplasms, parasites, poisoning (lead, mercury), with various types of leukemia (Hodgkin's disease, dysproteinemia).
Cotton-wool spots also occur with pheochromocytomas and in Wegener's granulomatosis (see page 184). Microemboli after cardiac surgery cause a similar picture.

Septic Retinitis

Sepsis may result in *metastatic ophthalmia* in the form of endophthalmitis, even panophthalmitis, or in *septic retinitis*. In septic retinitis, *small white retinal lesions* (Fig. 22.9) form, especially near vessel bifurcations. Small hemorrhages are also present. Vitreous clouding, papilledema and larger, fuzzy embolic lesions represent a transitional stage to metastatic ophthalmia.
Retinal damage due to septic emboli occurs

with cachexia, tuberculosis, diabetes, tumors, puerperal sepsis and endocarditis.

Tuberculosis

In tuberculosis (miliary tuberculosis, tuberculous meningitis), small fuzzy gray-white choroidal-retinal lesions may be scattered throughout the fundus (see page 215).

Choroiditis

Every active choroiditis (disseminated [Plate XV, Fig. 5, page 192 g]), juxtapapillary [Plate XVI, Fig. 1, page 192 h], diffuse chorioretinitis) (see page 215) leads to a chorioretinitis with localized gray retinal discoloration.

Medullated Nerve Fibers

Medullated nerve fibers are flame-shaped, pure white plaques usually obscuring blood vessels (Plate XXIV, Fig. 3, page 224 h). These are congenital anomalies generally located near the disc, but they may appear peripherally (Fig. 22.11). Normally, retinal nerve fibers are not myelinated until past the cribriform plate. With optic atrophy the medullation of retinal nerve fibers disappears completely.

White medullated nerve fibers can be confused with cotton-wool spots in grade IV hypertensive retinopathy. The normal vision, blood pressure and remainder of the fundus make the differential diagnosis easy. Branch artery occlusion looks similar, but the history of sudden vision loss is typical; furthermore, there is visual field loss, narrowed arteries and, later, optic atrophy.

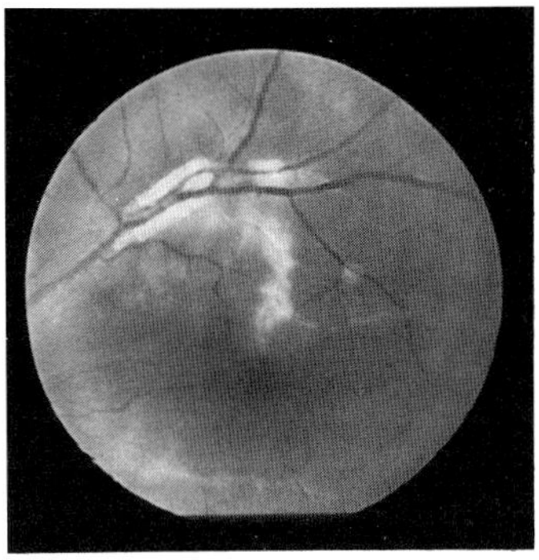

Fig. 22.9 Mycosis fungoides with exudations and ensheathing of the retinal arteries (♂ 37 yrs.)

Choroidal-Retinal Coloboma

(see page 213)

Choroidal colobomata are bilateral, usually inferior nasal, and result from a disturbance in closure of the embryonic fissure. A large gray-white (sclera) area of varying width extends from the periphery toward the optic disc (Fig. 22.12). The border of the coloboma is hyperpigmented. Anomalous retinal vessels cross the coloboma in increased number. The coloboma may be divided by a bridge of normal tissue.

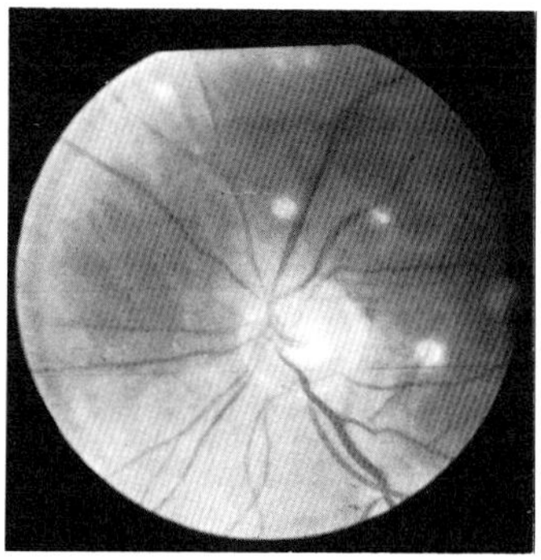

Fig. 22.10 Septicemia with gray disseminated retinal nodules (♂ 57 yrs.)

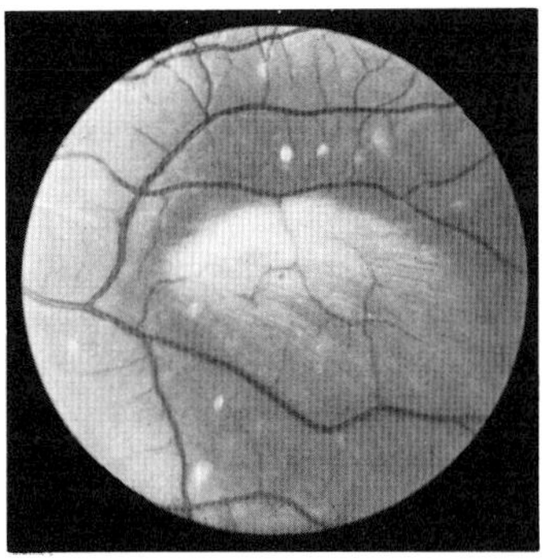

Fig. 22.11 Medullated nerve fibers (♀ 44 yrs.)

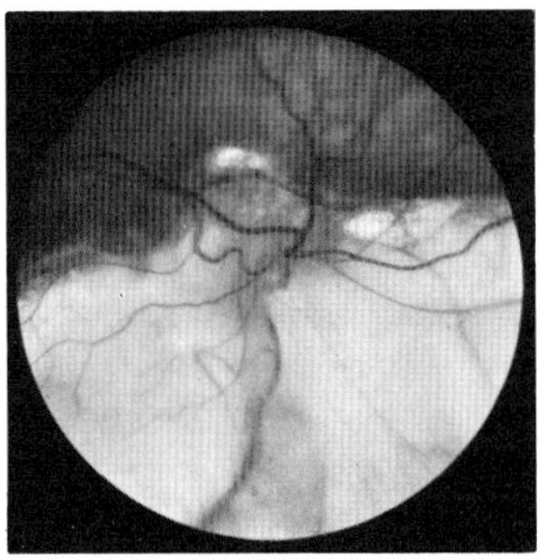

Fig. 22.12 Congenital coloboma of the choroid, retina and optic nerve (♂ 16 yrs.)

Choroidal colobomata are often combined with coloboma of the iris, optic disc and lens. Microphthalmos, hyperopia and amblyopia are common. Emmetropia or high myopia are possible.

Heredity is usually dominant.
Rarely, atypical colobomata present in some position other than the usual. "Macular colobomata" are almost always prenatal toxoplasmosis scars.

Diffuse Gray Discoloration of the Retina

Edema of any cause results in diffuse gray discoloration of the retina. This occurs with *interruption of the arterial blood supply* (central retinal artery occlusion, postmortem), *flat chorioretinitis, acute quinine poisoning,* and *trauma* (Berlin's edema). The retina appears somewhat gray in a fresh, *flat, retinal detachment.*
Oguchi's disease patients (see page 31) (a variation of essential congenital night blindness) develop a white-gray fundus color after one half to one hour of light adaptation. This discoloration particularly occurs in the peripapillary area and in the macula. The fundus color returns to normal after two to three hours of dark adaptation (Mizuo's phenomenon).
Gray central discoloration, especially with a cherry red spot (Plate XXVII, Fig. 6, page 288 c), results from lipid storage in metabolic disorders and may be associated with tapetoretinal degeneration. The various lipidoses (see page 365) have to be considered: Tay-Sachs disease, Niemann-Pick disease and Gaucher's disease.

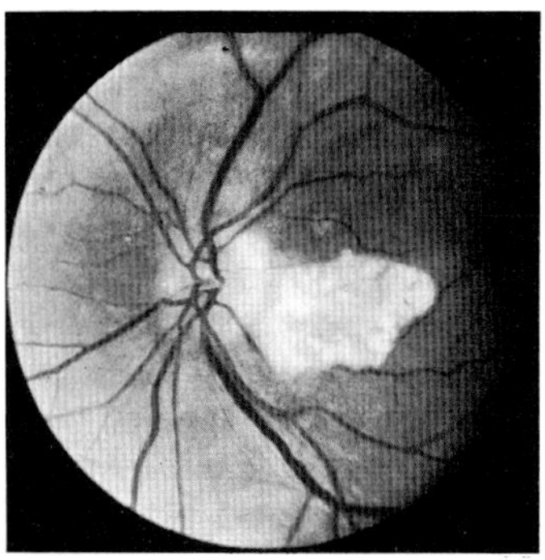

Fig. 22.13 Embolus of a cilioretinal artery (♀ 46 yrs.)

Retinal Artery Emboli

Central retinal artery emboli — Branch emboli, etiology of emboli — Endarteritis obliterans — Temporal arteritis — Periarteritis nodosa — Carotid occlusion, pulseless disease — Wegener's granulomatosis — True emboli — Fat emboli, Purtscher's retinopathy — Air emboli — Compression.

Central retinal artery emboli (Plate XXIV, Fig. 4, page 224 h): The history provides the diagnosis: "The light suddenly turned off in this eye." The pupil is amaurotic. Ophthalmoscopically the fundus appears gray. Interruption of nutrition results in edema of the inner retinal layers. Since Henle's fiber layer radiates away from the fovea, this area retains its normal red color, appearing as a cherry red spot one-quarter to one-third of the disc diameter in size. The arteries are narrowed, partly from lack of circulation, partly from obscuration by edematous tissue. Rouleaux formation of red blood cells results in a granular blood flow. The blood column is interrupted in places, simply moving back and forth in parts of the vessel. Since retinal vessels, like cerebral vessels, are end arteries, there is no restitution of function by anastomoses.
After three weeks the fundus color returns to normal (edema and degenerated nerve fibers have been removed via Nissl bodies). The optic disc is white, and retinal vessels are thin threads.
Branch emboli: A branch embolus causes the same clinical picture, but is limited to the appropriate fundus area (Fig. 22.13). A corresponding visual field defect is present. If a cilioretinal artery is present (Fig. 22.14), a small area between the disc and fovea may remain intact when the central retinal artery is occluded. A small tunnel of vision, potentially with normal central acuity, remains.

Etiology of emboli: The clinical picture of arterial emboli is usually not produced by actual emboli. In older patients, at least, it is generally due to *endarteritis obliterans* (Plate XXIV, Fig. 5, page 224 h), arteriosclerosis, hypertension, or rarely lues. Thromboarteritis can occur with orbital cellulitis.

Temporal arteritis: In temporal arteritis the vascular occlusion is due to giant cell arteritis. Severe optic neuritis results.

Temporal arteritis (giant cell arteritis [Horton, see page 311]) usually occurs in persons over the age of 60. The temporal arteries are tortuous, nodular, pulseless and painful to pressure. Low grade fever, elevated erythrocyte sedimentation rate, temporal headaches, and pain on mastication are common. Ischemic papillitis leads to optic atrophy, severe vision loss, and often complete blindness (see page 311). Besides the picture of papilledema (ischemic optic neuropathy), the picture of central retinal or branch artery occlusion is common.

Periarteritis nodosa: Ocular involvement is rare: small nodules on the walls of retinal arteries, floccular retinal infiltrates, branch artery occlusion (Hollwich 1963).

Carotid occlusion: Carotid thrombosis (occlusion of the internal carotid) (see page 315) must be considered with unilateral central artery or branch occlusion, central retinal vein thrombosis, papilledema, optic atrophy, cotton-wool spots, ocular muscle paresis, Horner's syndrome, exophthalmos, phthisis, *asymmetric ophthalmic artery pressure* (ophthalmodynamometry), homonymous hemianopsia, visual field loss and decreased acuity in combination with *contralateral hemiparesis.* Occlusion of the internal carotid artery (Seitz 1961) is rarely acute, is usually slow in onset and may lead to unilateral amaurosis with contralateral hemiplegia. Incomplete occlusion often causes acute painless unilateral vision loss (amaurosis fugax) on the side of the carotid insufficiency. Often headaches, hemiparesthesia, aphasia or cramps are the only symptoms (Hager 1962).

Takayasu's disease *(pulseless disease)* (see page 315) causes narrow retinal arteries, sausage-like dilatation of retinal veins with granular blood flow, peripapillary arteriovenous anastomoses, vascular obliteration in the retinal periphery, vitreous hemorrhages, retinitis proliferans, retinal detachment, dilatation of episcleral vessels, iris atrophy, annular vessel formation at the root of the iris, internal ophthalmoplegia, and cataracts developing with varying rapidity.

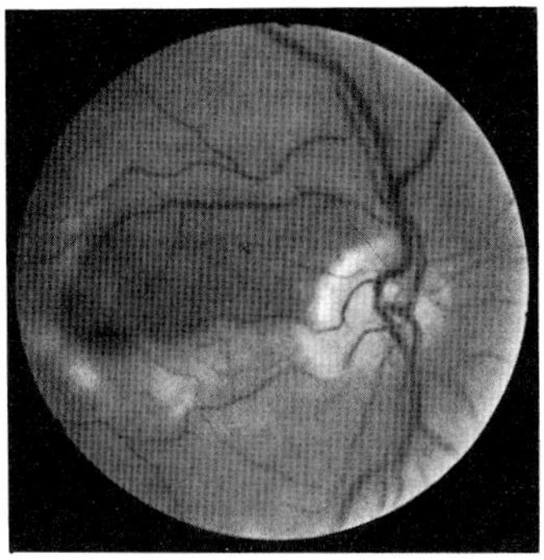

Fig. 22.14 Central retinal artery embolus with an intact cilioretinal artery (♂ 63 yrs.)

Ophthalmodynamography and *ophthalmodynamometry* are of value in the *differential diagnosis of carotid artery occlusion,* the *aortic arch syndrome* (pulseless disease) and *temporal arteritis.*

Ophthalmodynamometry measures the blood pressure in the ophthalmic artery (not the central retinal artery). The results reflect changes in intracranial and cerebrovascular resistance. *Ophthalmodynamography* (Hager 1963) is an oscillographic recording, an orbital oscillogram. This gives information about occlusion of the large arteries in the neck.

Ophthalmodynametrically measured ophthalmic artery pressure is decreased on the side of carotid occlusion or thrombosis. Ophthalmodynamography shows a reproducible reduction in pulse volume on the occluded side.

Dynamometry values are markedly reduced bilaterally in the aortic arch syndrome. Contrary to temporal arteritis, there may be no pulse in the upper extremities (Bettelheim 1968).

Wegener's granulomatosis can result in central retinal artery emboli, cotton-wool spots, rarely retinal detachment (see page 184 and 338).

True emboli: True emboli are more common in younger patients, for instance with valvular endocarditis, aortic aneurysms, etc. Embolic cholesterol plaques and platelet thrombi do occur in older patients and are a sign of arte-

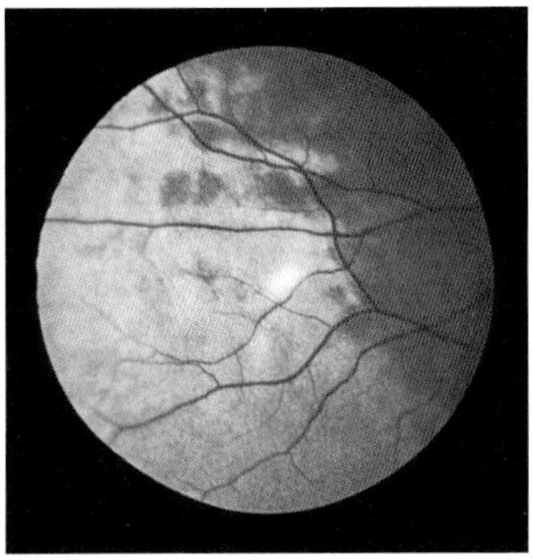

Fig. 22.15 Commotio retinae (Berlin's edema) 12 hours following contusion of the globe (♂ 9 yrs.)

riosclerotic plaques in the ipsilateral carotid artery.

Fat emboli usually occur after fracture of long bones, or as a result of thoracic or compression injury. These result in plaquelike exudates, usually near vessels and the optic disc. These exudates are gray-white, and may be floccular (cotton-wool-like) or sharply delineated. Flame-shaped or blot hemorrhages and retinal edema are common (Calmettes et al. 1967; Verin and le Rebeller 1967). Pulmonary and neurologic complications may occur.

Purtscher's traumatic angiopathy (Plate XXIV, Fig. 6, page 224 h; see page 285) has a characteristic fundus picture (Urbanek 1933) that differs from that of fat emboli. In contrast to fat emboli, Purtscher's retinopathy usually results in considerable permanent damage (Pape 1964) (see page 285).

Air emboli: Air emboli may appear as small bright interruptions of the blood column or as the cause of central or branch retinal artery occlusion (Sachsenweger 1957). Muscle paresis, nystagmus and pupillary disturbances occur. Symptoms are usually fleeting. In contrast, in caisson disease (the bends, decompression sickness), air emboli (nitrogen gas) allegedly appear in the veins (Kittel 1953) (see page 268). Air emboli are rare and occur primarily after neck surgery, after irrigation of sinuses, and with pneumothorax, soap irrigation of the uterus, arteriography, etc.

Compression: The clinical picture of emboli can be simulated by external compression as with orbital tumors, marked retrobulbar hemorrhages, etc.

Berlin's Edema

This occurs after direct trauma to the globe (Fig. 22.15). There is an immediate decrease in visual acuity. One hour later, gray-white retinal edema, occasionally with small petechial hemorrhages, occurs. When located centrally, a cherry red spot is present. The edema resolves after 24 to 36 hours.

Retinitis Proliferans

Recurrent vitreous hemorrhages, exudates, inflammation or injury can stimulate ingrowth of vascularized connective tissue from the retina into the vitreous. This results in localized traction detachments which become total.

Retinitis proliferans occurs most commonly in stage III diabetic retinopathy, untreated periphlebitis, recurrent or poorly resorbing hemorrhages as with arteriosclerosis, central vein thrombosis, anemia, leukemia, macroglobulinemia, dysparaproteinemia, sickle cell anemia, and lupus erythematosus. Circumscribed connective tissue proliferation, traction and star folds may occur after perforating injuries, retinal detachment or diathermy-light-cryotherapy. Severe inflammation (endophthalmitis, tuberculosis) can cause retinitis proliferans. Retrolental fibroplasia, occurring in premature infants given oxygen in incubators, is a form of retinitis proliferans.

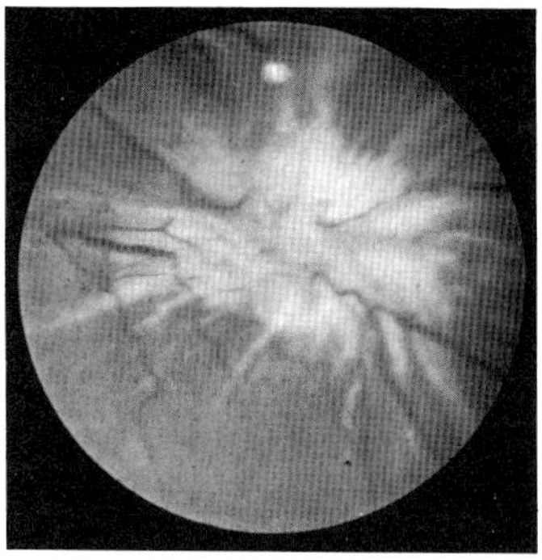

Fig. 22.16 Star traction folds in retinal detachment (♀ 40 yrs.)

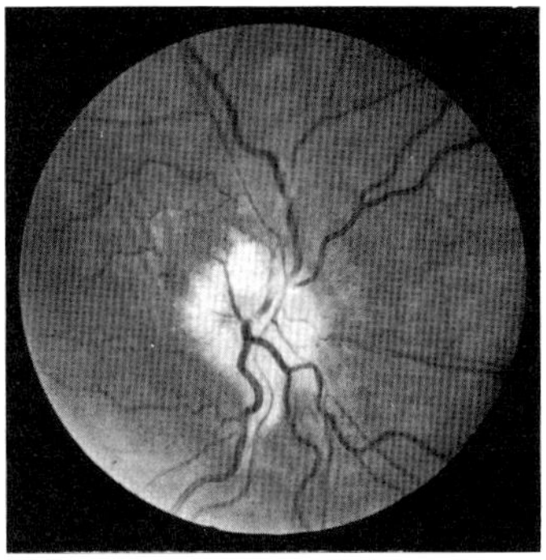

Fig. 22.17 Choroidal folds superior temporally to a swollen optic disk with beginning atrophy due to a retrobulbar tumor (♂ 46 yrs.)

Retinal Folds

These occur (Dellaporta 1954) as:

Traction folds with scarring after perforating injury, chorioretinitis, retinitis proliferans, retinal fibroplasia or star folds following retinal detachment (Fig. 22.16). Retinal damage through light-laser-diathermy-cryocoagulation causes retinal folds in some 3 percent of cases owing to development of preretinal membranes. A similar picture occurs with retinal holes and attached retina or after retinal detachment. This was called "epiretinal fibroplasia" by Gloor (1970) and "puckering syndrome" by Gass (1973).

Retinal folds with edema occur with: perforating injuries (contusio bulbi, especially in young patients), inflammation as with cyclitis, diffuse chorioretinitis (Förster), juxtapapillary chorioretinitis, papilledema, with marked hypotension (e vacuo – usually after perforating injury or fistulizing surgery) (Plate XXV, Fig. 1, page 288 a). Hypotensive retinal folds appear mainly at the posterior pole and are accompanied by papilledema. This occurs preferentially in younger patients, disappearing with normalization of the intraocular tension. With chronic hypotension, the retinal folds become fixed by connective tissue organization (Pau 1950).

Chorioretinal Folds
(Fig. 22.17)

These result from displacement of choroid and retina by intraocular tumors or pseudotumors and with external pressure on the globe by orbital lesions.

Retinoschisis and Cysts

Biomicroscopically cystoid degenerations can be demonstrated in any living eye after indentation of the ora. Both the typical or external and the reticular or internal cystoid degeneration of the peripheral retina increase in frequency and extent with increasing age. The picture of cystoid degeneration can also be produced artificially and postmortally (Pau 1976).

Retinoschisis can be categorized as (Hruby 1956):

1. Primary idiopathic retinoschisis. This belongs to the hyaloideoretinal degenerations (see page 233).
2. Primary retinoschisis with cyst formation
a) idiopathic
b) post chorioretinitis.

Hyaloideoretinal Degeneration

In hyaloideoretinal degeneration, three forms of vitreous, vitreous membrane and retinal changes can be distinguished (Ricci 1961;

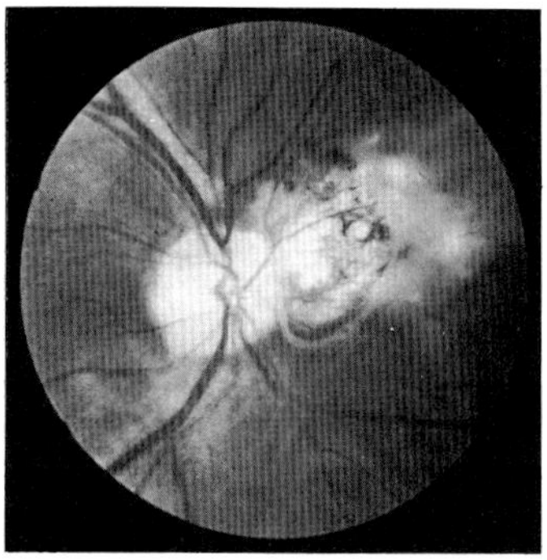

Fig. 22.18 Juxtapapillary chorioretinitis with posterior vitreous detachment

Hauschild et al. 1970; Bengtsson and Linder 1967) (see page 233):

a) **Primary idiopathic retinioschisis** with *inner layer holes* (see page 274): In this form of retinoschisis, delicate, perforated, vascularized membranes develop from the inner retinal layer. This condition occurs bilaterally, inferior temporally, in nonmyopic young males. It is a sex-linked recessive congenital anomaly usually beginning in early youth. The retinal splitting is symmetrical, bilateral, and easily mistaken for ora tears. There is a corresponding visual field loss. Macular changes causing vision loss are common. Gray gliotic patches form on the detached limiting membrane. The optic disk is often pale (Kleinert 1953). Tears in the inner leaf cause arcadelike lacunae and hemorrhage so that the detached portion can look like a vascularized vitreous membrane. Retinal detachments and cataracts can develop.

b) **Hereditary vitreous-retinal degeneration** *(Wagner's hyaloideoretinal degeneration)* (see page 233) is vitreous degeneration with the formation of peripheral avascular preretinal membranes. Retinoschisis is rare. Retinal pigment clumping and complicated cataracts are more common (Böhringer et al. 1960). Heredity is autosomal dominant.

c) **Recessive vitreous-tapetoretinal degeneration** *(recessive hyaloideo-tapetoretinal degeneration)* (Goldmann-Favre) (see page 233). Clinical findings include retinoschisis, preretinal vitreous membranes, macular edema or schisis, tapetoretinal degeneration with pigmentation, nyctalopia, abnormal ERG, cataract.

Primary Retinoschisis with Cyst Formation

Idiopathic form: In primary retinoschisis with cyst formation, unilateral or bilateral, circumscribed, flat to bullous transparent detachment of the inner retinal layer occurs, usually temporally. The diagnosis can be made by the parallactic shift of retinal vessels and the diffuse red-gray discoloration of the involved retina. The patients are usually emmetropes with good visual acuity. This form of retinoschisis may be sex-linked recessive in young patients or appear as an abiotrophy, especially inferior temporal, in older patients. Senile cystic retinoschisis is quite common (Charleux et al. 1969; Eisner 1973; Shea et al. 1960; Zimmerman and Spencer 1960). The condition is frequently asymptomatic and discovered only on routine examination.

Postinflammatory form: Choroidal scarring, intraretinal scars, retinal cysts, potentially with lamellar holes, develop after chorioretinitis. Self-healing localized retinal detachments present a similar picture.

Cysts in Detached Retina

Giant cysts may develop in detached retina.

Macular Cysts

Macular cysts are classified as (Hruby 1956):

a) Microcystic (Plate XXV, Fig. 2, page 288 a) – rarely macrocystic (Plate XXV, Fig. 3, page 288 a) – macular edema can be differentiated from a macular hole only with the aid of a slit lamp.

b) Cystlike serous detachment in central serous retinopathy (see page 283).

c) A circumscribed posterior vitreous detachment (Fig. 22.18) often because of, or with, localized hemorrhage.

d) Owing to enhanced contrast, the *foveola* may look *cystic* or *simulate* a *macular hole*, especially in darkly pigmented persons (Slezak 1967). Small, irregular, gray-white dots (Gunn's spots) on the retinal surface near the macular can be mistaken for cystic degeneration. A dark red foveolar spot or mottled disruption of the pigment epithelium may be difficult to differentiate ophthalmoscopically from a small cyst or hole. Variations in thickness, or defects of Bruch's membrane, impart a delicate marbling to the fundus.

Retinal Detachment (Amotio Retinae)

Subjective symptoms of recent retinal detachment include: flickering, flimmering vision; light flashes; a gray dark wall or curtain, appearing in part of the visual field, worse in the evening than in the morning. There is a corresponding visual field loss. Rapid clouding of vision (minutes to hours) occurs with vitreous hemorrhage.

Ophthalmoscopically the detachment is seen in the retinal area opposite the side of the subjective complaints. It appears as a gray-red discoloration, often wavy, with tortuous retinal vessels. Veins and arteries appear dark red to black because of retroillumination. The choroid is poorly visible.

The detachment progresses rapidly – hours to days – becoming more extensive and bullous with undulating folds.

Primary Retinal Detachment

Retinal tears (holes) appear as red (visible choroid) areas in the gray detached retina and are of utmost importance in the etiology, therapy and prognosis of the detachment.

Horseshoe tear — Peripheral holes — Ora tear — Macular hole — Causes of detachment — Differential diagnosis.

Horseshoe tears: *Flap tears* constitute 60 percent of retinal tears, are usually *superior temporal* and may be shaped like a *horseshoe* (Fig. 22.19). The legs of the horseshoe point peripherally, its apex centrally. Vitreous is usually adherent to the tip of the retinal flap. The edges of the tear may be flat or rolled over. Flap-horseshoe tears generally occur along areas of *sclerotic degenerated* retina. Most patients are moderate myopes – between 40 and 60 years – and are often aphakic, occasionally with a history of trauma.

Operculated and atrophic holes: Small isolated or multiple, round or oval peripheral holes occur in about 30 percent of retinal detachments.

Ora tears generally occur days, even years, after trauma and are preferentially located inferior temporal.

Macular hole: True macular holes (Fig. 22.20) are rare, occurring in high myopia, or as degenerative holes with age or after trauma. Macular cysts or partial-thickness holes are more common. With a true macular hole, the thin slit lamp beam has to be completely interrupted. Macular cysts retain a thin membrane covering. The small red foveola can appear like a retinal hole or cyst in the gray surrounding of a flat retinal detachment. A cherry red

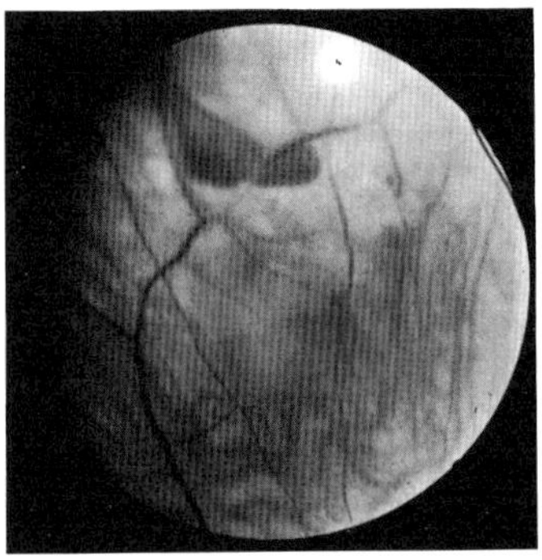

Fig. 22.19 Retinal detachment with horseshoe tear (♀ 50 yrs.)

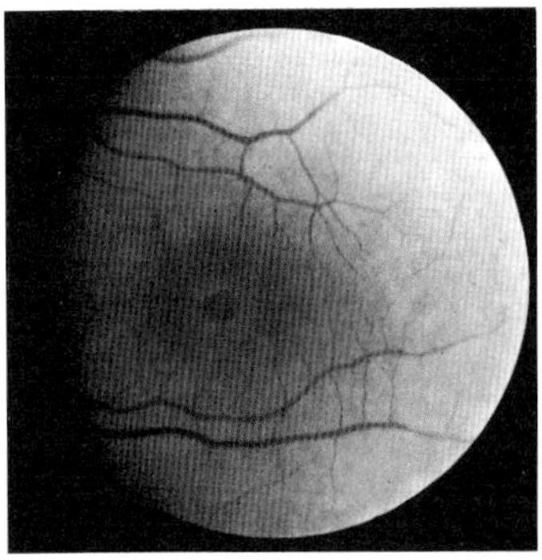

Fig. 22.20 Macular hole (♀ 66 yrs.)

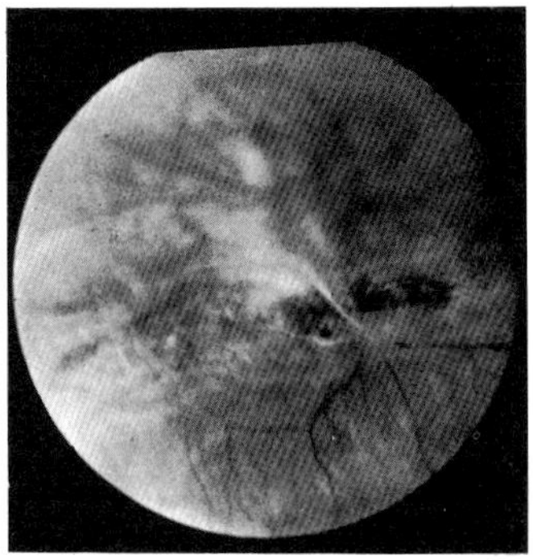

Fig. 22.21 Sclerotic retinal area (lattice degeneration) with vitreous adhesion (♂ 32 yrs.)

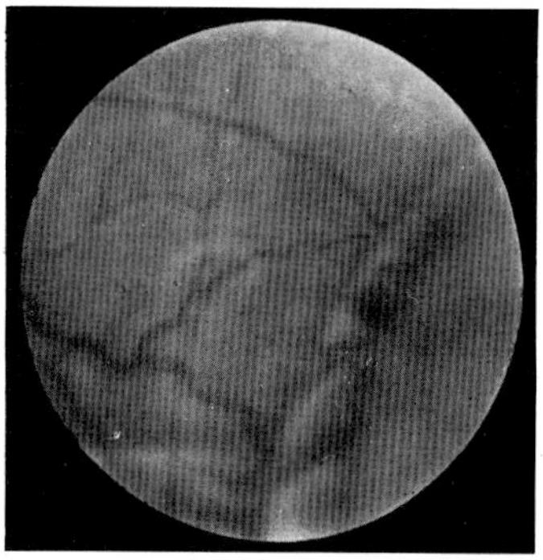

Fig. 22.22 Inflammatory retinal detachment in Harada's disease (♀ 49 yrs.)

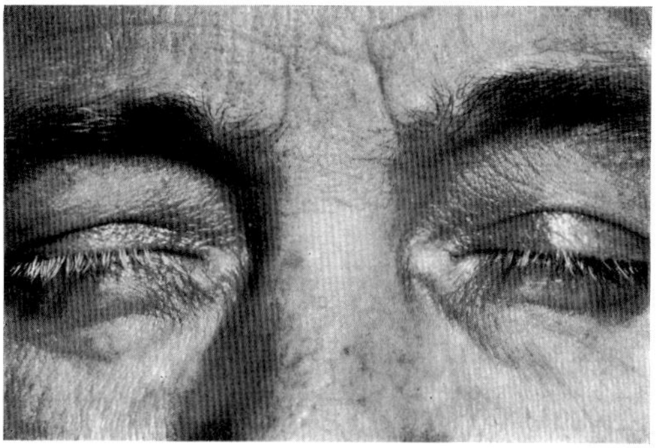

Fig. 22.23 Poliosis in Harada's disease

spot with macular edema from a central retinal artery embolus creates the same illusion.

Causes of primary retinal detachment: According to their etiology, retinal detachments appear in various forms:

Vitreous syneresis (myopia, senile, in aphakia, traumatic) is a requirement for the appearance of the most common type of retinal detachment from the pigment epithelium. The vitreous is particularly adherent to the retina at those locations where embryonal hyaloid vessels formerly attached. The retina is altered at this point by connective tissue derived from vitreoretinal border cells, perivascular connective tissue and pigment epithelium (Pau 1970, 1971, 1975, 1977). Between these sclerotic areas, (Fig. 22.21) the normal retina tears from vitreous traction. Sclerotic areas predisposing to detachment appear as snail tracts (Schneckenspuren) or lattice degeneration. The term "cystoid patches" is incorrect for lattice degeneration, which has little or no cyst formation. Blessig-Iwanoff edema (peripheral cystoid) is principally different.

Peripheral "paving-stone" degeneration differs from sclerotic areas in that it represents a degenerative fusion of choroid and retina. These are pale atrophic lesions with darkly pigmented borders. They do not predispose to retinal detachment, since the retina is firmly fused with underlying structures. As a retinal detachment from other causes expands, retina surrounding paving-stone areas may tear free, causing secondary holes.

Aphakia predisposes to retinal detachment, especially when vitreous was lost during surgery (Pau 1969).

In rare cases, a sudden tug from direct or indirect trauma is the final stimulus for detachment.

Besides retinal tears due to vitreoretinal adhesion, atrophic retinal holes with secondary tears occur. These are of special significance in hereditary vitreoretinal degeneration (see page 233):

1. Sex-linked congenital retinal detachment (Norrie's disease).
2. Sex-linked juvenile retinoschisis.
3. Dominant vitreoretinal degeneration (Wagner's disease).
4. Recessive vitreo-tapetoretinal degeneration (Goldmann-Favre).
5. Macrofibrillar vitreoretinal degeneration (Favre).

Differential diagnosis of idiopathic detachments, tumors, exudative uveitis, intraocular hemorrhages and intraocular foreign bodies is aided by echography and transillumination (Oksala 1964; Bronson 1973; Coleman 1972).

Secondary Retinal Detachment

Inflammatory exudate — Retinal detachment from alteration of vessel permeability — Exudative retinitis (Coats' disease) — Central serous retinopathy, tumors, parasites — Various forms of serous detachment of the pigment epithelium — Retinitis proliferans — Retrolental fibroplasia — Preretinal membrane formation, puckering syndrome — Falciform detachment.

Inflammatory exudate: Detachment of the retina from the pigment epithelium can result from serous or inflammatory exudate; with Harada's disease (Fig. 22.22, 22.23), Vogt-Koyanagi disease, sympathetic ophthalmia, scleritis, choroiditis, or *Toxocara canis* infection. The detachment may be total or circumscribed (see page 198).

Retinal detachment from alteration of vascular permeability: Renal disease, malignant hypertension, and eclampsia cause exudative detachment (Fig. 22.7).

Exudative retinitis (Coats' disease): This is a relatively rare form of exudative retinal detachment (Plate XXV, Fig. 4, page 288 a; Plate XXVIII, Fig. 5, page 288 d). Eighty percent of patients are males below age 25. The disease begins with numerous aneurysms of retinal vessels, hemorrhages and white exudates in and beneath the outer retinal layers (Reese 1956; François et al. 1956; Woods and Duke 1963), leading to detachment.

Birefringent lipid substances (cholesterol) are found in the subretinal exudate. There is pigment epithelium proliferation along with connective tissue formation and calcification. The cause is unknown. Toxic capillary processes are suspected.

Various Causes of Serous Retinal Detachment

Central serous retinopathy (see pages 283 and 216), *choroidal tumors* (melanoma), *retinal tumors* (retinoblastoma, angioma). *Parasites* in the retina or vitreous (cysticercus, ophthalmomyiasis).

Occasionally, serous detachment will occur with (see page 279 and following): *juvenile, presenile* and *senile disciform macular degeneration, idiopathic central serous pigment epithelial detachment, high myopia, angioid streaks, hereditary choroidal degenerations* (Doyne's honeycomb degeneration) (Gass et al. 1966).

Retinitis proliferans: Retinal detachment can result from vitreous traction: retinitis proliferans (see page 272) with organizing hemorrhages, diabetic retinopathy, retinal periphlebitis, arteriosclerotic hemorrhages, perforating injuries, after vitreous abscess, etc. Retrolental fibroplasia causes a similar picture. Preretinal membrane formation after surgery with diathermy, electrolysis, light or cryocoagulation can cause traction detachments. This is the same clinical picture as the puckering syndrome (see below).

Retrolental fibroplasia (see page 235) occurs in newborns, generally with a birth weight below 1,800 to 1,900 grams, who were given oxygen in the incubator. Peripheral retinal vessels dilate, and hemorrhages, edema, new vessel formation and proliferation occur within two to six weeks after birth. Sprigs of newly formed vessels extend, brushlike, into the vitreous, resulting in vascularized connective tissue, vitreous and retinal detachment (Fig. 20.3) (traction detachment).

After coagulation (diathermy, light, cryo surgery), gray retinal star folds leading to traction detachment can occur. These result from epi-

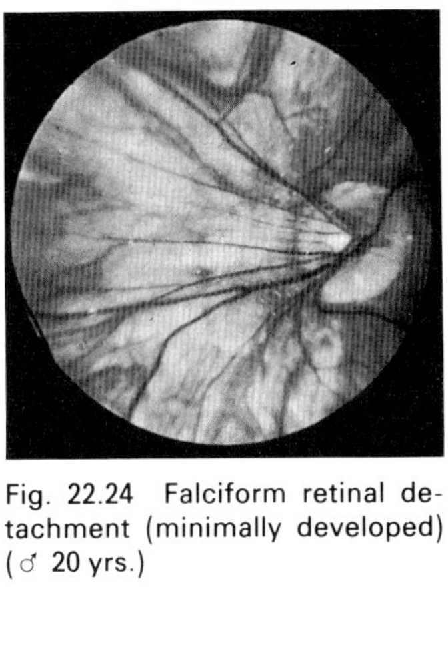

Fig. 22.24 Falciform retinal detachment (minimally developed) (♂ 20 yrs.)

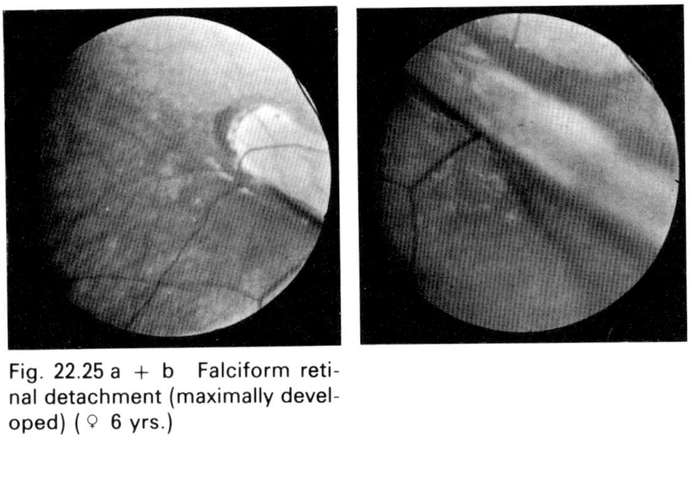

Fig. 22.25 a + b Falciform retinal detachment (maximally developed) (♀ 6 yrs.)

retinal membrane formation by proliferating vitreoretinal border cells. Gloor and Werner (1967) spoke of *internal retinal fibroplasia*, Gloor (1970) of *epiretinal fibroplasia* (Plate XXV, Fig. 5, page 288 a). Gass calls it *"puckering syndrome"* (see page 273).

Congenital falciform folds (detachment): This is a hereditary or congenitally acquired detachment (Weve 1935, Goldberg 1974) (Fig. 22.24, 22.25), usually consisting of reduplicated retina beginning at the optic disc and extending in a "fold" to the inferior temporal periphery where it connects with retrolental remnants of the hyaloid artery (Thiel 1968). The condition is usually bilateral.

Undoubtedly the picture of falciform folds can be acquired, as with retrolental fibroplasia, extensive star folds or traction folds with retinal detachment. Coats' disease can cause similar findings. *Form fruste retrolental fibroplasia (retinopathy of prematurity)* can result in peripheral retinal pigment dispersion, ectopic macula, falciform detachment, and congenital retinal folds (Lemmingson 1968). The relationship between retrolental fibroplasia and falciform folds has frequently been discussed (Planthen 1955, 1960; Schlitter 1957; Tasman 1975). In general it is considered to be healed retrolental, a transitional stage to retrolental, or a special form of retrolental fibroplasia.

Macular Diseases

Aplasia — Hypoplasia — Heterotopia of the macula lutea — Hereditary macular degeneration — Angioid streaks — High myopia — Microcystic macular damage, Irvine-Gass syndrome — Macular puckering — Macular holes — Light damage to the macula — Inflammatory macular damage — Camp amblyopia — Cherry red spot of the macula.

Aplasia/Hypoplasia of the Fovea

The fovea may be congenitally aplastic or hypoplastic. Besides poor central acuity, nystagmus is usually present. Other malformations such as albinism, aniridia, microphthalmos or marked hypermetropia are usually present.

Heterotopia of the Macula Lutea (Dragged Macula)

Heterotopia of the macula lutea may lead to pseudostrabismus or only a gamma angle. Heterotopia of the macula can be a congenital anomaly and is compatible with good vision. More commonly it occurs because of macular traction (dragged macula) by retinal scars (falciform detachment, inflammatory, traumatic, star folds).

Hereditary Macular Degeneration

Hereditary macular degeneration can have a variably early onset and be progressive (usually senile forms) or, once manifest, remain stationary (all forms except senile). Forms of juvenile macular degeneration can progress to complete destruction of the retina. Heredity varies, being more or less regular, irregular, dominant or recessive.

(Falls 1966; Deutmann 1971; Blach 1969; Hamilton et al. 1973; Maumenee and Emery 1972)

Hereditary macular degenerations can be divided into (Falls 1966):

Congenital macular degeneration

a) Best's disease (cystic macular degeneration, polymorphous macular degeneration, vitelliform macular degeneration)
b) Leber's congenital amaurosis
c) Achromatopsia

Juvenile macular degeneration (6–20 yrs.)

d) Stargardt's disease
e) Cone (rod) dystrophy
f) Juvenile retinoschisis
g) Vitreo-tapetoretinal degeneration (Favre-Goldmann)
h) Fundus flavimaculatus (dystrophia reticularis laminae pigmentosae retinae, dominant hereditary drusen)
i) Malignant myopia

Adult macular degeneration (20–50 yrs.)

j) Central choroidal sclerosis

k) Generalized choroidal sclerosis
l) Doyne's honeycomb degeneration
m) Tay's guttate "choroiditis"
n) Malattia leventinese
o) Sorsby's macular degeneration
p) inverse retinitis pigmentosa

Senile macular degeneration

q) Senile pigmentary macular degeneration
r) Senile disciform macular degeneration (Kuhnt-Junius)

Congenital Macular Degeneration

Best's macular degeneration, cystic macular degeneration, polymorphous macular degeneration, vitelliform macular degeneration. This begins as a round or oval egg-yolk-like transudate under the pigment epithelium (Plate XXV, Fig. 6, page 288 a) with relatively good visual acuity. Later various degrees of pigmentation and depigmentation occur in this region (Plate XXVI, Fig. 1, page 288 b).

Vitelliform cysts are hereditary, sharply delimited, yellow-orange elevated discs 1 to 2 disc diameters in size. Their contents are "semiliquid," at times with a fluid level, and located between Bruch's membrane and the pigment epithelium. The ophthalmoscopic picture reminds one of an egg yolk (un oeuf sur la plate). Vision is often decreased but may be normal.

Vitelliform cysts usually begin between ages 2 and 8. Resorption and rupture of the cysts in older persons (Remky et al. 1965) creates the picture of macular degeneration. Multiple vitelliform cysts can appear at the posterior pole (Denden 1966). Heredity is usually dominant (Sorsby et al. 1956; Hermann 1966; Krill et al. 1966).

Four stages occur in vitelliform macular degeneration (François et al. 1967):

1. The vitelliform stage
2. Pseudohypopyon or pseudocysts
3. Scarring
4. Atrophy

Vitelliform macular degeneration is indentical with Best's hereditary macular degeneration (Braley 1966; Duke-Elder 1967). Heredity is autosomal dominant (Thiel and Behnke 1971). The EOG is characteristically affected. The doubling in amplitude of the EOG standing potential that normally occurs with exposure to light is absent. The light peak – dark trough ratio remains at 1.0 (Francois et al. 1967; Deutman 1969). The ERG is normal but the foveal ERG and cortical VER may be variably affected. Fluorescein angiography fails to reveal any pathologic alterations with vitelliform cysts. In contrast, staining is reported in Best's macular degeneration (Ricci et al. 1969). Best's macular degeneration is the end stage of vitelliform cysts.

Leber's congenital amaurosis. Heredity: autosomal recessive. This is a generalized tapetoretinal degeneration with varying degrees of pepper and salt fundus pigmentation. A picture of retinitis pigmentosa or central pigmentary dispersion is rare. Cataracts and keratoconus may occur. Generally, chorioretinal and optic nerve atrophy develop with an absent b-wave on electroretinography.

In **achromatopsia** (see page 30), young patients are affected and develop fine pigmentary changes in the macula, with hyper- and hypopigmentation occurring. Visual acuity is in the range of 20/80 to 20/100 or worse. Heredity is sex-linked recessive.

Juvenile Macular Degeneration (6–20 yrs.)

Stargardt's macular degeneration is a familial macular degeneration with onset between ages 8 and 14. Central visual acuity is lost. Peripheral vision remains normal (Franceschetti et al. 1963). Within 12 months a normal ophthalmoscopic picture changes to bilateral, central, oval areas of pigment clumping and dispersion (Plate XXVI, Fig. 2, page 288 b). After years, chorioretinal atrophy develops. The macular ERG and VER are decreased. In contrast to vitelliform degeneration the EOG and mass response ERG remain normal for a long time (François et al. 1967; Deutman 1969).

Stargardt's macular degeneration is frequently associated with fundus flavimaculatus. The two diseases may be varying expressions of the same genetic disorder. As with vitelliform cysts, fluorescein angiography remains normal in the early stages of Stargardt's disease (François and de Laey 1969). In the late stage, Stargardt's disease resembles choroidal sclerosis.

Heredity: autosomal recessive or dominant.

Cone dystrophy usually begins before age 20. It can have the appearance of fundus flavimacu-

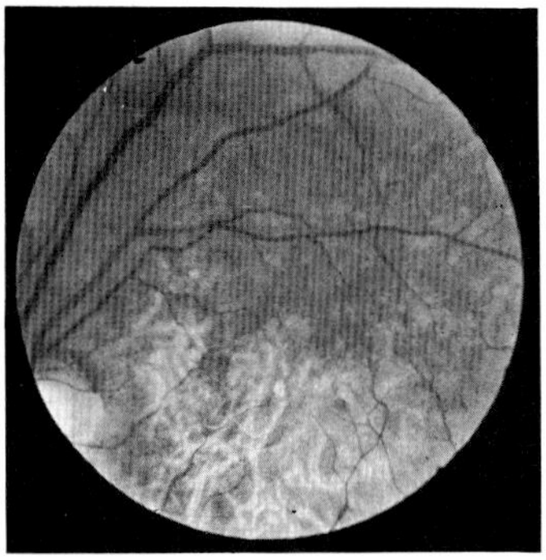

Fig. 22.26 Central choroidal sclerosis (♂ 51 yrs.)

latus, Stargardt's dystrophy, or "bull's eye" maculopathy. In contrast to Stargardt's dystrophy the photopic ERG in cone dystrophy is markedly affected early in the course of the disease (Krill and Deutman 1973). In advanced cases the scotopic ERG may also be affected. Heredity is autosomal dominant (can be recessive). If the rods are also affected, one speaks of cone-rod dystrophy.

Juvenile retinoschisis: In hereditary sex-linked juvenile retinoschisis (see page 274), radial stripes or folds develop in the macula at or before school age. Retinoschisis occurs peripherally. Vessels in the detached retinal layer cast a shadow on ophthalmoscopic examination, aiding in the diagnosis. Dehiscences of varying size develop in the inner retinal layer. Vitreous hemorrhage and retinal detachment can occur and have a poor prognosis. In the final stages there is a generalized chorioretinal atrophy. The EOG and ERG a-wave is usually normal with a depressed b-wave. The F – ERG is decreased and widened. Heredity is sex-linked recessive.

Vitreous-tapetoretinal degeneration: Favre-Goldmann vitreo-tapetoretinal degeneration (see page 233) has microcystic macular degeneration. At the same time gray, hyaline, preretinal bands, peripheral retinoschisis, atypical peripheral retinal pigmentation, tapetoretinal degeneration, sclerotic areas and small retinal holes develop.

Night blindness, ERG changes, myopia, cataracts.

Heredity: autosomal recessive.

In Wagner's vitreoretinal degeneration (see page 233), the macula is almost never affected. Heredity: dominant.

Fundus flavimaculatus, Sjögren's reticular dystrophy of the pigment epithelium, butterfly-shaped pigment dystrophy of the fovea, dominantly inherited drusen of Bruch's membrane.

Fundus flavimaculatus (Franceschetti 1965) (see page 287) leads to bilateral white-yellow pisciform spots throughout the retina (Plate XXVII, Fig. 4, page 288 c). The disease is usually stationary with a normal ERG. Heredity: autosomal recessive.

Sjögren's reticular dystrophy of the retinal pigment epithelium is a netlike retinal dystrophy developing in children (4–8 yrs.). The fovea becomes heavily pigmented, and pigmented lines resembling a fishnet develop especially paracentrally. With age, the pigment changes disappear. Vision is normal or minimally depressed. ERG, visual field and dark adaptation remain normal. Heredity is autosomal recessive.

Butterfly-shaped foveal pigment dystrophy (Deutman 1971) is symmetrical, bilateral, and appears in children between ages 1 and 15 years. Visual acuity, visual fields, dark adaptation, ERG and color vision are normal. Heredity is autosomal dominant.

Drusen of Bruch's membrane can be inherited in a dominant fashion (Deutman 1971).

Malignant myopia (see page 214) belongs in the realm of hereditary macular degenerations.

Macular Degeneration in Adults

Central choroidal sclerosis: Occurs between ages 20 and 50 (Fig. 22.26, page 219). It begins like an inflammatory macular edema followed by white-yellow spots with or without pigment clumping. This evolves into a sharply delimited gyrate-like central chorioretinal atrophy. The choroidal vessels within the area of depigmentation appear normal (Sorsby and Crick 1953).

Generalized choroidal sclerosis (see page 214): This will result in macular pigment dispersion. Optic nerve and retinal vessel may appear normal for a long period of time. The end stage resembles "choroidermia" (see page 219).

Doyne's honeycomb degeneration: This is a mosaic of giant macular drusen developing between ages 20 and 40. At first, visual acuity is normal. The lesions undergo various changes, including lipid and crystalline deposits. Even "fluid" levels develop. The result is a picture of central chorioretinal atrophy similar to Kuhnt-Junius senile macular degeneration. Heredity: dominant.

Tay's macular "guttate choroiditis": The clinical picture is similar to honeycomb macular degeneration. It begins as gray-white irregular spots in the region of the macula and optic disc. Pigment clumps, hemorrhages and finally a picture resembling choroidal sclerosis or Kuhnt-Junius degeneration follows.

Malattia leventinese: This was described by Klainguti and Wagner (1932, 1943) as an autosomal dominant hereditary macular degeneration appearing between ages 20 and 30. Bilateral gray-yellow spots appear in the macula and optic disc region. Varying degrees of pigment clumping and chorioretinal atrophy with visual deterioration and field loss follow. The ERG is normal.

Doyne's honeycomb degeneration, Tay's guttate choroiditis and Malattia leventinese probably represent the same clinical disease.

Sorsby's "inflammatory" macular degeneration: Between ages 20 and 40 exudative and/or hemorrhagic macular changes develop. The disorder resembles chorioretinitis and is bilateral. Similar changes in family members establish the diagnosis. With time the clinical picture is one of increasing chorioretinal atrophy. Heredity is autosomal dominant or recessive.

Inverse retinitis pigmentosa (see page 286) may cause primary macular pigment dispersion.

Senile Macular Degeneration

Senile pigmentary maculopathy: The clinical picture of senile pigmentary macular degeneration is highly variable. Usually pigment clumps or yellow flecks surrounded by pigment, often confluent, develop. The shape can be: oval (2 disc diameters in size), irregular, serpentine or maplike. At times multiple drusen (see page 260) are present.

Drusen arise by hyalinization of intracellular pigmentary substances or through extracellular deposition of hyaline on Bruch's membrane (Wolter 1957). Multiple retinal drusen occur in Urbach-Wiethe lipoid proteinosis (hyalinosis cutis et mucosae) (Marquardt 1962; see page 260).

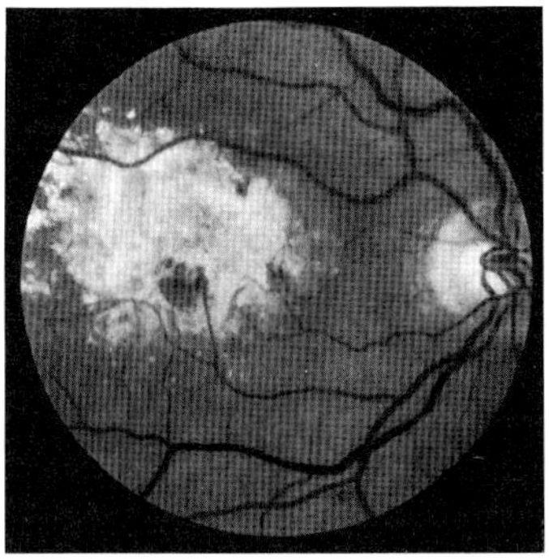

Fig. 22.27 Senile disciform macular degeneration (♀ 72 yrs.)

Senile disciform macular degeneration: The most important macular degeneration is that occurring after age 50, the relatively common *senile disciform* (Kuhnt-Junius) macular degeneration (Fig. 22.27). The disorder is bilateral, beginning with minimal macular pigmentary changes and progressing to gray circumscribed serous detachment of the retina. Recurrent subretinal hemorrhages cause scar tissue formation and vascular ingrowth. Finally the central retina is replaced by a gray-white, partially pigmented prominent connective tissue disc. The central area may be surrounded by small white exudates (circinate retinitis). Subjective symptoms begin with metamorphopsia and visual deterioration, leading to a complete central scotoma.

Circinate Retinitis

Circinate retinopathy is the annular arrangement of small white-yellow, at times confluent, hard exudates (Plate XXVI, Fig. 3, page 288 b). These exudates usually form a circle or semicircle around the fovea but may surround any area of hemorrhage or vessel proliferation in the retina. Typically, circinate retinitis is observed in connection with central *disciform macular degeneration* (Kuhnt-Junius). It also occurs in stage III diabetic retinopathy, with arteriosclerotic hemorrhage, Coats' disease or old central vein thrombosis. In these cases it is usually atypical in its location and often coalesces into a large white spot.

Angioid Streaks

"Angioid streaks" (Knapp) (see page 219) are tears in Bruch's membrane (Plate XV, Figs. 1, 2, page 192 g). These appear as red-brown or gray cracks beneath the retina, often radiating concentrically from a gray peripapillary ring. In the area of the streaks, gray-white connective tissue proliferation takes place, especially centrally and near the optic disc. The subretinal exudates and hemorrhages result in a picture similar to that of disciform macular degeneration (Plate XXVI, Fig. 4, page 288 b). Angioid streaks are part of the symptom complex of Grönblad-Strandberg syndrome. Pseudoxanthoma elasticum (Darier) is found in the skin at points of mechanical stress (neck, elbows, axillae, etc.). The disorder is systemic and affects elastic fibers of arteries, leading to peripheral vascular occlusion, calcification, angina pectoris and aortic-carotid artery aneurysms. Heredity is recessive or dominant, consanguinity is common.

Excessive myopia (see pages 25 and 214) results in two different types of macular change:

1. Lacquer cracks (Plate XXI, Fig. 5, page 224 e) and
2. Fuchs' black spot (Plate XXII, Fig. 2, page 224 f).

Lacquer cracks are tears in Bruch's membrane with surrounding areas of hyper- or hypopigmentation. The choroid may be atrophic in patches of varying size, exposing the underlying white sclera.
Reactive hyperpigmentation is directly adjacent. Lacquer cracks can cause decreased acuity, depending on their location. Fuchs' black spot occurs in high myopia, independent of age. The incidence increases with age. Onset is sudden visual loss from subpigment epithelium macular hemorrhage, usually about $^1/_4$ disc diameter in size. This becomes a round, sharply delineated black, pigmented spot (Fuchs' spot), which may turn slate gray with time.

Microcystic maculopathy: *Iridocyclitis* (see page 204), *tapetoretinal degeneration, retinal detachment, hypertensive retinopathy,* and *siderosis* can lead to rapid vision loss from microcystic macular edema (Plate XXV, Fig. 2, page 288 a; Plate XXVII, Fig. 2, page 288 c). The macula has a honeycomb appearance on ophthalmoscopic examination. Iridocyclitis may be associated with cystic macular edema, papilledema, peripapillary retinal edema and venous stasis (Pietruschka 1954).
Cystic macular edema is also seen in (François 1973): diabetes, arterial hypertension, retinal vein thrombosis, retinal telangiectasia, Coats' disease, after radiation, epinephrine maculopathy in aphakia, griseofulvin maculopathy.

Irvine syndrome: The Irvine-Gass syndrome occurs when vitreous strands attach to the wound after cataract surgery and cause macular irritation by traction. This results in macular cystic edema with vision loss (see page 233).

Internoretinal fibroplasia (Gloor and Werner 1967) (see page 278).

Epiretinal fibroplasia (Gloor 1970) (see page 278).

Macular "puckering" (Gass syndrome) (see page 273).

Macular Holes
(see page 275)

These appear as sharply delineated red foveal spots $^1/_4$ to $^2/_3$ disc diameter in size (Fig. 22.19). The retina around the hole may be slightly gray with fine punctate deposits. Vision is markedly decreased with a central scotoma. The etiology includes perforating or blunt injury. Macular holes also occur in a variety of ocular diseases – arteriosclerosis, thrombosis, cystic maculopathy with iridocyclitis, periphlebitis, and retinitis pigmentosa. They may appear spontaneously in a matter of weeks without any known cause, usually in older patients. The disorder is rarely bilateral. Macular holes in high myopia can cause retinal detachment. *Macular holes* appear secondarily in *retinal detachment* from other causes.
True macular holes are rare, usually being cysts or partial-thickness holes. The diagnosis "macular hole" requires a full-thickness defect on slit lamp examination.

Light Damage to the Macula
(Solar Retinitis)

Light (sun, photocoagulator, etc.) can cause macular burns. First there is gray-white macular edema followed by pigmentary dispersion and hyperplasia. Symptoms include vision loss, metamorphopsia, micropsia and permanent central scotomata.

Inflammatory Macular Damage

Toxoplasmosis — Histoplasmosis — Toxocara canis — Central serous retinopathy — Camp amblyopia.

Toxoplasmosis: Relatively large, heavily pigmented, "punched-out" central chorioretinal scars (formerly believed to be macular colobomata) (Fig. 22.28) caused by prenatal toxoplasmosis (see page 216).

Toxocara canis

Toxocara canis larvae can cause chronic endophthalmitis with secondary retinal detachment or granuloma (Duguid 1961; Braun-Vallon et al. 1964). *Toxocara canis* larvae can produce isolated tumorlike retinal changes often with circumscribed subretinal hemorrhage (Ashton 1960; Wilkinson and Welch 1971).

Histoplasmosis

Histoplasmosis is the presumed cause of punched-out peripheral depigmented spots and disciform, hemorrhagic central (Plate XXVI, Fig. 6, page 288 b) or circumpapillary choroiditis (Schlaegel 1964, Ryan and Smith 1974). In Europe such patients are histoplasmin skin test negative and the condition is called, among other things, *focal hemorrhagic choroiditis* and *hemorrhagic central serous chorioretinitis* (see below).

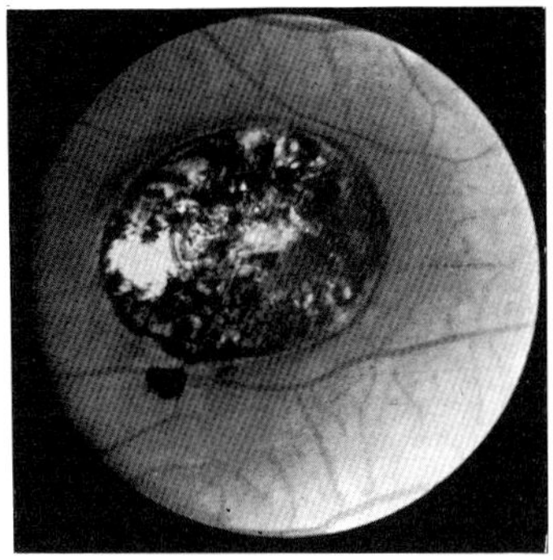

Fig. 22.28 Macular toxoplasmosis lesion (♀ 17 yrs.)

Central serous chorioretinitis: A central $^1/_2$ to 2 disc diameter-sized oval or round, serous retinal detachment develops relatively suddenly (Plate XXVI, Fig. 5, page 288 b). Frequently a small round gray spot that leaks fluorescein (Fig. 22.29) is seen in the area of detachment.

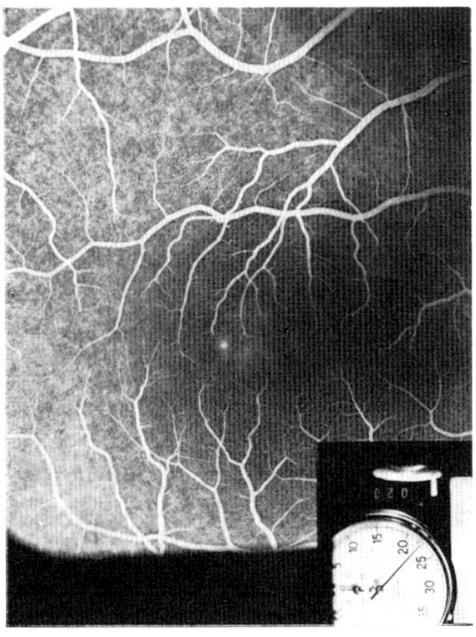

Fig. 22.29 Central serous retinopathy. Fluorescein angiography, early venous phase. Bright leakage point temporal to the foveola (♀ 35 yrs.)

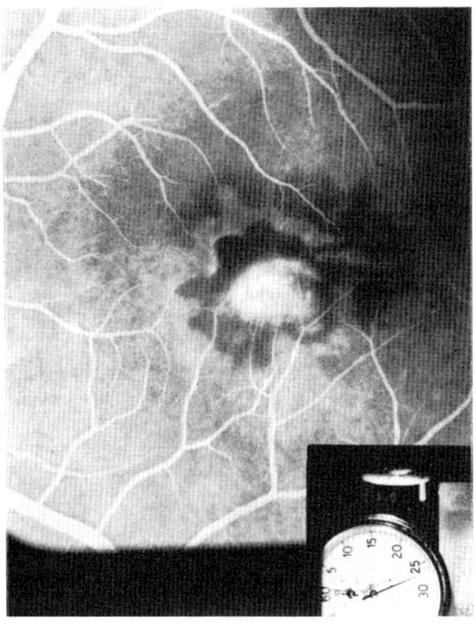

Fig. 22.30 Hemorrhagic central serous retinopathy. Presumed ocular histoplasmosis. Venous phase in fluorescein angiography. Area of central staining surrounded by dark blood (♀ 34 yrs.)

Subretinal precipitates may be visible. Subjectively there is a distinct positive scotoma, which is usually described as a gray oval spot. Micropsia, metamorphopsia and transient hypermetropia of 0.75 to 1.5 diopters occur. The process usually persists for 8 to 10 weeks and heals with or without pigmentary dispersion and minimum vision loss.

Males between 25 and 45 years are primarily affected. The etiology may be infectious, toxic or allergic. Central serous retinopathy can occur with vaccination (also central vein thrombosis) (see page 216).

If hemorrhage has occurred *(chorioretinitis centralis serosa hemorrhagica)* (Fig. 22.30) scarring and black pigmented lesions develop along with severe vision loss (Pau 1968). Such a clinical picture is also described as *focal hemorrhagic choroiditis* (Schildberg and Wessing 1975). In the U.S.A. it is known as *presumed ocular histoplasmosis,* and etiologically considered to be totally different from central serous retinopathy. If hemorrhages dominate rather than serous exudation, the disease is called chorioretinitis centralis hemorrhagica, also known as focal hemorrhagic choroiditis (Schildberg and Wessing 1975) or presumed ocular histoplasmosis (Schlaegel 1975).

Central hemorrhagic chorioretinitis. This is manifested by central bleeding with no or only slight serous subretinal exudation.

Camp amblyopia (see page 294): Camp amblyopia first appeared in Japanese prison camps on Java during 1942 to 1945. It is a nutritional deficiency disorder affecting the fovea and optic nerve. Chronic malnutrition (Heinsius 1950; Scholtyssek 1950; Siegert 1956) leads to macular edema, fine pigmentation and yellow spots. Peripheral yellow lesions, retrobulbar neuritis and optic atrophy also develop.

Visual disturbance: Acuity decreases to below 20/200 (will usually recover). A persisting central scotoma, which is often broken up into numerous islands, night blindness and photophobia exist.

Causes of camp eye: Individual predisposition. Protein-poor diet, avitaminosis B (pellagra), avitaminosis A (xerophthalmia) (Obal 1951). Hormonal disturbances. Photosensitization of the cones. Circulatory and permeability disruption in the retinal and choroidal capillaries. Camp amblyopia may first appear after normalization of the diet.

Cherry red macular spot

A cherry red macular spot occurs with any retinal edema. The thin retina allows the red choroid to shine through at that point. Causes include: central retinal artery embolus, Berlin's edema, fresh chorioretinitis and various storage diseases. A cherry red macular spot (Plate XXVII, Fig. 6, page 288 c) may be seen in the following storage diseases (Thiel and Wiedemann 1972) (see page 289):

1. Classic Tay-Sachs infantile disease (GM_2-gangliosidosis). Enzyme defect: β hexosaminidase A. Increased incidence among eastern European Jews.

2. A variant of infantile Tay-Sachs disease with visceral involvement (GM_2-gangliosidosis with visceral globoside accumulation) = Sandoff variant. Enzyme defect: hexosaminidase A + B. No ethnic predilection.

3. Generalized gangliosidosis (GM_1 gangliosidosis). Close similarity to Hurler's disease but without mucopolysaccharide excretion in the urine. Macular cherry red spot is common. The disease progresses rapidly, usually ending in death by age 2. Corneal opacities, retinal hemorrhage, and optic atrophy are rare. Enzyme defect: β galactosidase A, B, and C.

4. Mucolipidosis I (formerly lipomucopolysaccharidosis) resembles Hurler's syndrome. Corneal opacities are possible besides a cherry red spot.

5. Infantile form of Niemann-Pick sphingomyelinosis with cerebral involvement. This results in marasmic, deaf, blind, retarded children with hepatosplenomegaly and lymphadenopathy.

6. In metachromatic leukodystrophy (Grennfield-Scholz type) there is a central and peripheral demyelinization with motor disturbances and dementia. Besides a cherry red spot, optic atrophy is reported.

7. In Farber's lipogranulomatosis, granuloma containing ceramide and gangliosides develop. Optic atrophy, pepper and salt retinal pigmentation and a cherry red spot can occur.

Bull's Eye Macula

A bull's eye macula consists of a dark fovea surrounded by an area of pigmentary dispersion which transmits choroidal fluorescence on fluorescein angiography. A bull's eye macula can occur with (1) chloroquine retinopathy (see page 291), (2) cone dystrophy (Deutman 1971), (3) Spielmeyer-Vogt cerebroretinal dystrophy (see page 290), and (4) sporadically as dominant benign bull's eye macular dystrophy (Deutman and van Lith 1975).

Traumatic Retinal Damage

Commotio Retinae

Retinal edema develops within 24 to 36 hours after severe trauma to the globe (Berlin's edema). The edema can appear anywhere in the fundus. A cherry red spot develops when the macula is involved, and the clinical picture resembles that of a central retinal artery embolus. Commotio retinae resolves over a period of days with improvement in vision.

Retinal contusion: Retinal edema and hemorrhages can result from blunt trauma to the globe. In contrast to commotio retinae, pigmentary changes (Fig. 22.31), macular holes (see page 275), visual field loss and loss of visual acuity remain permanently (contusio retinae).

Birth trauma: Newborns frequently have retinal hemorrhages, which historically have been blamed for nonstrabismic amblyopia (untrue). The hemorrhages may be extensive and result from elevation of retinal venous pressure during birth.

Choroidal ruptures are situated concentrically around the disc. After resorption of the hemorrhage, they appear as white (sclera) halfmoons (Plate XV, Fig. 4, page 192 g; see page 214). A scotoma corresponding to the choroidal rupture develops because of the interruption of retinal nutrition in this area.

Retinitis sclopetaria: Very severe concussion injury, as from the impact of a bullet, causes retinal and choroidal tears and hemorrhages with scarring in sheets or strands: retinitis sclopetaria (Richards et al. 1968).

Perforating injury can cause direct trauma to the retina, potentially with secondary retinal detachment, traction detachment from retinitis proliferans, endophthalmitis, phthisis.

Purtscher's traumatic retinopathy (see page 272; Plate XXIV, Fig. 6, page 224 h) occurs as a remote complication of compression injuries to the chest or body or from blows to the head. Skin and conjunctival petechiae occur along with bright peripapillary spots and hemorrhages, usually near veins. A similar picture develops with fracture of long bones and fat emboli.

Retinal fat emboli are part of systemic fat embolization and usually resolve without late sequelae. In contrast, Purtscher's traumatic retinopathy has a short latent period and considerable permanent damage (Pape 1964).

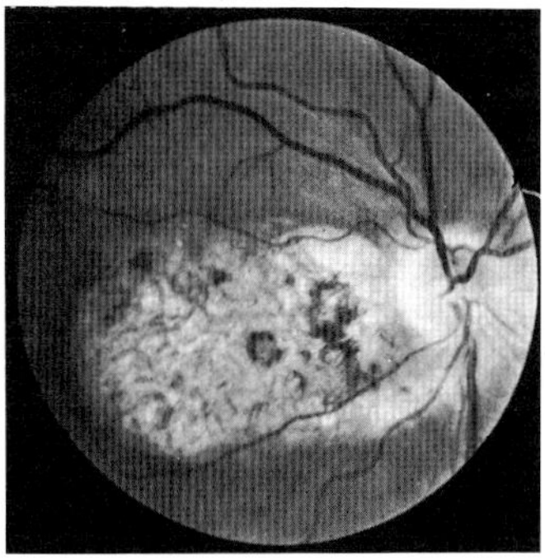

Fig. 22.31 Central scarring from a contusion injury (♂ 37 yrs.)

Retinal Pigmentation

(Waardenburg et al. 1963, Krill 1972, Carr et al. 1973, Franceschetti et al. 1974).

The most prominent symptom in all tapetoretinal degenerations is progressive night blindness. Such nyctalopia results from loss of peripheral rods. There is an appropriate ring-shaped visual field loss which progresses concentrically until only a small central field remains (Fig. 3.6, Fig. 3.4). Even this is often lost because of cystic macular degeneration and cataractous changes common in advanced cases. Heredity is autosomal recessive, rarely dominant or sex-linked recessive. Retinal pigmentary degenerations are hereditary diseases manifesting as early as the first decade of life, but may be considerably later.

Retinal pigmentary degeneration may be associated with glaucoma, cataracts, deafness, polydactyly and idiocy. Essential progressive choroidal atrophy (see page 215) is usually associated with tapetoretinal degeneration.

A depressed or absent *electroretinogram* (ERG) is the hallmark of all tapetoretinal degenerations. The standing retinal potential *(electro-oculogram,* EOG) is significantly lowered in tapetoretinal degenerations, and light-dark oscillations are missing (Krill 1972; François et al. 1974).

The difference of electric potential between the cornea and the posterior pole in the EOG appears to be dependent primarily on the pigment epithelium but also on the outer receptor layer and choriocapillaries. The oscillatory part of the EOG appears to develop in the outer rod and cone layers and adjacent pigment epithelium. The ERG results from the recording of shifts in electrical potential in the outer retinal layers. The ERG is a sum of electric potential producing activity of the rods and cones as well as proximal cells up to the bipolar level. The a-wave of the ERG originates in the receptors. The b-wave is dependent on the function of the bipolar cells. The scotopic b-wave and photopic a- and b-wave are examined in the ERG.

Central retinal stimulation (focal ERG) is responsible for the *light-evoked cortical potential* (visually evoked cortical response, VER).

Processes deep in the retina affect the a-wave and potentially the b-wave. Disorders more superficial in the retina (for example, retinal circulation) affect the b-wave with a normal a-wave. The light-dark oscillations of the EOG are decreased by disturbances of rod function (for example, pigmentary degeneration). A normal focal or macular ERG and absent VER imply damage to the optic nerve or visual pathways (Henkes and Deutman 1973). In macular (fovea) degeneration, the macular ERG and VER are altered while the total response ERG and EOG may be normal.

Retinitis Pigmentosa

At first only a few isolated, later many branching, bone corpuscle-like pigment clumps are seen ophthalmoscopically (Plate XXVII, Fig. 1, page 288 c). They are a dark black-brown color and are situated at the level of the equator surrounding macula and optic disc. The pigment clumps increase with time both centrally and peripherally until only a small central area is left free. Cystic macular degeneration and vitreous syneresis are common (Plate XXVII, Fig. 2, page 288 c). The optic disc develops a waxy yellow pallor and slightly blurred margins (Plate XXVII, Fig. 3, page 288 c).

Retinal vessels (arteries and veins) become thin and threadlike. The pigment epithelium is atrophic, with obliterated, sclerosed, choroidal vessels visible in advanced cases. Rarely, retinitis pigmentosa will be sectorial, usually involving the inferior nasal quadrant (Franceschetti et al. 1963; Haase and Hellner 1965). Unilateral or at least markedly asymmetric involvement is extremely rare. In inverse retinitis pigmentosa, the retinal pigmentation may begin in the macula. Visual acuity is further decreased by the common development of posterior polar (permeability) cataracts.

Retinitis pigmentosa can be combined with nystagmus and ptosis in Fröhlich's adiposogenital dystrophy, and with mental retardation, hypogenitalism and polydactyly *(Laurence-Moon-Bardet-Biedl syndrome).*

Recessively inherited retinitis pigmentosa is more frequently associated with deafness, mental retardation, vestibulo-cerebellar ataxia, polydactyly or other skeletal anomalies.

Recessively inherited retinitis pigmentosa with deafness is called Usher's syndrome.
Pigmentary degeneration can occur with: oligophrenia, progressive infantile hearing loss, spasticity, developmental retardation (long extremities, short trunk, kyphosis), progeria (due to lack of subcutaneous fat) *(Cockayne's syndrome)* (Fig. 22.32).

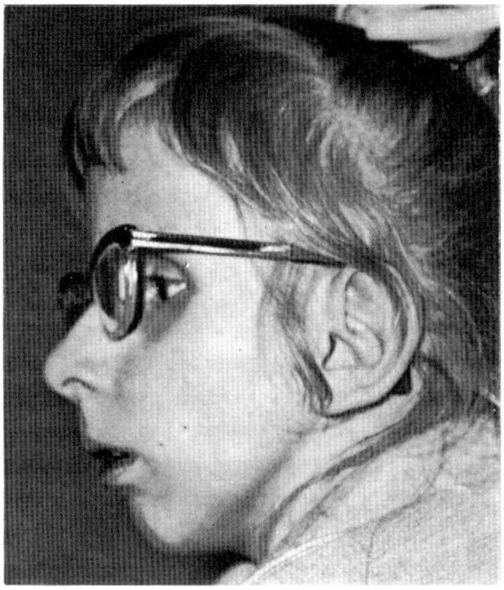

Fig. 22.32 Cockayne's syndrome with hearing loss, progeria, oligophrenia, and tapetoretinal degeneration (♀ 8 yrs.)

Atypical Retinal Pigmentary Degenerations

Besides the common forms of tapetoretinal degeneration, atypical forms occur:
Retinitis pigmentosa sine pigmento clinically has all the stigmata of retinitis pigmentosa (nyctalopia, concentric visual field loss, narrow vessels, yellow disc) except that there is little or no pigment.
Retinitis punctata albescens: Again there is no pigmentation but small round white retinal spots occur especially near the disc and macula. Otherwise the clinical picture is one of progressive retinitis pigmentosa.

Hereditary Retinitis Pigmentosa-Like Retinal Diseases

Fundus albipunctatus with night blindness — Fundus flavimaculatus — Fundus pulverulentus — Sjögren's reticular pigment dystrophy.

Fundus albipunctatus with night blindness: This is a congenital stationary night blindness with normal optic disc and vessels and is clearly separate from the progressive tapetoretinal degenerations.
Fundus flavimaculatus: Franceschetti (1965) used this term to describe yellow-white, round or oval, often pisciform (Plate XXVII, Fig. 4, page 288 c), sharply delineated lesions of varying size and color scattered throughout the fundus but most numerous at the posterior pole. One-half of the cases have macular degeneration and one-fourth are night blind. The ERG is maintained (Franceschetti and François 1965). Fundus flavimaculatus is a primary defect of the pigment epithelium, presumably with deposition of acid mucopolysaccharides. Drusen and *fundus albipunctatus* as well as *fundus flavimaculatus* appear to be primary diseases of the pigment epithelium (Klien and Krill 1967).
Bietti's crystalline fundus dystrophy (François and de Laey 1977). A rare condition is the incorporation of small glittering crystals into the inner layers of the retina (Fig. 22.33). If the central retinal area is involved, the visual acuity is lowered. The ERG is normal. Similar white disseminated crystalline deposits can be observed in *oxalate* retinopathy (Bullock and Albert 1975, Timm 1976).
Fundus pulverulentus: This is a familial disturbance of the pigment epithelium first de-

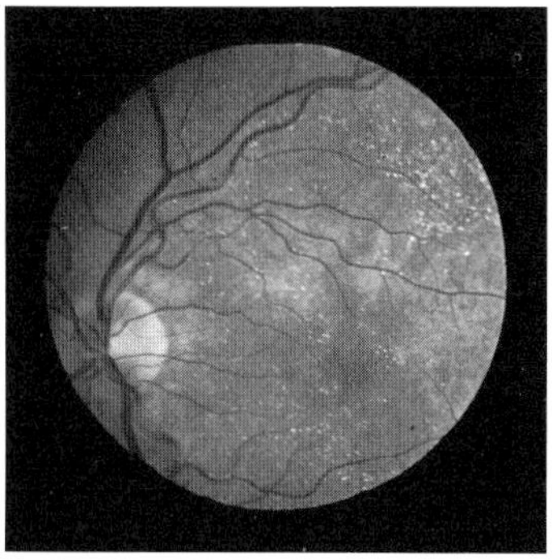

Fig. 22.33 Bietti's crystalline retinal degeneration with numerous fine glistening crystal deposits in the inner retinal layers. (♀ 38 yrs.)

scribed by Slezak and Hommer (1969). Retinal function is normal, but granules and spots of pigment develop at the posterior pole, around the optic disc and near the equator. The pigmentations fade peripherally.

Sjögren's reticular pigment dystrophy: Pigmentation in the form of a net develops at the posterior pole, without functional disturbances.

Tapetochoroidal Degeneration

(see page 219)

In *gyrate atrophy* of the choroid and retina, areas of both choroid and retina become atrophic. The retina develops small pigment spots, and atrophic choroidal vessels become visible against the white background of the sclera. The maplike choroidal areas do not coalesce completely.

If the choroid is totally atrophic, only a small central choroidal rest remains at the fovea and it is called *essential progressive choroidal atrophy* (choroideremia). Choroideremia (Plate XXVII, Fig. 5, page 288 c) can be congenital. If the disc is waxy yellow and retinal vessels are constricted, the choroidal and retinal gyrate atrophy belongs in the realm of tapetoretinal degeneration (with night blindness). Both gyrate atrophy and choroideremia belong to the hereditary tapetochoroidal dystrophies. Choroideremia is inherited in an intermediate sex-linked manner - only males are affected. Female carriers have granular pigment changes in the retinal periphery without functional loss.

Gyrate atrophy has a regular autosomal heredity. Myopia is part of gyrate atrophy; cataracts are common. There is night blindness with concentric constriction of the visual field. Hyperornithinemia has been reported (Takki and Simell 1974) and serves to identify heterozygotes.

Progressive chorioretinal atrophy can lead to early blindness. In some families, however, visual acuity is maintained into the forties. *Generalized choroidal sclerosis* creates a clinical picture very similar to choroideremia (see page 219).

If the optic disc and retinal vessels are not altered in gyrate atrophy, it does not belong to the hereditary tapetoretinal degenerations but is caused by occlusion of choroidal vessels (Neubauer 1955). There is no night blindness.

Tapetoretinal Degeneration in Childhood

Tapetoretinal degenerations can appear in childhood (Franceschetti 1963; Vinken and Bruyn 1972).

Congenital tapetoretinal amaurosis (Leber) — Congenital degenerative retinopathy (Alström-Olson) — Hereditary metabolic disorders with tapetoretinal degeneration: Congenital amaurotic idiocy (Norman-Wood) — Infantile amaurotic idiocy (Tay-Sachs) — Late infantile amaurotic idiocy (Dollinger-Bielschowsky) — Juvenile amaurotic idiocy (Batten-Mayou-Spielmeyer-Vogt-Stock) — Late amaurotic idiocy (Kufs) — Niemann-Pick disease — Farber's disease (disseminated lipogranulomatosis) — Refsum's syndrome (Hereditary ataxia with nyctalopia and polyneuritis) — Bassen-Kornzweig syndrome — Schilder's disease (metachromatic leukodystrophy) — Cockayne's syndrome — Urbach-Wiethe syndrome (lipid proteinosis).

With **Leber's congenital tapetoretinal amaurosis** (see page 279) vision is markedly reduced often to blindness at or shortly after birth. The children show the digito-ocular sign and nystagmus. The fundus picture can vary: The fundus may be normal with pigmentation occurring only after age 3. A sort of salt and pepper retinal pigmentation may be present. The fundus can appear albinotic with "choroidal sclerosis." With age the typical picture of retinitis pigmentosa can develop. The fundus can have polymorphous changes. The periphery may appear marmorized, or dustlike pepper and salt pigmentation, bone corpuscles or pigmented spots can develop. The ERG is depressed. Keratoconus is a common ancillary finding. Heredity is autosomal recessive.

Congenital degenerative retinopathy (Alström and Olson 1957): This is a congenital, autosomal recessive retinopathy similar to tapetoretinal amaurosis of Leber. Blindness or severely decreased vision may be present at birth. Vision may deteriorate in the early years of life. With time, enlarging pigmented lesions form in the retinal periphery. The sclera becomes visible through atrophic choroid. The retina may, however, remain intact. Retinal vessels are narrow; optic atrophy is present. In time the patients develop cataracts, keratoconus

Plate XXV (Chapter 22)

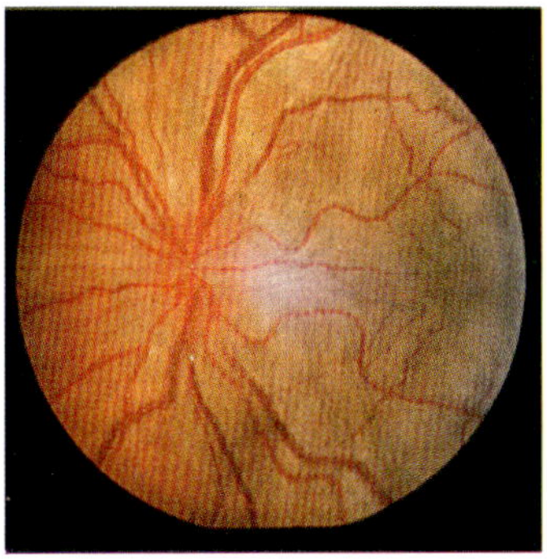

Fig. 1 Retinal folds, papilledema e vacuo, hypotony after a glaucomatous attack (♂ 42 yrs.) (see pages 273, 309)

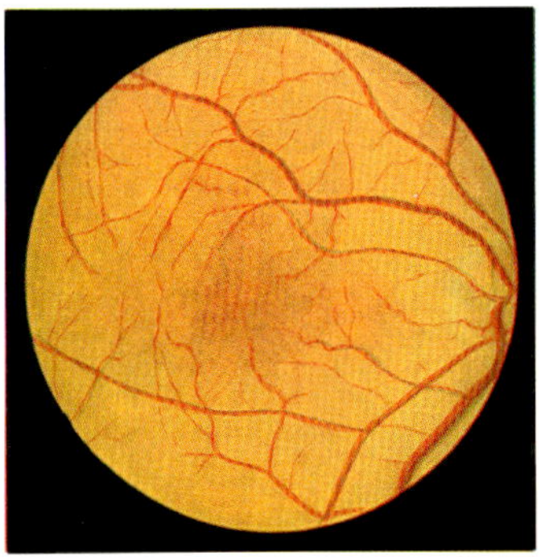

Fig. 2 Microcystic macular edema in cyclitis (♂ 49 yrs.) (see pages 197, 274, 282)

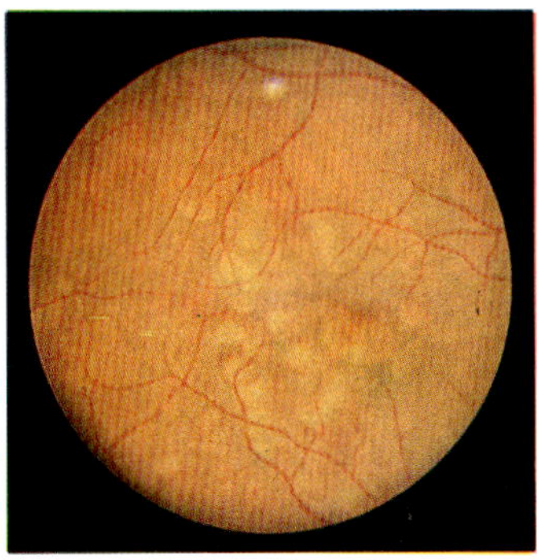

Fig. 3 Macrocystic macular edema (♀ 42 yrs.) (see page 274)

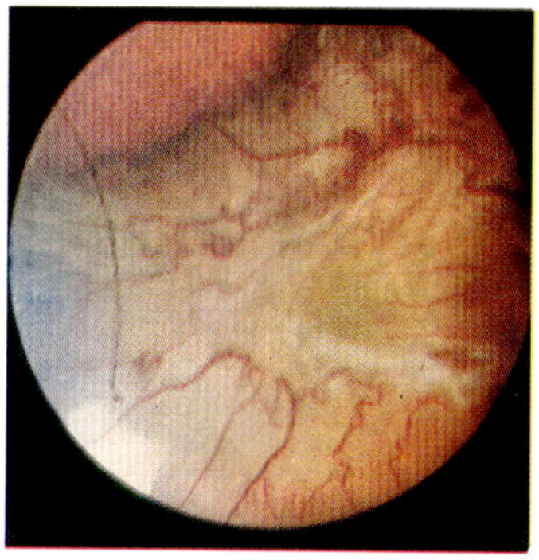

Fig. 4 Coats' disease (♂ 16 yrs.) (see pages 258, 277, 296)

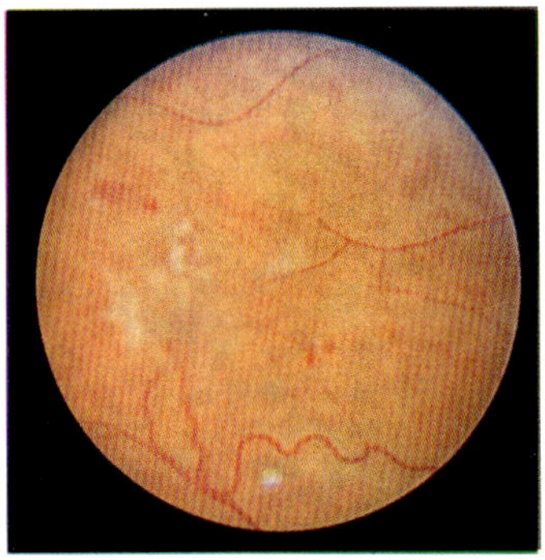

Fig. 5 Retinal fibroplasia with retinal traction and isolated hemorrhages (♀ 38 yrs.) (see page 278)

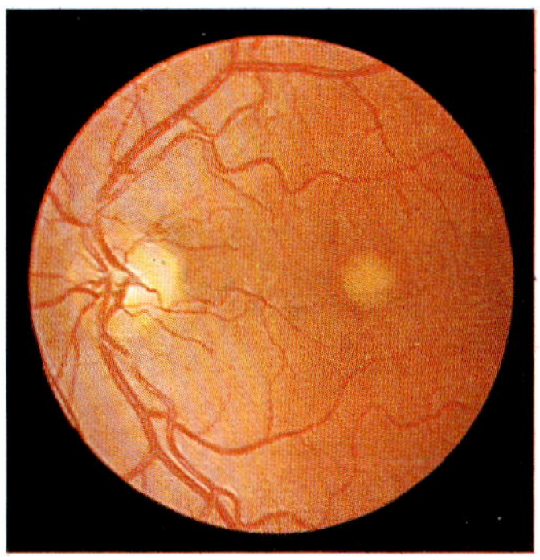

Fig. 6 Vitelliform macular degeneration (Best's disease) (♀ 12 yrs.) (see page 279)

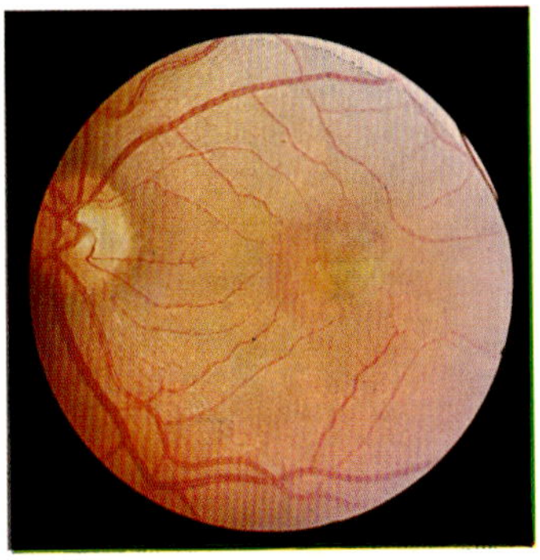

Fig. 1 Best's disease with irregular macular pigmentary dispersion (♀ 46 yrs.) (see page 279)

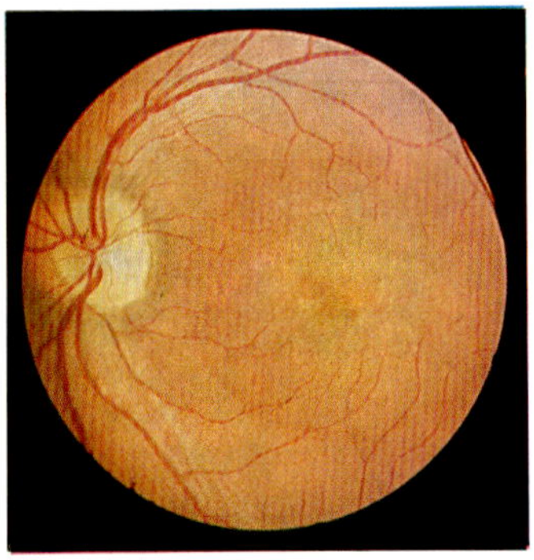

Fig. 2 Stargardt's macular degeneration with bilateral, symmetrical, expansive central retinal pigmentary changes (♂ 17 yrs.) (see page 279)

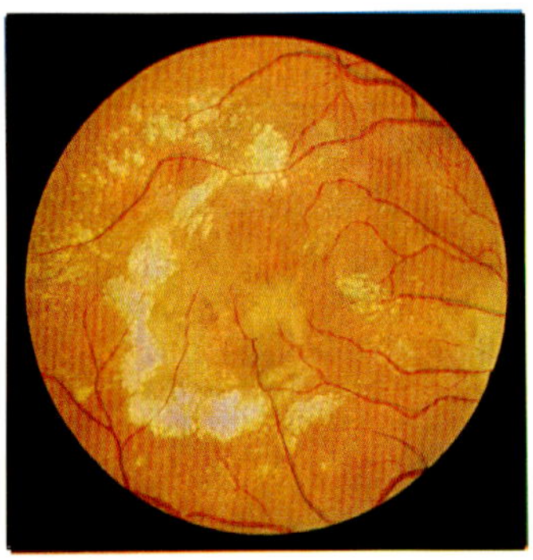

Fig. 3 Senile circinate retinopathy, early disciform macular degeneration (Kuhnt-Junius) (♀ 68 yrs.) (see page 281)

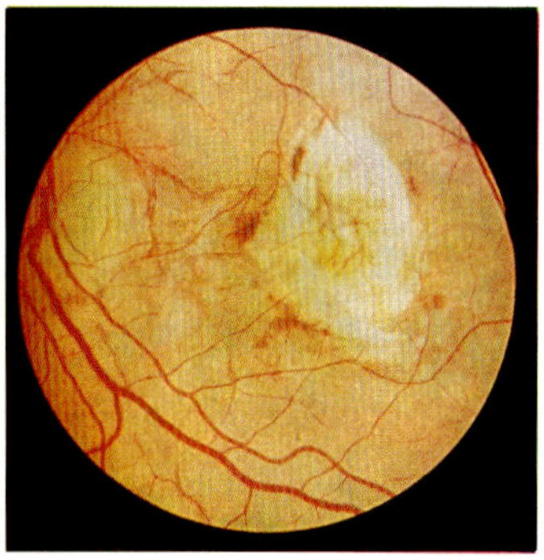

Fig. 4 Angioid streaks (simulating vessels) with central disciform retinopathy (♀ 40 yrs.) (see page 282)

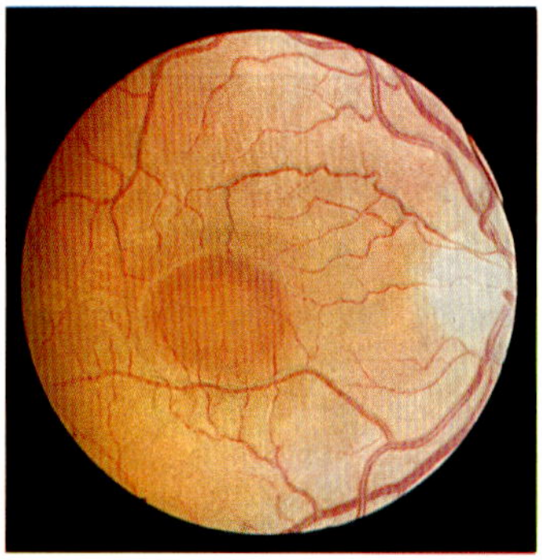

Fig. 5 Central serous chorioretinitis (♂ 20 yrs.) (see pages 216, 283)

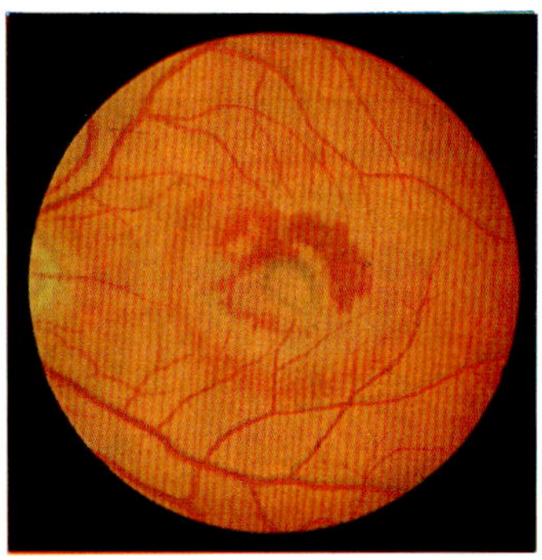

Fig. 6 Chorioretinitis centralis haemorrhagica (presumed histoplasmic chorioretinitis) with hemorrhages and early slate gray scar formation (♀ 35 yrs.) (see pages 216, 283)

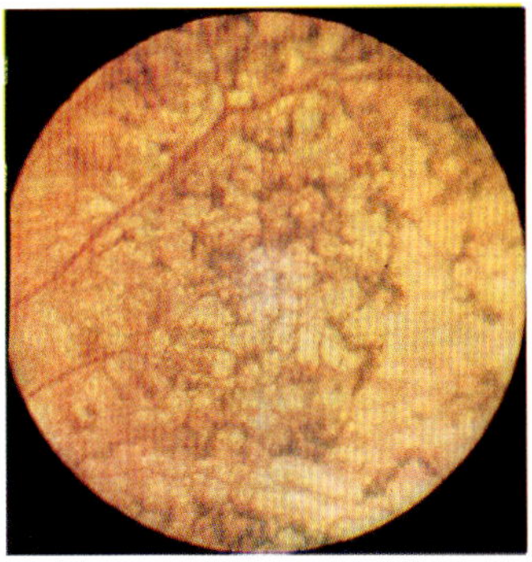

Fig. 1 Retinitis pigmentosa (periphery) with bone corpuscle-like pigment (♂ 20 yrs.) (see page 286)

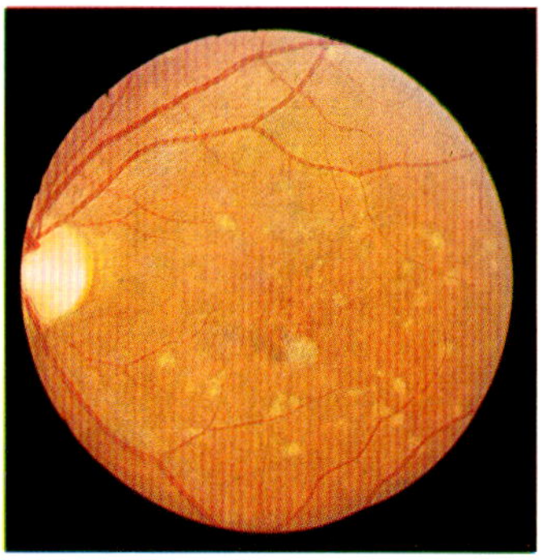

Fig. 4 Fundus flavimaculatus (♀ 38 yrs.) (see pages 280, 287)

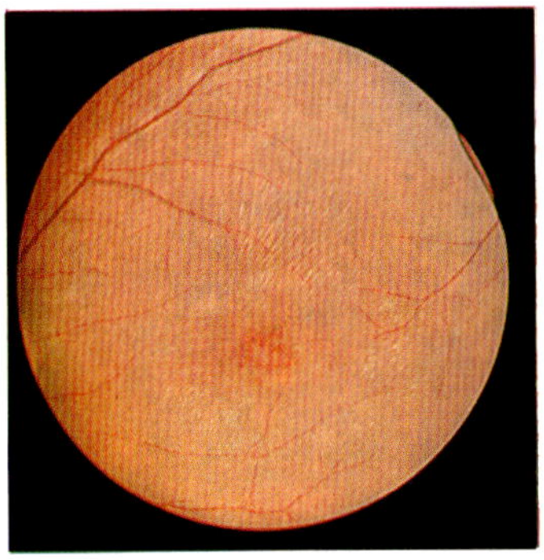

Fig. 2 Cystic macular degeneration in retinitis pigmentosa (♀ 9 yrs.) (see pages 282, 286)

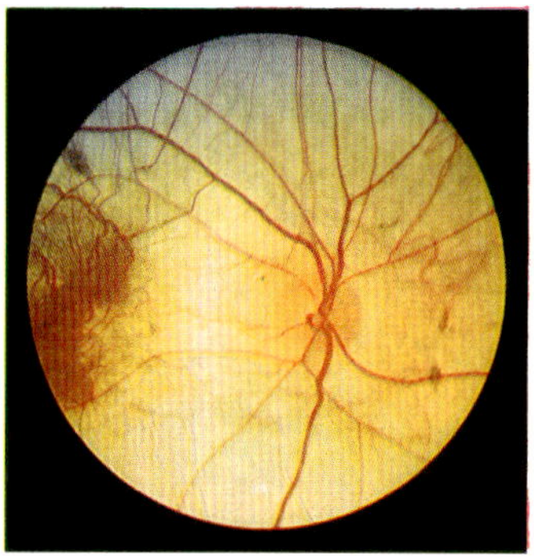

Fig. 5 Choroideremia ,Choroid is still present centrally (♂ 24 yrs.) (see pages 219, 288)

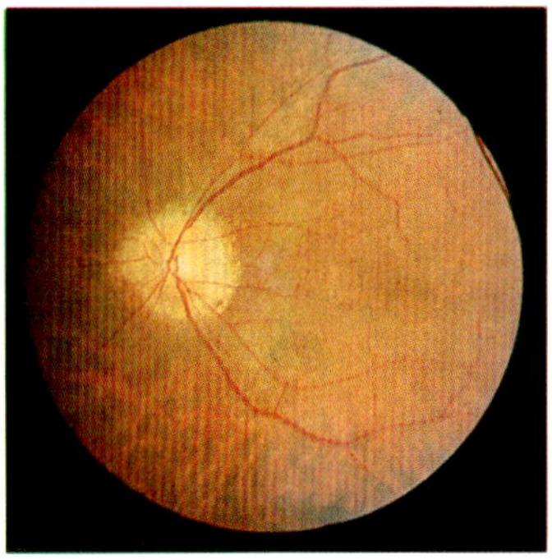

Fig. 3 Waxy-yellow disc and narrowed vessels in retinitis pigmentosa (♂ 49 yrs.) (see pages 286, 316)

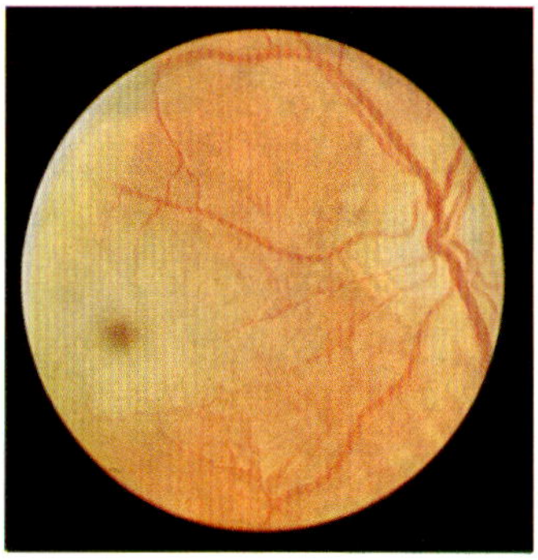

Fig. 6 Infantile amaurotic idiocy (Tay-Sachs). Gray retina with a cherry red foveolar reflex (♀ 1 yr.) (see pages 260, 270, 284, 289)

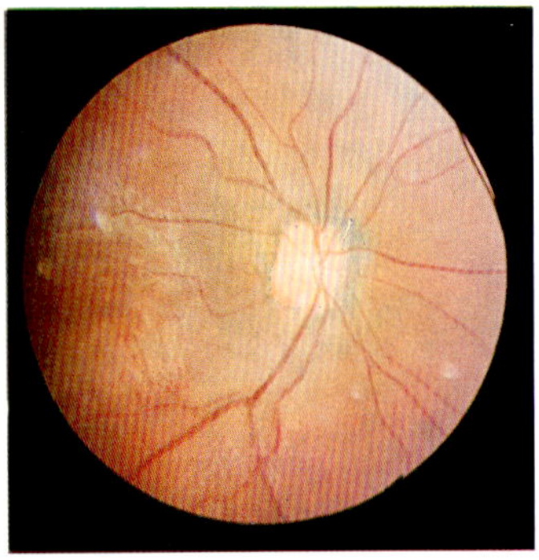

Fig. 1 Quinine amblyopia. Pale disc, narrow vessels, paracentral retinal edema (♀ 28 yrs.) (see pages 291, 311)

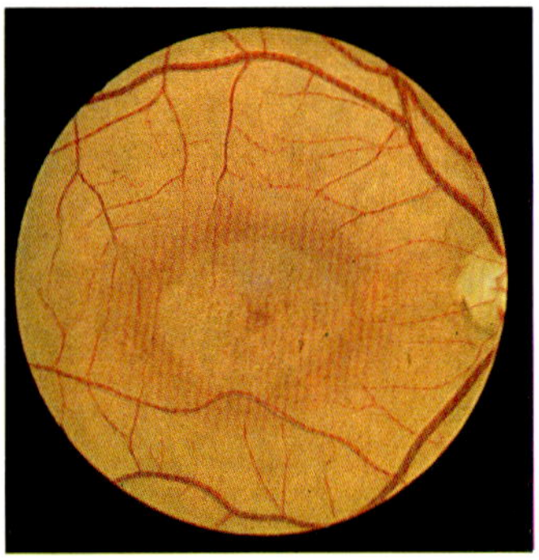

Fig. 2 Chloroquine retinopathy (bull's eye macula) (see page 291)

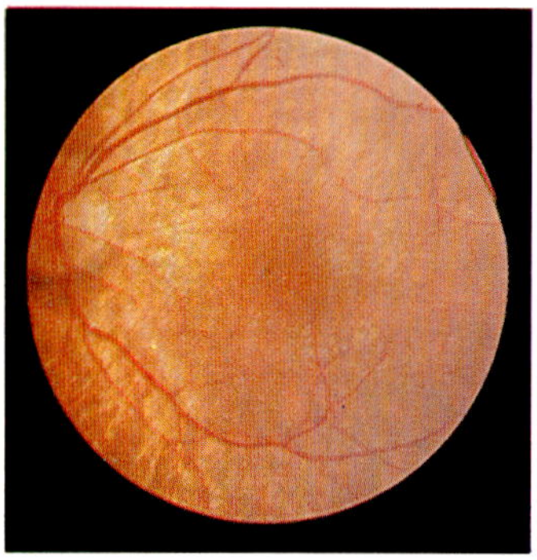

Fig. 3 Pseudoretinitis pigmentosa after measles (♂ 10 yrs.) (see page 292)

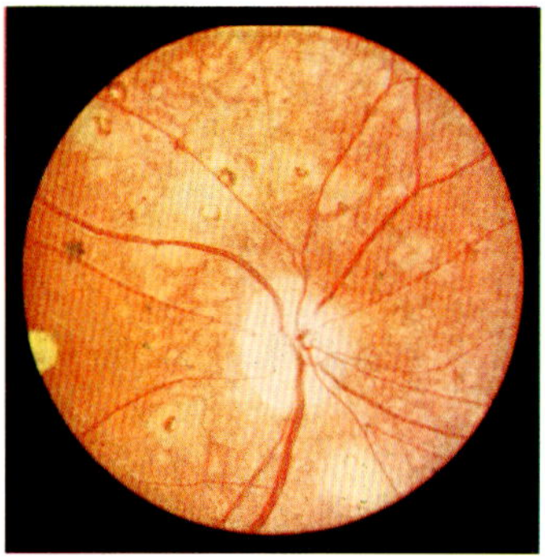

Fig. 4 Pepper and salt fundus, luetic chorioretinitis (♀ 15 yrs.) (see pages 156, 216, 293)

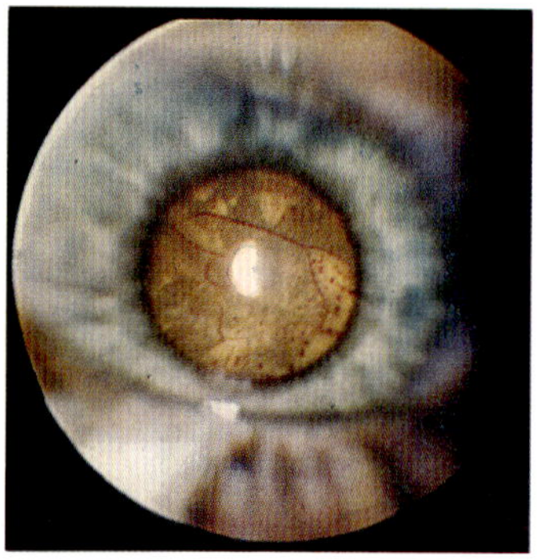

Fig. 5 Coats' disease, small aneurysms of retinal vessels, subretinal cholesterol (♂ 13 yrs.) (see pages 258, 277, 296)

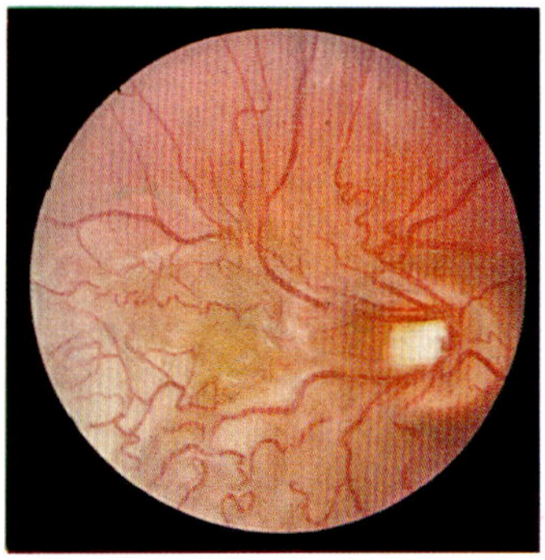

Fig. 6 Choroidal angioma with retinal vessel proliferation (♂ 13 yrs.) (see pages 220, 296)

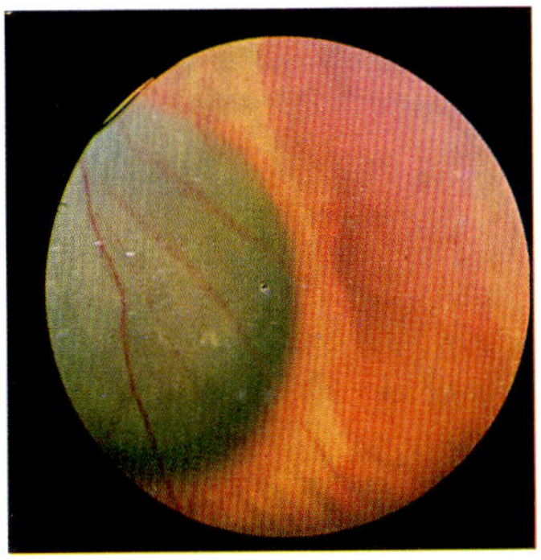

Fig. 1 Choroidal melanoma with retinal hemorrhage (♂ 37 yrs.) (see page 296)

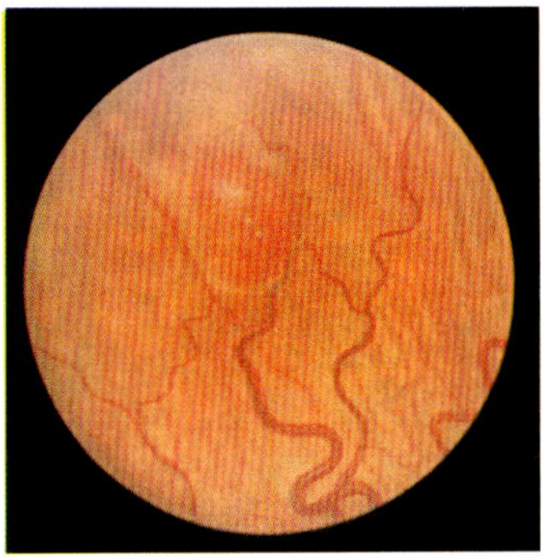

Fig. 2 Retinal angiomatosis (v. Hippel-Lindau) (see pages 257, 296)

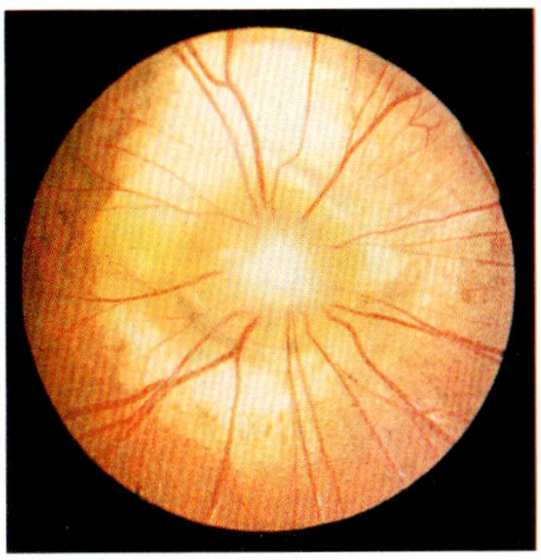

Fig. 3 Large coloboma of the optic disc (♂ 4 yrs.) (see page 305)

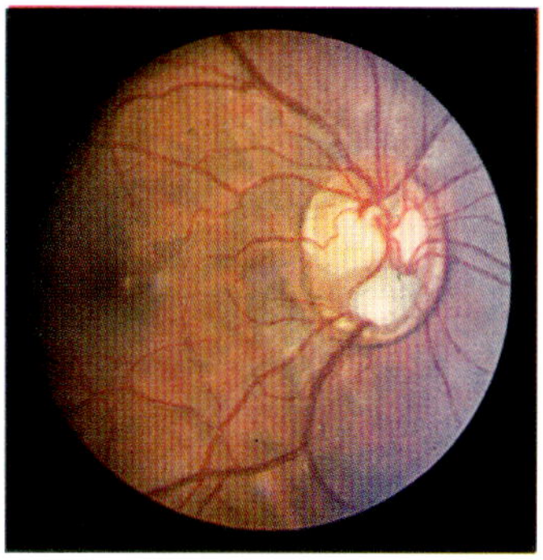

Fig. 4 Optic pit (♀ 18 yrs.) (see page 305)

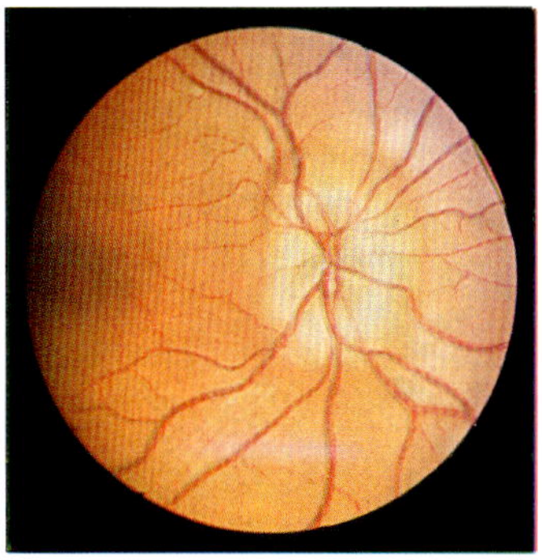

Fig. 5 Papilledema, 4 diopters (♀ 32 yrs.) (see pages 307, 308)

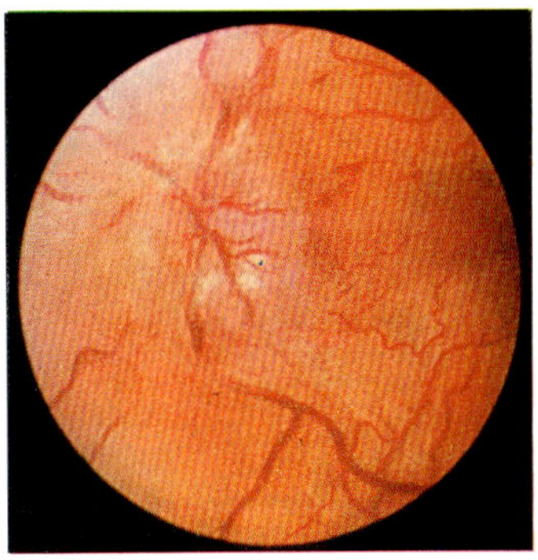

Fig. 6 Papilledema, 7 diopters (♀ 22 yrs.) (see pages 307, 308)

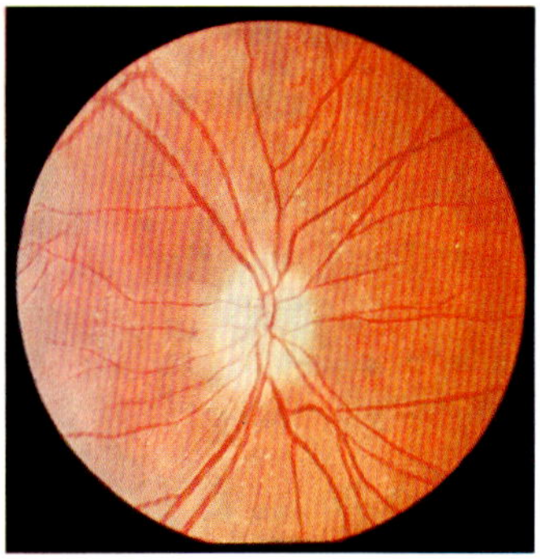

Fig. 1 Postpapillitic optic atrophy with blurred margins, white disc (see pages 308, 309, 316)

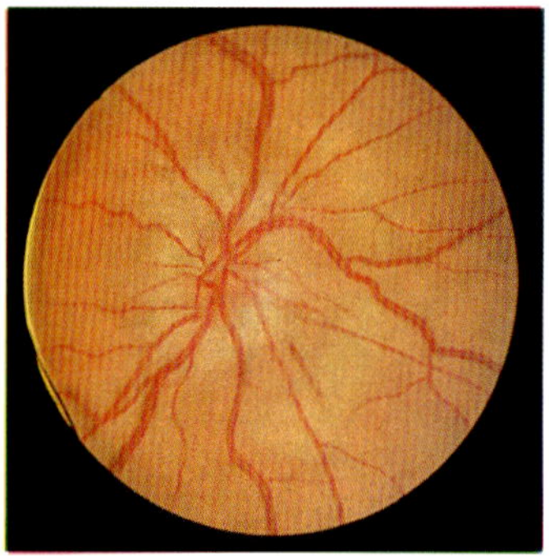

Fig. 2 Optic neuritis, blurred disc margins, prominent edematous papilla (♀ 32 yrs.) (see pages 307, 309)

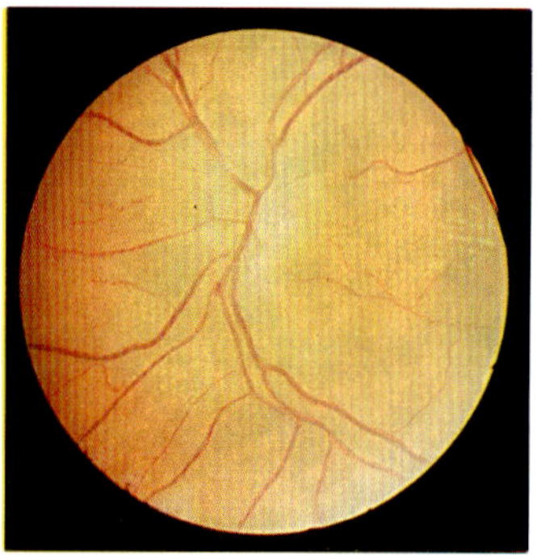

Fig. 3 Atrophy developing in optic neuritis with yellow retinal exudates and macular star figure (♀ 60 yrs.) (see page 309)

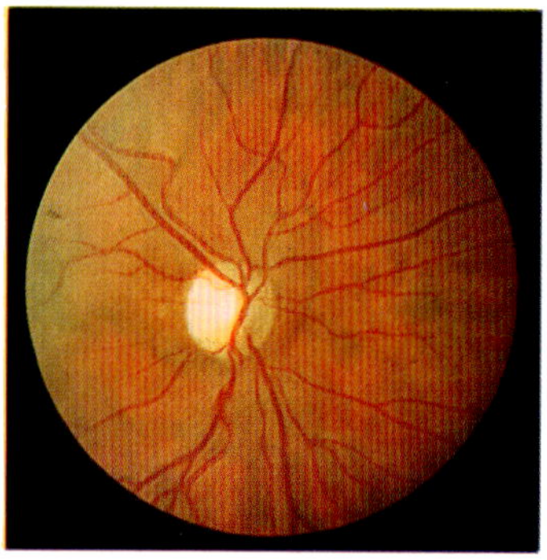

Fig. 4 Temporal pallor of the disc (♀ 28 yrs.) (see pages 310, 313)

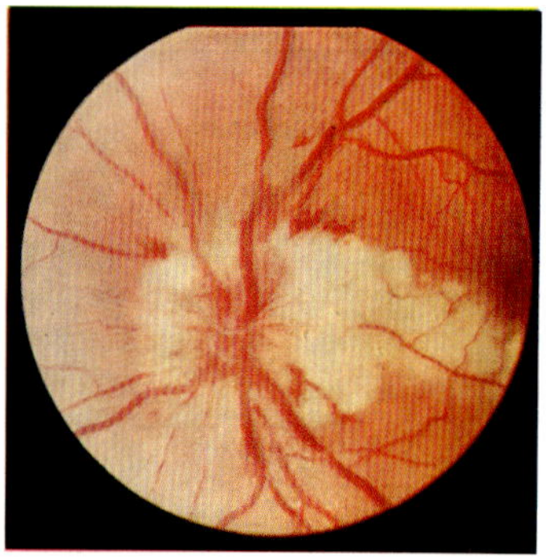

Fig. 5 Temporal arteritis with retinal branch artery occlusion (♂ 62 yrs.) (see pages 311, 312)

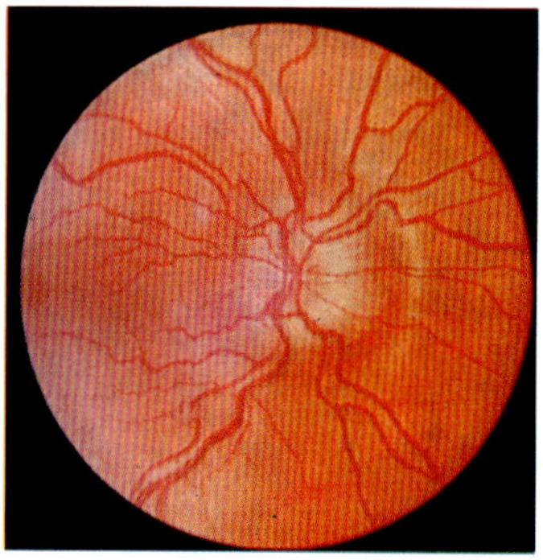

Fig. 6 Pseudopapillitis, sharp disc margins without edema (♀ 15 yrs.) (see pages 306, 308, 312)

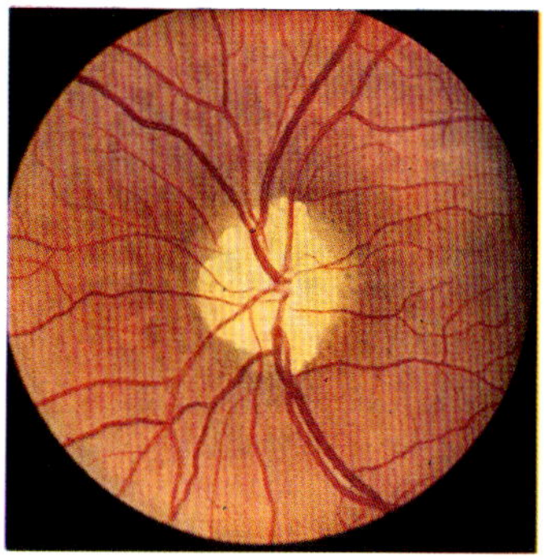

Fig. 1 Drusen of the optic disc (♀ 33 yrs.) (see pages 306, 308, 312)

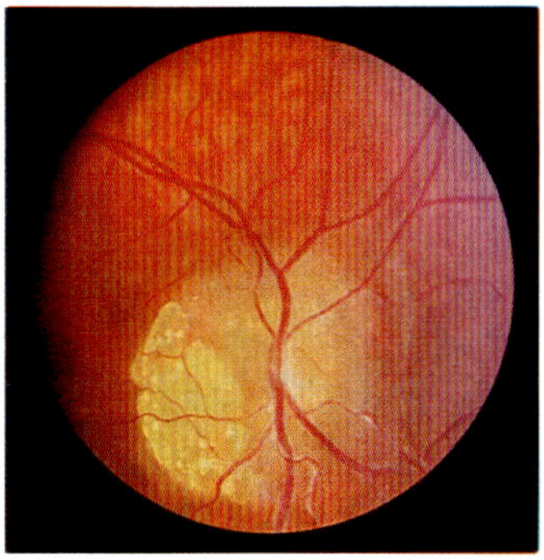

Fig. 2 Yellow-white drusen on and near the slightly elevated optic disc (♂ 24 yrs.) (see page 306)

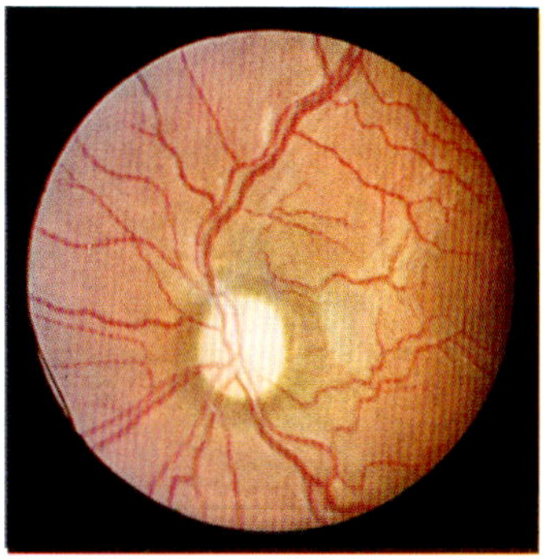

Fig. 3 Primary optic atrophy (Leber's optic atrophy) (♂ 20 yrs.) (see page 313)

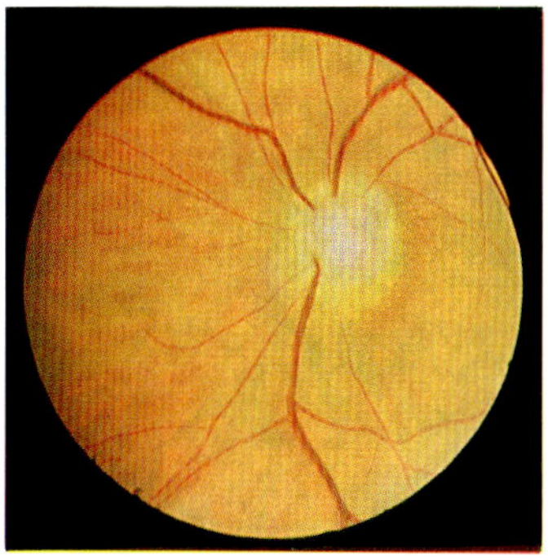

Fig. 4 Glaucomatous optic atrophy; deep excavation of the disc extending to the disc margin with nasal shift of vessels, narrow arteries (see pages 305, 316)

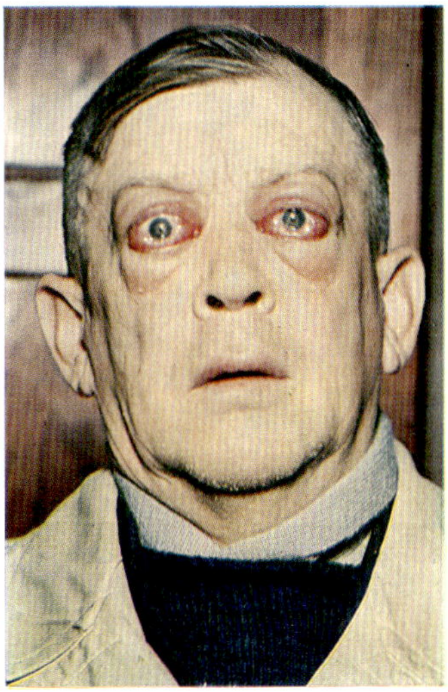

Fig. 5 Endocrine exophthalmos with conjunctival chemosis (see page 339)

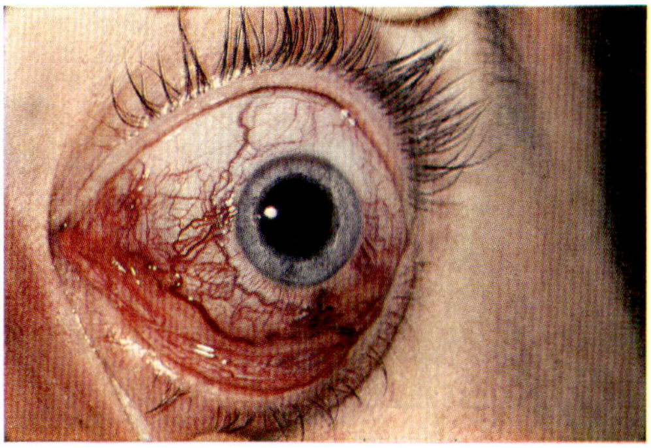

Fig. 6 Exophthalmos with caput medusae of episcleral and conjunctival vessels in pulsating exophthalmos (see page 340)

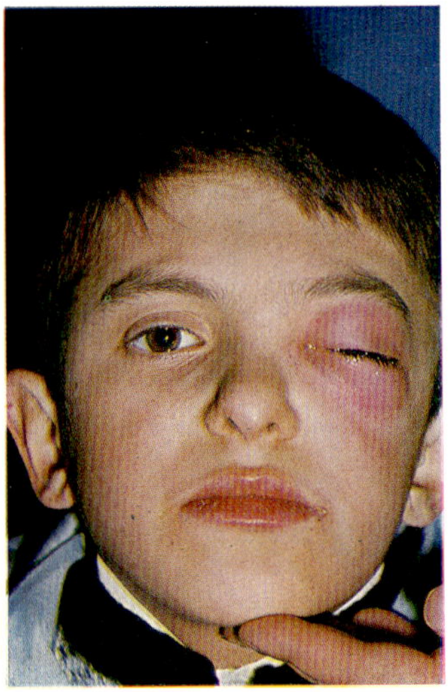

Fig. 1 Orbital cellulitis with pansinusitis (♂ 12 yrs.) (see page 348)

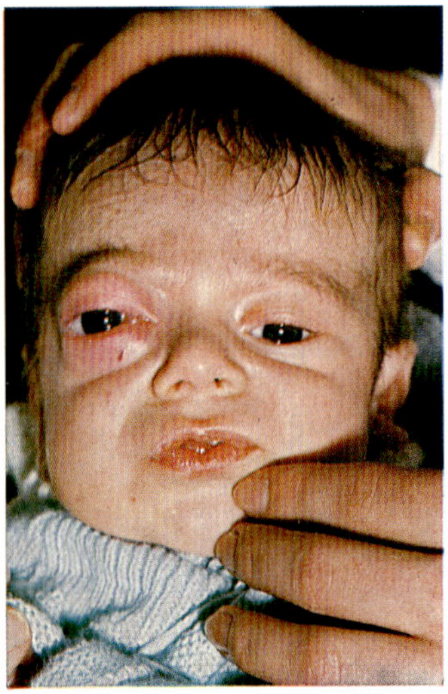

Fig. 2 Orbital cellulitis with maxillary osteomyelitis (♂ 1 month) (see page 349)

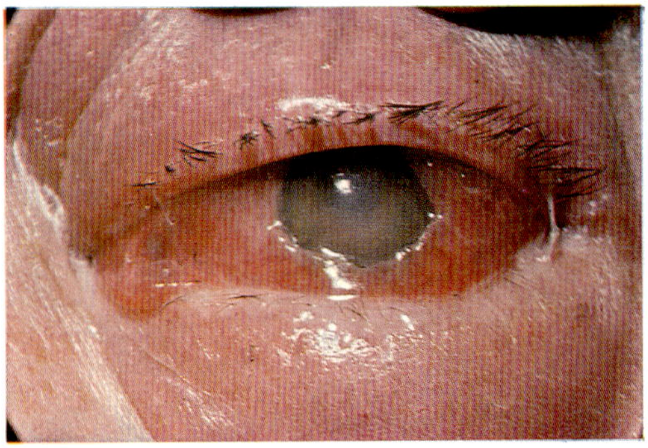

Fig. 3 Panophthalmitis with orbital cellulitis (see page 349)

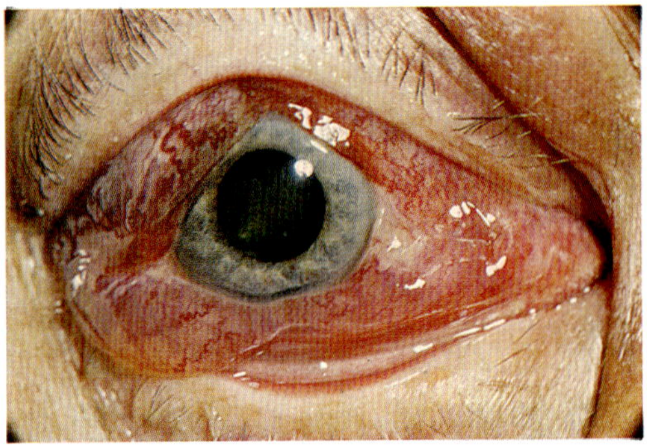

Fig. 4 Tenonitis with chemosis (♀ 65 yrs.) (see page 349)

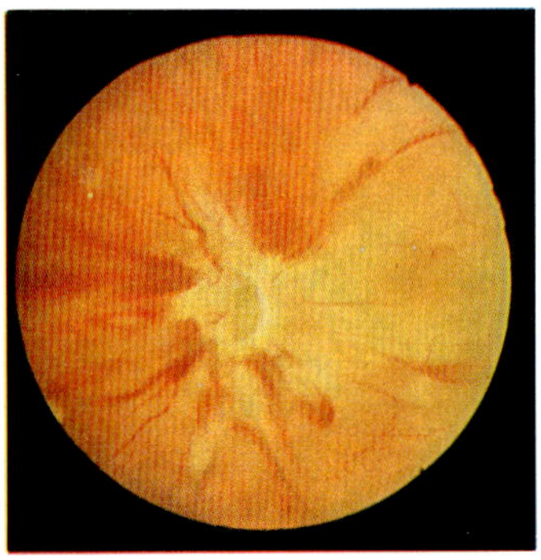

Fig. 5 Partial avulsion of the optic nerve head Vitreous hemorrhage; collapsed arteries, veins are identifiable. Hockey stick injury (♂ 28 yrs.) (see pages 313, 359)

and nystagmus. Ten percent of all blindness in Sweden is due to this disorder, with 21 percent of affected individuals totally blind before the age of 15.

Probably *Leber's congenital amaurosis* and the *progressive retinal aplasia* (Alström and Olson) *are the same disease*. There is marked pleomorphism. Many cases of "atypical retinitis pigmentosa" with various congenital syndromes belong in this category (Sorsby 1970): Laurence-Biedl syndrome (see page 286), Alström syndrome (with hypogenitalism, deafness, diabetes), Hallgren syndrome (mental retardation, deafness, cerebellar ataxia), Sjögren-Larsson syndrome (congenital cataract, mental retardation, spastic ataxia, ichthyosis). Inborn errors of metabolism are present in syndromes associated with very similar atypical retinitis pigmentosa: Refsum's disease (see page 290), Cockayne's syndrome (see page 290) and Bassen-Kornzweig disease (see page 290).

Differential diagnosis: Congenital (usually dominant heredity) optic atrophy begins slowly with gradual vision loss, whereas blindness or near blindness in recessively inherited retinal dysplasia (Leber-Alström-Olson) is present at birth or develops rapidly with slowly increasing retinal pigmentation.

Tapetoretinal Degeneration in Hereditary Metabolic Disorders (see page 365) Combined with Cerebral Disturbances

Recessively inherited lipidoses can be differentiated into those involving the macula and those of later onset with peripheral retinitis pigmentosa-like changes. In the macular form there is progressive amaurosis, secondary optic atrophy, dementia, paraplegia and death in the first years of life.

Three autosomal recessive lipidoses have to be considered. Tay-Sachs disease (infantile amaurotic idiocy with glycolipid deposition – ganglioside and cerebrosides) in the retina and central nervous system; Niemann-Pick disease with storage of phospholipids (especially sphingomyelins) in the retina and central nervous system; and Gaucher's disease with retinal and central nervous system accumulation of cerebrosides.

These three lipidoses also have juvenile and adult forms. Macula and retinal periphery are variably affected in those cases.

Amaurotic familial idiocy is a group of *cerebroretinal lipidoses*. As a result of some enzyme defect, gangliosides accumulate in ganglion cells of the central nervous system and retina. According to the age of onset, one can differentiate:

Congenital amaurotic idiocy (Norman-Wood-Landing syndrome) — Infantile amaurotic idiocy (Tay-Sachs) — Late infantile amaurotic idiocy (Dollinger-Bielschowsky syndrome) — Juvenile amaurotic idiocy (Batten-Mayou-Spielmeyer-Vogt-Stock syndrome) — Late amaurotic idiocy (Kufs' syndrome).

Infantile (and congenital) amaurotic idiocy (Tay-Sachs) (GM_2 type I): This tapetoretinal degeneration primarily involves children of eastern European Jewish descent. This most common form of cerebroretinal lipidosis manifests before age 4 to 6 months with a disciform gray-blue-white discoloration and slight prominence in the macular area (ganglioside storage in retinal ganglion cells). A cherry red spot is present (due to thinning of the retina and absence of ganglion cells at the fovea) (Plate XXVII, Fig. 6, page 288 c). The optic nerve develops progressive waxy yellow atrophy. Blindness, dementia, muscle palsies and generalized debility lead to death usually by the third year of life (van Bogaert and Klein 1965; Larsen and Ehlers 1965). According to Franceschetti (1963), consanguinity is present in 23 to 31 percent of Jewish and 55 to 66 percent of non-Jewish patients. The hereditary pattern is autosomal recessive (Klein and Ktenides 1954) or dominant (Badtke 1961). Tay-Sachs infantile amaurotic idiocy has been observed in a Negro child (Duke and Clark 1962).

The rare congenital amaurotic idiocy (Norman-Wood-Landing syndrome) (GM_1 type I) is clinically an early form of Tay-Sachs disease. Microcephaly is an additional finding.

Late infantile amaurotic idiocy: The Bielschowsky-Jansky-Dollinger syndrome has no higher incidence among children of Jewish extraction. Symptoms begin around the third to fourth year of life, generally leading to death 3 to 4 years later. Optic atrophy develops, and the atypical retinitis pigmentosa fundus changes are less pronounced than in the infantile form. Van Bogaert and Klein (1955) described the late infantile form in a pair of monozygotic twins. GM_2 type III and GM_1 type II gangliosidosis has been reported in some cases.

Juvenile amaurotic idiocy and late amaurotic idiocy (ceroid lipofuscinosis and GM_2 type III). Juvenile amaurotic idiocy manifests between ages 6 and 10 (Vogt-Spielmeyer-Stock syndrome or Batten-Mayou syndrome) and leads to blindness, dementia, clonic-tonic cramping, weight loss and death at the end of the second decade of life. Clinically *pigmentary dispersion appears in the macula* (macular type, cerebromacular degeneration, Batten-Mayou syndrome) or periphery (peripheral type, cerebroretinal degeneration, Vogt-Spielmeyer syndrome). Finally, the entire retina becomes atrophic, and the peripheral retina has a pepper and salt pigmentation. There is a correlation between amaurotic idiocy and vacuolization (lipoid degeneration) of lymphocytes (Rayner 1952; Julajo et al. 1956; Gilje and Nissen 1957).

The rare **late form of amaurotic idiocy** (Kufs' syndrome, Hallervorden-Kufs syndrome) manifests between 15 and 22 years of age. The disease resembles the juvenile form. Retinal changes are usually less pronounced. The ganglioside pattern is normal with presence of lipofuscin.

Other hereditary metabolic disorders with tapetoretinal degeneration include **Niemann-Pick disease.** Because of a hereditary enzyme defect, this rare phosphatide storage disease leads to sphingomyelin accumulation in the reticuloendothelial system (especially histiocytes). Liver, spleen, sometimes brain and retina are primarily involved. The retinal picture strongly resembles that of familial amaurotic idiocy.

Disseminated lipogranulomatosis (Farber's disease) is an inborn metabolic disorder leading to histiocyte accumulation of ceramide in early infancy. Ocular changes resemble those of Tay-Sachs disease.

Refsum's syndrome: Hereditary ataxia with nyctalopia and polyneuritic ataxia is associated with: Atypical retinitis pigmentosa, nyctalopia, visual field constriction, absent ERG, chronic polyneuritis with progressive paralysis of the distal extremities, pupillary changes, cataract, elevated cerebrospinal fluid protein and nystagmus. Heredity is autosomal recessive (Baum et al. 1965). Deafness, anosmia, and ichthyosis are less common. The disorder is due to a deficiency of phytanic acid α-hydrolase activity with impaired oxidation of ingested phytanic acid. The accumulation and storage of phytanic acid leads to neurotoxic symptoms.

Differential diagnosis includes: retinitis pigmentosa, Laurence-Moon-Bardet-Biedl syndrome with adiposogenital dystrophy, polydactyly and mental retardation, Cockayne's syndrome with progeria, dwarfism, paucity of fat and skin changes in the hands and face resembling striate porokeratosis of Mibelli. Acanthocytosis or abetalipoproteinemia with emphasis on distal polyneuropathy. The betalipoprotein fraction is missing in the serum. Erythrocytes are acanthotic (Hoffmann 1964).

Bassen-Kornzweig syndrome: This syndrome belongs to the retinal pigmentary and spinocerebellar degenerations. There is a lack of betalipoprotein in the serum with acanthocytosis of erythrocytes.

Schilder's disease: Schilder's disease or metachromatic leukodystrophy leads to central as well as peripheral retinitis pigmentosa-like changes, at times with white punctate deposits. This is an autosomal recessive inborn error of metabolism with storage of metachromatic sulfatides in the brain and retina (see page 366). The central nervous system damage leads to a clinical picture resembling multiple sclerosis.

Cockayne's syndrome (Coles 1969) (see page 290) includes retinal pigmentary degeneration with yellow-waxy optic atrophy and peripheral or central retinal pigmentary dispersion. Infantile deafness, dwarfism, oligophrenia, progeria (due to lack of subcutaneous fat) (Fig. 22.31, *"Mickey Mouse" syndrome*) are other hallmarks. There is a skin photosensitivity. Heredity is recessive (Ufermann, Heege-Dohr and Kosenow 1973).

Lipid proteinosis (Urbach-Wiethe syndrome) can present with a macular pseudopigment degeneration because of red-yellow drusen-like deposits beneath the pigment epithelium. This metabolic disorder (mucopolysaccharides and lipids are bound to a glycoprotein) leads to peculiar nodular and cystic changes on the lids (Fig. 10.37).

Mucopolysaccharidoses. Tapetoretinal degenerations are seldom observed in Hurler's, Hunter's, Sanfilippo's or Scheie's syndrome.

"Cystinosis" may lead to "pepper and salt" pigmentation (Fig. 22.34).

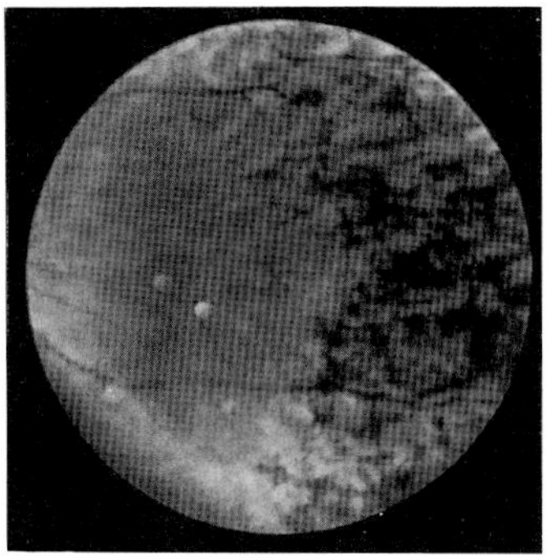

Fig. 22.34 Pseudoretinitis pigmentosa (posttrauma)

Retinitis Pigmentosa-like Phenocopies (Pseudoretinitis Pigmentosa)

Pseudoretinitis Pigmentosa after Trauma or Drugs

Retinitis pigmentosa-like phenocopies have often been observed, especially after retinal contusion injury (Fuchs 1935; Rieger 1947) (Fig. 22.35) and with retinal siderosis. Sodium hypoiodide (Scheerer 1926; Riehm 1927, 1929; v. Sallmann 1933 and others) and sodium iodide (Auricchio and de Vinventis 1950) and "Mp 20 Sandoz" (Verrey 1956) cause retinal toxicity with pseudoretinitis pigmentosa.

Mild *quinine toxicity* will cause blurred vision, tinnitus, nausea and generalized weakness.

With severe poisoning one sees vomiting, confusion, a drop in blood pressure and temperature, coma, respiratory arrest and even death. If the patient survives, quinine amblyopia may resolve over a period of hours to days.

Ophthalmoscopically, acute quinine poisoning can cause retinal edema (Plate XXVIII, Fig. 1, page 288 d) with a cherry red spot and blurred pale optic disc. In the end stage (after months or years) there is optic atrophy with thin threadlike retinal vessels. Rarely, pigmentary clumping in the sense of a pseudoretinitis pigmentosa occurs. Central visual acuity is usually relatively well maintained. The peripheral field may be markedly constricted. ERG a- and b-waves are varyingly altered. Quinine may have a direct toxic action on the retina (Hommer 1968; Cibis et al. 1974).

Toxic pseudoretinitis pigmentosa occurs after long-term phenothiazine or antimalarial therapy. There is vision loss with a ring scotoma. Pigmented granules and spots appear at the level of the pigment epithelium (Verrey 1947, 1956). Retinal pigmentation occurred (Plate XXVIII, Fig. 2, page 288 d) after chloroquine had been given for two years (Böke et al. 1967). It began in the macula, leading to a "bull's eye" configuration (François and de Becker 1965). As with measles retinitis, there is optic atrophy and narrowing of vessels. Visual acuity, dark adaptation and ERG are altered. Histologically, the rods and cones are degenerate with pigment hyperplasia (Heydenreich 1966). Areas of the macula hyperfluoresce on

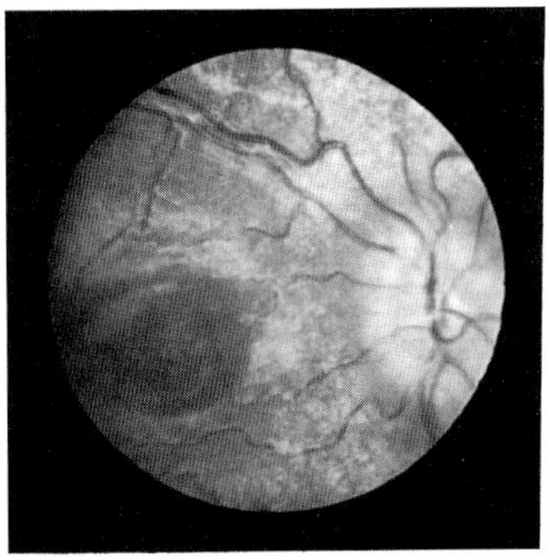

Fig. 22.35 Cystinosis: slightly prominent and blurred optic disk. There is a fine granular pigmentation of the entire fundus (except for the paramacular region) (♀ 6 yrs.)

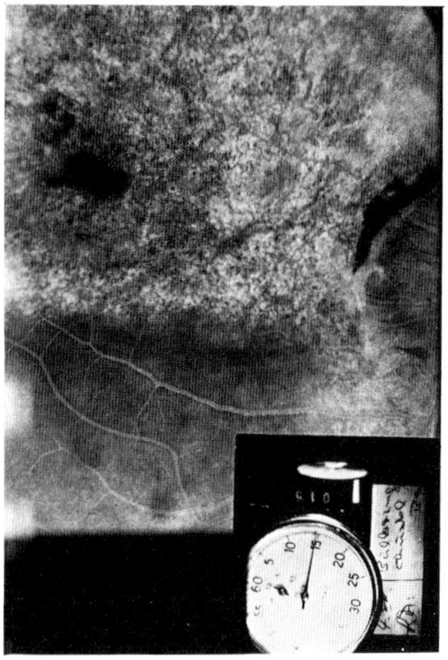

Fig. 22.36 Severe chloroquine damage with partial loss of pigment epithelium. Fluorescein angiography (after 15 seconds) shows marked fluorescence in this area

fluorescein angiography due to pigmentary dispersion (Kearns and Hollenhorst 1966).

A dosage of chloroquine greater than 250 mg/day can produce retinopathy (Fig. 22.36). A time period of 3 months to 5 years may be required (Bernstein 1968). Nylander (1967) found retinopathy before three years of treatment in one-fourth of patients with a total dose under 291 grams. In three-fourths of the cases, retinopathy occurred later at higher total doses.

Long-term *indomethacin* (Indocin) therapy can produce a similar picture (Burns 1968; Palimeris et al. 1972) (see page 168).

Of the *phenothiazines* (Alkemade 1968), piperazine and thiopropazate hydrochloride deserve special mention.

Pseudoretinitis pigmentosa also occurs after high dosages of chlorpromazine (Largactil, Megaphen, Thorazine, Hibernal, etc.). There is significant vision loss with black-brown retinal pigment deposits centrally or in a ring distribution (Baumann 1957; Wagner 1956).

Retinal damage not resembling retinitis pigmentosa has been observed with a variety of intoxicants. Chronic lead poisoning results in retinal neuritis with postneuritis optic atrophy. Chronic carbon monoxide poisoning can lead to retinal hemorrhages and neuritis. Retinal hemorrhages have also been observed with aromatic nitroamino compounds. Carbon disulfide can cause retinopathy (Jaensch 1963).

Pseudoretinopathy after Infectious Diseases

Infectious diseases can produce the picture of pseudoretinitis pigmentosa: smallpox (Germaix), typhus (Schupfer 1951), scarlet fever, mumps, encephalitis (Böck and Risak 1934; Maeder 1949 a and b). Measles encephalitis is particularly prone to cause retinal pigmentary changes (Bücklers 1942; Rieger 1944; Bedrossian 1955; Hentsch and Külz 1969), especially in the retinal periphery (Plate XXVIII, Fig. 3, page 288 d). Optic atrophy and vascular narrowing are present. Vision, visual field, and ERG are affected. In contrast, dark adaptation is minimally disturbed (Franceschetti 1963). According to Rieger (1944), measles retinopathy is due to selective damage to external retinal layers. As in central retinal artery emboli, there is sudden bilateral vision loss evolving into retinitis pigmentosa-like changes with permanent acuity and visual field deficits.

Other infectious diseases may produce a picture of pseudoretinitis pigmentosa: toxoplasmosis, syphilis, vaccinia, influenza virus, Newcastle virus, onchocerciasis, nematode endophthalmitis, Behçet-Gilbert syndrome (hypopyon iritis) and Harada's disease. Cytomegalovirus can cause retinal hemorrhages, perivascular exudates, vitreous clouding and retinal pigmentary changes (Aaberg, Cesarz and Rytel 1972). The cytomegalovirus is a DNA virus of the herpes virus group.

Embryopathies

Pseudoretinitis pigmentosa can be present at birth from intrauterine inflammation (see page 244): toxoplasmosis, syphilis, measles, typhus, scarlet fever, variola, varicella, and mumps. Primary damage is thought to be to the retinal vessels (Blum and Babel 1948).

Congenital viral *pseudoretinitis pigmentosa* morphologically resembles retinitis pulverulentus. The changes of rubella are associated with other malformations (congenital cataract, microphthalmos, deafness, etc.).

Choroideremia Carriers

Female carriers of choroideremia can have a fundus picture resembling pseudoretinitis pigmentosa. The granular-macular pigmentation is restricted to the periphery.

Pseudoretinitis Pigmentosa in Systemic Disease

A number of systemic diseases have retinitis pigmentosa-like fundus changes:

Turner's syndrome — Alport's syndrome — Alkaptonuria — Incontinentia pigmenti — Waardenburg's syndrome — Pulseless (aortic arch) disease.

Turner's syndrome: Besides pterygium colli there is infantilism, potentially pseudoretinitis pigmentosa, congenital cataracts and ptosis. The chorioretinal pigmentary dispersion occurs at the equator. This is a chromosomal anomaly (XO karyotype): chromatin-negative (see page 330).

Alport's syndrome: Hereditary nephropathy with lenticonus anterior and potentially pseudoretinitis pigmentosa (see page 252).

Alkaptonuria: Ochronosis (see page 364) can develop tapetoretinal degeneration and optic atrophy.

Incontinentia pigmenti: The Bloch-Sulzberger syndrome includes microcephaly, skin pigmentation, potentially corneal and lens opacification, retinal and choroidal pigmentary anomalies, optic atrophy, blue sclera and microphthalmos (see page 247).

Waardenburg's syndrome (see page 87) may also be associated with pseudoretinitis pigmentosa.

Pulseless disease (Takayasu's syndrome) may have retinal pigmentary dispersion (see pages 193 and 315).

Vitamin B deficiency (pellagra) rarely causes pseudoretinitis pigmentosa.

Peripheral pigmentary changes are seen in **cystinosis** (François et al. 1972). Cystinosis can develop pseudoretinitis pigmentosa.

Inflammatory Diseases of the Retina

Diffuse Chorioretinitis (or Neuroretinitis, Retinoneuritis, Retinochorioneuritis)

This appears in congenital *lues* in healed scarred form (Plate XXVIII, Fig. 4, page 288 d). With acquired syphilis, an acute or chronic, diffuse chorioretinitis with white edematous opacification of retina and optic disc occurs. Vitreous clouding, iritis and cyclitis are part of tertiary luetic chorioretinitis.

Edema, retinal hemorrhages and exudates, sheathing and narrowing of vessels are observed. Preretinal hemorrhages, venous thrombosis, or arterial occlusion are more rare.

Both congenital and acquired healed luetic chorioretinitis may be difficult to differentiate from retinitis pigmentosa. The optic disc in healed luetic chorioretinitis is pale white or red, not waxy yellow. The retinal vessels are narrowed and may be obscured by white perivascular sheathing. Pigment clumps are distributed throughout the fundus, not just at the equator, and are large and often extradense near the ora (anterior choroiditis). At other times the picture is of a fine pigment dust (pepper and salt fundus).

Virus infections (viral embolisms, often with encephalitis) may also cause a diffuse retinitis with speckled grey retinal infiltrations and narrowing of the retinal vessels, leading to the picture of pseudoretinitis pigmentosa: measles, rubella, infectious mononucleosis (Pfeiffer), parotitis epidemica, varicella, smallpox.

In about half the cases of epidemic typhus, hyperemic blurring of the disc margins appears around the tenth day of illness. Venous stasis and peripheral punctate retinal hemorrhages occur. Sectorial retinal edema and subretinal transudates are less common (Freusberg 1942).

Typhoid fever, scarlet fever and other general

diseases may also lead to diffuse retinitis. Diffuse chorioretinitis may after healing exactly resemble pseudoretinitis pigmentosa (see pages 216, 292).

Differential diagnosis: Compared with tapetoretinal degeneration, the most important differentiating points are lack of night blindness, normal ERG (electroretinogram), and usually lack of visual field loss. Sectorial or ring scotomata are the exception.

Juxtapapillary Chorioretinitis
(Jensen)

Jensen's juxtapapillary chorioretinitis (see page 215) occurs primarily in the third decade of life. Ophthalmoscopically one sees gray areas of retinal edema (Plate XVI, Fig. 1, page 192 h) 1 to 2 disc diameters in size, involving the inner retinal layers and therefore obscuring blood vessels. These tend to be near the optic disc but may be in other locations. Characteristically, the vitreous is very hazy with protein precipitates depositing on the posterior corneal surface. The inflammation tends to recur, beginning at the edge of the original lesion. Final healing leaves round, sharply demarcated, heavily pigmented chorioretinal scars. Depending on the clinical picture, various authors place the primary source of inflammation in either the choroid or retina. Nerve fiber bundle damage leads to characteristic scimitar-shaped visual field loss, which tends to be permanent. When the lesion abuts onto the optic disc, as it commonly does, the resultant scotoma connects with the blind spot (Fig. 3.12). If nerve fibers are interrupted more peripherally, the visual field defect does not connect with the blind spot (Fig. 3.12). Focal inflammation from syphilis, tuberculosis, or toxoplasmosis is the presumed cause.

Sepsis

Sepsis or bacteremia may result in metastatic ophthalmia due to infectious emboli in retinal vessels. These rapidly produce endophthalmitis (Fig. 16.20). Simple "septic retinitis" (Fig. 22.10) is a slow, more benign localized inflammation with sharply outlined white retinal lesions and hemorrhages resulting from septic emboli. There is no tendency for progression (see page 268).

Malnutrition Retinitis
(see page 284)

This was observed as "camp eye" (Spillare and Scott 1944; Dekking 1947) in malnourished war prisoners in combination with solar retinitis. Macular destruction and neuritis were present. Scholtyssek (1950) observed reversible retinal edema and retinal spots in 6 percent of returning dystrophic prisoners.

Inflammatory Macular Disease

(Toxoplasmosis, histoplasmosis, *Toxocara canis*, central serous retinopathy) (see page 283).

Chorioretinitis

Every choroiditis leads to simultaneous retinal involvement (chorioretinitis) (see page 215).

Pseudoretinitis Pigmentosa

Trauma, medications and infection can all produce a certain degree of retinal inflammation and pseudoretinitis pigmentosa (see page 291).

Retinal Tumors and Pseudotumors

Retinoblastoma

Retinoblastoma (retinal glioma, neuroepithelioma) is the most common *retinal tumor.*

This is a tumor of small children, with two-thirds of cases appearing before age two. Parents note a white pupillary reflex (Fig. 22.37) or seek medical advice because of strabismus. On examination there is a "cat's eye" (blind gray-white pupillary reflex). Ophthalmoscopy reveals a white mass lying free in the vitreous or covered by retina. Glaucoma and painful ocular inflammation follow. Left untreated, the rapidly growing tumor breaks through the wall of the globe anteriorly or posteriorly into the orbit and cranium. True metastasis occurs intracranially and to other parts of the body. Intraocular calcification may be visible ophthalmoscopically as white plaques or be visualized with special X-ray techniques. Since the tumor is derived from retinal neural cells which form rosettes, this tumor has been called neuroepithelioma (Wintersteiner 1897), retinocytoma or retinoblastoma (Mavas 1924).

Retinoblastomas have a tendency for spontaneous necrosis and collapse. This may delay the spread of the tumor, with manifestation at a later age. Temporary spontaneous remission occurs in 1 of 100 cases (Dollfus and Auvert 1953). Rare cases of spontaneous cure are reported (Wüstenberg 1950). Retinoblastomas are bilateral in 20 to 30 percent of cases (Dollfus and Auvert 1953), necessitating careful examination of the second eye. Tumor cells can accumulate in the anterior chamber, presenting the rare finding of a tumor "hypopyon."

Retinoblastomas have a dominant inheritance with irregular penetrance (about 80 percent) or represent spontaneous mutation or phenocopies (Rieger 1958; Falls and Neels 1951; Waardenburg et al. 1961, 1963; Goldberg 1974). Bilateral appearance of a retinoblastoma means that it is hereditary. The same is true for unilateral tumors when there is a second known case in the family. Eighty to eighty-five percent of sporadic unilateral cases are nonhereditary phenocopies, while the remainder are spontaneous new mutations with a dominant inheritance (Jaeger 1973).

Differential diagnostic considerations include pseudoglioma (see page 234) and retrolental fibroplasia (see page 277).

Pseudogliomatous malformations at the posterior pole can be hereditary (Pajtas 1950; Dahlberg-Parrow 1956).

Pseudoglioma

(see page 234)

Pseudoglioma must be considered when leukocoria (gray-white-yellow retrolental tissue or exudate) is present:

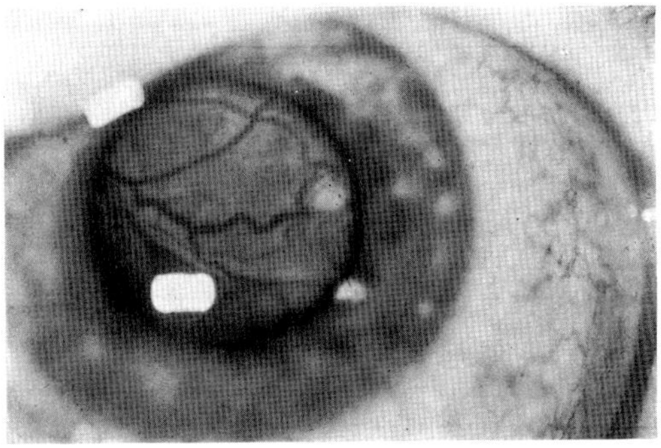

Fig. 22.37 Retinoblastoma (glioma retinae) (♀ 3 yrs.)

Persistent hyperplastic primary vitreous — Retrolental fibroplasia — Falciform fold — Endophthalmitis, vitreous hemorrhage — Exudative chorioretinitis — Coats' disease — Tumor — Retinal dysplasia — Phakomatosis.

Persistent hyperplastic primary vitreous: With so-called persistence or hyperplasia of the primary vitreous, specifically of the posterior tunica fibrosa (vasculosa) lentis, the hyaloid funnel is maintained behind the lens as white connective tissue. The posterior lens capsule is often ruptured, and posterior lens layers are opaque (see page 234). The condition is usually unilateral with microphthalmia of the affected eye. Retinoblastoma in a microphthalmic eye is virtually unheard of.

Retrolental fibroplasia (retinopathy of the newborn) (Fig. 20.3) generally appears only in prematurely born infants weighing less than 1,900 grams at birth and placed in an incubator (with over 40 percent O_2). The bilateral changes evolve after the child is removed from oxygen environment (see page 235, 277).

Congenital falciform folds pull the retina and retinal vessels away from the optic disc in a fold (Fig. 22.24 and 22.25) (see page 278).

Endophthalmitis, vitreous hemorrhage: Every severe endophthalmitis (infection, metastatic ophthalmia, injury) or vitreous hemorrhage can lead to connective tissue organization with vascular ingrowth. The history usually reveals: injury, severe inflammation, periphlebitis, diabetic retinopathy, etc. Normally the globe is hypotonic (mushy soft); rarely, secondary glaucoma is present. If the vitreous organiza-

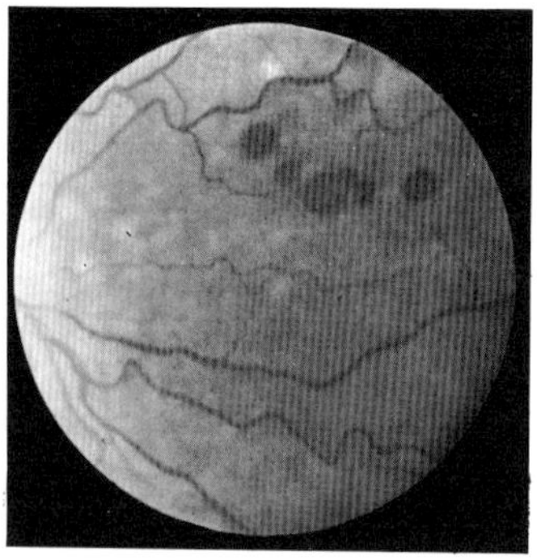

Fig. 22.38 Retinal nevi (♀ 42 yrs.)

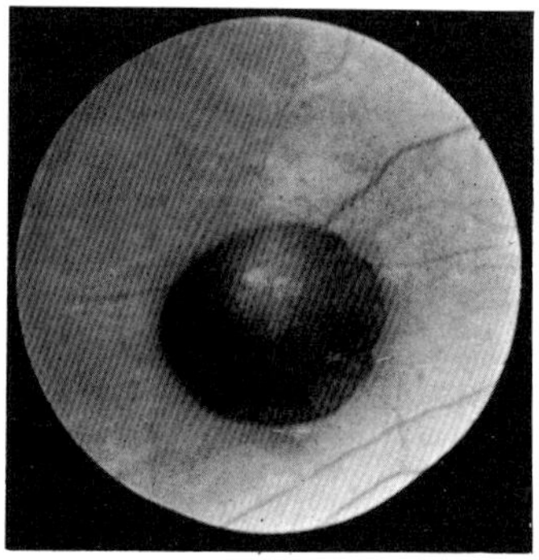

Fig. 22.39 Retinal nevus (♀ 54 yrs.)

tion occurred in utero or in the first months of life, the eye is generally microphthalmic. Retinoblastoma eyes are almost always normal in size with a normal anterior chamber. Lack of surface vasculature speaks in favor of a pseudoglioma. Inflammatory origin can be recognized by the presence of posterior synechiae. Retinoblastoma can, however, present with proliferation of tumor cells in the aqueous, precipitates, hypopyon, synechiae and iris atrophy.

Exudative chorioretinitis: Severe exudative retinitis or chorioretinitis can cause gray vitreous exudate as does *Toxocara canis* (see page 283).

Coats' disease (retinitis exudativa externa): The detached retina may be pushed directly behind the lens in this retinitis (Plate XXV, Fig. 4, page 288 a; Plate XXVIII, Fig. 5, page 288 d). There is a gray-yellow-white retrolental mass. Retinal vessels show aneurysmal dilatations (see page 277).

Retinal dysplasia: *Retinal dysplasia* (Krause 1946; Reese and Blodi 1950 [see page 235]) results from congenital malformations: bilateral retinal dysplasia with persistent primary vitreous, microphthalmos, systemic malformations (cerebral, cardiac, lung, gastrointestinal tract, skeletal, urogenital). The disorder occurs most commonly in trisomy D-1 (13–15), or E (18), less often with intrauterine cytomegalic or other viral infections (François and Neetens 1969).

Tumors: Other tumors may cause a pseudoglioma: sarcoma, metastatic carcinoma, diktyoma. Nevi (Figs. 22.38 and 22.39), like choroidal angiomas (Plate XXVIII, Fig. 6, page 288 d), raise the question of malignant melanoma (Plate XXIX, Fig. 1, page 288 e).

Phakomatoses

(van der Hoeve 1921, 1923)

Phakomatoses exhibit an incomplete dominant inheritance. They cause birthmarks on the skin and mucous membranes arising from undifferentiated embryonal cells.

The phakomatoses (François 1974), neuroretinal-cutaneous dysplasia, hereditary embryonal dysplasia, and hamartomas include:

Hemangioblastoma, specifically angiomatosis retinae (v. Hippel-Lindau) — Tuberous sclerosis (Bourneville) — Neurofibromatosis (v. Recklinghausen) (see page 103) — Trigeminocerebral angiomatosis (Sturge-Weber-Krabbe) (see page 103, 226) — Neuro-oculo-facial arteriovenous aneurysm (see page 257) — Klippel-Trenaunay syndrome (see page 226) — Turner's syndrome (see pages 89 and 330) — Louis-Bar syndrome (ataxia telangiectasia) (see page 257) — Nevus sebaceus (see page 189).

Retinal angiomatosis (von Hippel-Lindau disease): Cystic capillary hemangiomas develop in various organs – kidneys, ovaries, pancreas, etc. – with a predilection for the retina and cerebellum (v. Hippel 1904). A large feeding artery and vein stretch from the disc to the round hemangioma, which can appear at any retinal location (Plate XXIX, Fig. 2, page 288 e). The hemangiomas cause exudates within and under the retina, retinal detachment, retinitis proliferans, and sometimes, secondary glaucoma. Not only are the eyes threatened, but systemic tumors can be fatal (Lindau 1927). The angiomata are hereditary in one-fifth of cases (François and Coffyn 1951), with both eyes being involved in one-third of these.

Tuberous Sclerosis

Bourneville's disease (tuberous sclerosis) is a dominantly transmitted neuroectodermal dysplasia with skin tumors (sebaceous adenoma of Pringle) and is classified as one of the phakomatoses (van der Hoeve 1921, 1923) or hamartoses as per Albrecht (Purtscher 1935). Van der Hoeve first described the retinal tumors, which may vary in size (1 to 2 disc diameters) and are gray-white, yellow to gray-green, clearly demarcated round to oval nodules (Fig. 22.40).

Larger tumors are often found on or near the optic disc. One-third of these have a mulberry-like appearance (Hoffmann 1959). Vaas (1940) found 59 of 173 patients manifested the disease by 1 year of age and 90 percent by 12 years of age.

Schwab, in his extensive review of the literature, determined that the characteristic retinal lesions appear in over 20 percent of patients with tuberous sclerosis. The tumors (astrocytomas) arise in the retinal nerve fiber layer and may be in front of or below retinal vessels. Hyaline- and calcium-containing cystic structures also occur. Rupture of tumor cysts can cause vitreous clouding and droplet metastases (van der Hoeve 1921, 1923; Hoffmann 1959). Intracranial tumors can elevate cerebrospinal fluid pressure, causing papilledema (Schwab 1956).

Tuberous sclerosis is associated with sebaceous adenoma and cortical tumors, the latter causing seizure disorders. The tumors do not grow, and only symptomatic therapy is required.

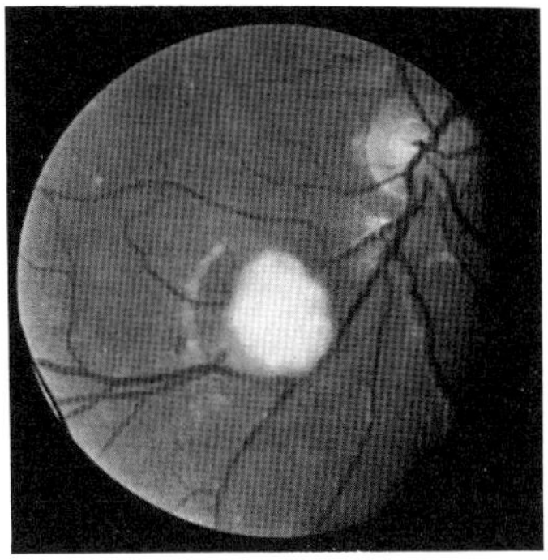

Fig. 22.40 Tuberous sclerosis (Bourneville) mulberrylike white retinal tumor (♂ 9 yrs.)

References

Aaberg, T. M., T. J. Cesarz, M. W. Rytel: Correlation of virology and clinical course of cytomegalovirus retinitis. Amer. J. Ophthal. 74 (1972) 407–415

Alkemade, P. P. H.: Phenothiazine-Retinopathy. Ophthalmologica 155 (1968) 70–76

Alpern, M., H. F. Falls, G. B. Lee: The enigma of typical total monochromacy. Amer. J. Ophthal. 50 (1960) 996–1012

Alström, C. H., O. Olson: Heredo-retinopathia congenitalis. Monohybrida recessiva autosomalis, a genetical-statistical study. Hereditas (Lund) 43 (1957) 1–177

Altenberger, cited by Velhagen: Augenkrankheiten und Allgemeinleiden. In: Der Augenarzt, Vol. VI, ed. by K. Velhagen. Thieme, Leipzig 1964

Amalric, P.: Fluorescein Angiography (International Symposium, Albi) S. Karger 1971

Ashton, N.: Central areolar choriodal sclerosis. A histopathological study. Brit. J. Ophthal. 37 (1953) 140–147

Ashton, N.: Larval granulomatosis of the retina due to toxocara. Brit. J. Ophthal. 44 (1960) 129–148

Auricchio, G., M. de Vincentis: Recherche esperimentali sulla patogenesi della degeneratione pigmentaria della retina da iodato di sodio. G. ital. Oftal. 3 (1950) 118–127

Aust, W., D. Kirsch, E. Herrmann: Glaskörper und Fundusveränderungen bei akuten Subarachnoidalblutungen. Ber. dtsch. ophthal. Ges. 168 (1968) 75–79

Baba, K., M. Hirayama: Vergleichende Betrachtungen der kongenitalen Netzhautfalte und der retrolentalen Fibroplasie. Paediat. Univ. Tokyo 1960 No. 5, 1–2, ref. in: Zbl. ges. Ophthal. 83 (1961) 303

Badtke, H.: Die Mißbildungen des menschlichen Auges. In: Der Augenarzt, Vol. IV, ed. by K. Velhagen. Thieme, Stuttgart 1961

Ballantine, A. J., J. C. Michaelson: The Fundus of the Eye. E. and S. Livingstone, Edinburgh and London 1970

Baum, J. L., M. Tannenbaum, E. H. Kolodny: Refsum's syndrome with corneal involvement. Amer. J. Ophthal. 60 (1965) 699–708

Baumann, H.: Treten nach langdauernder und hochdosierter Largactiltherapie Schädigungen des Sehorgans auf? Klin. Mbl. Augenheilk. 130 (1957) 769–793

Bedrossian, R. H.: Neuroretinitis following measles. J. Pediat. 46 (1955) 329–331

Bengtsson, B., B. Linder: Sex-linked hereditary juvenile retinoschisis. Acta ophthal. (Kbh.) 45 (1967) 411–423

Berneaud-Kötz, G.: Augenbeteiligung bei Dys- und Paraproteinanämien. Enke, Stuttgart 1959

Bernstein, H. N.: Ocular toxicity of chloroquine. Survey ophthal. 12 (1968) 415

Best, F.: Über eine hereditäre Maculaaffektion. Beitrag zur Vererbungslehre. Z. Augenheilk. 13 (1905) 199–212

Bettelheim, H.: Pulseless disease und bilaterale Karotisthrombose. Klin. Mbl. Augenheilk. 152 (1968) 487–501

Bettelheim, H.: Die klinische Bedeutung der Ophthalmodynamometrie und der Ophthalmodynamographie. Klin. Mbl. Augenheilk. 155 (1969) 769–791

Blach, R. K.: The hereditary hyalo-retinopathies. Brit. J. Ophthal. 53 (1969) 136–137

Blach, R. K., A. M. Hamilton: Symposium on the Macula. Trans. Ophthal. Soc. UK 92 (1973) 383–484

Blum, J. D., J. Babel: Diagnostic differentiel des rétinites et des pseudorétinites pigmentaires au point de vue histologique. Schweiz. med. Wschr. 1948, 696

Böck, J., E. Risak: Retinitis pigmentosa und Hochwuchs. Z. Augenheilk. 84 (1934) 48–58

Böhringer, H. R., P. Dieterle, E. Londolt: Zur Klinik und Pathologie der degeneratio-hyaloideo retinalis hereditaria (Wagner). Ophthalmologica 139 (1960) 330–338

Böke, W.: Augenerkrankungen bei entzündlichen Systemerkrankungen des Bindegewebes. Round-table-Gespräch. Ber. dtsch. ophthal. Ges. 70 (1970) 396–424

Böke, W., A. Bäumer: Klinische und histopathologische Augenbefunde beim akuten Lupus erythematodes disseminatus. Klin. Mbl. Augenheilk. 146 (1965) 175–187

Böke, W., A. Bäumer, W. Müller-Limmroth, M. Mludek: Zur Frage der Chloroquinschädigung des Auges. Klin. Mbl. Augenheilk. 151 (1967) 617–633

Bogaert, L. van, D. Klein: Observations sur l'hérédité des idioties amaurotiques et de la spléno-hépatomégalie lipidienne (11 familles). J. Génét. hum. 4 (1953) 23–78

Bonnet, P.: Tortuosité congénitale des vaisseaux de la rétine et sténose congénitale de l'isthme de l'aorte. Arch. Ophtal. (Paris) 14 (1954) 129–139

Braley, A. E.: Dystrophy of the macula. Amer. J. Ophthal. 61 (1966) 1–24

Braun-Vallons, S., N. Ashton, J. M. Duguid, P. Dhermy: Manifestations oculaires de l'infestation par toxocara. Ann. Oculist. (Paris) 197 (1964) 217–240

Bronson, N. R.: Recent developments in diagnostic ultrasound. Trans. Ophthal. Soc. UK 92 (1973) 149–159

Bruna, F.: Complicationi oculari nella porpora costituzionale di Werlhof. Boll. Oculist. 28 (1949) 41–56

Bücklers, M.: Retinitis pigmentosa nach Masern. Klin. Mbl. Augenheilk. 108 (1942) 380

Bullock, J. D., D. N. Albert: Flecked retina. Appearance secondary to oxalate crystals. Arch. Ophthalm. (Chicago) 93 (1975) 26–31

Burns, C. A.: Indomethacin reduced retinal sensitivity and corneal depots. Am. J. Ophth. 66 (1968) 825–835

Cagianut, B.: Das arterio-venöse Aneurysma der Netzhaut. Klin. Mbl. Augenheilk. 140 (1962) 180–191

Cagianut, B., W. Werner: Zum Krankheitsbild der familiären Tortuositas der kleinen Netzhautarterien mit Maculablutung. Klin. Mbl. Augenheilk. 153 (1968) 533–542

Calmettes, L., F. Deodati, G. Bechac: L'embolie graisseuse de la rétine. Arch. Opht. (Paris) 27 (1967) 209–220

Carr, R. E. et al.: Symposium: Pigmentary retinopathy. Summing up. Trans. Ophth. Soc. U. Kingdom 92 (1973) 173–301.

Charleux, J., L. Durand, B. Robert: Aspects ophtalmoscopiques et traitement du rétinoschisis kystique sénile. Bull. Soc. franç. Ophtal. 82 (1969) 223–238

Cibis, G. W., H. M. Burian, F. C. Blodi: Electroretinogram changes in acute quinine poisoning. Arch. Ophthal. (Chicago) 90 (1974) 307–309

Clifton, F., C. H. Greer: Ocular changes in acute systemic lupus erythematosus. Brit. J. Ophthal. 39 (1955) 1–10

Coleman, D. J.: Reliability of ocular and orbital diagnosis with B-Scan ultrasound. Amer. J. Ophthal. 73 (1972) 501–516

Coles, W. H.: Ocular manifestations of Cockayne's syndrome. Am. J. Ophth. 67 (1969) 762–764

Condon, P. I., G. R. Serjeant: Ocular findings in homozygous sickle cell anemia in Jamaica. Amer. J. Ophthal. 73 (1972) 533–543

Condon, P. I., G. R. Serjeant: Ocular findings in hemoglobin SC disease in Jamaica. Amer. J. Ophthal. 74 (1972) 921–931

Condon, P. I., G. R. Serjeant: Ocular findings in sickle cell thalassemia in Jamaica. Amer. J. Ophthal. 74 (1972) 1105–1109

Dahlberg-Parrow, R.: Congenital sex-linked pseudoglioma and grave mental deficiency. Acta ophthal. (Kbh.) 34 (1956) 250–254

Dekking, H. M.: Tropical nutritional amblyopia (campeyes). Ophthalmologica 113 (1947) 65–92

Dekking, H. M.: Pigmentary degeneration of the retina after quinine intoxication. Ophthalmologica (Basel) 118 (1949) 743–745

Dellaporta, A.: Über Fältelung der Netzhaut bei Hypotonie. Klin. Mbl. Augenheilk. 125 (1954) 672–678

Denden, A.: Über wenig bekannte multiple vitelliforme Retinalzysten des hinteren Fundusabschnittes. Klin. Mbl. Augenheilk. 149 (1966) 609–626

Deutman, A. F.: The hereditary dystrophies of the posterior pole of the eye. van Gorcum and Comp. Prakke, Assen the Netherlands, 1971

Deutman, A. F.: Electro-oculography in families with vitelliform dystrophy of the fovea. Arch. Ophthal. (Chicago) 81 (1969) 305–316

Deutman, A. F., G. H. M. van Lith: Differentialdiagnose der "Bull's Eye-Macula". 73 Zus. d. Deutsch. ophthal. Ges. 1975, 547–550

Dietzel, P. B., H. G. Willert: Morphologie und Histochemie der harten und weichen Exsudate der Retina bei Diabetes mellitus und essentieller Hypertonie. Klin. Mbl. Augenheilk. 139 (1961) 475–491

Doden, W.: Zur Klinik und Ätiologie der Periphlebitis retinae. Entwicklung und Fortschritte in der Augenheilkunde. Enke, Stuttgart 1963 (pp. 152–178)

Dollfus, M. A., B. Auvert: Le gliome de la rétine, Vol. VIII. Masson, Paris 1953

Doyne, R. W.: Quoted in Falls. 1966

Duguid, J. M.: Chronic endophthalmitis due to toxocara. Brit. J. Ophthal. 45 (1961 a) 705–717

Duguid, J. M.: Features of ocular infestation by toxocara. Brit. J. Ophthal. 45 (1961 b) 789–796

Duke-Elder, Sir St.: Diseases of the retina. System of ophthalmology, Vol. X. Himpton, London 1967

Duke, J. R., D. B. Clark: Infantile amaurotic familial idiocy (Tay-Sachs disease) in the Negro race. Amer. J. Ophthal. 53 (1962) 800–805

Dunphy, E. B.: Ocular conditions associated with idiopathic hyperlipemia. Amer. J. Ophthal. 33 (1950) 1579–1586

Eisner, G.: Biomicroscopy of the peripheral fundus. Springer, Berlin, Heidelberg, New York 1973

Ericson, L. A.: Lipaemia retinalis. Acta ophthal. 33 (1955) 79–91

Falls, H. F.: A classification and clinical description of hereditary macular lesions. Trans. Amer. Acad. Ophthal. Otolaryng. 70 (1966) 1034–1046

Falls, H. F., J. V. Neel: Genetica of retinoblastoma. Arch. Ophthal. 46 (1951) 367–389

Favre, M.: A propos de deux cas de dégénérescence hyaloideo-rétinienne. Ophthalmologica 135 (1958) 604–609

Filbry, G.: Zur diskontinuierlichen reversiblen Arteriopathie (Kyrieleis) bei Uveitis. Klin. Mbl. Augenheilk. 139 (1961) 577–582

Franceschetti, A.: A curious affection of the fundus oculi, helicoid, peripapillar chorioretinal degeneration, its relation to pigmentary paravenous chorioretinae degeneration. Docum. ophthal. 16 (1962) 81–110

Franceschetti, A.: Über tapeto-retinale Degeneration im Kindesalter. Dritter Fortbildungskurs der Dtsch. Ophthal. Ges. Hamburg 1962. In: Entwicklung und Fortschritt in der Augenheilkunde, ed. by H. Sautter. Enke, Stuttgart 1963 (pp. 107–120)

Franceschetti, A.: A special form of tapetoretinal dégéneration: Fundus flavimaculatus. Trans. Amer. Acad. Ophthal. Otolaryng. 69 (1965) 1048–1053

Franceschetti, A., J. François: Fundus flavimaculatus. Arch. Ophthal. 25 (1965) 505–530

Franceschetti, A., D. Klein: Hérédo-ataxies spino-ponto cérébelleuses. Rev. Oto-neuro-ophtal. (B.-Aires) 20 (1948) 109–166

Franceschetti, A., D. Klein: Démonstrations de la clinique ophtalmologique universitaire de Genève. Ophthalmologica (Basel) 125 (1953) 340–347

Franceschetti, A., J. François, J. Babel, A. de Rouck, P. Dieterle, G. Forni, D. Klein, A. Ricci, G. Verriest: Les hérédo dégénérescences chorio-rétiennes. Masson, Paris 1963

François, J.: Ocular manifestations of chloroquine intoxication. Trans. Ophthal. Soc. U. K. 85 (1966) 407–425

François, J.: Phakomatoses. Ann. Oculist. (Paris) 207 (1974) 497–515

François, J., L. de Becker: Les manifestations oculaires de l'intoxication chloroquinique. Ann. Oculist. 198 (1965) 513–544

François, J., J. Coffyn: Angiomatose rétino-cérébello-viscérale de Hippel-Lindau. Ann. Oculist. (Paris) 184 (1951) 206–213

François, J., M. Haussers, R. Coppieters, L. Evers: Cystinosis, Amer. J. Ophthal. 73 (1972) 643–650

François, J., J. J. de Laey: Dégénérescences maculaires juveniles et fluoro-angiographie rétinienne. Bull Soc. franç. Ophtal. 82 (1969) 417–431

François, J., J. J. de Laey: Bietti'sche kristalline Fundusdystrophie. Klin. Mbl. Augenheilk. 170 (1977) 353–362

François, J., A. Neetens: Dysplasie rétinienne de Reese et maladie a inclusions cytomégaliques. Bull. Soc. franç. Ophtal. 81 (1969) 523–534

François, J., M. Rabaey: Dystrophie cornéenne et paraprotéinémie. Bull. Soc. belge Ophtal. 125 (1960) 1007–1017

François, J., A. de Rouck, D. Fernandez-Sasso: Electrooculography in vitelliform degeneration of the macula. Arch. Ophthal. (Chicago) 77 (1967) 726–733

François, J., A. de Rouck, E. Cambie, A. Zanen: L'électrodiagnostic des affections rétiniennes. Masson, Paris 1974

François, J., G. Verriest, A. de Rouck: Hérédo-dégénérescence maculaire juvénile avec atteinte prédominante de la vision photopique. Ann. Oculist. 195 (1962) 1137–1191

François, J., M. Rabaey, L. Evens, E. de Vos: Etude histo-pathologique d'une rétinite de Coats probablement toxoplasmique. Ophthalmologica (Basel) 132 (1956) 1–12

François, J.: Das zystoide Ödem der Macula. Klin. Mbl. Augenheilk. 162 (1973) 125–138

Freusberg, O.: Über Erkrankungen des A. H. bei Fleckfieber. Klin. Mbl. Augenheilk. 108 (1942) 621–625

Fuchs, A.: Über seltene pathologische Befunde nach Verletzungen. Klin. Mbl. Augenheilk. 95 (1935) 721–738

Gärtner, J.: Klinische Beobachtungen über Glaskörperadhaerenzen am hinteren Augenpol. Klin. Mbl. Augenheilk. 140 (1962) 161–180

Gass, J. D., E. W. Norton, J. Justice: Serous detachment of the retinal pigment epithelium. Trans. Amer. Acad. Ophthal. Otolaryng. 70 (1966) 990–1015

Gass, D.: Das Puchering-Syndrom. 73. Tagung der Dtsch. Ophth. Ges. Heidelberg, 1973

Gavey, C. J.: The eye and blood diseases. Trans. ophthal. Soc. U. K. 83 (1964) 315–344

Germaix: Cited in Rieger

Giles, C. L.: Retinal hemorrhages in the newborn. Amer. J. Ophthal. 49 (1960) 1005–1011

Gilke, K., A. J. Nissen: The early diagnosis of juvenile amaurotic idiocy. Lipoid lymphocyte degeneration. Acta ophthal. (Kbh.) 35 (1957) 184–189

Gloor, B., H. Werner: Postkoagulative und spontan auftretende internoretinale Fibroplasie mit Maculadegeneration. Klin. Mbl. Augenheilk. 151 (1967) 822–845

Gloor, B. P.: Epiretinale Fibroplasie und massive präretinale Retraktion. Ophthalmologica (Basel) 161 (1970) 227–236

Godde-Jolly, D., P. Bonnin: La lipémie rétinienne. Ann. Oculist. (Paris) 194 (1961) 673–693

Goldberg, M. F.: Genetic and metabolic eye disease. Little, Brown and Co., Boston 1974

Haase, W., K. A. Hellner: Über familiäre bilaterale sektorenförmige Retinopathia pigmentosa. Klin. Mbl. Augenheilk. 147 (1965) 365–375

Hager, H.: Die Diagnose der Karotisthrombose durch den Augenarzt. Klin. Mbl. Augenheilk. 141 (1962) 801–840

Hager, H.: Die Ophthalmo-Dynamographie als Methode zur Beurteilung des Gehirnkreislaufes. Klin. Mbl. Augenheilk. 142 (1963) 827–846

Haimböck, K.: Augenerkrankungen bei Endangiitis obliterans. Klin. Mbl. Augenheilk. 140 (1962) 56–64

Hartmann, E., M. Massin: Les manifestations rétiniennes de la lupo-érythémato-viscérite malique. Ann. Oculist. (Paris) 189 (1956) 973–987

Hauschild, E., H. Hiller, A. Heydenreich: Beitrag zum Krankheitsbild der vitreo-retinalen Degeneration. Klin. Mbl. Augenheilk. 156 (1970) 628–643

Heimann, K., K. W. Jacobi, S. Kramer, H. G. Terheggen: Augensymptome beim Louis-Bar-Syndrom (Ataxia teleangiektasia). Ber. Verein Rhein.-Westf. Augenärzte, 120 (1969) 101–108

Heinsius, E.: Über Hornhautbeteiligung bei Agranulocytose. Ophthalmologica (Basel) 118 (1949) 69–75

Heinsius, E.: Über Augenhintergrundsveränderungen als Folge von Mangelernährung. Klin. Mbl. Augenheilk. 117 (1950) 19–28

Heinsius, E.: Retinopathia diabetica bei Kindern. Klin. Mbl. Augenheilk. 129 (1956) 499–505

Henkes, H. E., A. F. Deutman: Electrodiagnostic procedures in drug-induced ocular diseases. Documenta Ophthalm. 34 (1973) 209–219

Hentsch, R., J. Külz: Beitrag zur sekundären Pigmentdegeneration der Netzhaut nach Masern. Klin. Mbl. Augenheilk. 154 (1969) 706–712

Hentsch, R., G. Weißbach: Ophthalmologische Befunde bei der Pachymeningeosis haemorrhagica interna im frühen Kindesalter. Klin. Mbl. Augenheilk. 149 (1966) 323–328

Hermann, J. S.: Vitelliform degeneration of the macula. Amer. J. Ophthal. 61 (1966) 461–465

Heydenreich, A.: Chemisch-toxische Schäden der Augen. Klin. Mbl. Augenheilk. 149 (1966) 145–165

Hill, D. W. et al.: Symposium of diabetic retinopathy. Trans. Ophthal. Soc. UK 92 (1973) 59–130

Hiller, H.: Morbus Coats-Miliaraneurysmenretinitis Leber. Klin. Mbl. Augenheilk. 158 (1971) 225–234

Hippel, E. v.: Über eine sehr seltene Erkrankung der Netzhaut. Albrecht v. Graefes Arch. klin. exp. Ophthal. 59 (1904) 83–106

Hoeve, J. van der: Augengeschwülste bei der tuberösen Hirnsklerose (Bourneville). Albrecht v. Graefes Arch. klin. exp. Ophthal. 105 (1921) 880–898; 111 (1923) 1–16

Hoffmann, W. A.: Zur Kenntnis des Refsum-Syndroms. Ber. dtsch. ophthal. Ges. 65 (1964) 288–293

Hofmann, H.: Tuberöse Hirnsklerose. Albrecht v. Graefes Arch. klin. exp. Ophthal. 161 (1959) 122–143

Hollwich, F.: Erkrankungen von Netzhaut und Papille. In: Der Augenarzt, ed. by K. Velhagen. Thieme, Leipzig 1963 (pp. 593–836)

Hommer, K.: Über die Chininvergiftung der Netzhaut mit einer Bemerkung zur experimentellen Chlorochinvergiftung. Klin. Mbl. Augenheilk. 52 (1968) 785–805

Hruby, K.: Über cystische Veränderungen im Augenhintergrund. Albrecht v. Graefes Arch. klin. exp. Ophthal. 158 (1956) 87–105

Jaeger, W.: Vererbung von Augenleiden und Anomalien des Auges. In: Lehrbuch und Atlas der Augenheilkunde, ed. by Axenfeld-Pau. Fischer, Stuttgart 1973 (p. 640)

Jaensch, P.: Verletzungen, physikalische Schädigungen und Giftwirkungen. In: Der Augenarzt, Vol. V, ed. by K. Velhagen. Thieme, Leipzig 1963 (pp. 837–946)

Jochmus, J., H. Jochmus: Zum Krankheitsbild der tuberösen Hirnsklerose. Psychopathologische u. ophthalmologische Beobachtungen. Z. Kinderheilk. 85 (1961) 543–568

Julaio, O. F., H. M. Canelas, N. A. Longo: Juvenile amaurotic idiocy. Clinical and laboratorial study of three cases. Arch. Neuro-psiquiat. (S. Paulo) 14 (1956) 136–157

Kearns, Th. P.: Changes in the ocular fundus in blood diseases. Med. Clin. N. Amer. 40 (1956) 1209–1216

Kearns, T. P., R. W. Hollenhorst: Chloroquine retinopathy: Evaluation by fluorescein fundus angiography. Trans. Amer. ophthal. Soc. 64 (1966) 216–231

Keith, N. M., H. P. Wagener, N. W. Barker: Some different types of essential hypertension their cause and prognoses. Amer. J. med. Sci. 197 (1939) 332–343

Kittel, V.: Überraschendes Spiegelbild bei experimentell caissonkrank gemachten Tieren. Ber. dtsch. ophthal. Ges. Heidelberg, 58 (1953) 331–332

Klainguti, R.: Die tapeto-retinale Degeneration im Kanton Tessin. Klin. Mbl. Augenheilk. 89 (1932) 253–254

Klein, D., M. A. Ktenidès: Au sujet de l'hérédité de l'idiotie amaurotique infantile. J. Génét. hum. 3 (1954) 184–202

Kleinert, H.: Eine rezessiv-geschlechtsgebundene Form der idiopathischen Netzhautspaltung bei nichtmyopen Jugendlichen. Albrecht v. Graefes Arch. klin. exp. Ophthal. 154 (1953) 295–305

Klien, B. A., A. E. Krill: Fundus flavimaculatus. Clinical, functional and histopathologic observations. Amer. J. Ophthal. 64 (1967) 3–23

Krause, A. C.: Congenital encephalo-ophthalmic dysplasie. Arch. Ophthal. 36 (1946) 387–444

Krebs, W., G. Jäger: Netzhautblutungen bei Neugeborenen und Geburtsverlauf. Klin. Mbl. Augenheilk. 148 (1966) 483–490

Krill, A. E., P. A. Morse, A. M. Potts, B. A. Klien: Hereditary vitelliruptive macular degeneration. Amer. J. Ophthal. 61 (1966) 1405–1415

Krill, A. E.: Hereditary retinal and chorioidal diseases. Harper and Row, Hagerstown, Md. 1972

Krill, A. E., A. F. Deutman: The cone degenerations. Docum. ophthal. (The Hague) 35 (1973) 1–80

Kropp, R., H. Neubauer, V. Heimroth, K. Heimann: Der Augenhintergrund bei jugendlichen Hypertonikern. Klin. Mbl. Augenheilk. 156 (1970) 479–487

Kyrieleis, W.: Hyperergische Reaktionen an den Netzhautarterien bei Uvealerkrankungen. Ber. dtsch. ophthal. Ges. Heidelberg, 61 (1958) 78–82

Larsen, H. W., N. Ehlers: Ocular manifestations in Tay-Sachs and Niemann-Pick's disease. Acta ophthal. 43 (1965) 285–293

Leber, Th.: Das Aneurysma racemosum der Netzhautgefäße. In: Handbuch der gesamten Augenheilkunde, 2nd Ed., Vol. VII, ed. by A. Graefe, Th. Saemisch, C. v. Hess. Springer, Berlin 1915 (pp. 37–42)

Lemmingson, W.: Semiologie der Defektheilungen bei Retinopathia praematurorum. Ber. dtsch. ophthal. Ges. 69 (1968) 488–495

Lemmingson, W., G. Stark: Zur Klinik und Ätiologie der Netzhautblutungen bei Neugeborenen. Geburtsh. u. Frauenheilk. 17 (1957) 548–557

Lewine, R. A., A. M. Kaplan: The ophthalmoscopic findings in C-S disease. Amer. J. Ophthal. 59 (1965) 37–42

Lieb, W. A., W. J. Geeraets, D. Guerry: Retinopathie bei der Sichelzellenerkrankung. Klin. Mbl. Augenheilk. 137 (1960) 60–72

Lindau, A.: Zur Frage der Angiomatosis retinae und ihrer Hirnkomplikationen. Acta ophthal. (Kbh.) 4 (1927) 193–226

van Lith, G. M. H., A. F. Deutman: Elektro-Ophthalmologie der juvenilen Makuladegenerationen. 73. Bericht Dtsch. Ophth. Ges. 1975, 108–115

Lund, O. E.: Vergleichende histologische Untersuchungen bei Veränderungen der Netzhaut- und Hirngefäße. Ber. dtsch. ophthal. Ges. 62 (1960) 367–371

Maeder, G.: Rétinite pigmentaire après encéphalite. Ophthalmologica (Basel) 117 (1949 a) 192

Maeder, G.: Rétinite pigmentaire après maladies à virus. Ophthalmologica (Basel) 118 (1949 b) 746–750

Marquardt, R.: Augenveränderungen bei maligner Lymphogranulomatose (Morbus Hodgkin). Klin. Mbl. Augenheilk. 138 (1961) 535–544

Marquardt, A.: Augenveränderungen bei der hyalinosis cutis et mucosae. Ber. dtsch. ophthal. Ges. Heidelberg, 64 (1962) 458–459

Maumenee, A. E., J. M. Emery: An anatomic classification of diseases of the Macula. Amer. J. Ophthal. 74 (1972) 594–599

Mawas, J.: Les cancers de la rétine optique. Bull. Soc. franç. Ophtal. 37 (1924) 512–515

Merté, H. J.: Arbeitsmedizinische Fragen in der Ophthalmologie. Karger, Basel 1969

Merté, H. J.: Arbeits- und Sozialmedizin. In: Lehrbuch der Augenheilkunde, ed. by T. Axenfeld, H. Pau. Fischer, Stuttgart 1973

Munro, St., C. Walker: Ocular complications in sicklecell haemoglobin C disease. Brit. J. Ophthal. 44 (1960) 1–24

Neubauer, H.: Progressive Aderhautatrophie. Albrecht v. Graefes Arch. klin. exp. Ophthal. 156 (1955) 577–589

Neubauer, H.: Die gegenwärtigen diagnostischen Möglichkeiten bei Retinopathia hypertonica. Sitzungsber. Versamml. f. Rhein.-Westf. Augenärzte 116 (1967) 73–89

Nylander, U.: Ocular damage in chloroquine therapy. Acta Ophthal. Suppl. 92 (1967) 1–71

Obal, A.: Alimentäre und endokrine Einflüsse auf die Trophik des Auges. Albrecht v. Graefes Arch. klin. exp. Ophthal. 151 (1951) 623–661

Oksala, A.: Bisherige Erfahrungen über die Ultraschalldiagnostik von Augenkrankheiten. Klin. Mbl. Augenheilk. 144 (1964) 347–360

Oye, L. van: Contraceptifs oraux. Bull. Soc. Belge d'Ophtalm. 160 (1972) 297–317

Pajtáš, J.: Cas de pseudogliome familial héréditaire dans trois générations (Retinitis exsudativa Coats). Ophthalmologica (Basel) 120 (1950) 411–415

Palimeris, G., J. Koliopoulos, P. Velissaropoulos: Ocular side effects of indomethacin. Ophthalmologica 164 (1972) 339–353

Pape, A. R.: Angiopathia retinae traumatica Purtscher und retinale Fettembolie. Albrecht v. Graefes Arch. klin. exp. Ophthal. 167 (1964) 585–606

Pau, H.: Stauungspapille und Netzhautfalten nach operativer Hypotonie beim Glaukom. Klin. Mbl. Augenheilk. 117 (1950) 591–597

Pau, H.: Chorioretinitis exsudativa centralis (haemorrhagica). Klin. Mbl. Augenheilk. 152 (1968 a) 348–357

Pau, H.: Phlebitis und Periphlebitis retinae bei Lymphogranulomatose (Hodgkin). Klin. Mbl. Augenheilk. 152 (1968 b) 655–657

Pau, H.: Zur Prognose der Aphakieamotio. Klin. Mbl. Augenheilk. 154 (1969) 786–792

Pau, H.: Pathogenese und Histologie von sklerotischen Arealen und Netzhauteinrissen bei idiopathischer Netzhautablösung. Bücherei des Augenarztes, 53. Enke, Stuttgart 1970 (pp. 94–108)

Pau, H.: Histologie von zum Einriß disponierenden degenerativen bzw. sklerotischen Arealen der Netzhaut. Symposium der dtsch. Ophthalm. Ges. 1970 Vienna: Die Prophylaxe der idiopathischen Netzhautabhebung. Bergfann, Munich 1971 (pp. 26–40)

Pau, H.: Hohlraumbildungen in der Netzhautperipherie. Docum. Ophthalmologica 41 (1976) 241–256

Pau, H.: Gitterfiguren bzw. dendritische Streifen der Netzhautperipherie. Ophthalmologica 174 (1977) 2–9

Pau, H.: Entstehung und Histologie der degenerativsklerotischen zum Netzhauteinriß disponierenden peripheren Netzhautareale 74. Ber. dtsch. ophthal. Ges. 1977, 269–288

Pau, H., W. Tillmann, G. Goerz: Mycosis fungoides mit Befall des Auges und innerer Organe. Klin. Mbl. f. Augenheilk. 168 (1976) 706–712

Paufique, L., M. P. Ravault, M. Bonnet, M. Istre: L'angiomatose miliaire rétinienne de Leber. Ann. Oculist. (Paris) 197 (1964) 937–955

Pietruschka, G.: Über klinische Beobachtungen bei Iridocyclitis, insbesondere hinsichtlich der Fundusveränderungen. Klin. Mbl. Augenheilk. 124 (1954) 309–326

Pillat, A.: Über allergisch-hyperergische Gefäßerkrankungen der Netzhaut. Wien. klin. Wschr. (1955) 506 und Ber. dtsch. ophthal. Ges. 61 (1958) 66–77

Planten, J. H.: A case of retrolental fibroplasia terminating in an ablatio falciformis. Ophthalmologica (Basel) 130 (1955) 214–216

Putschar, W.: Über Angiomatosis des Zentralnervensystems und der Netzhaut (v. Hippel-Lindau'sches Syndrom) mit besonderer Berücksichtigung der Pankreasveränderungen. Münch. med. Wschr. 82 (1935) 1084–1088

Rayner, S.: Juvenile amaurotic idiocy. Diagnosis of heterozygotes. Acta genet. (Basel) 3 (1952) 1–5

Reese, A. B.: Tumors of the eye. Hoeber, New York 1953

Reese, A. B.: Teleangiectasis of the retina and coats disease. Amer. J. Ophthal. 42 (1956) 1–8

Reese, A. B., F. C. Blodt: Retinal dysplasia. Amer. J. Ophthal. 33 (1950) 23–32

Remky, H., J. Rix, K. F. Klier: Dominant autosomale Maculadegeneration (Best, Sorsby) mit zystischen und vitelliformen Stadien (Huymans, Zanen). Klin. Mbl. Augenheilk. 146 (1965) 473–497

Ricci, A.: Clinique et transmission génétique des différentes formes de dégénérescences vitréo-rétiniennes. Ophthalmologica 139 (1960) 338–343

Ricci, A.: Clinique e transmission héréditaire des dégénérescenses vitréo-rétiniennes. Bull. Soc. Fr. Ophtal. (1961) 618–662

Ricci, A., K. Psilas, Tracopoulos: Le diagnostic des dégénérescences maculaires par angiofluorescence: est il possible? Bull. Soc. franç. Ophtal. 82 (1969) 432–444

Richards, R. D., C. E. West, A. A. Meisels: Chorioretinitis sclopetaria. Trans. Amer. Ophthal. Soc. 66 (1968) 214–233

Rieger, H.: Ein Beitrag zur Kasuistik der tapeto-retinalen Degeneration (Heredodegeneration der Macula mit Beteiligung der Peripherie bei 3 Brüdern). Nebst Bemerkungen über den Erbgang der Heredodegeneration der Macula. Z. Augenheilk. 57 (1925) 429–463

Rieger, H.: Retinitis pigmentosa und Masern. Albrecht v. Graefes Arch. klin. exp. Ophthal. 147 (1944) 105–120

Rieger, H.: Über eine Sippe mit unregelmäßig-dominant erblicher atypischer Retinitis pigmentosa. Klin. Mbl. Augenheilk. 112 (1947) 203–213

Rieger, H.: Erbpathologie des Auges. In: Der Augenarzt, Vol. I, ed. by K. Velhagen. VEB Thieme, Leipzig 1958

Riehm, W.: Über Presojod-Schädigung des Auges. Klin. Mbl. Augenheilk. 78 (1927) 87

Riehm, W.: Akute Pigmentdegeneration der Netzhaut nach Intoxikation mit Septojod (zehnfach konzentrierte Preglsche Jodlösung). Arch. Augenheilk. 100/101 (1929) 872–882

Rintelen, F.: Der Augenhintergrund bei Hypertonie. Ophthalmologica 135 (1956) 389–411

Rodger, F. C., H. M. Sinclair: Metabolic and nutritional eye diseases. Charles C. Thomas, Springfield, Illinois 1969

Rosen, E.: Fluorescence photography of the eye. Butterworth, London 1969

Rummeld, R.: Fundusveränderungen bei Haemoglobinopathie. Ber. Dtsch. Ophthal. Ges. 72. Sitzung in Hamburg 1972

Ryan, S. J., R. E. Smith: The eye in systemic disease. Grune and Stratton, New York, London 1974

Sachsenweger, R.: Luftembolie und Auge. Klin. Mbl. Augenheilk. 130 (1957) 813–823

Sallmann, L. v.: Über Netzhautschädigung durch Salze der unterjodigen, unterbromigen und unterchlorigen Säure. Ein Beitrag zur Frage der Septojodintoxikation. Z. Augenheilk. 80 (1933) 342–351

Scheerer, R.: Akuter Zerfall des retinalen Pigmentepithels nach intravenöser Injektion von Septojod im Wochenbett. Klin. Mbl. Augenheilk. 76 (1926) 524–528

Schildberg, P., A. Wessing: Die fokale hämorrhagische Chorioiditis. Klin. Mbl. Augenheilk. 166 (1975) 651–659

Schlaegel, T. F.: Ocular histoplasmosis. Internat. ophthal. diseases, Vol. 15. Little, Brown & Co., Boston 1975

Schlitter, K.: Zur Frage der retrolentalen Fibroplasie. Klin. Mbl. Augenheilk. 131 (1957) 544–547

Schmidt, B., H. J. Trojan: Augenhintergrundsbefunde und histologische Untersuchungen bei der Pachymeningeosis haemorrhagica interna des Kindes. Klin. Mbl. Augenheilk. 157 (1970) 239–244

Scholtyssek, H.: Beobachtungen über tiefe Augenveränderungen nach Mangelernährung. Klin. Mbl. Augenheilk. 117 (1950) 1–18

Schreck, E.: Veränderungen des Sehorgans bei Haut- und Geschlechtskrankheiten. In: Dermatologie und Venerologie, Vol. IV, ed. by H. A. Gottron, W. Schönfeld. Thieme, Stuttgart 1960 (pp. 831–945)

Schupper, F.: Retinite pigmentose consecutive a malattie infettive acute. Boll. Oculist. 30 (1951) 424–432

Schwab, F.: Die Augenhintergrundsveränderungen bei tuberöser Hirnsklerose. Klin. Mbl. Augenheilk. 128 (1956) 257–296

Seitz, R.: Die Genese und Ätiologie des Kreuzungsphänomens und seine Bedeutung für die Diagnostik von Netzhautgefäßerkrankungen. Klin. Mbl. Augenheilk. 139 (1961) 491–512

Seitz, R.: Augenhintergrunderkrankungen bei arteriellen Allgemeinerkrankungen, Entwicklung und Fortschritt in der Augenheilkunde. Enke, Stuttgart 1963 (pp. 130–152)

Shea, M., C. L. Schepens, S. R. v. Pirquet: Retinoschisis. Arch. ophthal. (Chicago) 63 (1960) 1–9

Siegert, P.: Über Augenerkrankungen bei mangelernährten Spätheimkehrern. Klin. Mbl. Augenheilk. 129 (1956) 3–13

Simell, O., K. Takki: Raised plasma ornithine and gyrate atrophy of the choroid and retina, Lancet 1, 1031 (1973)

Sjögren, H.: Dystrophia reticularis laminae pigmentosae retinae. Acta ophthal. (Kbh.) 28 (1950) 279–295

Slezak, H.: Über loch- und cystenähnliche Befunde des hinteren Augenpols. Albrecht v. Graefes Arch. klin. exp. Ophthal. 173 (1967) 168–174

Slezak, H., K. Hommer: Fundus pulverulentus. Albrecht v. Graefes Arch. klin. exp. Ophthal. 178 (1969) 177–182

Sorsby, A.: Ophthalmic genetics. Butterworth, London 1970

Sorsby, A., M. E. Joll Mason: A fundus dystrophy with unusual features. Brit. J. Ophthal. 33 (1942) 67–97

Sorsby, A., R. P. Crick: Central areolar choriodal sclerosis. Brit. J. Ophthal. 37 (1953) 129–139

Sorsby, A., M. Savory, J. B. Davey, R. J. L. Fraser: Macular cysts: a dominantly inherited affection with a progressive course. Brit. J. Ophthal. 40 (1956) 144–158

Stucchi, C. A., J. D. Geiser: Manifestations oculaires de la sclerodermie généralisée. Docum. ophthal. (The Hague) 22 (1967) 72–110

Stucchi, C. A., W. Höpping: Varix aneurysmaticus vicarians retinae et manifestations cérébrales. Traitment. Bull. Soc. franç. Ophtal. 79 (1966) 90–101

Tasman, W.: Retinal detachment in retrolental fibroplasia. Albrecht v. Graefes Arch. Klin. exp. Ophthal. 195 (1975) 129–139

Thannhauser, G. J.: Lipidoses. Oxford University Press, London 1950

Thiel, H. J.: Beitrag zur Klinik und Genese der Ablatio falciformis congenita. Klin. Mbl. Augenheilk. 152 (1968) 46–50

Thiel, R.: Augenhintergrundsveränderungen bei arterieller Hypertonie und Nierenkrankheiten. Dtsch. med. Wschr. 75 (1950) 1495–1500

Thiel, H. J., H. Behnke: Klinik und Vererbung der vitelliformen Maculadegeneration. Klin. Mbl. Augenheilk. 158 (1971) 235–246

Thiel, H. J., H. R. Wiedemann: Der kirschrote Fleck der Macula als Ausdruck einer Speicherkrankheit. Klin. Mbl. Augenheilk. 161 (1972) 174–182

Timm, G.: Das Krankheitsbild der Retinopathia oxalogenica. Klin. Mbl. Augenheilk. 168 (1976) 537–543

Ufermann, K., R. Heege-Dohr, W. Kosenow: Augenbeteiligung beim Cockayne-Syndrom. Klin. Mbl. Augenheilk. 162 (1973) 655–658

Urbanek, J.: Über Fettembolie des Auges. Albrecht v. Graefes Arch. klin. exp. Ophthal. 131 (1933) 147–173

Vaas, J.: Klinik und Erbgang der tuberösen Sklerose. Arch. Psychiat. Nervenkr. 111 (1940) 1, 547–614

Velhagen, K.: Augenkrankheiten und Allgemeinleiden. In: Der Augenarzt, Vol. VI, ed. by K. Velhagen. Thieme, Leipzig 1964

Verin, P., M. J. le Rebeller: Les embolies graisseuses. Arch. Ophtal (Paris) 27 (1967) 123–144

Verrey, F.: Dégénérescence pigmentaire de la rétine en secteurs symétriques. Schweizer med. Wschr. 1947, 859

Verrey, F.: Dégénérescence pigmentaire de la rétine d'origine médicamenteuse. Ophthalmologica (Basel) 131 (1956) 296–303

Viefhues, T. K.: Einseitige Makulaaplasie, Myopie und markhaltige Nervenfasern bei einem eineiigen Zwilling. Klin. Mbl. Augenheilk. 132 (1958) 104–106

Viefhues, T. K., W. Strobel: Zur Klinik der Retinopathie bei Anämien. Klin. Mbl. Augenheilk. 134 (1959) 643–654

Vinger, P. F., B. A. Sachs: Ocular manifestations of Hyperlipoproteinemia. Amer. J. Ophthal. 70 (1970) 563–573

Vinken, P. J., G. W. Bruyn: Handbook of clinical neurology, Vol. 13, Neuroretinal degenerations. North-Holland Publishing Co., Amsterdam, Elsevier Publishing Co., New York 1972.

Waardenburg, P. J., A. Franceschetti, D. Klein: Genetic and Ophthalmology. Royl van Corcum Assen, Netherlands. Blackwell Scientific Publications. Oxford, Charles C. Thomas, Vol. I 1961, Vol. II 1963

Wagner, P.: Untersuchungen über die Wirkung von Phenothiazinderivaten auf den Augenhintergrund des Tieres. Klin. Mbl. Augenheilk. 129 (1956) 772–781

Wagner, H., R. Klainguti: Weitere Untersuchungen über die Mallatia leventinese. Ophthalmologica 105 (1943) 225–228

Walma, D., T. F. Schlaegel: Presumed histoplasmic chorioiditis. Amer. J. Ophthal. 57 (1964) 107–110

Weigelin, E.: Die Arteriosklerose vom Standpunkt des Augenklinikers. Med. Wschr. 12 (1958) 218–221

Wernecke, Th.: Angioma papillae nervi-optici (caput medusae). Klin. Mbl. Augenheilk. 104 (1940) 434–436

Weve, H.: Über ablatio falciformis cong. Arch. Augenheilk. 109 (1935) 371–394

Weve, H.: The origin and relationship between anterior dialysis, retinal cysts, retinal folds and retrolental fibroplasia. Trans. ophthal. Soc. Aust. 13 (1954) 35–46

Wilkinson, C. P., R. B. Welch: Intraocular Toxocara. Amer. J. Ophthal. 71 (1971) 921–930

Wintersteiner, H.: Das Neuroepithelioma retinae. F. Deuticke, Vienna 1897

Witmer, R.: Augenveränderungen bei Autoimmunerkrankungen. Bericht über die 70. Zusammenkunft der Deutschen Ophthalmologischen Gesellschaft. Bergmann, München 1970 (pp. 301–306)

Wolter, J. R.: Die Histogenese der Drusen im Pigmentepithel der Netzhaut des menschlichen Auges. Klin. Mbl. Augenheilk. 130 (1957) 86–95

Wolter, R.: Die Natur der baumwollflockigen Herde der Netzhaut. Klin. Mbl. Augenheilk. 138 (1961) 83–91

Woods, A. C., J. R. Duke: Coats disease. Brit. J. Ophthal 47 (1963) 385–434

Wüstenberg, W.: Über zwei Fälle von spontan geheiltem Netzhautgliom. Klin. Mbl. Augenheilk. 117 (1950) 423–426

Zanen, J., R. Hermans: Le disque vitelliforme de la macula. Nouvell observation. Bull. Soc. belge Ophtal. 129 (1961) 462–484

Zanen, J., G. Rausin: Kyste vitelliforme congénital de la macula. Bull. Soc. belge Ophtal. 96 (1950) 544–549

Zimmerman, L. E., W. H. Spencer: The pathologic anatomy of retinoschisis. Arch. ophthal. (Chicago) 63 (1960) 10–19

23 Optic Nerve

Visual Pathway

Since the retina is an extension of the brain, the optic nerve is not a true nerve but a cerebral tract. The optic nerve begins in the eye at the 1.5 to 1.7 mm wide optic disc. The nerve is surrounded by a dural sheath which arises from the periosteum of the bony optic canal and merges with the sclera at the globe. A pial layer surrounds the nerve directly, and the delicate arachnoid lies in the intervening space.

The central retinal artery arises from the ophthalmic artery and with the vein enters the optic nerve from below or inferior nasally 10 to 15 mm behind the globe.

Fibers from the nasal, retinal half (temporal visual fields) cross at the chiasm while temporal retinal fibers (nasal visual fields) remain uncrossed. From the chiasm the optic tracts course to the lateral geniculate body. Here the second neuron ends and the third neuron begins as Gratiolet's visual radiation to the upper and lower lips of the calcarine fissure.

Ophthalmoscopy of the Normal Optic Disc

The optic disc has a diameter of 1.5 to 1.7 mm. It is more oval vertically than round. The normal disc has a mildly blurred, often slightly thickened nasal border. Frequently, there is a white sickle-shaped temporal crescent adjacent to the disc. This is an area devoid of pigment epithelium and choroid with the underlying sclera exposed. Occasionally it represents an area of connective tissue hyperplasia.

The delicate pink color of the disc depends on age, vascular perfusion and visibility of the lamina cribrosa. The optic disc of nonpremature newborns is normal in color or pale-gray in 50 percent. After four months the color becomes more normal.

Retinal hemorrhages are present immediately after birth in one-fourth of newborns. Arteries and veins enter and leave the optic disc near its center. Cilioretinal arteries (from the choroid) may be seen at the temporal edge of the disc extending towards the macula. Optico-ciliary vessels may form secondarily after central retinal vein occlusion.

Visible Vascular Pulsations

Venous-Arterial Pulsations

Spontaneous *venous pulsations* are seen in 70 percent of all people. Pulse synchronous collapse of veins with systole can be observed at the optic cup or near the edge of the disc (see page 308). *Arterial pulsations* appear with any elevation of intraocular tension above the diastolic blood pressure, e.g., with glaucoma. Space occupying orbital lesions may cause arterial compression and pulsation. Aortic insufficiency can also lead to spontaneous arterial pulsations.

The gradient between mean retinal artery pressure and intraocular pressure is important for retinal and optic disc circulation. For example, while there is no circulatory disturbance with aortic insufficiency there is a severe disruption of retinal and optic nerve circulation with "pulseless disease."

The retinal artery pressure is measured with an ophthalmodynamometer. Weigelin (1954) used ophthalmodynamometry to differentiate various cerebral circulatory disturbances and dilatory and spastic vasomotor headaches. Remky (1951) calculated the percentage change of mean retinal arterial pressure between the lying and sitting positions (modified Schellong test) and used this to diagnose changes in arterial wall tonus and carotid circulation.

Optic Disc Cupping

Physiologic cupping: The optic disc is normally cupped. There is a variable degree of central excavation up to exposure of the stippled lamina cribrosa. In *senile cupping* the optic disc sinks below the level of the retina and there is a gray-yellow discoloration. *Atrophic cupping* occurs with *optic atrophy*, for example, from syphilis, trauma, or secondary to optic nerve compression by tumors, especially of the hypophysis, etc.

Glaucomatous cupping leads to bayonetlike kinking of vessels at the disc margin (Plate XVI, Fig. 6, page 192 h), and a nasal shift of vessels. The excavation is deep and can extend to the disc margin. With time, the disc takes on a white-gray color (Plate XXXI, Fig. 4, page 288 g). A small irregular glaucomatous halo (zone of chorioretinal atrophy) surrounds the disc. Glaucomatous cupping may not develop in high myopia with glaucoma, but instead a posterior staphyloma may be present.

Congenital Anomalies of the Optic Nerve

Hypoplasia, aplasia of the disc — Supertraction of the disc, megalopapilla — Optic disc coloboma — Double papilla — Other malformations of the disc — Drusen.

Hypoplasia and Aplasia of the Disc

The *optic nerve* and *vessels* can be entirely absent, e.g., the *optic disc* is *aplastic* (with microphthalmos, severe cranial malformation), or the disc may be small on one or both sides. The *hypoplastic optic disc* is gray-white with decreased visual acuity. Hypoplasia or aplasia of the optic disc or nerve usually appears in combination with other malformations (Streiff 1962): anencephaly, hydrophthalmos, colobomata, and aniridia. The optic disc may be *oval* in the horizontal direction or its insertion may be inverse. Rarely, there is a *duplication* of the optic disc.

Cilioretinal arteries extending from the edge of the optic disc towards the retinal center occur in 25 percent of hypoplastic discs. Vascular tortuositiy is common. Hypoplasia and aplasia of the disc can appear without other ocular malformations, neurologic signs, or family history (Smith 1954). In Turner's syndrome the disc is often smaller (or larger) (see pages 89, 330). The large variation in disc size and differences induced by the refractive error of the eye must always be considered before a diagnosis of *hypoplasia* or *megalopapilla* may be made (Streiff 1961).

Supertraction of the Disc; Megalopapilla

Conus and oblique insertion of the disc with *supervolution* (supertraction) (Fig. 23.1) can simulate increased size. True *megalopapilla* is often associated with *optic pits* or excavation of the disc.

Optic Nerve Coloboma

Various forms of optic nerve colobomata (Fig. 23.2; Plate XXIX, Fig. 3, page 288 e) almost always appear in conjunction with retinal and choroidal colobomata. *Congenital pits* $\frac{1}{8}$ to $\frac{1}{2}$ disc diameter across are usually situated in the temporal half of the disc (Plate XXIX, Fig. 4, page 288 e). They may cause no visual disturb-

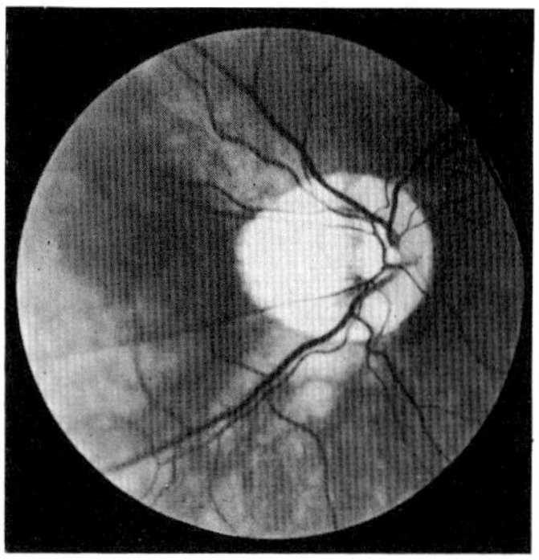

Fig. 23.1 Supertraction of the papilla with temporal crescent and posterior staphyloma (♂ 30 yrs.)

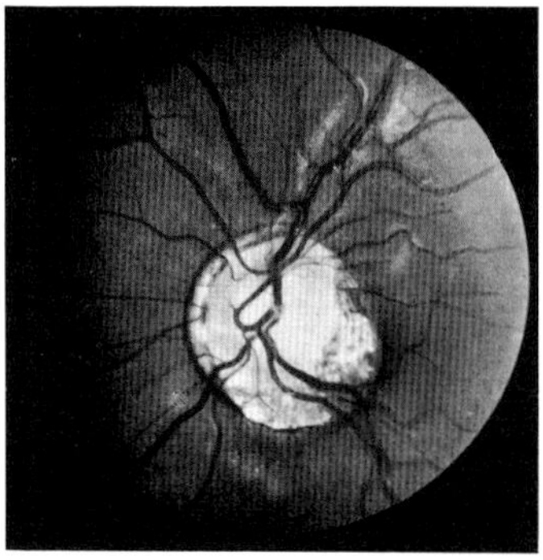

Fig. 23.2 Small coloboma of the optic disk (♀ 18 yrs.)

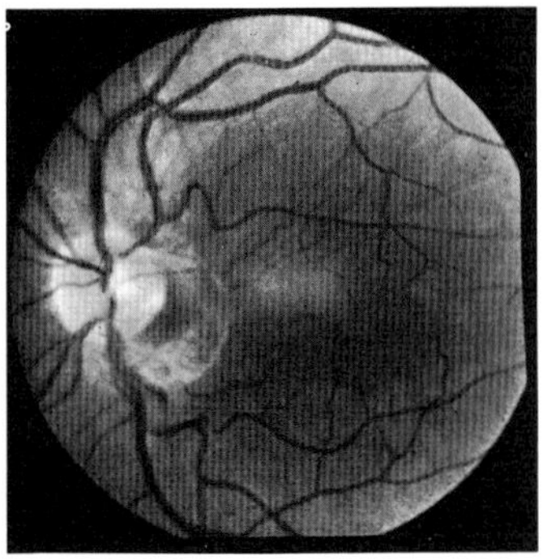

Fig. 23.3 Epipapillary membrane (♀ 31 yrs.)

ance or be associated with central serous retinal detachments usually developing later in life (30 percent; Badtke and Bauermann 1964; Meyer 1969; Andersen 1953; Paffenbach and Walsh 1972). Central pigmentary changes, retinal folds and subretinal fluid frequently develop (Vogel and Wessing 1974).

Double Papillae

Two optic discs in an eye are possible (Collier 1958).

Other Hereditary Malformations of the Disc

Harmless congenital disc malformations include: *pseudopapilledema* (Plate XXX, Fig. 6, page 288 f) (*epipapillary membrane* may sometimes be confused with papilledema) (Fig. 23.3), *inferior conus, cilioretinal vessels, vascular tortuosity* (Plate XX, Fig. 2, page 224 d). These changes are more common with hyperopia and astigmatism and less so with myopia (Beeler 1929; Rieger 1956; Badtke 1959; Rogahn 1956). *Nasal supertraction* (supervolution) (Fig. 23.1) and posterior staphyloma are common in high myopia and may simulate pseudoneuritis with myopic conus.

Optic Disc Drusen

Papillary drusen (Plate XXXI, Fig. 1 and 2, page 288 g) can cause optic disc prominence (over five diopters) (Hoeg 1909; Löhlein 1931). Peripheral visual field loss and enlargement of the blind spot may be present owing to pressure atrophy of the nerve fibers. Optic disc drusen can be hereditary and, among other conditions, are associated with pituitary adenomas, retinitis pigmentosa and pseudoxanthoma elasticum. The pathogenesis of drusen of the optic disc is obscure, but they may be a degeneration product of the non-myelinated nerve fiber axons (Seitz 1968).

anterior lenticonus, and retinal pigmentation may occur in Alport's syndrome along with familial nephropathy and hearing loss (see page 252).

Persistent hyaloid artery (Plate XVII, Fig. 5, page 224 a) occurs as a congenital anomaly. Most congenital anomalies present little problem in terms of differential diagnosis.

Pigmentation in the Region of the Optic Disc

Pigmented changes on or near the optic disc are *usually not melanomas but benign processes*. These consist of:

Pigmented nevi – Proliferation of retinal pigment epithelium – Melanocytoma – Hemosiderin deposits – Malignant melanoma.

Pigmented Choroidal Nevi

These are more or less round, barely elevated, and have a slate gray color. Secondary degeneration of the overlying sensory epithelium can cause small localized scotomata.

Retinal Pigment Epithelium Proliferation

The retinal pigment epithelium can proliferate in a *pseudoneoplastic* manner. Frequently this involves dispersed, dustlike pigment totally or partially covering the disc. The pigmented center may be surrounded by a halo of thickened gray-white retina. Visual field loss is possible. Histologically there is a filigreelike proliferation of retinal pigment epithelium beginning at the optic disc margin. The retina may be gliotic and thickened at this point (Vogel 1969).

Melanocytoma

Melanocytoma is frequently mistaken for melanoma. Melanocytomas are common in pigmented races, appearing as dark black tumors directly on or adjacent to the disc. They have slightly feathery borders and a mossy appearance. A melanocytoma may occur at the level of the lamina cribrosa and not reach the disc surface. It appears as a dark crest deep in the papilla (Fig. 23.4). Melanocytomas are benign; change to a malignant melanoma, however, has been reported. Histologically they are pigmented cells with relatively uniform, round to oval nuclei (visible only after bleaching). A deep melanocytoma may be mistaken for an optic pit. With optic pits the disc is slightly depigmented or brown-green at the depth of the excavation.

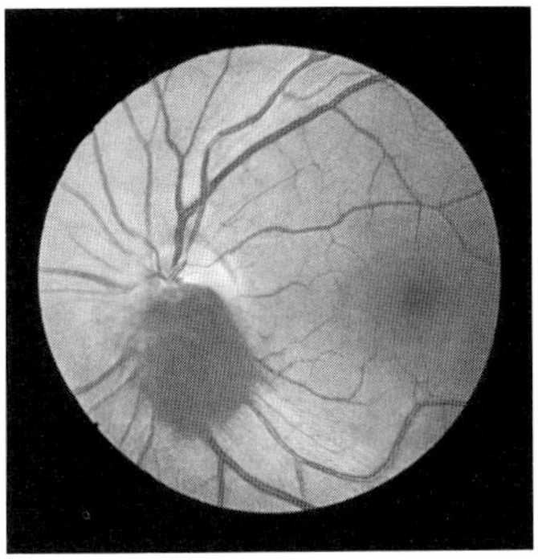

Fig. 23.4 Melanocytoma of the optic disk (♀ 46 yrs.)

Hemosiderin Deposition

Hemosiderin crystals can accumulate on the *optic disc*, for example, after vitreous hemorrhage.

Malignant Melanoma

Malignant melanomas have a brown to slate gray color and a smooth-knobby surface with a distinct tendency to grow. Often there is an overlying serous retinal detachment.

Papillitis (Optic Neuritis) and Papilledema

Differential Diagnosis of Neuritis, Pseudopapillitis, Papilledema, Malignant Hypertension

Subjective symptoms — Ophthalmoscopy — Vitreous involvement.

The patient's subjective symptoms are of great differential *diagnostic importance*. Optic neuritis usually results in immediate decreased acuity, always with varying visual field loss. With papilledema visual acuity remains normal for a long period of time.

Ophthalmoscopy

Both *optic neuritis* (Plate XXX, Fig. 2, page 288 f) and *papilledema* (Plate XXIX, Figs. 5, 6, page 288 e) cause a gray-red swelling of the optic disc.

Usually the edema of papilledema is more glassy and transparent; that of papillitis more opaque gray-red. The disc margins are blurred

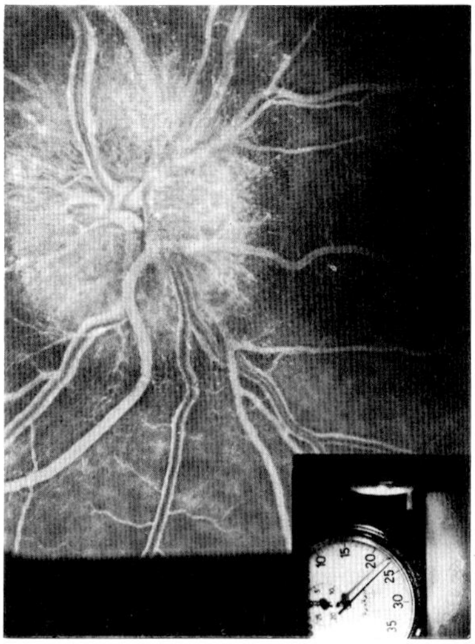

Fig. 23.5 Papilledema. Early fluorescein venous phase. Microaneurysmalike capillary changes, fluid leakage (♂ 46 yrs.)

in either case. Hemorrhages and yellowish-white exudates develop. The arteries appear slightly narrowed while the veins are dilated owing to compression and obstruction. Capillaries on the disc are hyperemic. White perivascular inflammatory sheathing accompanies vessels near the disc, especially with papillitis. The peripapillary retina shows striate edema.

Disc elevation in a fully developed case is considerably less with papillitis than with papilledema. Retinal venous pulsation usually disappears with the onset of papilledema. The value of this sign to diagnose early papilledema is controversial. Superficial radial hemorrhages and cotton wool spots are more common with papilledema. Macular stars (lipid exudates) can occur. The appearance of the disc in papilledema and *malignant hypertension* (Fig. 22.7) is the same. When this is the case the diagnosis may be made by observing the peripheral retinal arteries. These are *maximally constricted* in hypertension with cotton-wool spots, hemorrhages and exudates (see page 263). The blood pressure should be measured in either case. Papilledema may occur with *marked hypotony* (after glaucoma surgery, with choroidal detachment, perforating injury, etc.). The mechanism is possibly similar to that with choroidal detachment. Papilledema owing to ocular hypotony *(papilledema e vacuo)* generally heals without optic atrophy. In time, papilledema results in optic atrophy.

Optic disc drusen (Plate XXXI, Fig. 1, page 288 g) and *pseudopapilledema* (see page 312; Plate XXX, Fig. 6, page 288 f) simulate papilledema. However, true edema, hemorrhages and exudates are missing; the blood vessels remain normal and there is no late staining on fluorescein angiography (Fig. 23.5).

Vitreous Involvement

Optic neuritis, in contrast to papilledema, may cause vitreous opacities (exudates) near the disc.

Papilledema

Transient amaurosis — Ophthalmoscopy — Optic atrophy and visual field loss — Papilledema and myopia, absence of papilledema in small children with optic atrophy — Causes of papilledema.

Transient Amaurosis

At first, vision is normal with papilledema, but in time can black out momentarily (for 10 to 30 seconds) on rising from a prone to standing position or with bending owing to a momentary lack of perfusion.

Ophthalmoscopy

(Plate XXIX, Fig. 5 and 6, page 288 e)

High-grade papilledema presents little diagnostic difficulty. The gray-red disc projects into the vitreous like a mushroom. Peripapillary retinal edema accentuates the radial nerve fiber layer, elevating the dark congested veins along with it. Striate hemorrhages may be few or numerous. Long-standing papilledema results in glistening degeneration exudates. Papilledema with optic atrophy in the other eye constitutes the *Foster-Kennedy syndrome (see page 313).*

Optic Atrophy and Visual Field Loss

Optic atrophy results when papilledema owing to elevated intracranial pressure is present for a variable length of time (weeks to months) (Plate XXX, Fig. 1, page 288 f). At the same time, the *visual field* undergoes *concentric constriction.* Once optic atrophy has begun, it is progressive in the majority of cases, even if the intracranial pressure is normalized. The disc elevation decreases with increasing optic atrophy until the surface of the optic disc is level with the retina. The disc is then pale white, with blurred margins. Such a disc cannot be differentiated from *postneuritic* optic atrophy. Vision is lost or markedly decreased in both cases (Plate XXX, Fig. 1, page 288 f).

Minimal Papilledema with Myopia

It must be pointed out that papilledema is less marked in *highly myopic* and *senile* eyes.

Papilledema in Infants and with Optic Atrophy

Infants with open cerebral sutures develop a hydrocephalus with cerebral compression but *do not* have papilledema.
Regardless of the cause (see page 313), once *optic atrophy* is present *papilledema is no longer possible.*

Etiology of Papilledema

Papilledema, like sixth nerve paresis, headache and vomiting is a *nonlocalizing sign of raised intracranial* pressure.
In two-thirds to three-fourths of cases, the cause is a space-occupying lesion – primarily *brain tumors* (Tönnis 1955; Huber and Blodi 1974; Walsh and Hogl 1969; Bonamour et al. 1968). Posterior fossa tumors near the cerebellum, the quadrigeminal plate or in the pons exhibit early onset of high-grade papilledema. In contrast, tumors at the base of the skull or in the region of the hypophysis lead to papilledema much less commonly. Posterior fossa tumors (astrocytoma, medulloblastoma, ependymoma) and the resultant marked papilledema appear more commonly in children under the age of ten. Meningiomas, glioblastomas and neuromas (cerebellar pontine angle tumors) occur most commonly in middle age. Children tend to have cranio-pharyngiomas in the region of the chiasm. Rapidly growing and infiltrating gliomas and paragliomas lead to papilledema more readily than slowly expanding meningiomas. It is disputed whether or not asymmetry of papilledema between eyes is of significance in localizing the lesions to the side with greater elevation. Olfactory meningiomas may cause papilledema of one disc and primary optic atrophy of the other (Foster-Kennedy syndrome); other signs in these cases include hypoanosomia, bossing of the frontal bone, and symptoms of raised intracranial pressure.
Vitamin A intoxication (from prolonged therapy, self-medication) can cause papilledema and pseudotumor cerebri with intracranial pressure elevation, hair loss and dermatoses. *Pseudotumor cerebri* (benign intracranial hypertension) is seen most commonly in young obese females with no known cause for the intracranial pressure elevation.
Further causes of papilledema are: *encephalitis, meningitis, arachnoiditis, brain abscess, intracranial hemorrhage, apoplexy,* intracranial *aneurysm, subdural hematoma* (delayed onset), optic nerve *sheath hematoma, syphilitic gumma, tuberculous granuloma, Cysticercus, Echinococcus, oxycephaly,* and *cranio-facial dysostosis.* The same picture may occur unilaterally with orbital lesions that occupy space, e.g., *orbital tumors, hematoma, phlebitis, optic nerve tumors,* and *central retinal vein thrombosis.* Papilledema is also seen with grade IV *hypertensive retinopathy, leukemia, anemia,* and *polycythemia.*
Iridocyclitis can cause edema of the optic disc (see page 197). Sudden marked hypotony can result in "papilledema e vacuo". Hypotony may occur after filtering operations, glaucoma, pressure drop after treatment of a glaucomatous attack, perforating injury, or contusion injury (Plate XXV, Fig. 1, page 288 a) etc.

Optic Neuritis

Optic neuritis (Plate XXX, Figs. 2, 3, page 288 f) has to be differentiated into *retrobulbar neuritis* where the ophthalmoscopic picture is normal, at least at first, and *papillitis.* The similarity between papillitis and early papilledema has been stressed. With neuritis, the optic disc is more hyperemic and the edematous exudate less transparent. Striation of the peripapillary retinal nerve fibers is more prominent. Perivascular spaces are dilated and infiltrated resulting in perivascular sheathing near the disc. A fine vitreous haze may develop in front of the disc. The immediate, marked visual deterioration with papillitis is a major differential point from papilledema. Various types of visual field defects may be seen, e.g., paracentral scotoma, central scotoma, concentric constriction, and sectorial defects, etc.

Retrobulbar Neuritis

Besides rapid deterioration of vision (hours to days), signs of retrobulbar neuritis include central scotoma and pain on pressing or moving the globe. The optic disc is normal at first. After about three weeks, vision more or less recovers. Since the maculopapillary bundle is involved, temporal pallor frequently becomes visible about this time (Plate XXX, Fig. 4, page 288 f).

Differential diagnosis: Retrobulbar neuritis is readily differentiated from simulated visual loss by the presence of an afferent pupillary defect in the involved eye (swinging flashlight test, Marcus Gunn pupil).

Etiology of Papillitis and Retrobulbar Neuritis

Multiple sclerosis, meningitis, encephalitis — Infectious disease, focal involvement, leukemia — Intoxications, tobacco alcohol amblyopia, methanol, quinine, anti-tubercular medications — Autointoxication, optico-chiasmatic arachnoiditis — Chorioretinitis, iridocyclitis — Leber's optic atrophy.

Multiple sclerosis is one of the major causes of retrobulbar neuritis. Conversely, retrobulbar neuritis may be the first sign of multiple sclerosis. Other symptoms may be delayed for months or years, or may never occur at all. Other etiologies include meningitis, encephalitis, various **infectious diseases,** e.g., scarlet fever, typhus, measles, diphtheria, syphilis, tuberculosis, etc.

Malaria can cause optic atrophy with narrow retinal vessels. Paresis of ocular muscles, neuralgias, keratitis, iridocyclitis, and retinal hemorrhages may be observed. The keratitis is generally related to concurrent herpes virus infection.

Papillitis and retrobulbar neuritis are occasionally caused by paranasal sinusitis, anemia, leukemia, orbital cellulitis or local inflammation.

Intoxications: Inflammation of the optic nerves is seen in a variety of intoxications (Jaensch 1958; see page 316): chromic acid and chromates can cause optic atrophy. Chronic lead poisoning may cause transient central amaurosis or retinitis with optic atrophy and visual field loss. A modern source of lead toxicity is high concentrations of leaded gasoline (tetraethyl lead or "anti-knock" compounds). Subacute or chronic thallium poisoning produces conjunctival hyperemia, cataracts, hair loss and potentially partial optic atrophy with a central scotoma. Chronic exposure to manganese dust (manganese dioxide mines) causes encephalopathy with retrobulbar neuritis. Acute carbon monoxide poisoning produces severe systemic symptoms (headaches, nausea, vomiting, even death). Chronic carbon monoxide poisoning may cause hemianopsia, central scotomata, concentric visual field constriction, optic neuritis, retinal hemorrhages, ocular muscle paresis, accommodative paresis and flickering vision. With chronic carbon disulfide poisoning, the symptoms resemble multiple sclerosis, e.g., neuritis, partial optic atrophy, central scotoma, concentric visual field loss, and ocular muscle paresis. Various halogenated aliphatic hydrocarbons (dissolving, extracting agents) produce neuritis and pupillary disturbances.

Various aromatic nitro- and amido-compounds (dinitrophenol, dinitrobenzol, etc.) absorbed through the skin or lungs or ingested can cause retrobulbar neuritis, papillitis and late optic atrophy.

Optic atrophy and visual field loss have been observed with pentavalent organic arsenicals.

Slowly increasing vision loss with a central scotoma and temporal pallor occur in so-called *tobacco-alcohol amblyopia.* Apparently, poorly fermented tobacco, the smoking of cigarette butts (and heavy alcohol intake) play a role in older patients with generalized debility. Tobacco-alcohol amblyopia is actually an incorrect term. Tobacco and methyl alcohol poisoning damage the optic nerve (Silvette et al. 1960). However, there is no known primary optic nerve damage from ethyl alcohol. The damage with chronic alcoholism seems to be based on a lack of nutrition in the sense of subclinical pellagra (Harrington 1962; Silvette et al. 1960). Hydroxocobalamine deficiency appears to play a decisive role in tobacco-alcohol amblyopia (Kommerell and Castillón-Oberndorfer 1968).

Methyl alcohol (methanol) poisoning causes severe systemic acidosis with vomiting and coma leading to potentially permanent loss of vision or blindness after two to three days. The optic disc is edematous and rapidly becomes atrophic. If any vision is retained at all, a central scotoma remains. Temporal pallor or total optic atrophy result.

Severe *quinine poisoning* (Plate XXVIII, Fig. 1, page 288 d) leads to retinal edema with a cherry red spot (as in central retinal artery occlusion). The retinal vessels are maximally constricted. Optic atrophy, narrowed retinal vessels and a tubular visual field result. At first, there is miosis followed by a nonreactive amaurotic pupillary dilatation. Quinine also causes hearing loss, even total deafness (Jaensch 1958).

A similar picture is seen with intoxication from optochin, ergot, and filix mas.

Tuberculous meningitis results in *optic atrophy* in 35 to 50 percent of cases. Optic nerve disease has increased with the introduction of intrathecal isoniazid, i.e., streptomycin therapy (Böke 1955). Optic atrophy is observed with nearly all anti-tubercular drugs (see page 316). Retrobulbar neuritis and optic atrophy with temporal pallor are particularly common (in about 1.5 % with long-term (over 4 months) ethambutol therapy (Myambutol 25 mg/kg/day) (Pau 1974). *Bilateral optic neuritis* has been observed with numerous medications: isoniazid = INH (Neoteben, Rimifon), chloramphenicol and cytostatic vinca rosacea derivatives (vinblastin, vincristin).

The use of *halogenated hydroxyquinol* derivatives (enterovioform, mexaform, intestopan, enterosept, etc.) for gastroenteritis has resulted particularly in Japan in subacute myelo-optic neuritis (S.M.O.N.). Apparently the resultant retrobulbar neuritis can clear completely. It is not clear whether the damage is caused by hydroxyquinol derivatives or other agents (viruses?) (Dralands and Garin 1972).

Autointoxication: Autointoxication, as with pregnancy, lactation, diabetes, dermal burns, carcinomatous cachexia, camp amblyopia, and pellagra can result in *toxic optic nerve damage.*

Optico-chiasmatic arachnoiditis *can cause the picture of retrobulbar neuritis.* The most prominent findings with optico-chiasmatic arachnoiditis are various forms of visual field loss: central scotoma, concentric constriction, and irregular, peripheral, binasal, bitemporal or uncharacteristic field defects. Visual acuity deteriorates slowly (at times rapidly) without remission. Usually there is increasing optic atrophy or temporal pallor. Preceding papilledema is rare. All other neurologic findings are negative.

Optico-chiasmatic arachnoiditis (leptomeningitis chronica proliferans) cannot clearly be differentiated from retrobulbar neuritis either by history or clinical findings. Because of its bilaterality, it resembles intoxication amblyopia and Leber's optic atrophy. With time, the unrelenting clinical deterioration of chiasmatic arachnoiditis makes the differentiation from retrobulbar neuritis possible by exclusion. Optico-chiasmatic arachnoiditis is not a single entity. Surgical exploration of the chiasm may reveal membranes or bands mechanically constricting blood supply to the nerves and chiasm. The etiology of chiasmatic arachnoiditis includes trauma, sinusitis, encephalitis, tuberculosis, syphilis and alcohol intoxication.

Chorioretinitis and iridocyclitis: *Papillitis* may occur with chorioretinitis, for example, with syphilitic neurochorioretinitis. Other forms of intraocular inflammation (iridocyclitis, especially with *sympathetic ophthalmia)* may cause the picture of papillitis.

Leber's optic atrophy (see page 314) develops as a retrobulbar neuritis. Its heredity is modified sex-linked. The disease, which occurs primarily in men, manifests after puberty, around age 20, and leads to temporal pallor with a central scotoma. Visual acuity declines rapidly within a few months to 20/200 or less. In contrast to retrobulbar neuritis, there are no remissions.

Ischemic optic neuropathy (vascular papillitis) (François et al. 1961) occurs mainly with arteriosclerosis and temporal arteritis (Plate XXX, Fig. 5, page 288 f), less often with diabetes mellitus, periarteritis nodosa, Raynaud's disease, essential polycythemia (Vaquez), internal carotid artery emboli, endarteritis, pulseless disease, and posthemorrhagic blindness.

Temporal arteritis (Horton) (Hutchinson-Horton-Magath-Brown syndrome [Plate XXX, Fig. 5, page 288 f]) has a serious prognosis. It appears in older patients with sudden unilateral (occasionally bilateral) vision loss. The optic nerve head is pale gray and swollen. Sometimes a retinal branch artery is occluded. Various types of visual field loss may occur, e.g., altitudinal scotoma, arcuate scotoma, central scotoma, etc. The eyes are affected in 38 to 70 percent of cases of temporal arteritis. Vascular optic atrophy equivalent to opticomalacia results (Kreibig 1959). Retinal vessels are narrowed but the temporal arteries are usually thickened, tortuous and painful. There may be a low-grade fever, leukocytosis and increased alpha-2 globulin and glycoprotein. Usually the erythrocyte sedimentation rate is markedly elevated. Cerebral, cardiovascular complaints and symptoms of pain, fever, night sweats, headaches, malaise, and muscle pain appear. Histologically there is a giant cell arteritis. Although onset is unilateral, the disease usually becomes bilateral unless treated with systemic steroids in high doses.

Arteriosclerosis: This can result in an ophthalmoscopic picture similar to that of temporal arteritis. Arteriosclerosis can also produce opaque-milky edema of ischemic optic neuropathy. Fine peripapillary hemorrhages may be present. Arteriosclerosis has to be considered with optic neuritis in older persons having hypertension and systemic arteriosclerosis (Peters 1958). Temporal arteritis and arteriosclerotic ischemic optic neuropathy end with a white, relatively sharp, atrophic disc with narrow vessels. Both discs are frequently affected in these disorders resulting in severe vision loss or blindness.

Pseudopapillitis or Pseudopapilledema

Pseudopapillitis (Plate XXX, Fig. 6, page 288 f) causes a picture resembling papilledema. With pseudopapillitis the optic disc may appear prominent, blurred and hyperemic. In contrast to true papilledema or papillitis, edema, hemorrhages, exudates and venous stasis are not present.

The optic disc is more elevated centrally with pseudopapilledema, whereas in true papilledema the disc margins are more prominent. Frequently, pseudopapillitis is associated with venous tortuosity. The blind spot is not enlarged on visual field examination with pseudopapilledema as it is with true papilledema. Fluorescein angiography is useful in the differential diagnosis. Fluorescein leaks from vessels in papilledema (Fig. 23.5) causing "staining" of the disc, whereas with pseudopapilledema the vessels are normal and do not leak dye. Nonetheless, cases still exist where the differential diagnosis cannot readily be made. Such eyes should be followed, ideally with photographs, for months to determine any change in the ophthalmoscopic picture. Pseudopapillitis occurs mainly with hyperopia or astigmatism and rarely with myopia.

Optic disc drusen (Plate XXXI, Fig. 1, page 288 g): These may cause pseudopapilledema or appear without it. The diagnosis is easy when one or more, highly refractile, yellow-white, tapiocalike nodules of varying size are visible. An irregular nodular disc with scalloped edges should raise the suspicion of buried disc drusen. The deep drusen glow on indirect illumination best performed with a slit lamp beam. Optic disc drusen are usually pale yellow-red. Visual field defects can occur with increasing size and number of drusen: enlarged blind spots, concentric constriction, paracentral scotomata, irregular peripheral defects. Drusen of the optic disc appear to be axonal degeneration products of nonmyelinated nerve fibers (Seitz and Kersting 1962).

Optic Atrophy

The white, atrophic optic nerve may have *sharp* or *blurred* margins. With *sharp margins*, the lamina cribrosa is usually clearly visible.

Temporal pallor — Simple optic atrophy — Glaucomatous atrophy — Postinflammatory atrophy (atrophy after papilledema or papillitis) — Retinal (yellow) atrophy.

Temporal Pallor

Partial atrophy, usually temporal pallor from involvement of the maculo-papillary bundle (Plate XXX, Fig. 4, page 288 f) can occur in a nerve head with sharp borders. It usually results from retrobulbar neuritis. *Leber's optic atrophy* (Plate XXXI, Fig. 3, page 288 g) resembles that of retrobulbar neuritis - optic atrophy with sharp disc margins. This hereditary disorder primarily affects males. It begins between ages 18 to 20 with sudden visual deterioration and central scotoma. Both optic discs are hyperemic at first. Later, bilateral temporal pallor or total optic atrophy results. Visual acuity declines to less than 20/200 within a few months. Lack of remission differentiates this hereditary disorder from retrobulbar neuritis.
Partial or sectorial optic atrophy associated with a sectorial visual field loss can be caused by branch artery occlusion.

Simple Optic Atrophy

The entire optic nerve is *white* and *sharply outlined.*
Simple optic atrophy (Plate XXXI, Fig. 3, page 288 g).

Tabetic optic atrophy — Optic nerve injury — Pressure atrophy — Optic nerve tumors — Following blood loss — Arteriosclerosis — Hereditary optic atrophy: Leber's optic atrophy; Behr's complicated optic atrophy; dominant hereditary optic atrophy, dominant hereditary optic atrophy with nystagmus and recessive congenital optic atrophy; Leber's congenital blindness.
Carotid thrombosis — Aortic arch syndrome, pulseless disease — Incontinentia pigmenti — Central retinal artery emboli — Poisonings.

Tabetic Optic Atrophy

Optic atrophy occurs as part of tertiary lues or tabes dorsalis. Usually the visual field is concentrically constricted or shows sectorial defects, especially to colored test objects. The patients develop night blindness. The bilateral affliction can lead to blindness within months or two to three years.

Injury to the Optic Nerve

This may be caused by injury to the optic nerve as an **optic canal syndrome.** A severe blow to the head, usually face or occiput, can result in unilateral blindness (rarely bilateral) with amaurotic pupillary paralysis and normal ophthalmoscopic findings. Optic atrophy develops 10 to 14 days later. The optic canal syndrome appears in 1 to 5 percent of cases of severe blunt trauma to the head (Seitz 1963). The pathogenesis is a shearing or tearing injury to the nerve at the transition point from where it is fixed in the optic canal and the free intracranial portion. In contrast, damage from bony fragments, hemorrhage, torn nutrient blood vessels or optic nerve edema tends to show some improvement.
Optic nerve edema probably played a major role in those cases of amaurosis showing marked improvement (Seitz 1963). Trauma to the head can cause *sudden* loss of acuity and visual field constriction, or it may result in *slowly progressive* vision loss with optic atrophy and a variety of visual field defects owing to opticochiasmatic arachnoiditis. On rare occasions, the optic nerve will be avulsed by severe trauma (Plate XXXII, Fig. 5, page 288 h).

Pressure Atrophy

This may be caused by pituitary tumors, basilar skull tumors, orbital tumors, meningiomas, and pressure in the region of the chiasm. Unilateral papilledema with primary optic atrophy in the other eye (and anosmia on that side) is called the Foster-Kennedy syndrome. Two-thirds of these cases are caused by tumors (frontal, olfactory groove, sphenoid). Other causes include vascular or inflammatory processes (ateriosclerosis, arachnoiditis). Pressure atrophy also results from narrowing of the optic canal (craniofacial dysostosis, oxycephaly, Paget's disease, fibrous dysplasia, etc.) and hydrocephalus. Optic atrophy is seen in marble bone disease.

Synonyms for marble bone disease are: osteopetrosis, osteosclerosis fragilis generalisata, and diffuse congenital osteosclerosis. The reduction in bone marrow stimulates extramedullary hematopoiesis. Erythroblasts appear in the blood.

Chondrodystrophia congenita punctata (synonyms: chondrodystrophia fetalis hypoplastica of Conradi, universal calcinosis, congenital calcifying chondrodystrophy, Conradi's or Conradi-Hünermann syndrome) includes bilateral cataracts and, potentially, optic atrophy (Badtke 1961). Primary optic atrophy with papilledema in the other eye, also the Foster-Kennedy syndrome with anosmia, indicates an olfactory groove meningioma. The Foster-Kennedy syndrome is found more frequently with frontal and middle cranial fossa tumors as well as with tumors near the sella or sphenoid. Mainly meningiomas, but also vascular and inflammatory processes are at fault.

Tumors of the Optic Nerve

Optic nerve tumors cause slowly developing axial exophthalmos. The visual field is concentrically constricted or, when the chiasm is involved, shows bilateral field cuts. The visual acuity deteriorates. Papilledema followed by optic atrophy may be present. The fundus is normal or shows choroidal folds (Nover and Zielinski 1957). Optic nerve gliomas are the most common cause by far, meningiomas being much more rare. Gliomas (spongioblastomas) appear mainly in children and young adults, over 90 percent before age 20 (Jaensch 1958). On X-ray the optic canal on the involved side is concentrically enlarged (up to five times normal) with sharp edges. While gliomas are seen more commonly in children, meningiomas predominate in adults. One-tenth of true primary optic atrophy is due to meningiomas (Kittel et al. 1961). Fibromas, fibrosarcomas, and angiomas, etc. involving the optic nerve have rarely been described. The differential diagnosis includes orbital tumors. These displace the globe, alter bone, cause motility disturbances and occur mainly in older persons (fifth to seventh decade).

After Blood Loss

Severe, recurrent blood loss (G.I. bleeding, metrorrhagia, bleeding from an amputation stump, etc.) can result in partial optic atrophy. The visual field loss is usually an inferior altitudinal hemianopsia (Fig. 3.28, page 22).

Arteriosclerosis

Large arteriosclerotic vessels (internal carotid artery) can directly compress the chiasm, causing optic atrophy (and binasal hemianopsia). *Arteriosclerotic optic atrophy*, however, denotes the gray-yellow discoloration of the sharply outlined optic disc which may be observed with age. This is usually associated with other changes, especially of the retina (depigmentation, pigmentation circinate retinopathy, drusen, gray degenerative patches).

Hereditary Optic Atrophies

These can be differentiated into (Jaeger 1954; Lodberg and Lund 1950; Kjer 1956; Vinken and Bruyn 1972):

1. *Leber's optic atrophy* (see page 311). Males are primarily affected. Optic atrophy develops after an initial episode of hyperemia of the optic disc. Visual acuity usually falls below 20/200. A central scotoma is present. Age of onset is overwhelmingly between ages 18 and 25 with rapid vision loss. Heredity is classically thought to be x-linked recessive. Females (carriers), however, constitute 15 percent of the patients in Europe and 35 percent in Japan. Since affected males almost never pass the gene on to their offspring, it is implied that the paternally derived gene, as opposed to the maternal one, causes some difficulty with fertilization or embryogenesis. Incomplete dominant inheritance is also considered (Jaeger 1954).

2. *Behr's complicated optic atrophy* is similar to Leber's except that it may be present at birth or manifest before puberty. Mental retardation, neurogenic bladder, mild ataxia, and cerebrospinal disturbances causing difficulty in walking are other findings

3. *Dominant optic atrophy*. Visual acuity is moderately affected: 20/100–20/200 (0.2–0.1). The visual field is concentrically constricted, especially to colored test targets (blue-yellow more than red). Onset is in the early years of

life (early childhood form of dominant optic atrophy).

4. *Dominant optic atrophy with nystagmus* is similar to dominant optic atrophy. The entire optic disc is atrophic, retinal vessels are narrowed. Nystagmus, severe vision loss and concentric visual field constriction are present. The disease is congenital and visual acuity is usually less than 20/200 (Lodberg and Lund 1950). The same is true for *congenital, hereditary recessive optic atrophy*. Parental consanguinity is usual. Infantile optic atrophy may be inherited or sporadically acquired as with cranial dysostosis, hydrocephalus, extensive chorioretinitis or prolonged hypoxia at birth (Harcourd and Wybar 1966).

Blindness beginning in childhood includes *Leber's congenital blindness* (see page 288). In Holland, this accounts for 18 percent of blind children (Schappert-Kimmigser et al. 1959). Blindness or severely decreased vision is present at birth or has its onset in the first months of life, potentially with nystagmus and photophobia. The pupillary light reflex is decreased or lost. The fundus may be normal or show only minimal pigmentary dispersion in the macula and possibly a slightly pale optic disc. Later the picture becomes one of atypical tapetoretinal degeneration with narrowed arteries and optic atrophy. Heredity is autosomal recessive. The ERG is usually lost. In contrast the ERG generally remains normal with cerebral damage, macular disease or albinism. The ERG may be minimally decreased in congenital lues (pepper-and-salt fundus). Other signs of syphilis (interstitial keratitis, iritis, etc.) are usually also present. In *mentally retarded children* who have a normal fundus it may be difficult to determine if they are also blind.

Carotid Thrombosis

(see page 271)

Postinflammatory or simple optic atrophy may occur in the *aortic arch syndrome* (pulseless disease).

A variety of vascular disorders can result in *occlusion of the internal carotid artery*, e.g., arteriosclerosis, arterial thrombosis, giant cell arteritis, syphilitic granuloma, endangiitis obliterans, etc. Occlusion is usually incomplete or transient leading to repeated momentary attacks of blindness (amaurosis fugax) (Hollenhorst 1960).

Complete acute occlusion results in unilateral blindness and contralateral hemiplegia (Weigelin and Lobstein 1962; Hager 1963). With amaurosis fugax the fundus is usually normal but central retinal artery emboli may be seen. In the end optic atrophy often results, potentially with hemianopsia.

Ocular findings with carotid thrombosis are: decreased vision, visual field loss (potentially homonymous), papilledema, central retinal artery emboli, optic atrophy, and intraocular pressure changes. Neurologic symptoms include hemiparesis or nuclear palsies. Internal carotid artery thrombosis may also occur with Urbach-Wiethe's lipoproteinosis (hyalinosis cutis et mucosae) (Jütte 1962). According to Hager (1963) the diagnosis can be established in 80 percent of patients by use of ophthalmodynamography. Dynametrically there is a marked difference between the two sides. In contrast to migraine and giant cell arteritis, internal carotid artery occlusion occurs without either prodrome or pain (Seitz 1969).

Aortic Arch Syndrome, Takayasu's Disease, Pulseless Disease, or Arteritis of Young Females

The external carotid and subclavian arteries occlude. Ocular *ischemia* develops. This manifests as vision loss on walking or exertion and improves when the patient lies down. Reference has, therefore, been made to "visual claudications" (Frowig 1946). Retinal vessels may be segmented. *Degenerative areas* and *pigmentary changes* appear in the retina. Sequelae include *optic atrophy, peripapillary arteriovenous anastomoses, retinal hemorrhages, cotton-wool spots, pupillary dilatation, stromal iris atrophy* and *cataracts*. The patients tend to faint on standing or with exertion. It becomes difficult to raise the hypothermic, poorly-diffused arm. Trophic muscle atrophy of the face and head develops. There is cranial hypotension but distal hypertension (see page 193, 258, 271). Overwhelmingly the patients are young, generally females with luetic, tuberculous, rheumatoid, auto-immune, or nonspecific arteritis and endarteritis. Aortic artery aneurysms, cervical arteriovenous fistulas or congenital dysplasia of the aortic arch vessels may also play a role (Seitz 1969).

Incontinentia Pigmenti

Optic atrophy and rarely papillitis may be seen in incontinentia pigmenti (Bloch-Sulzberger syndrome) (see page 247).

Central Artery Emboli

Optic atrophy with sharp disc borders combined with marked *arterial vessel narrowing* appears two to three weeks after central artery emboli.

Poisoning

Optic atrophy with narrowed retinal vessels may be seen after poisoning (see page 310) with *quinine* (see page 311), *optochin, filix mas,* and *arsenicals*. In all these cases, the visual fields are markedly constricted. Intoxication from leaded gasoline, etc. may also cause simple optic atrophy. *Occupational diseases* with optic nerve damage include (Merté 1969):

Arsenicals – neuritis with central scotomata, and retinal pigmentation as in pseudoretinitis pigmentosa; corneal and conjunctival inflammation.
Benzene – retrobulbar neuritis, retinitis, conjunctival and corneal inflammation.
Nitro and amino benzene compounds (methemoglobin formers):
Nitro- and dinitrobenzol – retrobulbar neuritis, transient amaurosis with subsequent optic atrophy or temporal disc pallor.
Nitronaphthalene – neuritis, papilledema followed by optic atrophy, central scotoma, retinal hemorrhages, severe corneal and conjunctival inflammation.
Carbon disulfide – papilledema, neuritis, partial optic atrophy, central scotoma or peripheral visual field loss, conjunctival and corneal burns.
Hydrogen sulfide – optic nerve damage, conjunctival and corneal inflammation.
Lead (leaded gasoline, tetraethyl lead, "anti-knock" compounds): Vision can diminish to blindness within hours; toxic optic nerve damage with or without papilledema and postinflammatory optic atrophy, specifically, temporal pallor or retinal vessel constriction.
Chromate: optic atrophy.
Manganese: retrobulbar neuritis.
Thallium: toxic optic nerve damage with resultant atrophy and varying degrees of vision loss. Hemianopsia (binasal) is possible.
Carbon monoxide: papilledema, postpapillitic atrophy, central scotoma, concentric visual field constriction, retinal hemorrhages.

Most *anti-tuberculous medications* have toxic side effects for the retina (Honegger and Genée 1969) with optic atrophy. *Streptomycin* can cause optic atrophy, transient ocular muscle paresis, accommodative paresis, transient myopia, xanthopsia and vestibular damage with dizziness and vomiting. *Isoniazid* can cause optic atrophy, accommodative disturbances, neuralgias, peripheral neuritides, psychic disturbances, and epileptic seizures. *Para-aminosalicylic acid* (PAS) causes blepharitis, accommodative paresis, gastrointestinal disorders and rarely, hepatitis, agranulocytosis, polyneuritis, or goiter. *D-Cycloserine* (Roche) leads to optic atrophy, accommodative paresis (central nervous system); *Myambutol* (Lederle) causes optic neuritis.

Glaucomatous Optic Atrophy

(Plate XXXI, Fig. 4, page 288 g)

This is a special form of noninflammatory optic atrophy. There is deep optic cupping and atrophy to the edge of the disc with nasal shift of vessels, bayonet-shaped kinking of vessels at the disc margin and, potentially, glaucomatous halo (gray-white rim of choroidal atrophy around the disc).

Postinflammatory (Postpapillitic) Optic Atrophy with Blurred Disc Margins

(Plate XXX, Fig. 1, page 288 f)

The optic disc is white or gray-white. The lamina cribrosa is not visible. The disc margins are blurred. The optic cup is effaced. The arteries are narrowed. There is usually a narrow, gray-yellow halo around the disc resulting from irregularity of the pigment epithelium in the formerly edematous region.

Optic atrophy after papilledema or optic neuritis (papillitis) (Plate XXX, Fig. 1, page 288 f): Edema and venous dilatation decrease as optic atrophy develops in papilledema.

Retinal (waxy yellow) **optic atrophy** is between sharply outlined and blurred optic atrophy. Retinal optic atrophy is part of the picture of *tapetoretinal degeneration* (Plate XXVII, Fig. 3, page 288 c). The optic disc develops a waxy yellow color and lies in the plane of the retina. The lamina cribrosa is not visible. The disc borders are minimally blurred. All vessels (arteries and veins) are markedly constricted. In retinitis pigmentosa, bone-corpuscle-like pigmentations spread centrally from the equatorial region. Night blindness is present early in the disease. The differential diagnosis includes, first of all, the various forms of tapetoretinal degeneration (see page 286). A similar picture may occur with *retinitis,* specifically *chorioretinitis* affecting large retinal areas (diffuse chorioretinitis, serpiginous *maplike chorioretinitis).* Concentric visual field constriction and night blindness are not present in these cases; the ERG remains normal. *Excessive myopia* with marked pigmentary changes throughout the fundus produces a similar picture.

Optic Disc Tumors

Primary tumors of the papilla are overwhelmingly melanocytoma, less often fibromas, neurocytoma, endothelioma or glioma. Sarcoma may metastasize to the optic disc at a late stage (Weisse 1965). Neurofibromas, gliotic tumors and angiomas may occur on the optic disc in the phakomatoses (Lund 1960/61).

Swelling of the papilla can be inflammatory, e.g., caused by syphilis, tuberculous granulomas and cysticercus cysts. These can usually be diagnosed by the accompanying inflammation.

References

Andersen, O. C.: Grubenbildungen auf der Papille mit Gesichtsfeldausfällen. Klin. Mbl. Augenheilk. 122 (1953) 159–168

Badtke, G.: Über die Pseudoneuritis und Pseudostauungspapille bei Myopie nebst Bemerkungen zur Genese dieser Veränderungen. Klin. Mbl. Augenheilk. 126 (1955) 546–561

Badtke, G., D. Bauermann: Über die Gruben oder Lochbildungen der Sehnervenscheibe, ihre Differentialdiagnose und formale Genese. Klin. Mbl. Augenheilk. 145 (1964) 641–657

Badtke, G.: Die Mißbildungen des menschlichen Auges. In: Der Augenarzt, Vol. IV, ed. by K. Velhagen. Thieme, Leipzig 1961

Beeler, A.: Der heterotypische Konus, insbesondere der Konus nach unten und die Ausbuchtung des angrenzenden Augenhintergrundes. Albrecht v. Graefes Arch. klin. exp. Ophthal. 122 (1929) 342–358

Böke, W.: Neuritische Sehnervenveränderungen bei der Meningitis tuberculosa. Klin. Mbl. Augenheilk. 126 (1955) 678–684

Bonamour, G., P. Bregeat, M. Bonnet, P. Juce: La papille optique. Masson, Paris 1968

Collier, M.: Les doubles papilles optiques. Bull. Soc. franç. Ophtal. 71 (1958) 328–354

Dralands, L., P. H. Garin: Médicaments anti-infectieux. Soc. Bull. d'Ophtalm. Belge 160 (1972) 326–389

Dubois-Poulsen, A.: Le champ visuel. Topographie normale et pathologique de ses sensibilités. Masson, Paris 1952

Duke-Elder, S.: Neuroophthalmology. System of ophthalmology XII. Kimpton, London 1971

François, J., G. Verriest, A. Neetens, A. de Rouck: Pseudo-papillites vasculaires. Bull. Soc. belge Ophtal. 129 (1961) 413–427

Guillaumat, L., P. V. Morax, G. Offret: Neuro-ophthalmologie. Masson, Paris 1959

Hager, H.: Die Ophthalmo-Dynamographie als Methode zur Beurteilung des Gehirnkreislaufes. Klin. Mbl. Augenheilk. 142 (1963) 827–846

Harcourt, R. B., K. Wybar: The determination of blindness in infancy. Trans. ophthal. Soc. U. K. 86 (1966) 37–48

Harrington, D. O.: Amblyopia due to tobacco, alcohol and nutritional deficiency. Amer. J. Ophthal. 53 (1962) 967–972

Hoeg, N.: Über Drusen im Sehnervenkopf. Albrecht v. Graefes Arch. klin. exp. Ophthal. 69 (1909) 355–389

Hollenhorst, R. W.: Neurologic aspects of temporal arteriitis. Neurology (Minneapolis) 10 (1960) 490–498

Honegger, H., E. Genée: Akkommodationsstörungen bei Behandlung mit Tuberkulostatika. Klin. Mbl. Augenheilk. 155 (1969) 371–380

Horton, B. F., F. R. Magath, G. E. Brown: An undescribed form of arteriitis of the temporal vessels. Proc. Staff. Meet. Mayo-Clin. 1932, 700–701

Huber, A.: Augensymptome bei Hirntumoren. Huber, Bern 1956

Huber, A., F. C. Blodi: Eye symptoms in brain tumors. Mosby, St. Louis 1971

Jaeger, W.: Dominant vererbte Opticusatrophie (unter besonderer Berücksichtigung der dabei vorhandenen Farbsinnstörung). Albrecht v. Graefes Arch. klin. exp. Ophthal. 155 (1954) 457–484

Jaeger, W.: Vererbung von Augenleiden und Anomalien des Auges. In: Lehrbuch der Augenheilkunde, ed. by T. Axenfeld, H. Pau. Fischer, Stuttgart 1973

Jaensch, P. A.: Sehnervengeschwülste. Klin. Mbl. Augenheilk. 132 (1958) 617–625

Jütte, A.: Thrombose der Arteria carotis interna bei Hyalinosis cutis et mucosae. Ber. ophthal. Ges. 64 (1962) 459–465

Jütte, A.: Verletzungen, physikalische Schädigungen und Giftwirkungen. In: Der Augenarzt, Vol. V, ed. by K. Velhagen. Thieme, Leipzig 1963 (pp. 837–946)

Kittel, V., G. Goder, E. Kittel: Zur Klinik und Histologie der Opticusmeningeome. Klin. Mbl. Augenheilk. 138 (1961) 664–672

Kjer, P.: Hereditary infantile optic atrophy with dominant transmissions: preliminary report. Dan. med. Bull. 3 (1956) 135–141

Klein, D., A. Franceschetti: Mißbildungen und Krankheiten des Auges. In: Humangenetik IV/5, ed. by P. E. Becker. Thieme, Stuttgart 1964 (pp. 1–241)

Kommerell, G., W. L. Castrillon-Oberndorfer: Tabak-Amblyopie. Klin. Mbl. Augenheilk. 153 (1968) 551–562

Kreibig, W.: Diagnostische Möglichkeiten der Augenhintergrunduntersuchung bei Arteriosklerose. Dtsch. med. J. 8 (1957) 295–297

Kreibig, W.: Über Aplasie und Hypoplasie der Papilla nervi optici. Klin. Mbl. Augenheilk. 135 (1959) 212–223

Lodberg, C. V., A. Lund: Hereditary optic atrophy with dominant transmission. Acta ophthal. 28 (1950) 437–468

Löhlein, W.: Über die kegelförmige Papille mit Drusenbildung. Klin. Mbl. Augenheilk. 86 (1931) 433–445

Lund, O. E.: Histologische und morphogenetische Untersuchungen am Auge und Hirn bei Phakomatosen. Albrecht v. Graefes Arch. klin. exp. Ophthal. 162 (1960/61) 369–399

Mansour, F., M. D. Armaly: Ocular involvement in chondrodystrophia calcificans congenita punctata. Arch. ophthal. 57 (1957) 491–502

Merté, H. J.: Arbeitsmedizinische Fragen in der Ophthalmologie. Karger, Basel 1969

Merté, H. J.: Arbeits- u. Sozialmedizin. In: Lehrbuch der Augenheilkunde, ed. by T. Axenfeld, H. Pau. Fischer, Stuttgart 1973

Meyer, H. J.: Grubenpapille mit zentraler Netzhautablösung. Klin. Mbl. Augenheilk. 154 (1969) 797–806

Nover, A., H. W. Zielinski: Zur Differentialdiagnose der Orbita- und Optikustumoren. Klin. Mbl. Augenheilk. 131 (1957) 577–598

Pau, H.: Augenschädigung durch Myambutol (Ethambutol). Klin. Mbl. f. Augenheilk. 165 (1974) 121–126

Pau, H., H. Wahl: Myambutolschädigung des Auges. Ber. Dtsch. Ophthal. Ges. (1972) 176–181

Peters, W.: Über die Neuritis optici arteriosklerotischer Genese. Klin. Mbl. Augenheilk. 132 (1958) 363–377

Pfaffenbach, D., F. B. Walsh: Central pit of the optic disk. Amer. J. Ophthal. 73 (1972) 102–106

Pietruschka, G.: Über die Marmorknochenkrankheit (Albers-Schönbergsche Krankheit) nebst Bemerkungen zur Differentialdiagnose. Klin. Mbl. Augenheilk. 123 (1953) 189–201

Remky, H.: Über den Nachweis von Regulationsstörungen des Netzhautkreislaufes. Albrecht v. Graefes Arch. klin. exp. Ophthal. 151 (1951) 597–622

Remky, H.: Grundlagen der neuroophthalmologischen Diagnostik. In: Der Augenarzt, Vol. V, ed. by K. Velhagen. VEB Thieme, Leipzig 1963

Rieger, H.: Neues aus der Erbpathologie des Auges. Klin. Mbl. Augenheilk. 128 (1956) 513–526

Rogahn, E. J.: Über nasale Coni bei Myopie. Ein Beitrag zur Myopiegenese. Berl. Med. 7 (1956) 298–301

Schappert-Kimmijser, J., H. E. Henkes, J. van den Bosch: Amaurosis congenita (Leber). Arch. Ophthal. 61 (1959) 211–218

Schönenberg, H., K. Frohn: Das Cockayne-Syndrom. Mbl. f. Kinderheilkunde 117 (1969) 103–108

Schroeder, H., A. Schauer: Das sog. Melanozytom des Sehnervenkopfes. Klin. Mbl. Augenheilk. 146 (1965) 593–597

Seitz, R.: Ätiologie und Genese der akuten Erblindung als Folge stumpfer Schädelverletzungen. Klin. Mbl. Augenheilk. 143 (1963) 414–429

Seitz, R.: Die intraokularen Drusen. Klin. Mbl. Augenheilk. 152 (1968) 203–211

Seitz, R.: Erkrankungen der Netzhaut und ihrer Gefäße bei Allgemeinleiden. In: Almanach für die Augenheilkunde, ed. by H. J. Küchle. Lehmann, München 1969 (pp. 75–92)

Seitz, R., G. Kersting: Die Drusen der Sehnervenpapille und des Pigmentepithels. Klin. Mbl. Augenheilk. 140 (1962) 75–88

Silvetta, H., H. B. Haag, P. S. Larson: Tobacco amblyopia. Amer. J. Ophthal. 50 (1960) 71–100

Smith, H. E.: Aplasia of the optic nerve. Amer. J. Ophthal. 37 (1954) 498–504

Streiff, B.: Über Megalopapille. Klin. Mbl. Augenheilk. 139 (1961) 824–827

Streiff, B.: L'hypoplasie papillaire. Bull. Soc. franç. Ophtal. 75 (1962) 333–338

Tönnis, W.: Augensymptome bei 3033 Hirngeschwülsten. Ber. dtsch. ophthal. Ges. 59 (1955) 6–27

Vinken, P. J., G. W. Bruyn: Handbook of clinical neurology, Vol. 13. Neuroretinal degenerations. North Holland Publishing Co., Amsterdam, American Elsevier Publishing Co., New York 1972

Vogel, M.: Klinische und histologische Differentialdiagnose epi- und peripapillärer pigmentierter Veränderungen. Vers. Rhein.-Westf. Augenärzte, 119 (1969) 13–16

Vogel, M. H., A. Wessing: Makulaveränderungen bei Grubenpapille. Klin. Mbl. Augenheilk. 164 (1974) 90–97

Waardenburg, P. J.: Genetics and Ophthalmology, Vol. II. Beford-Assen, NL-Springfield 1963

Walsh, F. B., W. F. Hogt: Clinical neuroophthalmology, 3. Ed. Williams & Wilkins, Baltimore 1969, I–III

Weigelin, E.: Beurteilung des intracraniellen Kreislaufs mit Hilfe der Netzhautarteriendruckmessungen. Docum. ophthal. 7–8 (1954) 183–245

Weigelin, E., A. Lobstein: Ophthalmodynamometrie. Karger, Basel 1962

Weigelin, E., P. Niesel: Die Bedeutung des Therapietest für die Behandlung des vasomotorischen Kopfschmerzes und der Beschwerden von Hochdruckerkrankungen. Ber. Dtsch. ophthal. Ges. 60 (1956) 232–235

Weisse, U.: Tumor der Papilla nervi optici. Klin. Mbl. Augenheilk. 146 (1965) 65–69

Witmer, R.: Arteriitis temporalis. Ophthalmologica 121 (1951) 160–163

24 Pupil

Physiologic Changes in Pupillary Diameter
(Fig. 24.1)

The pupillary diameter is physiologically small during the first months of life (around 2 mm). It then increases to *3.4 to 4 mm* and decreases in senility to around 2 mm. The pupil displays a constant physiologic unrest which is more active in youth and less extensive with age.
Physiologic pupillary *constriction* (miosis) occurs with:
Light (retina-optic nerve-lateral geniculate body – brachium of the superior colliculus – synapsing in the pretectal nucleus – the Edinger-Westphal division of the oculomotor nucleus – ciliary ganglion – pupillary sphincter).
Close distances (convergence). Like the convergence impulse, pupillary constriction for close distances comes from the cortex via the oculomotor nucleus to the pupillary sphincter.
Forcible lid closure (orbicularis reflex), also when the lids are forcibly held open during attempted closure (Piltz-Westphal phenomenon). Irritation of the nervus vestibularis and (seldom) deep expiration produce miosis.
The pupil *dilates* in darkness; can be dilated with *mydriatics*, strong stimuli (fright, fear, epileptic attacks).
Severe *pain* and *deep inspiration* which, because it is a voluntary exertion, can cause pupillary dilatation.

Drug-Induced Changes in the Pupillary Diameter

The pupillary diameter (pupilla = doll) is controlled by parasympathetic innervation from the third nerve nucleus to the pupillary sphincter in the iris stroma and by sympathetic innervation to the dilator muscle situated in the most anterior portion of the iris pigment leaf.

Miotics

Contraction of the sphincter (by *miotics*) constricts the pupil: *parasympathomimetics* (cholinergic) = acetylcholine, carbachol, pilocarpine, physostigmine, prostigmin, mintacol, weak concentrations of nicotine, etc. *Dilator paresis* results in miosis. *Sympathicolytic agents* = guanethidine, reserpine, alpha-methyldopa, and phentolamine also cause pupillary constriction as do ergotamine preparations, opiates and histamine.

Mydriatics

Conversely, the pupil can be dilated by sphincter paresis (*parasympatholytics:* atropine, scopolamine, etc.) or by *contraction of the dilator* (sympathomimetics: subconjunctivally injected adrenalin, L-glaucosan, cocaine, etc.). Parasympatholytics are frequently used to dilate the pupil for diagnostic purposes (Homatropine, Mydriacyl, Cyclogyl, Mydriatikum [Roche]) or adrenergic agents which act rapidly and for only a short period.
Some mydriatic action occurs with: bromides (K^+, Na^+), salicylates (alkylide), Para-aminosalicylic acid, overdose of paraldehyde, antimalarials (Atabrin), antihistamines, chlorpromazine, etc.

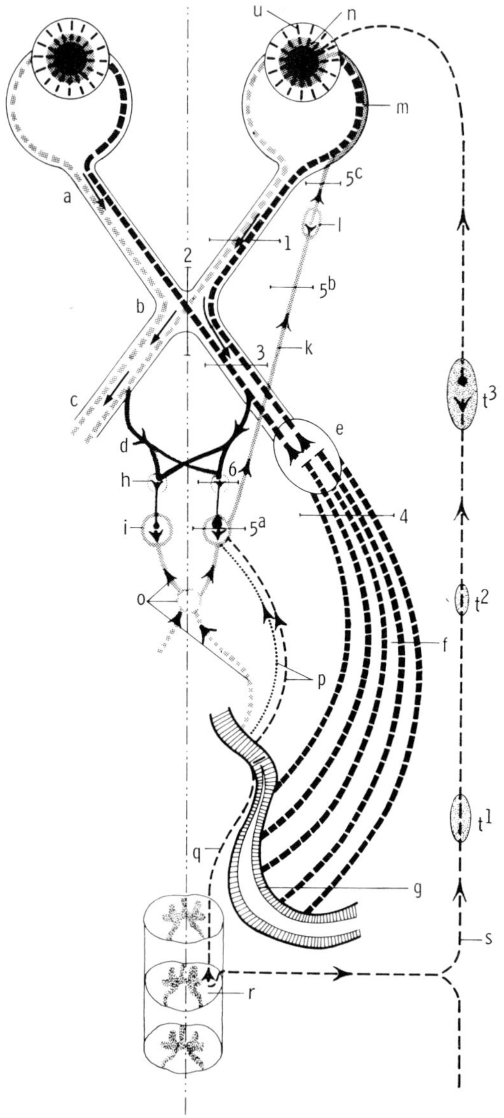

right retinal halves and visual pathways
left retinal halves and visual pathways
nucleus and pathway to the pupillary sphincter muscle
calcarine (fissure) cortex with line(s) of Gennari
ascending pupillomotor pathway
corticonuclear pathway of inhibition to the sphincter nucleus (psychosensory dilation)
central and peripheral sympathetic pathways

Fig. 24.1 Visual and pupillary reflex pathways (after C. Behr from: R. Thiel, Atlas of Diseases of the Eye, 6th Ed., Thieme, Stuttgart 1963)

Legend to fig. 24.1

a optic nerve
b chiasm
c optic tract
d ascending pupillary pathway in the brachium of the superior colliculus after leaving the visual pathway
e lateral geniculate body
f internal capsule and optic radiations
g visual cortex in the calcarine fissure
h pretectal nucleus
i Edinger-Westphal nucleus
k oculomotor nerve pathway to the sphincter
l ciliary ganglion
m intraocular sphincter pathway (posterior ciliary nerves between choroid and sclera)
n pupillary sphincter muscle
o subcortical center and pathway for the reaction to near (convergence)
p corticonuclear pathway of inhibition of the sphincter
q central sympathetic pathway
r ciliospinal center (Budge)
s sympathetic trunk
t_1 t_2 t_3 inferior, medial and superior cervical ganglia
u pupillary dilator muscle

1. Lesion in the optic nerve: amaurotic pupil
2. Lesion in the chiasm: pupillary hemiakinesia, bitemporal hemianopsia, optic atrophy.
3. Lesion in the optic tract: pupillary hemiakinesia, homonymous hemianopsia, optic atrophy
4. Lesion in the optic radiations: homonymous hemianopsia
5. (a, b, c) Lesion in the sphincter nucleus or sphincter pathway: fixes dilated pupil
6. Lesion in the pretectal nucleus or intercalary pathway between sensory and motor nucleus: light-near dissociation (Argyll Robertson)

Pathologic Pupillary Diameter

Anisocoria – Spastic miosis – Paralytic miosis – Spastic mydriasis – Paralytic mydriasis.

Anisocoria

The pupil is unilaterally constricted with iritis, enlarged during an acute glaucoma attack and with pupillary ectropion.

A difference in size between right and left pupils *(anisocoria)* in otherwise normal eyes raises the possibility of Horner's syndrome (see page 321, 322). Anisocoria may also be hereditary (dominant) (Kyrieleis 1951). Anisocoria of varying degrees can be seen with *all forms* of pathologic *miosis, mydriasis,* and *pupilloplegia.*

Spastic Miosis

Parasympathomimetics cause spastic miosis. Spastic miosis can also occur with *meningitis, encephalitis, and hemorrhage into the ventricle* (poor prognosis). Spastic miosis is also caused by *intoxications* with morphine or opium derivatives and certain insecticides (anticholinesterases). Miosis and sometimes voluntary nystagmus (see page 65) are seen with *hysterical spasm* of convergence.

Paralytic Miosis

Sympatholytic agents (see page 319) produce paralytic miosis.

Paralytic miosis is also produced by *sympathetic paresis* (usually sympathetic trunk lesions in the region of the neck) and is part of *Horner's syndrome* (miosis, ptosis, and anhidrosis) (see page 86) (Fig. 10.8). If such a lesion occurs in infancy *heterochromia* may result, i.e., a lighter colored iris on the side of the Horner's.

Förster and Gagel (1932) developed cocaine-adrenalin testing for pharmacodynamic proof of Horner's syndrome (Claude Bernard-Horner syndrome, Passow syndrome, oculopupillary syndrome). This test was thought to aid in differentiating central and peripheral damage (Horner's).

Peripheral Horner's can be further differentiated into preganglionic (intermediolateral gray column C_8–T_2 [= ciliospinal center of Budge] to the superior cervical ganglion) and postganglionic (superior cervical ganglion to the eye) lesions. See schema of Förster and Gagel.

The test works as follows: Norepinephrine released by the sympathetic nerve endings is promptly reabsorbed into the nerve endings. Cocaine blocks this reuptake, thereby heightening the adrenergic effect of the normally released noradrenalin. With interruption of the sympathetic pathway (central, pre- or postganglionic), cocaine is ineffective. Adrenalin and phenylephrine are direct-acting sympathomimetics. With denervation, their action is heightened (denervation supersensitivity). Indirect-acting sympathomimetics, OH-amphetamine (Paredrine 1 percent), release endogenous norepinephrine. Since Paredrine has no direct action on adrenergic receptors, the pupil can only dilate with an intact postganglionic sympathetic pathway (superior cervical ganglion - eye). See schema of Thompson: Page 322.

Spastic Mydriasis

Sympathomimetics cause *spastic mydriasis* (see page 319) which also occurs with sympathetic

Schema of Förster and Gagel (1932)

	Central	Preganglionic	Postganglionic
Cocaine	normal mydriasis	no dilatation	no dilatation
Adrenalin (1:1000)	no dilatation	no dilatation	mydriasis

Schema of Thompson (1972)

Drug	Normal	Central	Preganglionic	Postganglionic
Cocaine 2–10 % (2 drops)	Mydriasis	Impaired dilation	No dilation	No dilation
Epinephrine 1:1000 (several drops)	No dilation	No dilation	Moderate dilation	Dramatic dilation
Phenylephrine 1 % (2 drops)	Slight dilation	Slight dilation	Moderate dilation	Dramatic dilation
Phenylephrine 10 % (1 drop)	Dramatic dilation	Normal dilation; pupils become equal	At least normal dilation; Horner's pupil may become slightly larger	Horner's pupil dilates sooner, faster, and more than normal; becomes noticeably larger
Hydroxyamphetamine 1 % (2 drops)	Mydriasis	Normal dilation; pupils become equal	At least normal dilation; Horner's pupil may become slightly larger	No dilation

irritation as in *epileptic seizures* and *schizophrenia*.

Such an irritative mydriasis also occurs as a precursor to parasympathetic miosis with *irritation of the sympathetic trunk,* specifically the *stellate ganglion* by *tumors* or *enlarged glands in the neck* and with inflammation in the *superior posterior lung segment*.

Paralytic Mydriasis

Parasympatholytic agents – Brain diseases – Trauma – Accommodative paresis with diphtheria – Oculomotor paresis – Aortic arch syndrome – Occupational disease.

Parasympatholytic agents

The most common cause of paralytic mydriasis is with internal ophthalmoplegia usually caused by parasympatholytic agents (atropine, homatropine, scopolamine) used topically, or with systemic use of belladonna derivatives. Such an internal ophthalmoplegia may take up to eight days to resolve.

Bilateral mydriasis results from *poisoning* with *belladonna, botulism,* or *carbon monoxide.*

Botulism (agent: Clostridium botulinum) has an incubation period of 12 to 36 hours, usually appearing after the consumption of improperly pasteurized canned foods. Ophthalmic symptoms may include internal ophthalmoplegia, ocular motor palsies, nystagmus and optic neuritis, combined with gastroenteritis, dry mouth and, rarely, gaze palsies.

Brain diseases: The most common etiology for true internal ophthalmoplegia is central nervous system lues, tabes dorsalis or general paresis. It is also present in other brain disorders (encephalitis lethargica, polioencephalitis, tumors, etc.).

Traumatic iridoplegia: Blunt trauma to the globe can, without subluxation of the lens or tearing of the pupillary sphincter, result in paralytic mydriasis. *Photocoagulation* of *the iris* causes pupillary dilatation.

Diphtheria: Isolated accommodative paresis with pupillary sparing is occasionally seen four to six weeks after diphtheria.

Oculomotor nerve paresis: Oculomotor nerve damage (see page 54) from intracranial pressure usually affects the pupillary fibers causing mydriasis and a decreased pupillary reaction at first, then ptosis. Extraocular muscle paresis appears last. Progressive pupillary paresis (dilatation) is an important lateralizing sign with epi- or subdural brain tumors.
Aortic arch syndrome (pulseless disease): This disorder frequently results in pupillary dilatation on the diseased side (see pages 271, 315) because of ocular hypoxia.
Occupational diseases recognized to cause pupillary disturbances include (Merté 1973):
Arsenicals: Pupillary disturbances, ocular muscle paresis, retinal and optic nerve damage.
Nitro and amino benzenes (methemoglobin formers).
Nitronaphthalene: pupillary disturbances, nystagmus, optic nerve neuritis. *Aniline* (aminobenzene), *chlor-* and *nitroaniline:* pupillary disturbances and optic nerve damage.
Lead: Pupillary disturbances, ocular muscle paresis, optic neuritis.
Carbon disulfide: internal and external ophthalmoplegia, nystagmus, optic neuritis.
Fixed dilated pupil, ocular muscle paresis, retinal and lid hemorrhages may appear in *caisson disease* (rapid decompression of atmospheric pressure).

Differential Diagnosis of the Widely Dilated Fixed Pupil

The differential diagnosis of a widely dilated fixed pupil includes drugs similar to atropine, oculomotor paresis and Adie's syndrome. Instillation of one drop of 1 percent pilocarpine will constrict both the normal pupil and the pupil dilated by pre- or postganglionic parasympathetic damage. The action of pilocarpine is actually enhanced with damage to the parasympathetic innervation. The weak 1 percent pilocarpine solution fails to cause constriction with atropine mydriasis (Thompson, Newsome, Loewenfeld 1971).

Various Forms of Pupilloplegia

Amaurotic and amblyopic pupilloplegia — Hemianopic pupilloplegia — Light near dissociation — Pupillotonia — Isolated pupilloplegia with convergence — Absolute pupilloplegia.

Amaurotic and Amblyopic Pupilloplegia

With *unilateral blindness* both pupils react normally on illuminating the seeing eye (direct and consensual reaction). This bilateral pupillary constriction is absent when the blind eye is illuminated. Bilateral peripheral blindness results in loss of the light reaction, while pupillary constriction on convergence is maintained. With *amblyopic pupilloplegia,* visual *acuity* is *depressed,* but not lost from retinal or optic nerve damage (inflammation, trauma, tumor). The direct light reaction of this eye (and consensual reaction of the other eye) is correspondingly decreased. The consensual light reaction on illuminating the sound eye remains normal. Diagnostically the swinging flashlight test takes advantage of this difference.
Differential diagnosis: Unilateral amaurotic pupilloplegia in a comatose patient following cerebral injury indicates damage to the retina or optic nerve. A normal pupillary light reaction in an allegedly blind eye excludes organic blindness.

Hemianopic Pupilloplegia (Pupillary Hemiakinesia)

Bitemporal chiasmal hemianopsia or *homonymous hemianopsia* from optic tract lesions cause loss of the pupillary reaction from the blind visual field (pupillary hemiakinesis). Because of stray light such a pupillary hemiakinesia is difficult to diagnose. Hemianopic pupilloplegia would indicate a lesion in the optic tract prior to the lateral geniculate.
A true differential diagnosis between tract and optic radiation hemianopsia cannot be made with the aid of hemianopic pupilloplegia be-

cause the pupillary hemiakinesia is independent of the location of the hemianopsia (Harms 1951).
Using weak light stimuli, Schaknowitsch and Burdenko (1960) found that pupillary hemiakinesia with hemianopsia is caused by lesions in the optic radiations.

Light Near Dissociation

Argyll Robertson pupil — Light near dissociation with mydriasis = quadrigeminal pupilloplegia — Pseudo light near dissociation (pseudo Argyll Robertson).

Argyll Robertson phenomenon: Light near dissociation (as seen in the Argyll Robertson phenomenon) implies lack of or a very *poor light reaction* (direct and consensual) with a nearly *normal or intensified convergence response.* Argyll Robertson pupils are usually markedly miotic and irregular and fail to show physiologic hippus or dilatation to stress, especially pain and fright. The pupils do not dilate well with mydriatics. (For the differential diagnosis from tonic pupil see page 325).
Classically Argyll Robertson pupil was considered pathognomonic for *tabes,* specifically *tabetic paralysis.* The site of the lesion appears to be in the pretectal neurons above the Edinger-Westphal nucleus. Other causes (10 percent; Küchle 1969) of Argyll Robertson pupil in addition to lues (tabes dorsalis, progressive paralysis, cerebrospinal lues) include: encephalitis, multiple sclerosis, postencephalitic parkinsonism, syringomyelia, trauma, acute-chronic alcoholism, hemorrhages, diabetes, herpes zoster, and brain tumors near the third ventricle, the aqueduct, or the quadrigeminal region (pinealoma).

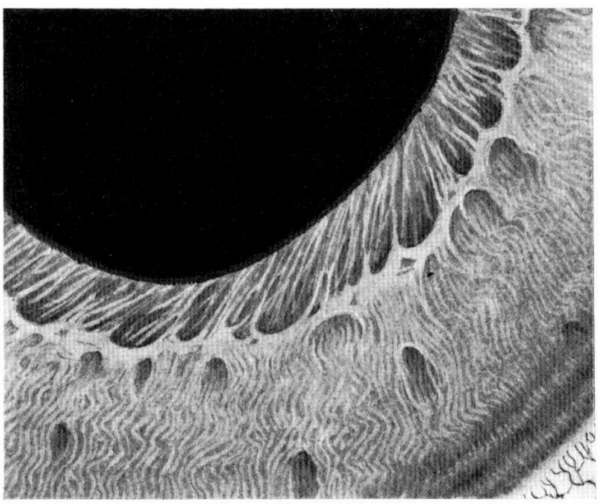

Fig. 24.2 Distortion of stromal fibers in Adie's syndrome (from: R. Thiel, Atlas of Diseases of the Eye, 6th Ed., Thieme, Stuttgart 1963)

Light near dissociation with mydriasis = quadrigeminal pupilloplegia (see page 59): Loss of the light reaction with normal near reaction and mid-dilated pupils occurs with tumors (pinealomas) or circulatory disturbances in the quadrigeminal region. Papilledema and vertical gaze paresis may be present. The pupil is more than mid-dilated with both unilateral or bilateral quadrigeminal pupilloplegia. The near reaction is normal or considerably better than the decreased or lost reaction to light. If the former is not the case, one can only speak of an incomplete absolute pupilloplegia.
Pseudo Argyll Robertson pupil can occur with aberrant third nerve regeneration after oculomotor paresis. With a poor light reaction there is synkinetic pupillary constriction on adduction simulating Argyll Robertson pupil. The abduction phenomenon (Behr) is observed with absolute pupilloplegia in neurosyphilis. After a considerable latent period the pupil of the abducted eye constricts.

Tonic Pupil

Clinical picture — Site and cause — Pharmacodynamic proof — Accommodation — Differential diagnosis.

Clinical picture: The tonic pupil, like the Argyll Robertson pupil, shows a light near dissociation (for differential diagnosis see page 325). It appears most commonly in the second and third decades of life but can occur in children. Often there is an associated *loss of the patellar and Achilles reflexes;* this constitutes *Adie's syndrome* (Markus-Holmes or Weill-Reys syndrome). Pupillary involvement is unilateral in two-thirds of cases. The pupil is more than mid-dilated and fails to react to light or reacts segmentally with vermiform movements. However, it reacts tonically (several to many seconds) but extensively on convergence and lid closure. Redilatation of the constricted pupil takes even longer (up to 1 min.).

The affected dilated pupil is often slightly distorted with iris stroma fibers running towards the most curved portions of the pupil (Fig. 24.2). The direct and consensual light reactions are absent in the involved eye. Segmental "vermiform" reactions (of those areas to which the stromal fibers are directed) still occur with bright illumination (Kyrieleis 1951). The pupillary diameter is different at various times. Accommodation is tonic in about 20 percent.

Site and etiology: Tonic pupil has been explained by dysfunction of the autonomic nervous system, damage to central pupillary fibers in the thalamus, diencephalon, or sympathetic irritation. Primary damage to the ciliary ganglion is most likely (Kyrieleis 1951; Küchle 1969; Loewenfeld and Thompson 1967). Of the neurons originating in the ciliary ganglion, 97 percent go to the ciliary body. Aberrant regeneration after primary ciliary ganglion injury would favor fibers which served accommodation reaching the sphincter (Loewenfeld and Thompson 1967).

Pharmacodynamic testing: Peripherally acting agents are enhanced in tonic pupils. Dilatation with cocaine and constriction by pilocarpine are more rapid and extensive.

Adler and Scheie found the tonic pupil contracted with 2.5 percent Mecholyl (acetyl-β-methacholine), whereas the normal pupil only reacted with 10 to 20 percent concentrations. The Mecholyl test may be positive, however, in absolute pupilloplegia (Kyrieleis 1951) and in many other conditions with small, poorly reacting pupils.

According to Kyrieleis (1959), 0.125 percent to 0.25 percent pilocarpine can be used instead of 2.5 percent Mecholyl.

Accommodative tonicity: In addition to pupillary constriction, accommodation may be *tonic*.

It may take several seconds when switching from near to distance fixation before a young patient sees clearly.

Differential diagnosis: The differential diagnosis may be difficult because of the number of atypical cases of tonic pupil. The disease is bilateral in about one-third of cases and may, therefore, resemble Argyll Robertson pupil.

Light near dissociation (Argyll Robertson, quadrigeminal plate) is almost always bilateral; the Argyll Robertson pupil is miotic and reacts promptly to convergence but not to light, and reacts *poorly* to drugs. The tonic pupil usually occurs unilaterally, is widely dilated, shows tonic miosis on convergence, and is supersensitive to pilocarpine. Slit lamp observation of the segmental, vermiform reactions to light suggests the diagnosis.

With incomplete absolute pupilloplegia, constriction on convergence is rapid but incomplete, as is redilatation. In contrast, constriction on convergence in the tonic pupil is slow but extensive. Drugs such as pilocarpine and cocaine have little effect in incomplete, absolute pupilloplegia compared to the tonic pupil which reacts strongly to these agents.

The light reaction of the tonic pupil may be relatively well maintained. It too, however, reacts tonically. The *tonic nature of the pupillary reaction*, no matter how obtained, is of great differential diagnostic importance.

Inverse Argyll Robertson pupil signifies a normal light reaction with lack of constriction on accommodation. It is rare but may occur with epidemic encephalitis, specifically postencephalitic parkinsonism.

Absolute Pupilloplegia

Clinical picture — Incomplete absolute pupilloplegia — Pseudo light near dissociation — Poisoning — Brain diseases — Tumors — Aneurysm, trauma, glaucomatous attacks, hemorrhages — Stupor, epileptic attacks.

Clinical Picture

With absolute pupilloplegia, the pupil is *dilated* and *fails* to react (either directly or consensually) to light or near. Pupilloplegia is usually unilateral, and the wider the pupillary dilatation the more peripheral the causal lesion. Rarely, as with epidemic encephalitis, the pupil may be small. The pupil reacts neither to light nor on convergence but does respond to drugs (especially miotics) and lid closure.

The *lid closure* or orbicularis reflex (Westphal-Piltz reaction) consists of pupillary constriction on lid closure. The lid closure reflex has little diagnostic significance since it is present in practically all forms of pupilloplegia.

If the lid closure reaction is missing, as with atropine or traumatic mydriasis (Küchle 1969), one speaks of total pupilloplegia.

Incomplete absolute pupilloplegia: The pupillary reaction is reduced and incomplete. The pupil is more than mid-dilated, but still reacts somewhat to light convergence and drugs.

Pseudoreflectory pupilloplegia (see page 324): This also belongs in the group of incomplete, absolute pupilloplegia. Etiology: residual of total oculomotor paresis (especially after trauma), post herpes zoster ophthalmicus. In contrast to loss of the light reaction, miosis on convergence is maintained.

Unilateral pupillary disturbances speak in favor of a peripheral etiology.

Poisoning: Absolute pupilloplegia can result from localized or systemic action (poisoning) of belladonna preparations, scopolamine and botulism. Strong sympathomimetics can cause absolute pupilloplegia.

Diseases of the brain: Absolute pupilloplegia can be caused by disturbances in the Edinger-Westphal nucleus, the oculomotor nerve, ciliary ganglion or pupillary sphincter. The primary central nervous system cause of absolute pupilloplegia is syphilis (cerebrospinal, vascular, progressive paralytic, meningitic). After *lues*, the most common etiology is *epidemic encephalitis* (lethargica) which is also a common cause of postencephalitic parkinsonism.

Congenital ciliary ganglion damage from varicella or zoster can lead to pupillary and accommodative paresis.

Tumors and aneurysm can lead to absolute pupilloplegia through damage of the oculomotor nerve.

Other etiologies of absolute pupilloplegia include **trauma** to the globe (potentially with iris sphincter tears) and **acute glaucoma.** Usually, *accommodation is paralyzed* (internal ophthalmoplegia) with the pupil.

If damage to the oculomotor nerve (see page 55) develops gradually, e.g., from intracranial pressure, the pupillary fibers are usually the first to be affected causing pupillary dilatation and decreased reactivity. This is followed by ptosis, then by paresis of other ocular muscles. Intracranial pressure elevation may cause transient irritative miosis before paralytic mydriasis occurs because of the sensitivity of the parasympathetic fibers. An example would be the appearance of a clivus edge syndrome with increasing stupor 12 to 36 hours after injury. This phase is followed by a fixed dilated pupil. In the case of a fresh head injury neurosurgical decompression should be done before the pupil becomes fixed and dilated.

Progressive pupilloplegia is an important sign in lateralizing an *epi-* or *subdural hematoma*. In traumatic head injuries, with a unilateral, fixed dilated pupil a clear sensorium is diagnostically significant. This indicates that the loss of muscle functions regulated by the third nerve is due to oculomotor nerve paresis and not a clivus edge syndrome. With damage in the region of the cavernous sinus (aneurysms, thrombosis) or superior orbital fissure (tumors) the sympathetic nerve supply (miosis, poor dilatation) may be involved in addition to the more usual loss of internal and external ocular muscle function (ophthalmoplegia totalis).

Stupor, epileptic fits: A catatonic pupil may develop in advanced degress of *stupor*. There is a *variable degree* of *pupillary dilatation* and no light reaction. The pupil may be slightly distorted. During an *epileptic* seizure the pupil is markedly dilated (spastic) and nonreactive to light.

Coma: in diabetic, uremic, apoplectic, meningitic, or alcoholic coma the pupils may be widely dilated and nonreactive to light.

Hippus

Hippus is a rhythmic variation of several millimeters in the pupillary diameter taking place over a few seconds. It may be caused by increased irritability of the autonomic nervous system.

Distorted Pupil

Inflammatory anterior and posterior synechiae with iritis or iridocyclitis cause pupillary distortion. Traumatic tears of the iris sphincter, specifically with iridodialysis and pupilloplegia, also result in a distorted pupil. The pupil also tends to be distorted after an acute glaucoma attack. The pupil is usually distorted to some extent with varying types of pupilloplegia (absolute, Argyll Robertson, Adie's pupil). Pupillary ectropion (supertractio uveae iridis) as occurs with rubeosis iridis, leads to pupillary distortion, as does iridoschisis and progressive mesodermal iris atrophy. Benign and malignant tumors of the iris (and anterior portion of the ciliary body) lead to localized pupillary distortion, potentially with loss of mobility in the involved sector.

References

Behr, C., in Wilbrand and Saenger: Die Neurologie des Auges. Ergänzungsband Part 1 p. 214, Bergman München 1927

Duke-Elder, Sir St.: The Pupillary and Ciliary Systems. System of Ophthalmology XII. Henry Kimpton, London 1971 (pp. 597–711)

Förster, O., O. Gagel: Die Vorderseitenstrangdurchschneidung beim Menschen. Zeitschr. ges. Neurol. Psychiatr. 138 (1932) 1–92

Harms, H.: Hemianopische Pupillenstarre. Klin. Mbl. Augenheilk. 118 (1951) 133–147

Küchle, H. J.: Pupillenstörungen. Almanach für die Augenheilkunde. Lehmann, München 1969 (pp. 93–106)

Kyrieleis, W.: Pupillotonie und Adie-Syndrom. Sammlung. Zwangl. Abhandlungen Augenheilk. VEB Marhold, Halle 1951

Kyrieleis, W.: Familiäre Anisokorie. Klin. Mbl. Augenheilk. 133 (1958) 769–776

Kyrieleis, W.: Die Pupille. In: Augenarzt, Vol. 2, Velhagen. Thieme, Leipzig 1959

Loewenfeld, J. E., H. St. Thompson: The tonic pupil; a re-evaluation. Amer. J. Ophthal. 63 (1967) 46–87

Merté, H. J.: Arbeitsmedizinische Fragen in der Ophthalmologie. Karger, Basel 1969

Merté, H. J.: Arbeits- u. Sozialmedizin. In: Lehrbuch der Augenheilkunde, ed. by T. Axenfeld, H. Pau. Fischer, Stuttgart 1973

Schaknowitsch, A. R., N. N. Burdenko: Hemianopic reactions of the pupils of the pathways at different levels. Vop. Neurochir. 5 (1960) 20–25

Thompson, H. S., D. A. Newsome, I. E. Loewenfeld: The fixed dilated pupil. Sudden iridoplegia or mydriatic drops? A simple diagnostic test. Am. Arch. Ophthalm. 86 (1971) 21–27

Thompson, H. S.: Medikamentöse Pupillendiagnostik. Symposium Dtsch. Ophth. Ges. Bad Nauheim, 1972: Die normale und die gestörte Pupillenbewegung. Bergmann, München 1973

25 Orbit and Globe

Variations in Orbital Contents

Using the cornea, normal values for protrusion of the globe anterior to the outer orbital rim are between 11 and 24 mm, as measured with a Hertel exophthalmometer. Exact values depend on orbital anatomy and age.

Exophthalmos — Enophthalmos — Anophthalmos and microphthalmos — Cyclopia — Methods of examination.

Exophthalmos (see page 331)

Protrusio bulbi (exophthalmos) is caused by an increase in orbital contents as with adipose tissue, blood, inflammation, tumors or bony hypertrophy. Laxity of the rectus muscles which normally retract the globe also results in exophthalmos.
Tumors and all other causes of exophthalmos create mechanical (or paretic) restriction of mobility with resultant diplopia (see Disturbances of extraocular muscles).

Enophthalmos

Loss of orbital content from fat atrophy, fluid loss or traumatic displacement of bone results in enophthalmos. *Etiology:* orbital fat atrophy with age. Fluid loss accompanies cholera, cachexia, age and starvation. Cicatricial scarring of orbital fat follows trauma and hemorrhage. Fractures with bony wall displacement (traumatic enophthalmos) occur, often with diplopia (for example, blow-out = entrapment of inferior rectus = restriction of upgaze). Sympathetic lesions: Horner's syndrome (miosis, ptosis, enophthalmos).

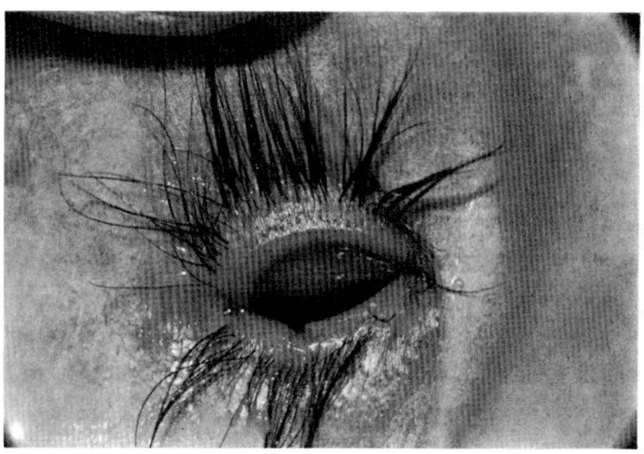

Fig. 25.1 Anophthalmus, coloboma of the lower lid, long eyelashes (♂ 6 yrs.)

Anophthalmos, Microphthalmos, Cryptophthalmos

Anophthalmos or microphthalmos can simulate enophthalmos. In cryptophthalmos the lids, cilia and lid fissure are absent. Microphthalmos or "incomplete anophthalmos" is usually present. The defect is generally bilateral. If unilateral, the other eye is frequently microphthalmic with a narrowed interpalpebral fissure.

Heredity — Embryopathies — Systemic diseases — Retrolental fibroplasia — Chromosomal anomalies (trisomies, etc.) — Phthisis bulbi.

Heredity: Anophthalmos (Fig. 25.1) and microphthalmos can be *inherited* (Scouras et al. 1970).
Embryopathies (see page 244) have to be considered with anophthalmos or microphthalmos.
The most common findings in the rubella syndrome are: cataracts, microphthalmos, glaucoma, pepper and salt fundus (retinopathy), posterior synechiae, nystagmus, strabismus (Alfano 1966).
Thalidomide embryopathy caused by ingestion of the drug 40 to 42 days after the last menstruation causes microphthalmos, anoph-

thalmos and severe malformations of the extremities.

Maternal vitamin A deficiency can lead to colobomas and microphthalmos in the fetus.

Microphthalmos, corneal and lens opacities, persistent hyaloid artery, and systemic malformations occur in familial hemolytic icterus.

Systemic diseases: Microcephaly is frequently associated with microphthalmos, optic atrophy, cataract, colobomata and chorioretinitis.

Bilateral microphthalmos may be seen in mandibulo-facial dysostosis (Hallermann-Streiff) (see page 332), oculo-dento-digital dysplasia (Meyer-Schwickerath et al. 1967) (see page 334), Marinesco-Sjögren syndrome (which also includes spinocerebellar ataxia, oligophrenia, strabismus, and cataracts), oculo-vertebral dysplasia (Weyers and Thier) and the oculo-auricular vertebral syndrome (Goldenhar).

Besides myopia, ocular findings include microphthalmos. The Pierre-Robin syndrome consists of micrognathia and glossoptosis.

Norrie's disease is described as sex-linked, recessive, congenital, hereditary retinal detachment (see page 235) with subsequent development (two months) of anterior and posterior synechiae and iris atrophy. There is a gray vascularized membrane behind the lens. The cornea becomes opaque within one year and cataract forms within two years. The globe finally atrophies. Mental retardation and deafness are common (Warburg 1963; Townes and Roca 1973).

Besides progressive aplastic anemia, Fanconi's anemia includes: microencephaly, skin pigmentation, vitiligo, cardiac anomalies, deafness and, in the eye, strabismus and microphthalmos (Badtke 1961).

Ocular changes in incontinentia pigmenti (Siemens-Bloch-Sulzberger syndrome) include (Krümmel and Rausch 1955): strabismus, cataract, pseudoglioma, retinal neovascularization, phthisis bulbi, blue sclera, and optic atrophy.

Retrolental fibroplasia can lead to microphthalmos (see page 235).

Chromosomal aberrations are frequently associated with microphthalmos.

Chromosomal disorders (Zellweger 1965; François et al. 1974):

Autosomes

Numerous trisomies are possible; the majority, however, are lethal. The three most common clinically are: trisomy 13–15 or Patau's syndrome, trisomy 17–18 or Edward's syndrome, and trisomy 21 or Down's syndrome (mongolism).

1. *Mongolism* (Down's syndrome), *trisomy 21* (G-trisomy, 13–15/21), translocation (D/G), translocation 21/22 and 21/21 (G/G), mosaic mongolism is the most common autosomal aberration. Incidence is 1:600 births.

Ocular findings include: *epicanthus, iris hypoplasia, cataract, strabismus, myopia, keratoconus, also acute hydrops.*

2. *Trisomy D* (13–15) (Patau's syndrome) and trisomy 18 (E) lead to severe changes in the central nervous system, heart, intestinal tract, polydactyly, etc. These children usually die within the first weeks of life.

Ocular findings with trisomy D include: *microphthalmos, iris coloboma, cataracts, retrolental membranes* (PHPV), *anophthalmia, retinal dysplasia, hypo- and aplasia of the optic nerve,* intraocular cartilage.

3. With *E trisomy* (18) (Edwards' syndrome): *ptosis* and *rarely ocular changes as with trisomy D.* Other findings include micrognathia, pigeon breast, and ventriculum septal defects.

4. *Monosomy* 21: *antimongoloid fissures,* micrognathia, mental retardation, *malformation* and *aplasia of the eyes,* heart, urogenital and skeletal systems.

5. *Cri-du-chat syndrome, Lejeune's syndrome (cat's cry syndrome):* lack of the short arm of chromosome B 5 (5p-), microcephaly, moon facies, micro- and retrognathia, *hypertelorism,* deep pinnae, catlike cry, muscular hypotony and idiocy (Howard 1972).

6. *De Grouchy syndrome:* lack of the short arm of chromosome E 18 (18p-), retarded growth, *ptosis,* large low projecting ears, micrognathia, caries, and idiocy.

7. *Hirschhorn-Cooper syndrome:* loss of the short arm of chromosome B 4 (4p-): microcephaly, brain malformations, *iris coloboma, hypertelorism, ptosis,* dysplastic pinnae, micrognathia and mental retardation.

Aberrations of the sex chromosomes (gonosomes) can be determined by the "Barr test."

Table 25.1 Most Important Alterations of the Eye Possible in Chromosomal Anomalies (from Schade)

	Trisomy 21 Down's Syndrome	Trisomy D Patau's Syndrome	Trisomy E Edward's Syndrome	Chromosome B 5 Deletion Lejeune's Syndrome	C/F Translocation	XO Ullrich-Turner Syndrome	XXX	XXY Klinefelter's Syndrome	XXXXY
1. Position of the palpebral fissures	↗	↗		↘		↘			
2. Hypertelorism	+	+	+	+					+
3. Epicanthus	+		+	+					+
4. Anophthalmia/ microphthalmia		+!			(+)				
5. Strabismus	+			+		+			+
6. Coloboma		(+)	(+)						
7. Myopia	(+)					(+)	(+)		+
8. Cataracts	+	+	+			+			
9. Blepharitis	+!								
10. Brushfield's spots	+!								
11. Ptosis			(+)						

Aneuploidy of the sex chromosomes results in the following:

8. *Klinefelter's syndrome* (XXY): chromatin positive, male phenotype, eunuchoid appearance, potentially mental retardation or even idiocy. XXXXY Klinefelter's syndrome patients often demonstrate *hypertelorism, epicanthus, strabismus* and *myopia.*

9. *Turner's syndrome* (XO): chromatin (Barr body) negative, secondary sex characteristics absent, female phenotype. *Hypoplastic optic discs* and *retinal vascular anomalies* occur (see pages 89, 305).

10. *The triple X syndrome* (XXX): chromatin double positive, female phenotype, may lead to debility and seizures.

11. *Testicular feminization* (XY): chromatin negative, female phenotype, female external genitalia, lack of uterus and ovaries.

12. XYY, male phenotype, chromatin negative, tall, debilitated, antisocial behavior.

Phthisis bulbi: acquired microphthalmos occurs with phthisis bulbi resulting from panophthalmitis, endophthalmitis, intraocular hemorrhage, perforating injuries, surgery, etc.

Cyclopia

There are varying degrees of fusion of orbit and globe.

Methods of Investigation

The degree of protrusion of the eyes is measured with the exophthalmometer (Hertel). Examination of ocular motility is important (see page 47). Space-occupying lesions and bony fractures located anteriorly in the orbits may be palpated. The ability to push the globe backwards in the orbit can be measured with a piezometer (for example as per Jaeger), also known as an orbitonometer. In this test pressure is exerted on the eye of the recumbent patient who is looking straight ahead. Nover (1959) found backward displacement of the globe to range between 2.25 and 12.75 mm. The amount the globe can be displaced backward is elevated with pulsating exophthalmos or orbital varices. It is somewhat increased with paresis of the ocular muscles but is decreased with elevated intraocular pressure over 60 mm of mercury and in axial myopia. Retrobulbar tumors (pseudotumor) or inflammatory orbital infiltrates (for example, orbital cellulitis) may be present when, in the face of a normal refraction, the globe cannot be displaced posteriorly.

Besides standard X-rays, useful radiological examination includes visualization of the bony optic canal (as per Rhese), stereo views, and tomography.

Of great importance is the EMI scan. In some cases orbital phlebography may also be helpful.

Carotid angiography is particularly important with intracranial tumors, aneurysms, or arterial venous fistulas.

According to Ossoinig and Seher (1967), echography (A- and B-) is the most reliable method for the diagnosis of orbital tumors. (See examination of tumors, page 341).

Non-Inflammatory Exophthalmos with Developmental Anomalies and Systemic Diseases

(Waardenburg 1961, 1963; Goldberg 1974)

Mandibulofacial dysplasia — Dyscranio-pygophalangea — Oculo-dento-digital dysplasia — Cranial facial dysostoses — Meningeal-encephalocele, Mucocele — Hydrocephalus — Systemic diseases — Wegener's granulomatosis.

Mandibulofacial Dysplasia

Of the mandibulofacial dysplasias, i.e., malformation in the first branchial arch segment, those important to the ophthalmologists include (Thier 1959):

Mandibulofacial dysostosis (Franceschetti-Zwahlen) — Ocular-auricular dysplasia (Goldenhar) — Oculo-vertebral dysplasia (Weyer-Thier) — Oculo-mandibulofacial dysmorphia (Hallermann) — Oculo-mandibulofacial dyscephaly.

Mandibulofacial dysostosis (Franceschetti-Zwahlen 1944) (Treacher Collins):

Mandibulofacial dysostosis has a fishlike facies or "Greek profile" (Fig. 25.2).

The lid fissure is slanted from up to down and outward (anti-mongoloid slant). A coloboma of the lower lid is located at the outer third of the lid (Fig. 25.3). Zygomatic hypoplasia, high gums, macrostomia, and dental anomalies are other findings. Malformations near the ear include fistulas, pre-auricular tags, malformations of the pinna and mandibular hypoplasia. A lid coloboma may be the only finding in incomplete forms of the syndrome. Heredity: irregular dominant.

Oculo-auricular dysplasia: Findings in the oculo-auricular dysplasia syndrome of Goldenhar (1952) (Fig. 25.4) include epibulbar dermoids or fibrodermoids located subconjunctivally near the limbus as well as pre-auricular fistulas or tags (Fig. 25.4). Malformations of the pinna of the ear and lid colobomas occur in some cases (see Heimann 1968; Holl-

Table 25.2 Clinical findings of dysplasias in the region of the embryonic first branchial arch (after C. J. Thier)

without involvement of the globe			with involvement of the globe		
mandibular dysostosis	oculo auricular dysplasia	mandibulo facial dysostosis	Oculo mandibulo facial dysmorphia	extensive form → oculo-mandibulo-facial dyscephaly	oculo vertebral dysplasia
Nager and de Reynier 1948	Goldenhar 1952	Franceschetti and Zwahlen 1944	Hallermann 1948; and Streiff 1950	Ullrich and Fremerey-Dohna 1953	Weyers and Thier 1958
1. antimongoloid lid fissures 2. malformations of the pinna of the ear 3. hypoplasia of the ascending mandibular ramus 4. aplasia of the mandibular joint	1. epibulbar dermoids 2. macrostomia 3. pre-auricular fistulas 4. pre-auricular skin tags 5. malformations of the pinna	1. antimongoloid lid slant 2. lower lid colobomata 3. zygomatic hypoplasia 4. macrostomia 5. malpositioned teeth 6. micrognathia 7. malformation of the pinna 8. pre-auricular fistulas 9. pre-auricular tags	1. microphthalmos 2. congenital cataract 3. hypotrichosis 4. parrot's beak nose 5. extreme micrognathia 6. malpositioned teeth	1–6 as in the Hallermann-Streiff syndrome 7. dyscephaly 8. nanism 9. atrophic skin 10. cranial suture anomalies	1. microphthalmos 2. maxillary hyperplasia 3. macrostomia 4. malpositioned teeth 5. vertebral and rib anomalies

wich and Verbeck 1969). This syndrome is usually unilateral; other findings may include: mandibulofacial dysostosis, lid coloboma, choroidal coloboma, microphthalmos, etc.

The **oculo-vertebral syndrome** (oculo-vertebral dysplasia) (Weyers and Thier 1958) belongs in the group of the mandibulofacial dysplasias. There is usually a unilateral (rarely bilateral) microphthalmos, rarely enophthalmos, unilateral maxillary hypoplasia and facial asymmetry, macrostomia and vertebral anomalies (kyphoscoliosis, wedge-shaped vertebrae, hemivertebrae).

Oculo-mandibulo facial dysmorphia (bird facies) (Hallermann 1948; Streiff 1950) (Fig. 25.5): there is bilateral microphthalmia with congenital cataracts or, sometimes, late-acquired cataracts (Pau 1950) along with extreme micrognathia, dental anomalies and a protruding parrot-beak-like nose.

Oculo-mandibulofacial dyscephaly (Ullrich and Fremerey-Dohna 1953): dyscephaly, microphthalmos, dwarfism, proportional nanism, vertebral anomalies, hypertrichosis and skin atrophy accompany bird facies, microphthalmos and, potentially, blue scleras and cataracts.

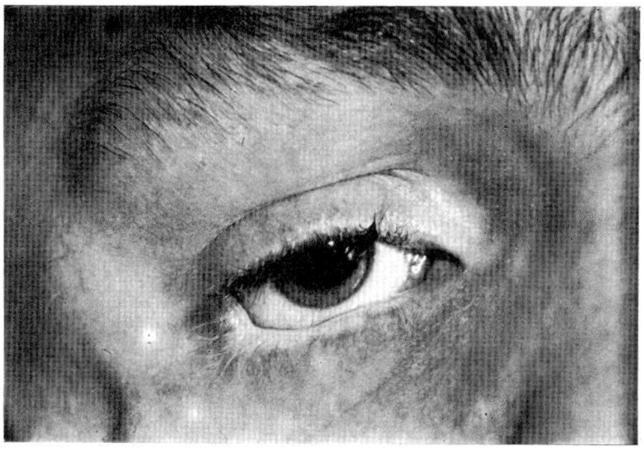

Fig. 25.3 Dysostosis mandibulofacialis, lid axis antimongoloid orientated, lateral coloboma of the lower lid (same patient as in Fig. 25.2)

Dyscranio-Pygo-Phalangea

In this group Ullrich includes (Badtke 1961):

1. Ullrich-Turner syndrome
2. Typus- amstelodamensis = Cornelia de Lange syndrome
3. Typus-Rostockiensis = dyscranio-pygo-phalangea
4. Cranio-carpo-tarsal dystrophy (Freeman-Sheldon)

Ocular findings in *Turner's syndrome* (see chromosomal anomalies) include *hypoplasia of the optic disc* and *retinal vascular anomalies.* There is an abnormal sex chromosome (XO) karyotype.

Cornelia de Lange's syndrome (typus amstelodamensis = de Lange 1938) includes *brachy-*

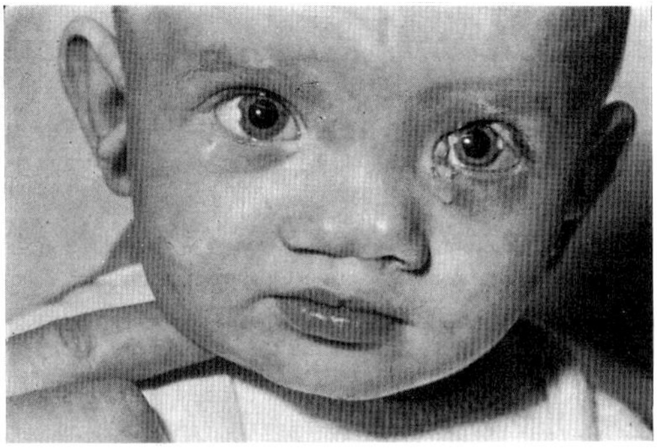

Fig. 25.4 Dyplasia oculo-auricularis (Goldenhar), bilateral epibulbar dermoids, colobomata of the lids, bilateral preauricular appendices (6 months)

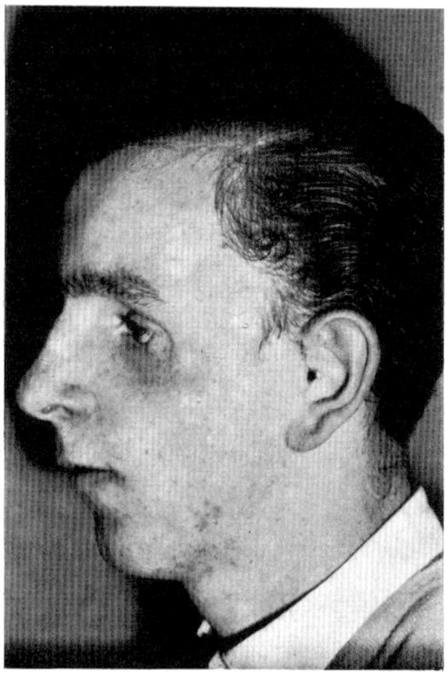

Fig. 25.2 Dysostosis mandibulo-facilis (Franceschetti) = fishlike face (♂ 16 yrs.)

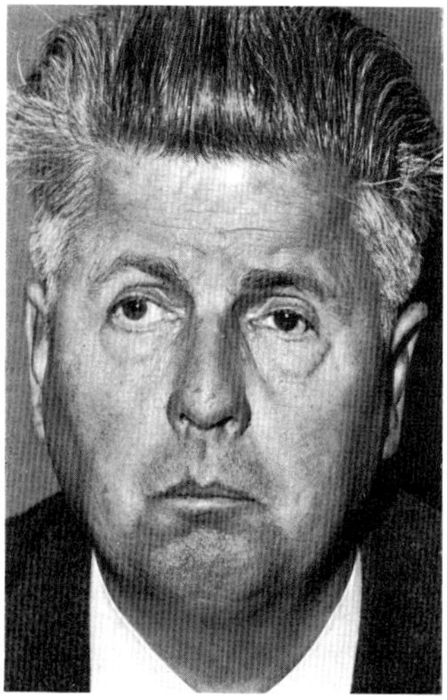

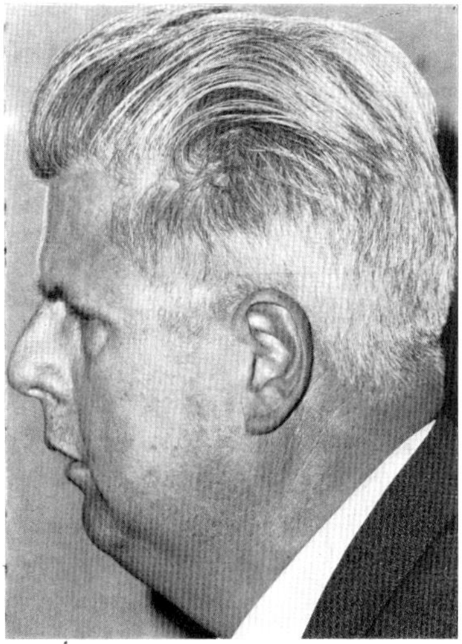

Fig. 25.5 a and b "Birdlike face" with cataract and micrognathia

cephaly, fusion of the eyebrows, long lashes, epicanthus, hypertelorism, anti-mongoloid slant, a small nose, hypoplastic mandible and syndactyly.

The *typus rostockiensis,* or marked *dyscranial pygo-phalangea* (Meyer-Schwickerath et al. 1957), includes microphthalmos, enophthalmos, small lid fissure, iris coloboma, pre-auricular tags, malformation of the ear, tower skull or shortened skull, micrognathia, polydactyly (rudimentary sixth finger or toe), cryptorchism, vaginal septa, cardiac anomalies and malformations of the brain. As a rule, this condition is incompatible with life. There is a parallelism to the recessively inherited aplastic anemia with multiple malformations – the so-called Fanconi's anemia.

The *cranio-carpo-tarsal dystrophy* of Freeman and Sheldon shows a picture similar to the typus amstelodamensis. In addition, there is a keratinized thickening of the skin and subcutaneous tissue on the dorsal surface over the first phalanges.

Acrocephalo-syndactyly of Apert (Badtke 1961) includes: pointed head, maxillary hypoplasia and syndactyly. Ocular findings may include: exophthalmos, exotropia, hypertelorism, papilledema and optic nerve atrophy.

Oculo-Dento-Digital Dysplasia

Oculo-dento-digital dysplasia as described by Meyer-Schwickerath et al. (1957) includes bilateral ocular malformation (microphthalmos), dental anomalies (hypoplasia of the tooth enamel) and malformation of the extremities (syndactyly, polydactyly). Heredity may be autosomal dominant (Pfeiffer et al. 1968).

Cranio-Facial Dysostoses

Cranio-facial dysostoses, or tower skull group, have shallow orbits.

Tower skull with Crouzon's disease — Scaphocephaly — Triangular head — Slanting head — Hypertelorism.

Tower skull and Crouzon's disease: Premature synostosis of all cranial sutures, particularly the coronal suture, results in a compensatory vertical growth of the skull leading to a tower skull or oxycephaly, pygocephaly, as well as the cranio-facial dysostosis of Crouzon. Exophthalmos appears by ages two to five years in 50 percent of cases of *tower skull.* Rarely, this may be so severe as to lead to luxation of the globe in front of the lid. Exophthalmos, nystagmus and papilledema with secondary optic atrophy are more common. In one-third of the cases there is a varying degree of vision loss, rarely total blindness. Men are predominantly affected (four-fifths of all cases).

A special form of *cranio-facial dysostosis* is that of *Crouzon* (Figs. 25.6, 25.7). Ocular findings are the same as with tower skull. Crouzon's disease is differentiated from the other forms of tower skull by a more marked dystrophy of the maxilla and face with prognathism. The hooked nose resembles a parrot's beak.

In the hereditary cranio-facial dysostoses (Crouzon) with brachycephaly one can also find increased separation of the globes (hypertelorism). Mental retardation is common.

Crouzon's disease usually begins within the first months of life. Heredity is generally dominant.

Tower skull may be associated with syndactyly (acrocephalic syndactyly of Apert) and potentially with skeletal anomalies.

Keel-shaped head, scaphocephaly: Premature ossification of the sagittal suture results in a keel- or boat-shaped (scaphocephalic or sphenocephalic) skull. Brachycephaly (the short skull) and dolichocephaly (the long skull) can be categorized in this group.

Triangular head: A triangular head results when the frontal suture is prematurely synostosed = trigonocephaly (with the peak extending anteriorly and excessive protrusion of the back of the head).

Slant head: A slant head oriented to one side or the other occurs when there is variable premature closure of the sutures (plagiocephaly). Flat head is called platycephaly or clinocephaly.

Hypertelorism (Figs. 25.6, 7, 9), or the Greig syndrome (Greig 1924; Gross 1956), is an abnormal separation of the orbits.

Hypertelorism may lead to separation of the medial canthi of up to 50 mm (normal 18 to 30 mm). The eyes appear as if they were pressed towards the side of the face. The root of the nose is flat and broad, and the skull is short and broad with a low, protruding forehead (Günther 1943/44; Friede 1954). The disorder is commonly inherited (Bojlen and Brehms 1938), possibly in a dominant fashion. Hypertelorism is regarded as a symptom of craniocerebral dysraphia and the tower skull craniodysostoses.

Hypertelorism and epicanthus are common in reno-facial dysplasia (Potter's syndrome) (see page 89).

Hypertelorism also occurs in chromosomal disorders: Turner's syndrome includes pterygium colli, lymphangectatic edema of the hands and feet, III, VI, VII, XII nerve pareses, hypertelorism, epicanthus and syndactyly. Hypertelorism is also observed in: cat's cry syndrome, Hirschhorn-Cooper syndrome, and Klinefelter's syndrome (see page 330).

Meningeal Encephalocele, Mucocele

Meningeal encephalocele owing to bony defects (Fig. 25.8) is rare in the region of the orbits. These usually lie superior nasally and are a soft elastic flocculent protrusion. Frequently they pulsate with the brain and increase in size on straining or crying. The bony defects can often be seen radiologically. Mucoceles (Fig. 25.16) can result from entrapment of secretions in the sinuses. This results in bony erosion and extension of the mucocele, which causes exophthalmos or displacement of the globe.

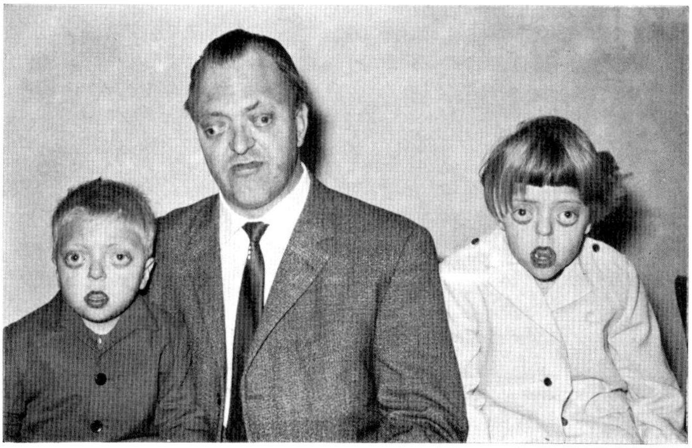

Fig. 25.6 Craniofacial dysostoses of Crouzon in a father (41 yrs.), daughter (6 yrs.) and son (3 yrs.). Hypertelorism, exophthalmos, exotropia, optic atrophy

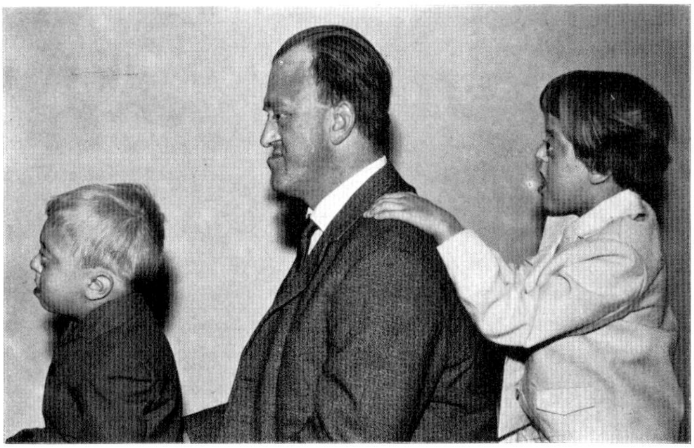

Fig. 25.7 (see Fig. 25.6)

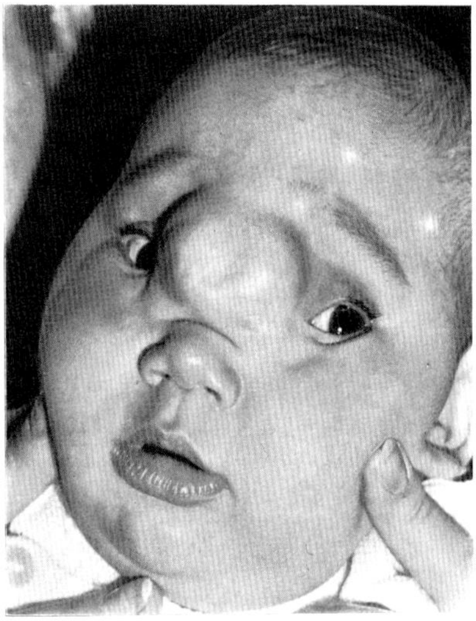

Fig. 25.8 Meningeal encephalocele with narrowing of the orbit and hypertelorism (♀ 6 months)

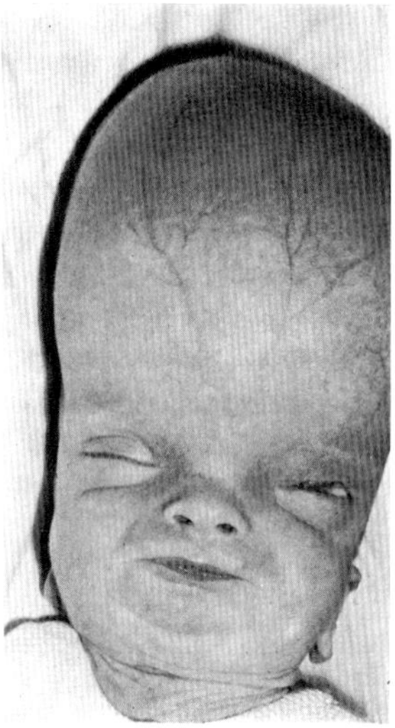

Fig. 25.9 Hydrocephalus with decrease in size of the orbit, hypertelorism and exophthalmos

Internal Hydrocephalus

This leads to a decrease in the size of the orbit. The orbital roof acquires a lower position in hydrocephalus and may result in exophthalmos (Fig. 25.9). Pressure exerted by the distended third ventricle can lead to optic nerve atrophy.

Systemic Diseases

Cystic fibrous osteitis — Osteitis deformans Paget — Polyostotic fibrous dysplasia — Marble bone disease (Albers-Schönberg) — Hand-Schüller-Christian disease — Eosinophilic granuloma — Niemann-Pick disease.

The rare **cystic fibrous osteitis** (Recklinghausen) is a generalized systemic disease probably of endocrine origin. Women between ages twenty and forty are primarily affected.

In contrast, **osteitis deformans,** or Paget's disease, afflicts older persons (60 to 70 yrs.) with localized changes even in those cases with polyostotic involvement. The bones of the skull are involved in approximately 30 percent of cases (leontiasis ossea) (Fig. 25.10). Radiologically there is a typical spotty cottonlike appearance to the markedly thickened bones of the skull. Exophthalmos, exotropia, extraocular paresis and optic nerve atrophy are further findings.

Exophthalmos may also occur with **polyostotic fibrous dysplasia** (fibrous osteodystrophy, disseminated fibrous osteitis, familial polyostotic osteodystrophy). When round or maplike skin pigmentations and precocious puberty occur, the Albright-McCune-Sternberg syndrome or Albright syndrome is the case. Besides exophthalmos, optic atrophy and zonular cataracts may occur (Badtke 1961).

Marble bone disease (Albers-Schönberg) or *osteopetrosis,* specifically *osteosclerosis congenita fragilis generalisata* frequently leads to bilateral optic atrophy, divergent strabismus, exophthalmos and facial asymmetry (Pietruschka 1953).

Radiologically, one finds osteosclerosis as well as bony fragility, anemia, hypersplenism, dwarfism, inner ear deafness and anomalies of the nails. Heredity is dominant.

In the **Hand-Schüller-Christian disease,** a typical triad occurs: exophthalmos, caput geographicum and diabetes insipidus.

There is a generalized accumulation of cholesterol in tissues and secondary granuloma formation. The granulomatous lipid infiltration of the orbital wall can lead to exophthalmos as well as paresis of extraocular muscles and papilledema. X-rays reveal translucent areas in the skull as well as the large bones (xantho-

Fig. 25.10 a–d Paget's disease (from: R. Thiel, Atlas of Diseases of the Eye, 6th Ed., Thieme, Stuttgart 1963)

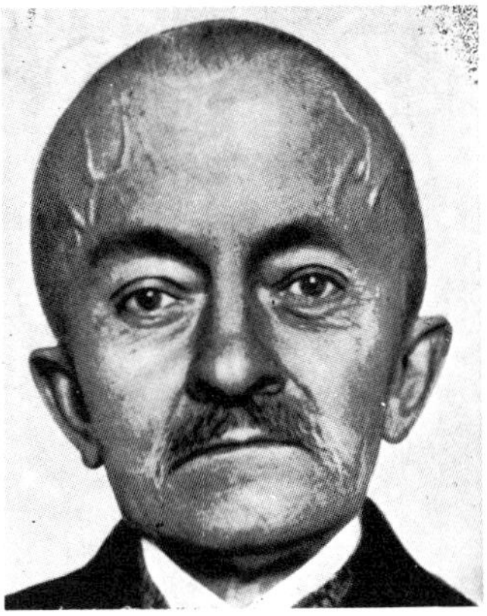

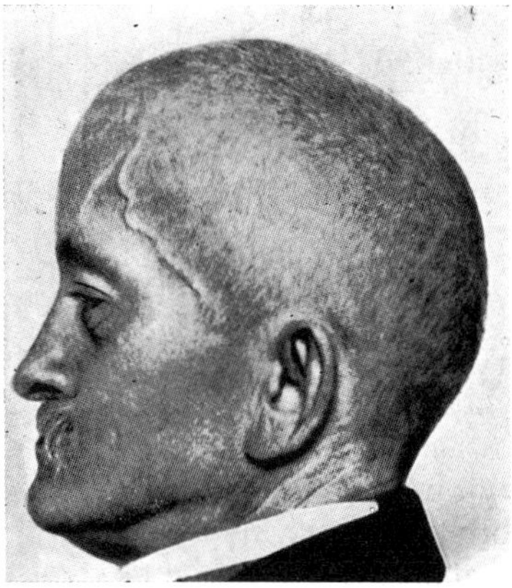

Fig. 25.10 a and b Diffuse symmetrical enlargement of the skull. Flat protrusions can be felt on the surface of the skull; distension and tortuosity of both temporal veins; early optic atrophy

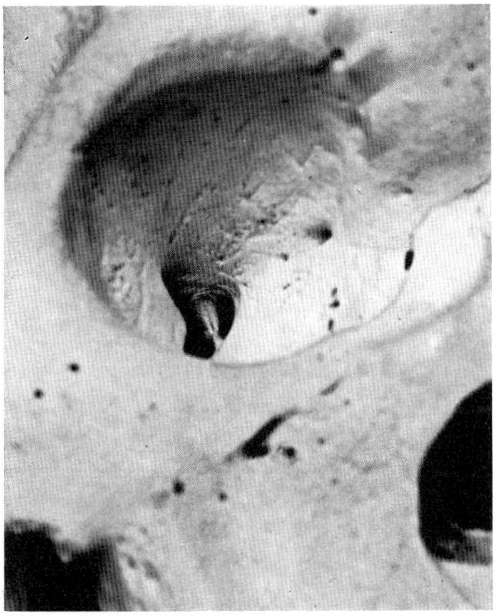

Fig. 25.10 c Autopsy specimen. Narrowing of the left bony optic canal owing to nodular bony thickening. Narrowing of the superior orbital fissure

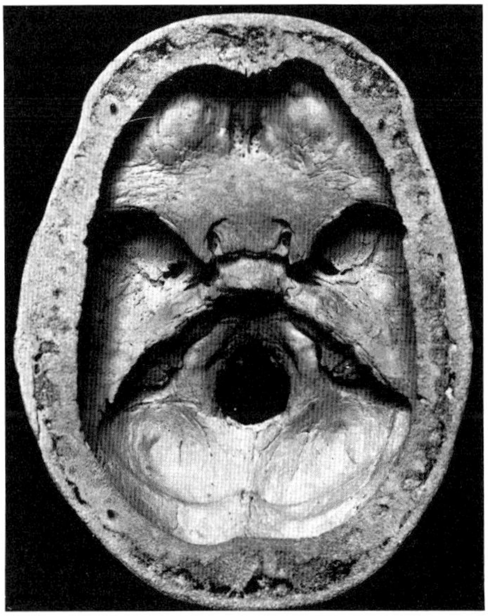

Fig. 25.10 d Base of the skull. Thickening of the wall of the skull, espacially between the cortical tables. The bones of the anterior and middle fossas show surface thickening and clumpy contours

matous granulomata). The young children afflicted with this disorder frequently exhibit unilateral exophthalmos (Fleischer 1942).

The **eosinophilic granuloma** (Jaffe and Lichtenstein) belongs in the group of chronic inflammations. It occurs preferentially in the cranial part of the facial bones. Eosinophilic granuloma consists of reticuloendothelial proliferation with deposition of eosinophilic leukocytes and multi-nucleated giant cells. Hemorrhages, necrosis, plasma cell and lymphocyte accumulation also occur. In three-fourths of cases, the eosinophilic granuloma begins at the upper orbital rim. According to Koenig et al. (1964), isolated orbital lesions occurred in 78 percent of cases and a further extraorbital location appeared in 22 percent of cases. Etiologically, viruses, trauma and local antigen-antibody reactions have been proposed. Eosinophilic granuloma is considered to represent a monofocal variant of the Hand-Schüller-Christian disease (Gornick 1968).

Ocular findings in **Niemann-Pick disease** (sphingomyelin lipidosis, phosphatide lipidosis) may include infantile amaurotic idiocy with a cherry-red macular spot and gray edema of the surrounding retina (similar to central retinal artery occlusion) (Plate XXVII, Fig. 6, page 288 c), nystagmus, and rarely exophthalmos (see page 365).

Wegener's Granulomatosis

Wegener's granulomatosis belongs more to the chronic inflammations (Böke and Reich 1967; Straatsma 1957). Ocular involvement may result from *direct extension* of the disorder to the orbit from the sinuses. This leads to exophthalmos, extraocular muscle disturbances and conjunctival chemosis. Papilledema may occur.

Ocular involvement secondary to *hematogenous spread:* granulomatous necrotizing inflammatory processes may appear as paralimbal infiltrates or ulcers which can progress to necrosis in the area of the conjunctiva and sclera with uveal prolapse. Less frequently, there is a uveitis and retinal involvement (emboli, cotton wool spots, retinal detachment). Wegener's granulomatosis belongs in the group of collagenoses or autoimmune disorders (see page 184).

Non-Inflammatory Pseudo Exophthalmos

Exophthalmos may be simulated (pseudo exophthalmos) by an abnormally long globe as occurs with high myopia or hydrophthalmos (buphthalmos = congenital glaucoma, see page 225). With Horner's syndrome the enopthalmos of the affected eye may lead to the mistaken diagnosis of exophthalmos of the sound eye. *Hemi-facial atrophy,* which is actually a failure of one side of the face to develop normally, may simulate exophthalmos on the normal side. A congenital cystic eye will also simulate exophthalmos (Dollfus et al. 1968). Retraction of the upper lid in endocrine ophthalmopathy may give the impression of a protruding globe. Paresis of one or more of the rectus muscles leads to anterior displacement of the globe.

Non-Inflammatory Exophthalmos with Retrobulbar Hematomas and Trauma

Retrobulbar Hematoma

Retrobulbar hematomas occur in a variety of conditions including hematologic disorders, hemophilia, Müller-Barlow-Scorbut disease, neuroblastoma, alterations in the vessel walls (arteriosclerosis, aneurysms, varices), trauma (birth trauma), retrobulbar injections, severe venous stasis from thoracic compression, strangulation, whooping cough, vicarious menstrual bleeding, etc.

Traumatic Exophthalmos

Traumatic exophthalmos may result from displacement of bone, or hemorrhage resulting from trauma. Sudden blindness is usually caused by fracture of the bony nerve canal, crushing of the optic nerve, or more or less commonly a hematoma of the nerve sheaths.

Bony fractures — Blow-out fracture — Luxation of the globe — Orbital foreign bodies — Orbital emphysema — Orbital apex syndrome.

Most **orbital fractures** as well as depressed fractures (through the sinuses, potentially with subcutaneous emphysema) result in exophthalmos and tissue edema owing to hemorrhage.

The question of possible brain involvement is important in all cranial fractures or penetrating injuries of the orbit: coma, vomiting, *cerebral signs* (cerebro-spinal fistula).

Classic periorbital ecchymosis attending *basi-*

lar skull fractures usually occurs after 24 hours. There may be no cerebral signs. Traumatic damage with the displacement of the globe and diplopia from extraocular muscle or nerve involvement is common. At first there is exophthalmos (retrobulbar hemorrhage) which usually evolves to enophthalmos over a period of weeks owing to loss of orbital fat and cicatricial scarring. It is surprising how binocular vision can be maintained by appropriate head turns in spite of severe displacement of the globe.

Blow-out fracture (see page 62) results from sudden elevation of intraorbital pressure owing to a blow from a fist, tennis ball, etc. This leads to herniation of orbital tissue into the maxillary sinus through fractures of the orbital floor. The inferior rectus and inferior oblique may or may not be included. Typically, the entrapment of orbital tissue leads to restriction of elevation above the mid-line (Fig. 8.22 a, b) and decrease in depression of the globe. X-rays, especially tomograms, may reveal clouding in the maxillary sinus. This may be obscured by hemorrhages and exudation (Hollwich et al. 1970; Smith and Reagan 1957).

Traumatic exophthalmos presents little differential diagnostic difficulty.

Luxation of the globe: This is a most marked exophthalmos. Mentally deranged patients may avulse their own eyes.

Orbital foreign body: Small orbital foreign bodies (stone, metal, glass) usually heal without irritation. Only large foreign bodies must be removed.

Orbital emphysema: *Non-inflammatory exophthalmos with orbital emphysema* (Fig. 10.31) usually occurs after trauma (lamina papyracea fracture). There is subcutaneous emphysema causing crepitance on palpation. Blowing the nose forces more air into the orbital tissues and under the skin.

Migraines in the region of the first division of the trigeminal nerve are common in the **orbital apex syndrome** (see page 60). This is followed by varying degrees of ophthalmoplegia with loss of the pupillary reaction (see the superior orbital fissure syndrome, page 60). There may be a loss of sensation in the area of the first division of the trigeminal nerve. Papilledema or simple optic atrophy may occur. Exophthalmos is possible. Etiology: tumor, syphilis, trauma (fractures), hemorrhages, sinusitis.

Endocrine Exophthalmos and Myxedema

The cardinal symptoms of Basedow's disease (Graves' disease) include goiter, hyperthyroidism, elevated metabolic rate, tachycardia, tremor and endocrine exophthalmos. Loss of regulatory control of the hypophyseal thyroid axis is at fault. Endocrine exophthalmos is a common finding (Plate XXXI, Fig. 5, page 288 g) and may be unilateral (10 to 20 percent). It is also seen frequently in children (Helmholtz 1926: 83 percent; Dinsmoor 1932: 76 percent; Schwartz 1945: 61.5 percent). In rare cases endocrine exophthalmos is already present at birth and is seen in the newborns of thyrotoxic mothers (Margetts 1950; Hoffmann and Lindquist 1957; and others). With endocrine exophthalmos, the intraocular pressure rises on upgaze, simulating glaucoma. Exophthalmos results from increased production of exophthalmos-producing substance by the hypophysis. Thyroxin retards the formation of the exophthalmos-producing factor. Exophthalmos is caused by edema of orbital tissues and extraocular muscles with cellular proliferation (lymphocytes, leukocytes, mast cells). On downgaze the upper lid lags behind the movement of the globe (Graefe's sign). The upper lid is retracted so that sclera is visible above the cornea (Dalrymple's sign) (this can be physiologic in infancy, Fig. 10.1). There is decreased blinking or lid stare (Stellwag's sign) and convergence is decreased (Möbius' sign). The closed lids are tremulous (Rosenbach's sign) and eversion of the upper lid is more difficult (Gifford's sign). On upgaze the normal contraction of the frontalis muscle is absent (Joffroy's sign). The radioactive iodine

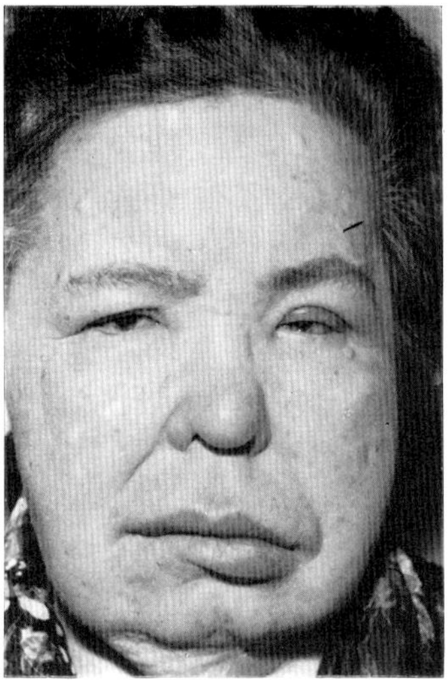

Fig. 25.11 Myxedema with dry scaly skin

uptake test has provided diagnostic help in many cases of endocrine exophthalmos (Horst and Ullerich 1958). Electromyography reveals a myopathy (see page 52). When the exophthalmos is so severe that the lids can no longer be closed (malignant exophthalmos) there is desiccation of the cornea with danger of corneal erosion, even perforation. Surgical, medical or radioactive damage to the thyroid gland can result in the acute appearance of "malignant exophthalmos." Furthermore, there is an increase in the restriction of the extraocular movements with diplopia and a decline in the extent to which the globe can be pressed back into the orbit. Loss of elevation of the eye followed by restriction of horizontal movements is the most common manifestation.

Lead poisoning can involve the thyroid gland resulting in exophthalmos as well as extraocular muscle paresis and optic neuritis.

Exophthalmos may also occur with *acute carbon monoxide poisoning*.

Myxedema (Fig. 25.11): Hypothyroidism can also lead to protrusion of the globe, strabismus, and papilledema. Myxedema is not a true edema because no depression remains after pressing. The skin and mucous membranes are dry and the skin is scaly.

Pulsating Exophthalmos

With pulsating exophthalmos (Plate XXXI, Fig. 6, page 288 g), the following must be differentiated:

1. vascular processes and
2. bony defects and encephaloceles.

1. Vascular processes are usually carotid cavernous sinus aneurysms (traumatic = 80 percent; spontaneous = 20 percent). Ophthalmic aneurysms, (racemose) orbital angiomas, or vascularized tumors (sarcoma) are less common.

2. With bony defects, those which are congenital (orbital roof – sphenoid wing, orbital encephaloceles) must be differentiated from those which are acquired (traumatic, post-surgical).

Vascular Processes

Pulse-synchronous pulsations of the protruding globe are visible in cavernous sinus carotid artery fistulas along with dilatation of retinal, conjunctival and episcleral veins (caput medusae). Subjectively, the patient hears a pulse-synchronous rushing "locomotive" noise which the physician can hear by auscultation over the globe and carotid arteries. Headaches, extraocular muscle paresis (oculomotor, trochlear, abducens), trigeminal nerve damage, vision loss and optic nerve atrophy are further clinical signs.

Etiology: Tearing or rupture of the wall of the internal carotid artery in the cavernous sinus results in an arterial venous aneurysm. This may occur spontaneously (arteriosclerosis, syphilis) or after injury (stab wound, gunshot). Ophthalmic artery aneurysms are rare. Congenital racemose angiomas can cause findings similar to those with carotid cavernous aneurysms. Any carotid angiographically highly vascularized tumor (especially a neoplasm) can lead to pulsations. *X-ray:* destruction of the bony orbit!

Bony Defects

Bony defects allow transmission of the brain's pulsations into the orbit. This results in pulsation of the globe (Bushy 1959). This is particularly true of congenital and acquired orbital encephaloceles.

Intermittent Exophthalmos

Exophthalmos occurs only on bending over, or with restriction of venous drainage by compression of the jugular veins (bending the head forward).
Etiology: congenital or acquired orbital varices. When the patient is upright the blood drains and the exophthalmos declines or disappears. Phleboliths in the orbital varices are occasionally seen radiographically. Retrobulbar cavernous hemangiomas may have an intermittent increase of the exophthalmos owing to temporary changes in their blood content. Radiographically, the involved orbit is usually enlarged both in congenital cavernous angiomas and lymphangiomas.
Rapid onset and progression of exophthalmos with a tumor generally indicates malignancy. Besides venous stasis (pressing, crying, etc.) systemic factors (menstruation, pregnancy) can lead to an increase in exophthalmos.

Orbital, Peri- and Retro-Orbital Tumors and Cysts

Symptomatology — Methods of investigation — Functional disturbances — Cysts and pseudotumor — Meningo-encephalo-mucocele — Teratoma, cholesteatoma, parasites — Orbital tumor.

Symptomatology

Displacement of the globe in the opposite direction from the tumor and mechanical restriction of ocular movement are symptomatic. Paresis of specific nerves or muscles occurs. Papilledema or optic atrophy secondary to pressure, and retinal folds which can be seen on ophthalmoscopy may occur.

Methods of Investigation

Systemic investigation for a primary lesion, hematologic examination for leukemia (leukemic infiltrate, lymphogranuloma, etc.) or syphilis is conventional. *X-ray* examination: calcified tumor – usually meningioma (sphenoidal, etc.); bony defect – malignancies; multiple myeloma – plasmacytoma; cloudy sinuses – suspect tumors of the sinus; circumscribed bony defects with round protrusions – mucocele, meningoencephalocele. The superior orbital fissure or the optic canal may be enlarged (Fig. 25.12, 25.13, 25.14, 25.15). Depending on the clinical findings other studies may be required: arteriography, phlebography of the ophthalmic vein and the angular vein, orbitography with injection of contrast materials behind the globe (or air injection [König 1954]), CAT scan (very important), diagnostic biopsy, neurosurgical investigation.
Ultrasonography of the orbit can differentiate between: various tumors, pseudotumors, cysts, infiltrates, hematomas, emphysema (Ossoinig 1969; Bronson 1973; Coleman 1972). The echogram of a diseased orbit is wider than normal. Orbital lesions are more homogeneous to ultrasound resulting in lower spike heights. Owing to improved conductivity of diseased tissues, the spike height of the abnormal echogram decreases more slowly from the left to right than does the normal. Abnormal orbital echograms are usually less mobile. The surfaces of circumscribed lesions may result in distinct "border" spikes.
Retrodisplacement of the globe using a piezometer becomes more difficult as the degree of exophthalmos increases. Of orbital tumors those nearer the apex provide the greatest resistance. With endocrine exophthalmos, the

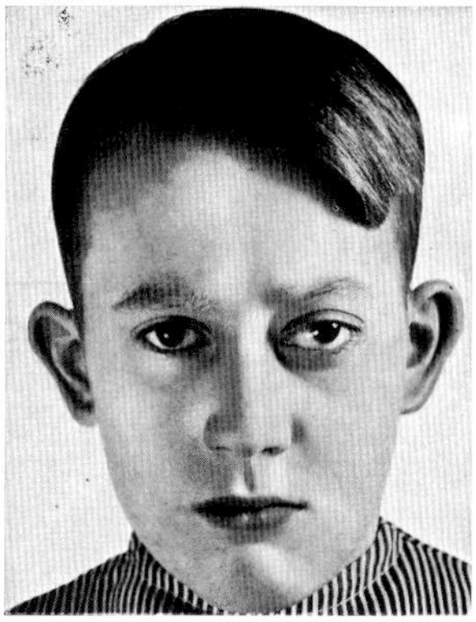

Fig. 25.12 Optic nerve glioma (Figs. 25.12–15 from: R. Thiel, Atlas of Diseases of the Eye, 6th Ed., Thieme, Stuttgart 1963).

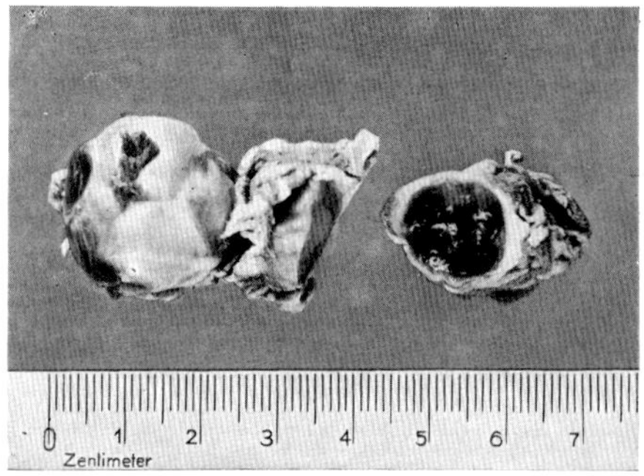

Fig. 25.13 Enucleated globe with a markedly thickened optic nerve

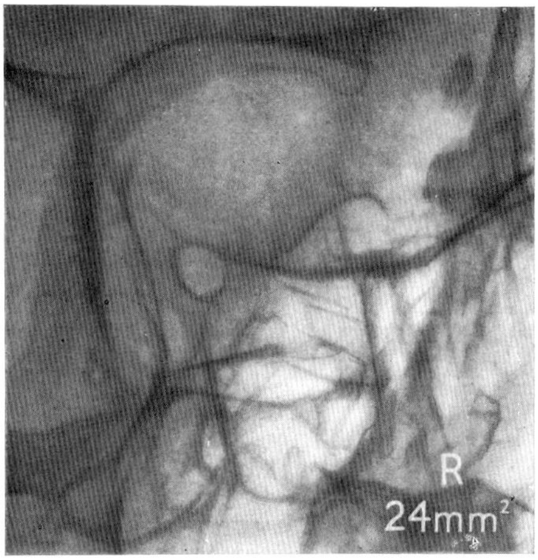

Fig. 25.14 Rhese-Goalwin view. Normal size and configuration of the right optic foramen

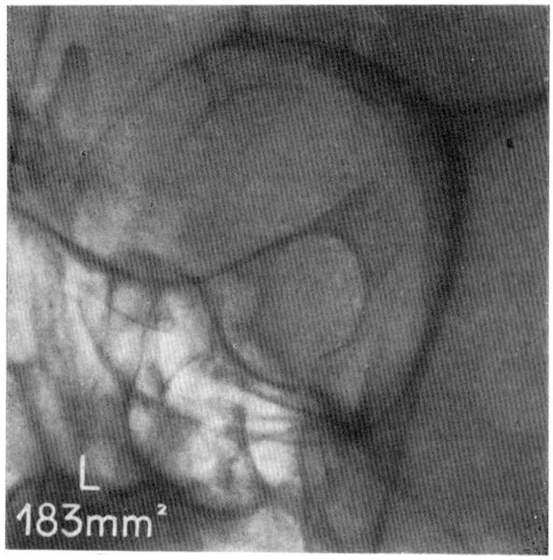

Fig. 25.15 Rhese-Goalwin view. Uniform enlargement of the left optic foramen

piezometer revealed only minimal differences between the two sides. With malignant exophthalmos, retrodisplacement of the globe was severely compromised (Nover et al. 1959) (see changes in orbital content, page 328). Primary intraorbital lesions tend to cause axial exophthalmos with restriction of movement whereas disorders involving the wall of the orbit, such as from the sinuses, lacrimal gland, sac, and periosteum tend to displace the globe. Benign processes tend to develop slowly without irritation and are practically symptom-free. Only rarely is there a feeling of tension or pressure. Findings on palpation are highly significant: One palpates between the orbital rim and globe using the small finger. Frequently, this allows determination of the size, location, consistency and flocculence of a lesion.

Steroids are a diagnostic test for pseudotumor. A pseudotumor improves rapidly after steroid therapy; this is usually true of endocrine exophthalmos or a lymphoma as well.

Symptomatology

Blurred vision can result from tumor pressure. The globe is displaced or flattened causing astigmatism. Slowly progressive vision loss can be caused by compression or infiltration of the optic nerve by tumor. This results in varying degrees of optic nerve atrophy. Diplopia which becomes progressively more severe may be caused by displacement of the globe, nerve palsy, infiltration or mechanical restriction of extraocular muscles.

Cysts and Pseudotumors

Cystic globes with microphthalmos or anophthalmos present no diagnostic difficulties. Acquired cysts may occur with *hematomas*, or be secondary to *laceration* of mucous membranes as well as caused by mucoceles (Fig. 25.16). *Dermoid cysts*, as well as *lipodermoids*, are most commonly found superior temporally, less often at the upper inner orbital rim. The content of dermoid cysts frequently includes hair and keratinized epithelium.

Meningo-Encephalo-Mucocele

Meningocele, or more specifically encephalocele (Fig. 25.8), has to be considered when the cystic structure lies superior nasally. These are white, elastic, frequently bilateral, thin-walled, transparent structures which are frequently pulsatile. Cerebral signs, such as vomiting and variation in pulse, can be elicited by pressure on the encephalocele.

Mucoceles (Fig. 25.16) are encapsulated accumulations of mucous in the sinuses. The surrounding bony walls ultimately become paper thin and may erode. There is painless displacement of the globe. Diplopia is rare in spite of what may be significant displacement of the globe. This is due to the slow progression, often over years, which allows compensatory adaptation. A history of sinusitis is common.

Teratoma, Cholesteatoma, Parasite

Other causes for cystic changes in the orbit include: *cholesteatomas* arising subperiosteally as well as the similar *pseudo cholesteatoma* and *teratomas* (usually in the region of the lacrimal gland, generally causing death in early childhood), and *parasites* (echinococcus, cysticercus). Parasites in the orbit are exceedingly rare. Eosinophilia and complement fixation reactions may aid in the diagnosis in some cases.

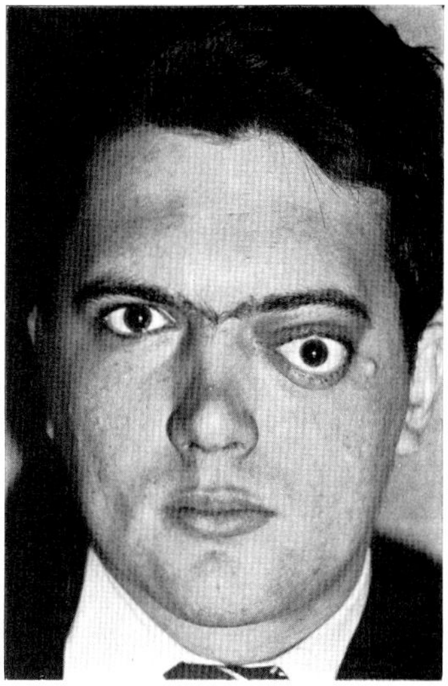

Fig. 25.16 Mucocele of the frontal sinus with inferior temporal displacement of the globe (♂ 20 yrs.)

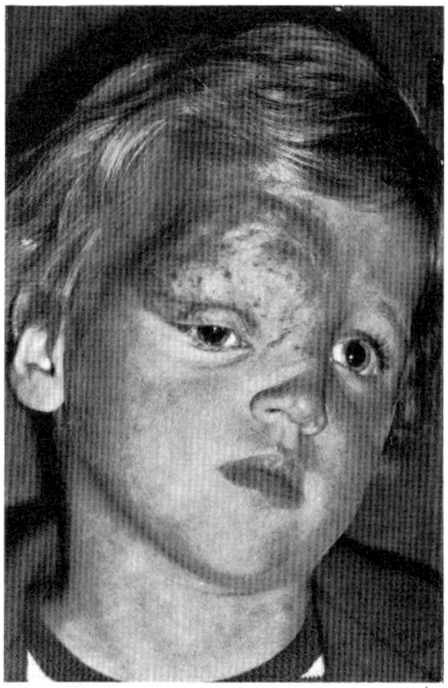

Fig. 25.17 Hemangioma of the orbit and forehead with inferior displacement of the globe (♀ 5 yrs.)

Orbital Tumors

(see page 113)

The most *common tumors* occurring in *children* (Bushe 1959) are: glioma of the optic nerve, venous hemangioma, rhabdomyosarcoma, round cell sarcomas and neuroblastomas metastatic to the orbit from the adrenal medulla.
In adults: fibromas, fibrosarcoma, osteoma, meningioma of the sphenoid, plasmacytoma, (brown) giant cell tumors. The primary choices for tumors metastatic to the orbit in adults include carcinoma, sarcoma and malignant melanoma (Henderson 1973; Offret and Haye 1971).

Benign orbital tumors — Malignant orbital tumors — Intracranial tumors — Pseudotumor and phakomatoses.

Benign orbital tumors: *Dermoid cysts* and *lipodermoids* are particularly common, usually appearing at the orbital rim superior temporally. Cavernous and capillary *hemangiomas* are not rare. Hemangiomas of the lid may extend behind the globe (Fig. 25.17), especially in small children, potentially destroying the eye (Kreibig 1961; Reese 1951). Cavernous hemangiomas located in the muscle cone may damage the optic nerve by pressure. Pulsation of the globe is common. These tumors grow slowly after age 20 and will, on occasion, reveal calcification on X-ray. The extent of a hemangioma may be determined by phlebography (du Boulay 1962). Lymphangiomas of the orbit are rare and are usually accompanied by similar changes in the conjunctiva, subcutaneously, or in the mucous membranes of the mouth. Lymphangiomas occur overwhelmingly in children around six years of age. There may be hemorrhage into the tumor. *Lipomas, fibromas, chondromas, myxomas, rhabdomyomas, leiomyomas, cholesteatomas,* and *juvenile xanthogranuloma* occur less commonly in the orbit.
Osteomas (Fig. 25.18) and *myxochondromas* may lead to severe unilateral exophthalmos. Osteomas can at times be palpated with the finger and are readily visible on X-ray. *Mixed tumors of the lacrimal gland* (Fig. 11.2) have to be considered with any non-inflammatory swelling in the region of the lacrimal gland.
Besides *plexiform neuromas* (see page 103) (Fig. 10.43) neurofibroma of von Recklinghausen's disease can also lead to elephantiasis, bony defects (with encephaloceles and pulsations) and enlargement of the orbit.
Optic nerve tumors (spongioblastomas, gliomas, meningiomas) appear in younger pa-

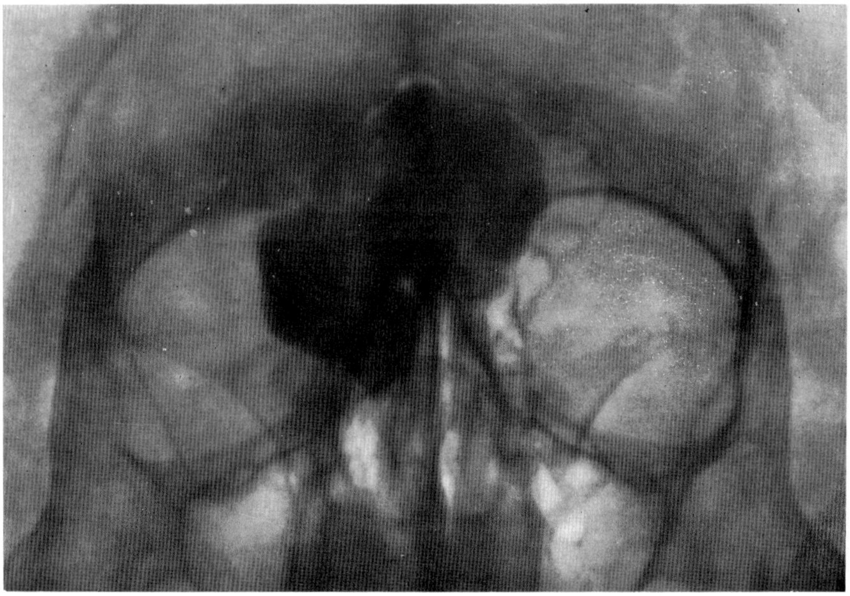

Fig. 25.18 Osteoma of the frontal sinus (from: R. Thiel, Atlas of Diseases of the Eye, 6th Ed., Thieme, Stuttgart 1963)

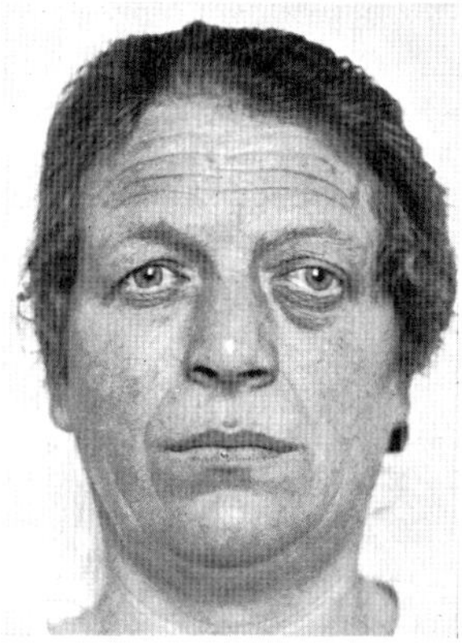

a

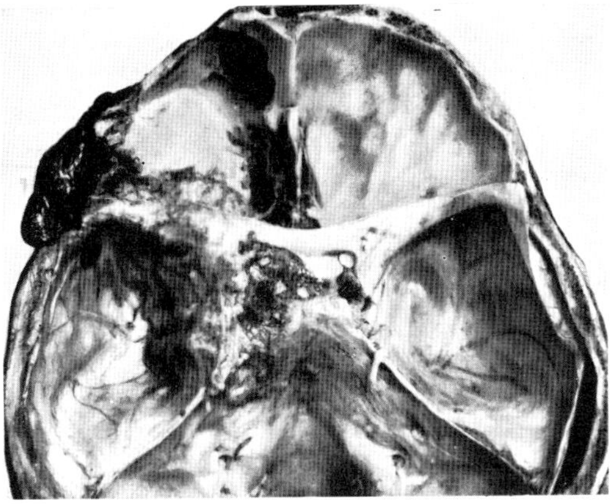

b

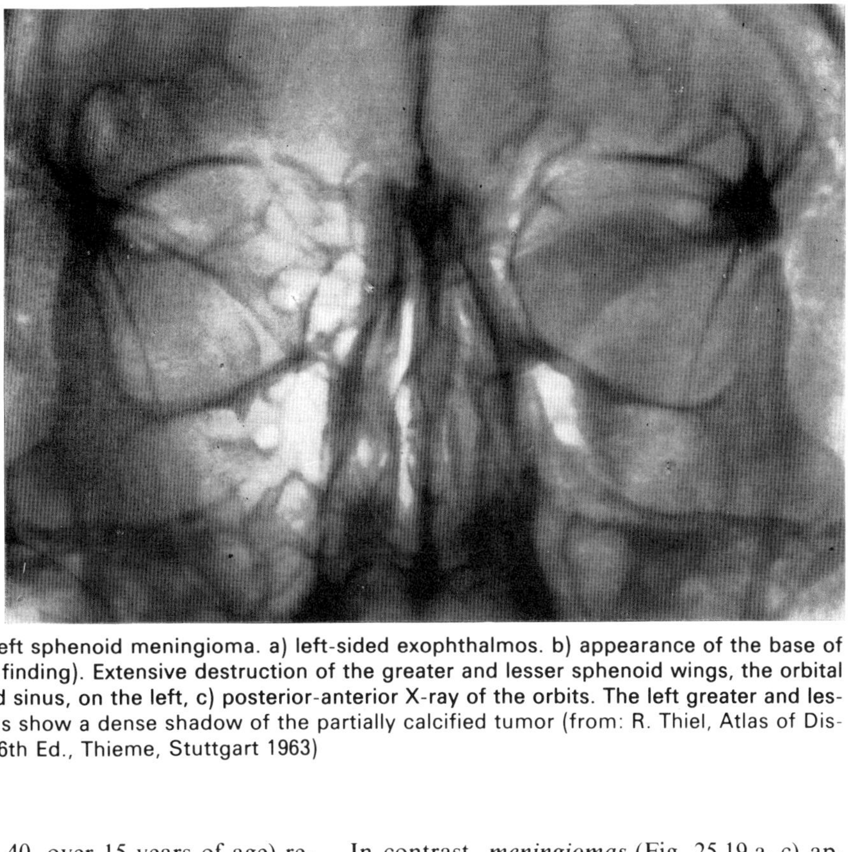

c

Fig. 25.19 a–c Left sphenoid meningioma. a) left-sided exophthalmos. b) appearance of the base of the skull (autopsy finding). Extensive destruction of the greater and lesser sphenoid wings, the orbital roof, and sphenoid sinus, on the left, c) posterior-anterior X-ray of the orbits. The left greater and lesser sphenoid wings show a dense shadow of the partially calcified tumor (from: R. Thiel, Atlas of Diseases of the Eye, 6th Ed., Thieme, Stuttgart 1963)

tients (under age 40, over 15 years of age) resulting in the early development of vision loss, papilledema, post-papillitic atrophy, as well as slowly progressive axial exophthalmos. Frequently an enlarged optic nerve foramen can be seen radiologically (Lundberg 1936; Gramberg-Danielsen 1955; Nover and Zielinski 1957) (Fig. 25.12, 25.13, 25.14, 25.15).

In contrast, *meningiomas* (Fig. 25.19 a–c) appear more rapidly. Mobility of the displaced globe is compromised early in the disease while vision is maintained.

Malignant orbital tumors. Primary and metastatic orbital malignancies (carcinoma, sarcoma) have to be considered when there is a rapid progression of tumor-induced exoph-

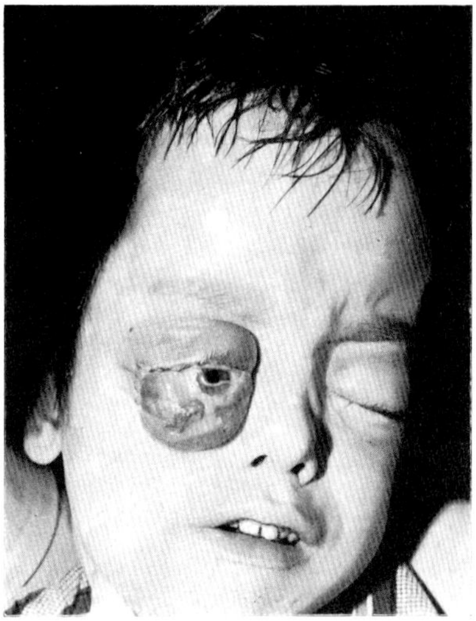

Fig. 25.20 Sympathicoblastoma (metastatic from the adrenal) (♂ 5 yrs.)

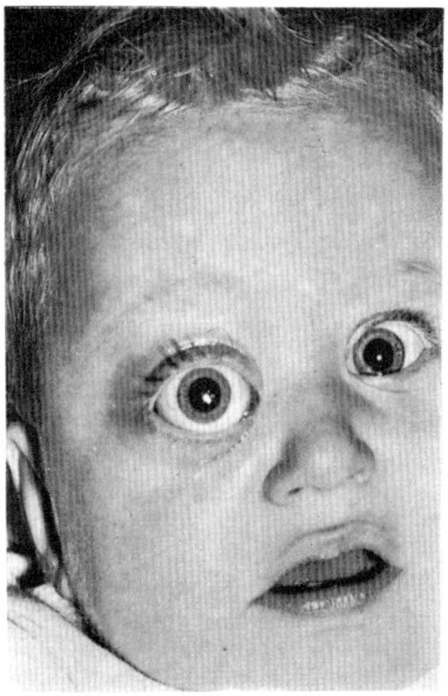

Fig. 25.21 Rhabdomyosarcoma exophthalmos (♂ 8 months)

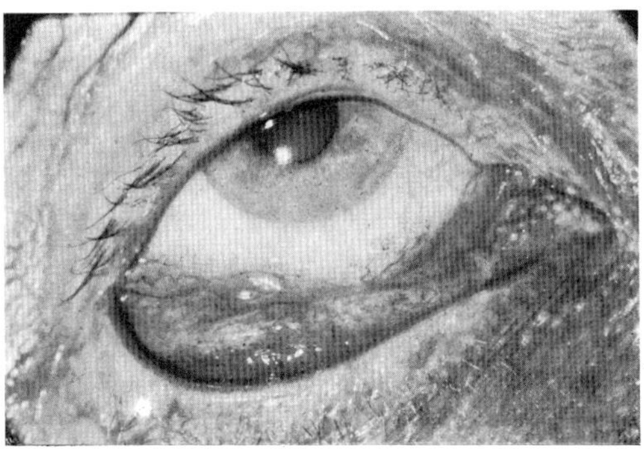

◄ Fig. 25.22 Nodular lesions (giant follicular lymphoblastoma of Brill-Symmers) in the conjunctiva (♂ 10 yrs.)

thalmos. In infants and *small children,* metastatic orbital tumors are most commonly *neuroblastomas,* specifically *sympathicoblastoma* (Fig. 25.20) (chromophobe cells of the sympathetic nervous system). One differentiates the *sympathicogonioma* composed of undifferentiated cells from the *sympathicoblastoma* composed of differentiated cells and from the *sympathicoganglioma* (which no longer metastasizes) composed of mature cells. Orbital metastases expand rapidly, freezing the globe. There is a predilection for hematoma formation. Also, metastases of Wilm's tumor (nephroblastoma) may appear in the orbita.

The rare orbital *teratomas* (derivative of all three embryonic cell layers) are usually already present at birth and rapidly lead to progressive exophthalmos.

Transscleral extension of *retinoblastomas* or *uveal melanomas* also leads to exophthalmos.

Carcinomas of the conjunctiva, caruncle, lacrimal sac, lid or sinuses can extend into the orbit. Mixed tumors of the lacrimal gland are not rare (see page 113). Sarcomas, retinoblastomas, carcinomas (breast, prostate, uterus, stomach, pancreas, lung, thyroid) will *metastasize* to the orbit.

Other considerations include: *sarcomas* (round cell sarcoma, fibrosarcoma, reticuloendothelial cell sarcoma and cylindroma). These often arise from the periosteum or the sinuses. *Hemangiosarcomas* are rare.

Sarcomas have been observed at birth (Felkel and Glowatzky 1941; Pŏstić 1944) and usually occur in small children. The most common malignant primary orbital tumor in childhood is *rhabdomyosarcoma* (Fig. 25.21). This rapidly growing tumor swiftly leads to unilateral exophthalmos, pain, vision loss, papilledema, optic nerve atrophy (enlargement of the optic canal) and generally occurs around ages seven to eight (Jones et al. 1966). Differentiated rhabdomyosarcomas are readily identified histologically by their muscle striations. The histological diagnosis is more difficult with embryonal rhabdomyosarcoma. Generally,

Fig. 25.23 a and b Plasmacytoma, multiple myeloma, Kahler's disease (from: R. Thiel, Atlas of Diseases of the Eye, 6th Ed., Thieme, Stuttgart 1963)

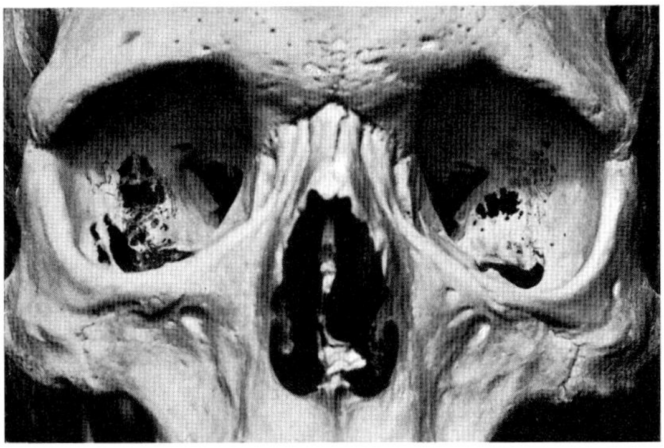

Fig. 25.23 a Postmortem specimen of the same skull shown in the X-ray below (Fig. 25.23 b). The marked destruction of the orbital walls explains the high degree of bilateral exophthalmos existing prior to death.

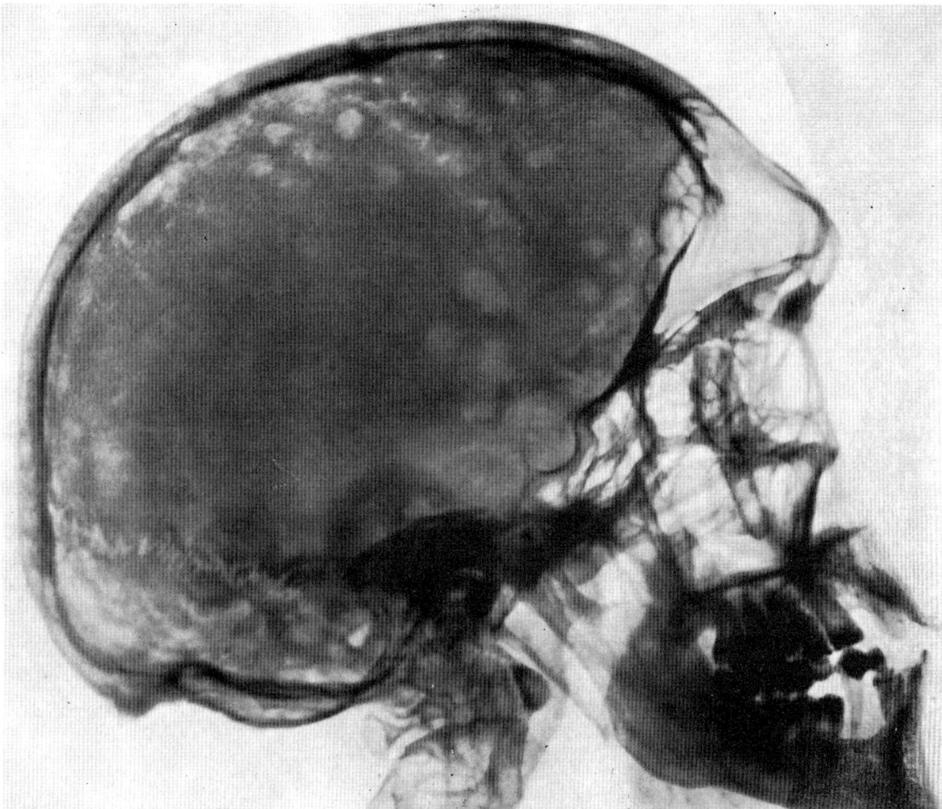

Fig. 25.23 b Lateral skull X-ray. Small punched out lesions scattered throughout the cranium

the erythrocyte sedimentation rate is normal with rhabdomyosarcoma.

On occasion, sarcomas have an explosive growth enlarging visibly wihtin a matter of days.

Transitional forms exist among the *myelomas* and *lymphomas* between benign *(lymphoid hyperplasia, small-, giant-follicle lymphoblastomas)* and malignant (lymph-reticulum cell sarcoma) tumors and pseudotumors.

Giant follicular lymphoma (Brill-Symmers) (Fig. 25.22) leads to hard nodular infiltrates in the lids and conjunctival folds. It occurs primarily in older patients but ultimately leads to a sarcomatous end stage. In the Brill-Symmers syndrome, one is dealing with a giant follicular lymphadenopathy or reticulum cell sarcoma which results in tumorlike lesions in the orbit, lacrimal gland, liver, bone marrow, lung, kidney, bladder and breasts. It occurs primarily during the fifth decade of life. The average length of involvement is five years (up to 12 years [Gärtner 1959]).

Multiple myeloma, plasmacytoma (Fig. 25.23 a, b) and *chloromas* (with myelogenous leukemia) can cause marked bony changes in the orbit and exophthalmos. *Leukemic infiltrates* appear most commonly in the region of the lacrimal gland. Leukemia must always be considered in childhood exophthalmos.

The majority of the relatively common *carcinomas* arise from the *sinuses* or *epipharynx*. These tumors can be detected by X-ray as can sphenoid meningiomas (see below).

Epipharyngeal carcinomas or sarcomas may not cause symptoms until they extend into the middle cranial fossa through the foramen lacerum. Symptoms include abducens paresis, visual loss, and neuralgias. Further extension into the orbit through the superior orbital fissure can produce an orbital apex syndrome (see page 339) with exophthalmos. There may be unilateral hearing loss and palpable cervical lymphadenopathy.

Intracranial tumors (cerebellum, brain stem, cerebellar pontine angle): besides papilledema these can also cause *bilateral exophthalmos*.

Generalized symptoms of **elevated intracranial pressure** indicate a brain tumor when combined with enlarged ventricles on ventriculography, lesions and endocrine disorders. Besides neuroligical examination, other diagnostic tests should include encephalography, arteriography, electroencephalography, echoencephalography, radioactive and CAT scanning.

Unilateral exophthalmos is primarily observed in basilar skull processes and those near the sella. Since sphenoid meningiomas usually grow through the superior orbital fissure, extraocular muscle paresis, corneal hypoesthesia, potentially papilledema, optic atrophy and visual field loss can occur. *Sphenoid meningiomas* leading to slowly progressing exophthalmos usually grow in the bones. This results in sphenoidal hyperostosis seen radiographically.

Phakomatoses and systemic diseases: exophthalmos owing to tumor occasionally results from one of the phakomatoses: *von Recklinghausen's neurofibromatosis* with optic nerve glioma and exophthalmos in children is usually associated with café-au-lait spots. Other possibilities include *tuberous sclerosis, von Hippel-Lindau angiomatosis, Sturge-Weber angiomatosis* and *Kaposi's disease*.

Hand-Schüller-Christian reticuloendotheliosis results in bony lesions especially in the skull and is often associated with diabetes insipidus. It occurs primarily in children. Round or oval rarefactions with eosinophilic granulomas can be seen in the bone. About two-thirds of the patients are under twenty years of age. *Osteofibrosis deformans juvenilis* (Jaffe-Lichtenstein-Uehlinger), marble bone disease, and Paget's disease can cause compression of the optic nerve at the foramen and exophthalmos. *Brown giant cell tumors*, like *sarcomas*, can produce osteolytic lesions.

Inflammatory Orbital Changes: Acute Inflammation

Sinusitis — Secondary orbital edema — Inflammatory exophthalmos in children (maxillary osteomyelitis, ethmoiditis, infectious diseases, etc.) — Abscess — Tenonitis — Dacryocystitis — Mycoses — Myositis, tendonitis, posterior scleritis — Cavernous sinus thrombosis.

Sinusitis

Sinusitis (frontal, ethmoid, sphenoid, and occasionally maxillary) frequently extend into the orbit (Rossberg 1966) (Plate XXXII, Fig. 1, page 288 h). Sinusitis can be present in children even before the sinuses are visible on X-ray. These inflammations may appear as *osteitis* or as *subperiosteal* abscesses or as true *orbital cellulitis*. The clinical picture is one of acute inflammation with restriction of movement of the globe, exophthalmos (the globe is usually displaced inferior temporally), conjunctival edema (chemosis), lid edema and generalized symptoms, such as fever (often very high, at times septic), debility, nausea and pain. Finally, the globe may be markedly proptotic and totally frozen. If the process occurs deep in the orbit there is danger of optic nerve involvement with optic neuritis causing atrophy and blindness. At times there is unilateral papilledema. The most dangerous complications are cavernous sinus thrombosis and meningitis.

Secondary Orbital Edema

Any inflammatory process near the eyes can lead to secondary lid and orbital edema. The most common causes are infected facial wounds, furuncles on the nose or upper lip, chalazion, herpes, dacryocystitis and infected insect bites.

Inflammatory Exophthalmos in Infants

Inflammatory exophthalmos in *infants* should lead one to consider *maxillary osteomyelitis* (Plate XXXII, Fig. 2, page 288 h) (Custodis 1931; Hallbrook 1964; Kittel and Ocklitz 1964). Other causes include *ethmoiditis* (in spite of radiologic lack of sinuses), and metastatic orbital cellulitis. In infants, inflammatory exophthalmos can occur as a rare complication of *scarlet fever, measles, syphilis* and *actinomycosis*. Acute dacryocystitis, paraorbital furuncles, orbital injury, as well as septic metastasis (sepsis, pyemia, furuncles, infectious diseases, cachexia) and panophthalmitis (Plate XXXII, Fig. 3, page 288 h) occur in infants as well as in adults.

Tendonitis (Plate XXXII, Fig. 4, page 288 h) leads to chemosis and kinesalgia, usually without general signs of illness.

Dacryocystitis, Erysipelas

With *dacryocystitis* (Plate IV, Fig. 5, page 128 d), edema, redness and pain are located nasally beneath the medial palpebral ligaments. With *dacryoadenitis* there is comma-shaped edema of the upper lid with redness and pain (superior temporally in the orbit).

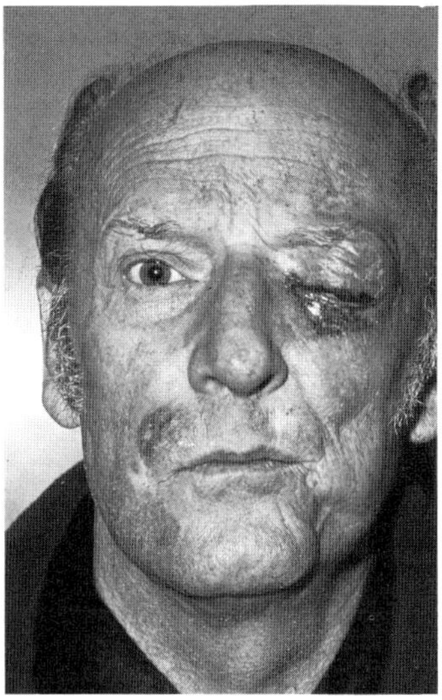

Fig. 25.24 Mycosis fungoides of the face, lids and orbit. Rockhard lid edema with chemosis, exophthalmos and optic atrophy (♀ 61 yrs.)

With *erysipelas* there is marked redness, sharply delineated edema and high fever.

Fungal Infections

Fungi can cause a variety of changes in the orbit (Hoffmann 1965; François 1968). Actinomycosis (gram-positive bacteria), aspergillosis, sporotrichosis and mucormycosis may lead to exophthalmos with firm orbital infiltrate, fistula formation, and bony erosion. The picture can resemble that of an inflammatory orbital tumor with paresis of extraocular muscles, papilledema and optic atrophy. The orbit becomes involved by extension from the sinuses, maxillary bone or directly from external invasion.

Myositis, Tendonitis and Posterior Scleritis

Myositis and *tendonitis* of the *extraocular muscles* leads to localized pain with ocular movement, diplopia (extraocular muscle paresis) and conjunctival edema. There are no major systemic findings. *Posterior scleritis* gives similar symptoms (see page 182).

Ocular neuromyositis can potentially cause an acute (sometimes bilateral) exophthalmos with lid edema and extraocular muscle paresis. The differential diagnosis includes exophthalmic myositis and endocrine ophthalmopathy (see page 53).

Cavernous Sinus Thrombosis

Progressive thrombophlebitis (furuncle of the face, orbital cellulitis) can lead to cavernous sinus thrombosis via involvement of the angular vein or can result from a sinusitis or orbital cellulitis. Cavernous sinus thrombosis results in a severe disturbance of circulation with bilateral exophthalmos, chemosis, frozen-immobile globes, venous stasis, and septic fever. The serious prognosis of septic cavernous sinus thrombosis has been improved by antibiotic and anti-coagulation therapy (Clune 1963).

Chronic Inflammation of the Orbit

Tuberculosis, syphilis, yaws – Pseudotumors (follicular lymphocytic infiltrates and leukemia – tumorlike, granulomatous processes) – Parasites.

Tuberculosis, Syphilis, Yaws

Chronic tuberculous inflammation of the bony orbital wall occurs (rare in this day and age) in children as *tuberculous periostitis* (Plate III, Fig. 1, page 128 c). This potentially leads to fistula formation and deep cicatricial scarring, especially in the region of the malar bone.

Tuberculoma and *syphilitic gumma* of the orbit and periosteum as well as periostitis from yaws were formerly more common than they are today.

Pseudotumors

Pseudotumors of the orbit which consist of a *lymphocytic infiltrate* with *follicles* can lead to an exophthalmos progressing over a period of weeks to months. Differentiation can be made between:

1. a diffuse lymphocytic infiltration throughout the entire orbital fatty tissue;

2. an inflammatory lymphocytic (round cell) infiltration limited to the periosteum of the orbit or to the lacrimal gland and its capsule (simulating a lacrimal gland tumor) or a markedly circumscribed lesion in the orbital fat; and

3. chronic lymphocytic myositis of the extraocular muscle.

True neoplasms or inflammations of other etiologies must be ruled out. Pseudotumors usually respond well to X-ray or steroid therapy.

Leukemia and aleukemic lymphadenopathy have also been described as causing tumor-like infiltrates of the orbit with exophthalmos (Schreck 1939; Bregeat and Hamard 1966).

The green color of a chloroma occurring with myelogenous leukemia is caused by hemoglobin breakdown products. Chloromas usually begin in the periosteum.

Disorders other than lymphomas and leukemia (Bregeat and Hamard 1966) which present as pseudotumors or tumor-like granulomatous involvement include: *tuberculoma, sarcoidosis* (see page 201), *gumma, leproma* (Holmes 1962), *foreign body granuloma, eosinophilic granuloma* (see page 337), *basophilic granuloma, Wegener's granulomatosis* (see page 184). The *mycosis fungoides* may lead to hard pseudotumorous infiltrations of the lids and the orbital fat as well as the extraocular muscles (Fig. 25.24) (Pau et al. 1976).

Myositis of the extraocular muscles can present as a tumor. Clinical findings include unilateral exophthalmos, chemosis, limitation of ocular movement and variable degrees of pain. Rarely, one also sees vision loss with post-inflammatory optic atrophy. In contrast to neurogenic paresis, electromyographic action potentials are maintained for a long period of time.

Recurrent, edematous *granulomatosis* of the *Melkersson-Rosenthal syndrome* has some relationship to sarcoidosis. Ptosis, lagophthalmos and periorbital edema may occur.

Parasites

Exophthalmos caused by parasites (echinococcus, cysticercus, trichina, ophthalmomyiasis) is exceedingly rare.

Orbital Pain

This appears to some extent in any inflammation (see page 348).

Oculonasal reflex neurosis (Charlin's syndrome, Sluder's syndrome) — Ciliary neuralgia — Trigeminal neuralgia.

Oculonasal Reflex Neurosis, Charlin's Syndrome, Sluder's Syndrome

Charlin's syndrome (see page 79) occurs as attacks of neuralgia in the region of the eyes, forehead, and jaw. There is lacrimation, lid edema, inflammation of the anterior segment of the eye (conjunctivitis, keratitis, iritis), rhinorrhea, as well as edema and sensitivity of the mucous membranes in the anterior third of the nose. This is assumed to be a neuritis of the naso-ciliary nerve. *Sluder's syndrome* (see page 78) is allegedly caused by irritation in the region of the sphenopalatine ganglion. There is pain behind the eyes and in the region of the upper jaw and root of the nose, lacrimation and rhinorrhea, attacks of sneezing, conjunctival hyperemia and photophobia.
Both Charlin's and Sluder's syndromes improve with cocaine-adrenalin anesthesia of the nasal mucous membranes.

Ciliary Neuralgias, Trigeminal Neuralgia

Ciliary neuralgias (for example with acute glaucoma [see page 73]) can be regarded as a referred pain. They may still be present after loss of sensitivity from destruction of the gasserian ganglion (Pau 1950). *Trigeminal neuralgias* may be localized solely in the orbit.

References

Alfano, J. E.: Ocular aspects of the maternal rubella syndrome. Trans. Amer. Acad. Ophthal. Otolaryng. 70 (1966) 235–266

Axenfeld, Th.: Zur Lymphombildung in der Orbita. Albrecht v. Graefes Arch. klin. exp. Ophthal. 37, IV (1891) 102–124

Badtke, G.: Die Mißbildungen des menschlichen Auges. In: Der Augenarzt, Vol. IV, ed. by K. Velhagen. Thieme, Stuttgart 1961

Bernoulli, R.: Über Pseudotumor der Orbita. Ophthalmologica (Basel) 127 (1954) 279–282

Birch-Hirschfeld, A.: Zur Diagnostik und Pathologie der Orbitaltumoren. Ber. dtsch. ophthal. Ges. 32 (1905) 127–135

Birch-Hirschfeld, A.: Die Erkrankungen der Orbita. In: Kurzes Handbuch der Ophthalmologie, Vol. III, ed. by F. Schieck, A. Brückner. Springer, Berlin 1930 (pp. 1–136)

Böke, W., H. Reich: Augenbeteiligung bei der Wegenerschen Granulomatose. Klin. Mbl. Augenheilk. 151 (1967) 802–822

Bojlén, K., T. Brems: Hypertelorism (Greig). Acta path. microbiol. scand. 15 (1938) 217–258

Boulay, G. H. du: Orbital phlebography in the diagnosis of intra-orbital haemangiomas. Trans. ophthal. Soc. U. K. 81 (1962) 245–259

Brégeat, P., H. Hamard: Manifestations oculaires des leucoses. Arch. Ophtal. (Paris) 26 (1966) 13–20

Bronson, N. R.: Recent developments in diagnostic ultrasound. Trans. ophthal. Soc. UK 92 (1973) 149–159

Bushe, K. A.: Zur Differentialdiagnose des einseitigen Exophthalmus. Klin. Mbl. Augenheilk. 135 (1959) 465–486

Clune, J. P.: Septic thrombosis within the cavernous chamber. Amer. J. Ophthal. 56 (1963) 33–39

Coleman, D. J.: Reliability of ocular and orbital diagnosis with B-Scan ultrasound. Amer. J. Ophthal. 73 (1972) 501–516

Custodis, E.: Über die entzündlichen Erkrankungen der Orbita bei Oberkieferosteomyelitis des Säuglings. Klin. Mbl. Augenheilk. 87 (1931) 631–637

Dinsmore, R. S.: Hyperthyroidism in children. J. Amer. med. Ass. 99 (1932) 636–638

Dollfus, M. A., P. Marx, J. Langlois, J. L. Clement, J. Forthomme: Congenital cystic Eyeball. Am J. Ophth. 66 (1968) 504–509

Duke-Elder, S.: The ocular adnexa. System of ophthalmology XIII. 1. diseases of the eyelids, XIII, 2. lacrimal orbital and para-orbital-diseases. Kimpton, London 1974

Fanconi, G.: Familiäre infantile perniziosaartige Anämie. Jb. Kinderkk. 117 (1927) 257–280

Felkel, R. K., F. Glowatzky: Über einen Fall von kongenitalem Rundzellensarkom der Orbita. Klin. Mbl. Augenheilk. 106 (1941) 582–585

Fleischer, B.: Über Hand-Schüller-Christiansche Krankheit. Klin. Mbl. Augenheilk. 108 (1942) 243–244

Franceschetti, A., D. Klein: The mandibulo-facial dysostosis, a new hereditary syndrome. Acta ophthal. (Kbh.) 27 (1949) 144–224

Franceschetti, A., P. Zwahlen: Un syndrome nouveau: la dysostose mandibulo-faciale. Bull. Acad. Suisse Sci. Méd. 1 (1944) 60–66

François, J.: Les mycoses oculaires. Masson, Paris 1968

François, J., R. Berger, H. Saraux: Les aberrations chromosomiques en ophthalmologie. Masson, Paris 1972

François, J., L. Haustrate: Anomalies colobomateuses du globe et syndrome du premier arc. Ann. Oculist. (Paris) 187 (1954) 340–368

Freeman, E. A., J. H. Sheldon: Cranio-carpo-tarsal dystrophy. Arch. Dis. Childh. 13 (1938) 277–283

Friede, R.: Über physiologische Euryopie und pathologischen Hypertelorismus ocularis. Albrecht v. Graefes Arch. klin. exp. Ophthal. 155 (1954) 359–385

Gärtner, J.: Orbitabeteiligung bei Brill-Symmersscher Krankheit. Klin. Mbl. Augenheilk. 135 (1959) 486–496

Goldberg, M. F.: Genetic and metabolic eye disease. Little, Brown and Co., Boston 1974

Goldenhar, M.: Associations malformatives de l'oeil et de l'oreille, en particulier le syndrome dermoide épibulbaire – appendices auriculaires – fistula auris congenita et ses relations avec la dysostose mandibulo-faciale. J. Génét. hum. 1 (1952) 243–282

Gornig, H.: Hypercholesterinämie und eosinophiles Granulom der Orbita. Klin. Mbl. Augenheilk. 152 (1968) 517–524

Gramberg-Danielsen, B.: Zur histopathologischen Einordnung der primären Opticustumoren. Confin. neurol. (Basel) 15 (1955) 240–250

Greig, D. M.: Traversing wounds of the orbit. Edinb. med. J. 31 (1924) No. 4, 241–262

Gross, H.: Der Hypertelorismus. Über Beziehungen des pathologisch weiten Augenabstandes zu den craniocerebralen Dysraphien und zu den turricephalen Schädeldysostosen. Ophthalmologica (Basel) 131 (1956) 137–156

Günther, R.: Über erbliche Gehörgangsatresie. Z. menschl. Vererb.- u. Konstit.-Lehre 27 (1943/44) 253–268

Hahlbrock, K. H.: Über die Oberkieferosteomyelitis des Säuglings. Klin. Mbl. Augenheilk. 145 (1964) 744–754

Hallermann, W.: Vogelgesicht und Cataracta congenita. Klin. Mbl. Augenheilk. 113 (1948) 315–318

Heimann, K.: Beitrag zur Klinik des Goldenhar-Syndroms. Klin. Mbl. Augenheilk. 152 (1968) 686–692

Helmholz, H. F.: Exophthalmic goiter in childhood. J. Amer. med. Ass. 87 (1926) 157–162

Henderson, J. W.: Orbital tumors. W. B. Saunders, Philadelphia, London, Toronto 1973

Herzau, W.: Über Osteomyelitis des Oberkiefers bei 3 Säuglingen. Klin. Mbl. Augenheilk. 90 (1933) 55–58

Hoffmann, D. H.: Pilzinfektionen des Auges. Fortschr. Augenheilk. 16 (1965) 63–217

Hoffmann, D., B. Lindquist: Kongenitaler endokriner Exophthalmus beim Neugeborenen einer thyreotoxischen Mutter. Klin. Mbl. Augenheilk. 130 (1957) 296–304

Hollwich, F., B. Verbeck: Zur Dysplasia oculo-auricularis (Franceschetti-Goldenhar-Syndrom). Klin. Mbl. Augenheilk. 154 (1969) 430–443

Hollwich, F., G. Jünemann, E. Damaske: Klinischer Beitrag zur Blowout-Fraktur. Klin. Mbl. Augenheilk. 156 (1970) 864–873

Holmes, W. J.: The eyes in leprosy. Trans. ophthal. Soc. U. K. 81 (1962) 397–420

Horst, W., K. Ullerich: Hypophysen-Schilddrüsenerkrankungen und endokrine Ophthalmopathie. Beiheft der Klin. Mbl. Augenheilk., 31. In: Bücherei des Augenarztes, ed. by R. Thiel. Enke, Stuttgart 1958

Howard, R. O.: Ocular abnormalities in the cri du chat syndrome. Amer. J. Ophthal. 73 (1973) 797–803

Jones, I. S., A. B. Reese, J. Kraut: Orbital rhabdomyosarcoma. Amer. J. Ophthal. 61 (1966) 721–736

Käfer, O.: Die Phlebographie der Orbita. Klin. Mbl. Augenheilk. 160 (1972) 419–429.

Kittel, V., H. W. Ocklitz: Der Exophthalmus beim Säugling. Klin. Mbl. Augenheilk. 145 (1964) 195–202

Koenig, F., Jr.: Zur Orbitographie. Ophthalmologica 127 (1954) 283–287

König, B., K. Vojáček, G. Zapletal: Eosinophiles Granulom der Orbita. Klin. Mbl. Augenheilk. 145 (1964) 212–221

Kreibig, W.: Das Auge und sein Hilfsapparat. Lehrbuch der speziellen Path. Anatomie von Kaufmann, Staemmler, Vol. III. Walter de Gruyter, Berlin 1961 (pp. 1107–1115)

Krümmel, H., L. Rausch: Anomalien des Auges bei der sog. Incontinentia pigmenti. Ophthalmologica 130 (1955) 31–53

Lange, C. de: Nouvelle observation du Typus Amstelodamensis et Examen anatomo-pathologique de ce Type. Arch. Med. Enf. 41 (1938) 193–203

Leonhardt, V. A.: Mitbeteiligung der Augen bei sequestrierender Zahnkeimentzündung im Säuglingsalter. Klin. Mbl. Augenheilk. 124 (1954) 560–567

Lundberg, A.: Über Oligodendrocystome des Sehnervs. Acta ophthal. (Kbh.) 14 (1936) 271–277

Margetts, B. M.: Thyrotoxicosis in a newborn infant. Proc. roy. Soc. Med. 43 (1950) 615

Meyer-Schwickerath, G., E. Grüterich, H. Weyers: Mikrophthalmus-Syndrome. Klin. Mbl. Augenheilk. 131 (1957) 18–30

Nover, A., H. W. Zielinski: Zur Differentialdiagnose der Orbita- und Optikustumoren. Klin. Mbl. Augenheilk. 131 (1957) 577–598

Nover, A., H. W. Zielinski, K. Josten: Zur Diagnostik und Verlaufskontrolle des Exophthalmus. Klin. Mbl. Augenheilk. 135 (1959) 32–52

Offret, G., C. Haye: Tumeurs de l'œil et des annexes oculaires. Masson, Paris, 1971

Ossoinig, K.: Die Ultraschalldiagnostik der Orbita. Klin. Mbl. Augenheilk. 149 (1966) 817–839

Ossoinig, K.: Der Beitrag der Echographie zur Diagnostik des Exophthalmus im Kindesalter. Ber. dtsch. ophthal. Ges. 69 (1969) 98–104

Ossoinig, K., K. Seher: Ergebnisse der Ultraschalldiagnostik orbitaler Tumoren. Klin. Mbl .Augenheilk. 151 (1967) 519–524

Papst, W.: Die oculäre Neuromyositis. Klin. Mbl. Augenheilk. 149 (1966) 663–673

Pau, H.: Vogelgesicht mit Permeabilitätskatarakt als Folge trophischer Störungen. Klin. Mbl. Augenheilk. 117 (1950) 529–532

Pau, H.: Kopfschmerzen aus augenärztlicher Sicht. In: Kopfschmerzen, ed. by J. Krischek. Karger, Basel 1958

Pau, H.: Die Ziliarneuralgie als vegetativer Schmerz. Klin. Mbl. Augenheilk. 116 (1950) 578–583.

Pau, H., W. Tillmann, G. Goerz: Mycosis fungoides mit Befall des Auges und innere Organe. Klin. Mbl. Augenheilk. 168 (1976) 706–712

Pfeiffer, R. A., H. Erpenstein, G. Jünemann: Oculo-dento-digitale Dysplasie. Klin. Mbl. Augenheilk. 152 (1968) 247–262

Pietruschka, G.: Über Marmorknochenkrankheit (Albers-Schönbergsche Krankheit) nebst Bemerkungen zur Differentialdiagnose. Klin. Mbl. Augenheilk. 123 (1953) 189–201

Pietruschka, G.: Weitere Mitteilungen über die Marmorknochenkrankheit (Albers-Schönbergsche Krankheit). Klin. Mbl. Augenheilk. 132 (1958) 509–525

Poštić, S.: Ein Fall von kongenitalem Sarkom der Orbita. Klin. Mbl. Augenheilk. 110 (1944) 84–86

Reese, A. B.: Tumors of the eye. Hoeber, New York 1951

Rossberg, G.: Orbitale Komplikationen bei Erkrankungen der Nase und ihrer Nebelhöhlen. Klin. Mbl. Augenheilk. 149 (1966) 761–800

Schade, H.: Korrelationen zwischen Chromosomenaberrationen und klinischem Status. In: Bücherei des Augenarztes, 50. Enke, Stuttgart 1968

Schreck, E.: Zur Klinik und pathologischen Anatomie der Orbitaltumoren. Klin. Mbl. Augenheilk. 103 (1939) 1–44

Schwartz, A. R.: Exophthalmic goiter in children. Arch. Pediat. 62 (1945) 214–218

Scouras, J., A. Catti, J. F. Cuendet: Les microphtalmies congenitales. Ann. Oculist. (Paris) 203 (1970) 953–970

Siegert, P.: Erkrankungen der Orbita. In: Der Augenarzt, ed. by K. Velhagen. Thieme, Stuttgart 1960 (pp. 653–816)

Smith, B., W. F. Regan: Blow-out-fracture of the orbit. Amer. J. Ophthal. 44 (1957) 733–739

Straatsma, B. R.: Ocular manifestations of Wegener's granulomatosis. Amer. J. Ophthal. 44 (1957) 789–799

Streiff, E. B.: Dysmorphie mandibulo-faciale (tête d'oiseau) et altérations oculaires. Ophthalmologica 120 (1950) 79–83

Thier, C. J.: Symptomenkomplexe im Rahmen der mandibulo-facialen Dysplasien. Mißbildungen im Bereich des ersten Kiemenbogensegmentes. Klin. Mbl. Augenheilk. 135 (1959) 378–388

Townes, P. L., P. D. Roca: Norries' disease. Amer. J. Ophthal. 76 (1973) 797–803

Ullrich, O., J. Fremerey-Dohna: Dyskephalie mit Cataracta congenita und Hypotrichose als typischer Merkmalskomplex. Ophthalmologica 125 (1953) 73–90; 144–154

Waardenburg, P. J., A. Franceschetti, D. Klein: Genetic and Ophthalmology. Royl van Corcum, Assen, Netherlands, Blackwell scientific publication, Oxford. Charles C. Thomas. Vol. I 1961, Vol. II 1963

Warburg, M.: Norrie's disease (atrofia bulborum hereditaria). Acta Ophthal. 41 (1963) 134–146

Weyers, H., C. J. Thier: Malformations mandibulo-faciales et délimitation d'un syndrome oculo-vertébral. J. Génét. hum. 7 (1958) 143–173

Wybar, K. C.: The nature of endocrine exophthalmus. Fortschr. Augenheilk. 7 (1957) 119–220

Zellweger, H.: Chromosomal aberrations and their significance for ophthalmo-otorhino-laryngology. Trans. Amer. Acad. Ophthal. Otolaryng. 69 (1965) 33–50

26 Damage from Light and Ionizing Radiation

Ultraviolet keratoconjunctivitis — Photocoagulation of the retina — Infrared cataract — Ocular damage from ionizing radiation — Photosensitivity.

Ultraviolet Keratoconjunctivitis

Ultraviolet rays are absorbed by surface tissues. With adequate exposure, multiple superficial corneal epithelial erosions in the form of a punctate keratopathy occur. There is a latent period of several hours between the irradiation and the onset of clinical symptoms. In severe cases there may even be slight clouding of the corneal stroma. This so-called *photoelectric keratoconjunctivitis* (ultraviolet keratoconjunctivitis) occurs with exposure to welding arcs, "snow blindness," and exposure to ultraviolet "sun lamps" without adequately protective absorbant glasses. There is severe pain, foreign body sensation, blepharospasms and lacrimation (see page 149) due to the marked irritation of the corneal involvement.

Retinal Photocoagulation

Sun gazing (usually during an eclipse or LSD trip) with inadequate protection results in retinal damage and edema with a central scotoma. Such heat coagulation heals with a pigmented scar. The coagulation effect of heat is used therapeutically in photocoagulation with the xenon-X-photocoagulator to treat retinal disease (periphlebitis, retinal tears, retinal tumors, etc.) (Meyer-Schwickerath 1959) (see page 282).

Infrared Cataract

Glassblowers and iron foundry workers exposed for more than ten years to short infrared wavelength light frequently develop a characteristic disciform central opacity under the posterior lens capsule. In addition, exposure in the same group of patients to heat frequently leads to exfoliation of the outer lamellae of the anterior lens capsule in the pupillary region (glassblower's cataract) (see page 242).

Ocular Damage from Ionizing Radiation

Excessive exposure to X-rays and radiation leads to erythema and loss of eyelashes. Conjunctiva and cornea can become edematous, even necrotic. A radiation cataract (see page 241) appears after a variable latent period (sometimes days, usually up to 1 to 2 years). Characteristically this is a central disciform posterior subcapsular opacity. A rapidly progressive intumescent to mature cataract can occur with markedly excessive radiation exposure.

Infrared and ultraviolet light damage around the eyes from atom bomb exposure can cause burns of the lid, cornea, conjunctiva and retina. The latter is similar to that occurring with sun gazing. Radiation damage from atom bombs can also cause fundus hemorrhages and exudates. Cataracts are observed as a late complication, more frequently in young than older patients. These usually appeared months to years after exposure in those patients who had a partial or total hair loss (usually about 14 days after exposure). The radiation cataracts were primarily posterior subcapsular plaques and remained stationary (Haye et al. 1965) (see page 242). Infrared (heat) cataracts and cataracts due to ionizing radiation (X-ray, radium, atom bombs) are morphologically very similar (complicated cataract, permeability cataracts).

Photosensitivity and Photodermatitis (see page 93, 135)

References

Haye, C., H. Jammet, M. A. Dollfus: L'œil et les radiations ionisantes, Vol. I, II. Masson, Paris 1965

Meyer-Schwickerath, G.: Lichtkoagulation. Bücherei des Augenarztes, 33. Enke, Stuttgart 1959

27 Thermal and Chemical Burns

Thermal burns (usually of the face) or chemical burns of the conjunctiva and cornea (see page 181) result in:

First degree burns with hyperemia, corneal stippling or erosion, lacrimation and blepharospasm.

Second degree burns with conjunctival chemosis, loss of corneal epithelium, stromal edema and blepharospasm.

Third degree burns with necrosis and coagulation. The conjunctiva is white, frequently anemic. Vessels can hardly be identified. The cornea is white (like a cooked fish eye) (Fig. 13.23) and anesthetic.

In acid burns, the resulting *coagulative necrosis* prevents further penetration of the acid, so there is a better prognosis for acid burns than for lye burns. The *liquefying necrosis* of alkali allows deeper penetration of the chemicals. Ammonia burns are among the most dangerous and often lead to corneal perforation after 8 to 10 days. Ocular lime burns are common. Both slaked and unslaked lime cause severe burns with deposition of calcium salt in the conjunctiva and cornea. These can be removed only superficially. The white corneal and conjunctival appearance in severe alkali burns leads to the term "boiled fish eye."

Ink pen injuries (Fig. 12.4) (methylviolet) are particularly common in children. There is a rapid discoloration of the conjunctiva with corneal erosion. Deposition of lime, ink, soap or various other foreign bodies into the conjunctiva by psychopaths or children results in an artificial conjunctivitis. Such a conjunctivitis is almost exclusively limited to the lower conjunctiva, with the remaining conjunctiva completely free of irritation. The diagnosis is confirmed by the rapid healing after removal of the foreign body and pressure patching. Tear gas and other chemical irritants fired at close range from self-defense devices result in a superficial chemical burn and imbedded foreign body material. Besides the superficial and deep corneal opacities, there is danger of a secondary iridocyclitis and glaucoma.

28 Traumatic Ocular Damage

Conjunctival foreign bodies — Corneal-scleral foreign bodies — Recurrent erosions — Perforating injuries — Blunt trauma — Intraocular foreign bodies — Sympathetic ophthalmia.

Conjunctival Foreign Bodies

These lead to corneal erosions, which are usually multiple, parallel, fluorescein-positive lines on the cornea. The foreign body is usually found beneath the upper lid. It is most easily found when in the lower lid conjunctiva, and most difficult to find when located in the upper cul-de-sac (double lid eversion).

Corneal Foreign Bodies

These are usually due to small imbedded iron foreign bodies (with rust ring), glass foreign bodies (windshields, glasses, exploded cookware), dust particles, insects (flies, mosquitoes), etc.

A hidden perforation has to be considered with any corneal or scleral injury after hammerblow, explosions, or use of high-speed machinery.

Recurrent Erosions (see page 149)

Perforating Injuries to the Globe and Penetration into the Orbit

The diagnosis of a perforated globe is readily made when the cornea is lacerated, and there has been loss of the anterior chamber, iris tissue incarceration in the cornea, specifically at the limbus, iris or lens perforation, posterior perforation, rosette cataracts, and marked hypotony or retinal holes. The diagnosis may be extremely difficult when these signs are not present. X-ray examination for foreign bodies is mandatory (localization after Comberg, bone-free exposure after Vogt). Ultrasound and electroacoustical methods are helpful.

Perforating injuries carry a risk of chronic endophthalmitis, sympathetic ophthalmia (see page 360), phthisis bulbi, secondary glaucoma, retinal detachment, siderosis, chalcosis, etc.

Careful slit lamp and X-ray examination are necessary. Since very small iron foreign bodies may hardly be visible on X-ray, an attempt at extraction should be made using a giant magnet.

Brain involvement always has to be considered when the orbit has been penetrated by stab injuries (spears, knives, sticks, knitting needles, etc.). Pieces of wood or other foreign bodies may be retained in the orbit. The globe itself is usually severely injured, but may be spared.

Blunt Trauma

Blunt corneal trauma — Alteration of the anterior chamber — Blunt trauma to the iris — Ruptured globe — Blunt lenticular trauma — Blunt retinal trauma — Choroidal rupture — Retrobulbar hemorrhage — Traumatic damage to the optic nerve.

Blunt trauma to the globe can cause transient circumscribed gray *corneal opacification, specifically swelling,* as well as ciliary injection, photophobia and lacrimation. Fibrous strands may be seen in the anterior chamber. These disappear within 24 hours. Sudden severe vision loss occurs with anterior chamber hemorrhage owing to rupture of iris vessels. The blood rapidly sinks in the anterior chamber, resulting in a horizontal fluid level (hyphema), and usually reabsorbs in a matter of days. There is always the danger of secondary glaucoma and, with poorly reabsorbing hemorrhage, of corneal hemosiderosis.

Blunt Trauma to the Iris

Pupillary dilatation — Sphincter tears — Iridodialysis.

Blunt trauma causes pupillary dilatation (traumatic mydriasis) with a decreased and incomplete pupillary reaction. Typical traumatic iris damage includes: the so-called *sphincter tears* (see page 189) with tears at the pupillary margin (Fig. 16.5) extending for a variable degree into the iris stroma.

Iridodialysis (see page 189) is a disinsertion of the peripheral iris (Fig. 16.6) leading to distortion of the pupil in the appropriate segment.

Rupture of the Globe

Blunt trauma can rupture the globe either directly or indirectly by pressing the globe against the bony orbit. The rupture occurs preferentially concentric to the limbus, or 2 to 3 mm from it (region of Schlemm's canal). Iris, lens, or other intraocular contents are often expressed from the globe. Posterior rupture of the globe is recognized by the marked hypotony, deep anterior chamber and intraocular hemorrhage. Laceration of the globe by a sharp instrument leads to varying degrees of intraocular damage, potentially with prolapse of intraocular contents (iris, vitreous, retina, etc.).

Lens

Dislocation of the lens — Posttraumatic late rosettes — Perforation rosette — Vossius' ring.

Lenticular damage with zonular tears from blunt trauma includes:

Subluxation or luxation (see page 252) (Fig. 21.22) with iridodenesis and prolapse of vitreous into the anterior chamber. Anterior luxation of the lens usually leads to an acute glaucomatous attack.

Posttraumatic late rosettes (see page 249) are white opacities located between the sutures that appear weeks to months after blunt trauma (Fig. 21.17). They occur beneath the anterior, less often posterior, lens capsule, are sharply delineated and with time are displaced deeper into the lens through newly formed clear lens fibers.

In contrast, the **perforation rosette** (see page 250) is a feathery opacity along the lens sutures and beneath the posterior capsule. It occurs acutely with injury to the lens capsule and disappears after a few weeks if the capsule seals itself (Fig. 21.18).

Pigment from the pupillary border can be pressed onto the lens capsule by blunt trauma where it remains as a *Vossius' ring,* which disappears after a few weeks (see page 249).

Blunt Retinal Trauma

Commotio-contusio retinae — Traumatic retinal detachment — Retinopathia sclopetaria.

Blunt trauma to the *retina* results in *commotio* or *contusio retinae* (see page 285). In both cases there is gray (edema) discoloration of the appropriate retinal area. When the lesion is centrally located, the macula appears as a cherry red spot (see page 285). Vision loss is severe. The differential diagnosis is important, since the edema of commotio retinae resolves spontaneously with full restitution of function, whereas contusio retinae results in varying degrees of scar formation with residual vision loss. Contusio retinae is commonly accompanied by retinal hemorrhage.

Ora tears (see page 275) with *retinal detachment* are overwhelmingly the result of blunt trauma. Macular *holes* are observed with myopia and retinal degeneration and at times following trauma. Potentially, trauma can prematurely precipitate a retinal detachment in patients so inclined (sclerotic-degenerative areas).

Retinopathia sclopetaria (see page 285) is due to indirect trauma to the globe from an orbital injury. This results in retinal tears and hemorrhages with severe "strandlike" connective tissue scarring.

Choroidal Ruptures

Choroidal rupture (see page 214) has to be considered when blunt trauma results in large areas of retinal hemorrhage. After reabsorption of the hemorrhage (Plate XV, Fig. 3, page 192 g), one sees white sickle-shaped areas located concentrically around the optic disc (Plate XV, Fig. 4, page 192 g). These are choroidal ruptures and are white owing to visibility of the underlying sclera. A few choroidal vessels are usually still visible in the area of the rupture.

Retrobulbar Hemorrhages

Retrobulbar hemorrhage (orbital fracture?) due to a contusion injury may lead to exophthalmos as well as periorbital hematomata. This may be followed by endophthalmos due to cicatricial scarring or fracture of the bony orbit (blow out fracture, see page 62). Onset of diplopia is usually delayed. Nose bleeds and subcutaneous emphysemas of the lid indicate a fracture in the nasal portion of the orbital wall. Fractures of the zygoma can be diagnosed by palpation or X-ray.

Traumatic Damage to the Optic Nerve

Sudden blindness after head injury can be due to *fracture in the bony portion of the optic canal* or *a hematoma in the optic nerve sheath,* or represent a *contrecoup action* of the mass of the brain *against the optic nerve.* Traumatic avulsion of the optic nerve head is possible (Plate XXXII, Fig. 5, page 288 h).

Intraocular Foreign Bodies

Siderosis – Chalcosis – Other foreign bodies.

Siderosis

Intraocular iron-containing foreign bodies lead to *siderosis*. Siderosis of the iris appears as a yellow-brown discoloration (Plate XIII, Fig. 6, page 192 e). Lenticular siderosis begins as brown anterior subcapsular spots in the region of the epithelium (Plate XIX, Fig. 6, page 224 c). These are followed by gray subcapsular opacities of the nature of a permeability cataract (cataracta complicata). Brown spots may appear in the vitreous. *Retinal siderosis* ultimately leads to retinal atrophy and yellow optic atrophy. The electroretinogram b-wave is extinguished.

Chalcosis

Intraocular copper leads to *corneal chalcosis* in the form of a limbus-parallel blue-gray ring-shaped deposit. *Chalcosis lentis* (Plate XX, Fig. 1, page 224 d) is a sunflower cataract on the anterior lens surface, particularly evident in those regions where the iris touches the lens. Red puncta may appear in the vitreous and on the retina.

Other Foreign Bodies

Intraocular *glass splinters* are often found in the inferior chamber angle. Here, sometimes after a period of years, they cause a progressive inferior sectorial keratopathy (edema, opacification, epithelial bullae) owing to mechanical endothelial trauma. Glass splinters in the vitreous present the danger of glaucoma and retinal detachment.

Because of the marked inflammation, intraocular vegetable matter usually has to be removed. The same is true of caterpillar hairs causing *ophthalmia nodosa*.

Sympathetic Ophthalmia

Iridocyclitis after perforating injury – potentially many years later – raises the crucial question of whether or not one is dealing with sympathetic ophthalmia. Inflammation of the uninjured, sympathizing eye occurs no earlier than 10 days, usually 4 to 8 weeks, but potentially many years, even decades, after the trauma.

Sympathetic ophthalmia is considered to be an autoimmune process appearing as chronic uveal inflammation after perforating injury. Usually there is the picture of a "plastic" iridocyclitis with aqueous flare, cells, extensive posterior synechiae, keratic precipitates and vitreous opacification. Histologically there is a lymphocytic infiltration of the uvea with epithelioid and giant cells. The uvea appears thickened. Involvement of the sympathizing eye results in disturbances of accommodation (young patients) with decreased dark adaptation as well as iridocyclitis, photophobia, ciliary injection, aqueous flare, cells, precipitates, and early marked posterior synechiae. Cyclitic vitreous exudates as well as small gray infiltrates appear at the posterior pole, especially in the periphery. The optic disc is hyperemic.

Besides the progressive iridocyclitic opacities, there is the danger of secondary glaucoma potentially leading to hypotony with phthisis bulbi and inflammatory retinal detachment.

The most important differential diagnosis is a phakolytic reaction (see pages 200, 217). This is always associated with release of lens protein and inflammation (bacterial). In contrast to sympathetic ophthalmia, aspiration of lens material in phakolytic ophthalmia leads almost immediately to an irritation-free eye.

Causes and Results of Ocular Injuries in Children (Holland 1965)

Table 28.1 Age and sex of injured children treated by hospitalization between 1950 and 1960

1	2	3	4	5	6	7	8	9	10	11	12	13	14	Age in years
7	12	18	22	20	26	34	24	19	33	39	33	37	33	Total number of patients = 357
4	5	15	16	16	16	30	19	14	27	34	27	29	30	282 boys = 79 %
3	7	3	6	4	10	4	5	5	6	5	6	8	3	75 girls = 21 %

Table 28.2 Number of various types of injury

Perforated globe	132 = 37 %
Lid laceration with perforation	8 = 2.2 %
Contusion of the globe	107 = 30 %
Lid injury and contusion	27 = 7.6 %
Lid injury	26 = 7.3 %
Burns	18 = 5 %
Chemical burns	14 = 3.9 %
Conjunctival injury	5 = 1.4 %
Corneal injury	18 = 5 %
Scleral injury	2 = 0.6 %

Table 28.3 Number of injuries due to the patient's own negligence

Injuries due to own negligence	160 = 44.8 %
Injuries due to outside factors	184 = 51.5 %
Unknown	13 = 3.7 %

Table 28.4 Incidence of various causes of injury

Cause of injury	Number	Total
A. Injuries from shots		68 = 19.3 %
1. catapult	21	
2. arrows	24	
3. rifles, etc.	23	
B. Injuries from thrown objects		41 = 11.5 %
1. stones	18	
2. potatoes	4	
3. dirt clump	3	
4. snow balls	3	
5. others	13	
C. Injuries from a blow		121 = 33.8 %
1. sticks	32	
2. pen or pencil	7	
3. scissors	9	
4. kitchen utensils	7	
5. knives	8	
6. wire	10	
7. others	48	
D. Injuries from foreign bodies entering the eye		46 = 12.8 %
1. glass	13	
2. hammering	14	
3. chopping wood	5	
4. others	14	
E. Injuries from objects snapped into the eye (whip, rubber bands, chains)		9 = 2.5 %
F. Injury from explosions and fire		24 = 6.7 %
1. powder, etc.	22	
2. oven	2	
G. Injury through chemical burns		14 = 3.9 %
1. alkali	10	
2. acid	2	
3. ink	2	
H. Injury from falling (roller skating, bicycle riding, etc.)		26 = 7.3 %
I. Injury from animals (dog bites, beaks)		4 = 1 %
J. Cause unknown		4 = 1 %

References

Duke-Elder, S.: Injuries. System of ophthalmology XIV, 1, 2, Kimpton, London 1972

Holland, G.: Augen- und Lidverletzungen beim Kinde. Klin. Mbl. Augenheilk. 145 (1965) 915–927

29 Hereditary Inborn Errors of Metabolism with Ocular Findings

The question of inborn errors of metabolism is commonly raised with any ocular disease that appears congenitally or in early childhood. The most important inborn errors of metabolism with ocular findings are reviewed (Rodger and Sinclair 1969; Goldberg 1974; Cotlier 1972; Warburg 1972; François 1975).
Heredity is generally autosomal recessive, rarely dominant, or sex-linked.

Table 29.1 Hereditary inborn errors of metabolism with ocular findings (Bickel 1969)

Disorders of amino acid metabolism	sphingomyelinosis (Niemann-Pick)
cystinosis	glucocerebrosidosis (Gaucher's disease)
homocystinuria	sulfatide lipidosis (metachromatic leukodystrophy)
albinism	Refsum's syndrome
alkaptonuria	glycosphingolipid lipidosis (Fabry)
Disorders of carbohydrate metabolism	Hand-Schüller-Christian disease
galactosemia	**Other metabolic disorders**
diabetes mellitus	Wilson's disease
mucopolysaccharidoses (Hurler and others)	Lowe's syndrome
Disorders of lipid metabolism	porphyria
hypercholesterolemia	hypophosphatasia
gangliosidoses (Tay-Sachs and others)	hypoparathyroidism (pseudo-)

Disorders of Amino Acid Metabolism

Cystinosis

Slit lamp examination of the cornea in cystinosis (page 171) reveals needle-shaped crystals appearing as a glassy bronze dust. These are distributed throughout the stroma near the limbus but involve only the anterior stromal third at the center of the cornea (Plate XI, Fig. 2, page 192 c).
Glistening crystals are also seen around conjunctival vessels, especially near the limbus and in the fornices. Crystal needles may also appear on the anterior iris surface. A pepper-and-salt-like granular pigmentation occurs in the retinal periphery. Gray dots, staining lightly with fluorescein, occur in the corneal epithelium.
Cystinosis (cystine storage disease) is an autosomal recessively inherited enzyme disorder of cystine metabolism. There is dwarfism with a doll-like facies and cystine deposition in the reticuloendothelial system, liver, spleen, lymph nodes and eye. There is progressive renal damage beginning in the proximal tubules and leading to renal atrophy. Clinical findings appear in the second year of life. The disorder is lethal.
Cystinosis also occurs in the Fanconi syndrome, which includes severe damage of the

proximal renal tubules, hyperaminoaciduria, glycosuria, and hyperphosphaturia.

Homocystinuria

Hereditary luxation of the lens occurs first of all in Marfan's syndrome (with dolichomorphia) and Marchesani's syndrome (with brachymorphia). Homocystinuria should be considered with any spontaneous luxation of the lens (Fig. 21.22). It is due to an enzyme defect for degradation of sulfur-containing aminoacids from methionine to cystine (homocystine to cystathionine = cystathionine synthesis).
Besides ectopia lentis, findings in homocystinuria include: ruddy cheeks (dilatation of blood vessels), thin blond hair, skeletal anomalies similar to Marfan's syndrome (arachnodactyly), and often mental retardation. Ocular findings may or may not be present and are similar to those of Marfan's syndrome. Ectopia lentis is found in 25 percent of cases with homocystinuria.
Heredity is autosomal recessive.

Albinism

Albinism (Plate XIII, Fig. 3, page 192 e) and *alkaptonuria* (Fig. 12.3) are amino acid disorders. Hypoplasia and aplasia of the central fovea occur with nystagmus in both *total* as well as *partial* and *ocular albinism* (page 192).
The lack of pigment (Plate XIII, Fig. 3, page 192 e) is particularly noticeable on transillumination of the iris with light reflected from the fundus (retroillumination). The ciliary processes and edge of the lens can be seen through the iris.
In albinism there is an absence of tyrosinase. This results in failure of melanin development.
Heredity:
Total albinism – autosomal recessive.
Partial albinism (leukodermia) – autosomal dominant.
Ocular albinism – X-chromosome recessive.
The Chédiak-Higashi syndrome includes: ocular albinism (potentially also oculocutaneous), photophobia, alacrimia, generalized lack of pigment, anemia, hepatosplenomegaly.
Ocular albinism is also associated with the Klein-Waardenburg syndrome (see page 87).

Alkaptonuria

Alkaptonuria (see page 173) results in circumscribed, semilunar, yellow-brown discolorations of the conjunctiva. These are located in the palpebral fissure area, halfway between the cornea and angle of the eye (Fig. 12.2). Dark corneal and scleral deposits may also develop in the interpalpebral fissure area. Occasionally a dark discoloration of the tarsus of the upper lid appears after the third to fifth decade of life. Tissues such as skin, cartilage, and mucous membranes become dark with time (ochronoses). Arthritic changes can develop. The depositon of homogentisic acid in alkaptonuria leads to inflammation with foreign body giant cells. Heredity is autosomal recessive. On exposure to air, the patient's urine becomes a brown-black owing to its homogentisic acid content.

Disorders of Carbohydrate Metabolism

Galactosemia

Galactosemia (see page 246) causes development of cataracts in the first days to weeks of life. Other findings include galactosuria, albuminuria, anemia, hepatosplenomegaly, mental retardation and digestive problems.

Diabetes Mellitus, Mucopolysaccharidoses

Diabetes mellitus causes a variety of ocular changes (see Chapters on lens, iris, vitreous, retina, optic nerve).
Mucopolysaccharidoses (Kenyon et al. 1972 [see page 170]). Certain congenital disorders of connective tissue metabolism excrete mucopolysaccharides in the urine. One differenti-

ates the mucopolysaccharidoses according to the type of mucopolysaccharide excreted in the urine (dermatan sulfate, heparin sulfate, keratin sulfate). There are seven types: Pfaundler-Hurler (autosomal recessive), Hunter (X-linked recessive), Sanfilippo (autosomal recessive), Morquio (autosomal recessive), late Hurler = Scheie (autosomal recessive), Maroteaux-Lamy β-glucuronidase deficiency.
With the exception of Hunter's and Sanfilippo's syndromes, all types have corneal clouding due to the deposition of mucopolysaccharide. Such deposition occurs primarily in Bowman's membrane and stroma. Tapetoretinal degenerations are primarily seen in Hurler's, Hunter's, Sanfilippo's and Scheie's syndromes. Hurler's syndrome (type I) patients develop gargoylism as well as corneal clouding (Fig. 13.49), dysostosis multiplex, stubby hands, polydystrophy, hepatomegaly, kyphosis, mental retardation and hearing loss. The Maroteaux-Lamy syndrome may lead to atrophy of the optic nerve.

Disorders of Lipid Metabolism

Hypercholesterolemia

Xanthelasma and arcus lipoides – embryotoxon – can occur with essential *hypercholesterolemia.*

Lipid Storage Diseases

Ocular findings in lipid storage diseases are mainly in the retina and optic nerve (see page 289). Macular changes occur in *Tay-Sachs, Niemann-Pick* and *Gaucher's* diseases. *Refsum's* disease has peripheral retinal changes of retinitis pigmentosa.
A cherry red macular spot surrounded by yellow or white retina is seen in *Tay-Sachs* and less often in *Niemann-Pick* disease (Plate XXVII, Fig. 6, page 288 c).
At the same time there is a varying degree of optic atrophy. Cherry red spots due to central retinal artery occlusion are usually unilateral, in contrast to bilateral involvement with storage diseases (Tay-Sachs, etc.). The differential diagnosis is readily made by the history and sudden onset of vision loss.
At first the ganglioside deposits occur almost exclusively in the ganglion cells. Later, pigment epithelium and retinal receptor cells become involved. There is development of a central scotoma, ultimately leading to blindness.
In *Tay-Sachs disease* the musculature is hypotonic at first, but spasms with contractures follow. The disease occurs primarily in Jewish families and has an autosomal recessive heredity. Historically one differentiates five types of familial amaurotic idiocy:

1. *congenital type* = Norman-Wood, appearing in newborns;
2. *infantile form* = *Tay-Sachs,* begins in the third to seventh month;
3. *late infantile form* = *Jansky-Bielschowsky,* occurring in the second to fourth year;
4. *juvenile form* = *Spielmeyer-Vogt,* maculocerebral degeneration, beginning in the fifth to seventh year;
5. *adult form* = *Kufs-Hallervorden,* develops after puberty.

All forms of amaurotic familial idiocy lead to varying degrees of retinal pigmentation, optic atrophy, athetosis, ataxia, attacks of cramping, vision loss and mental retardation. Heredity is autosomal recessive.

Gangliosidoses

Gangliosidoses can be differentiated biochemically into: GM_2-gangliosidosis Type I (Tay-Sachs), Type II and Type III with a defect of *hexosaminidase;* and GM_1, Types I and II with a defect in *β-galactosidase.* Retinal pigmentary changes occur in GM_1-gangliosidosis type II and GM_2-gangliosidosis type III. A *cherry red macula* occurs with GM_2-gangliosidoses types I and II.
Neuronal ceroidlipofuscinosis is apparently identical with juvenile and adult forms of

amaurotic idiocy (Batten-Spielmeyer-Vogt-Kufs). Autofluorescent lipopigment occurs in neurons and blood leukocytes. The etiology of late infantile amaurotic idiocy (Jansky-Bielschowsky) is still unclear.

Sphingomyelinosis

A cherry red macula is occasionally seen with Niemann-Pick disease. This autosomal recessive disorder is due to a lack of metabolism of sphingomyelins and is associated with developmental retardation, hepatosplenomegaly, spasticity, athetosis, cramping and anemia. Death results by age 4 years.

Glucosyl Ceremide Lipidoses (Gaucher)

Gaucher's disease may cause a cherry red spot in the macula and brown pinguecula-like conjunctival changes. This recessively inherited disorder of *cerebroside* metabolism leads to hepatosplenomegaly, panmyelopathy and developmental retardation.

Sulfatide Lipidosis

Ocular findings in *metachromatic leudodystrophy* include tapetoretinal degeneration, a cherry red macula and optic atrophy. In this recessively inherited disorder there is a disturbance in the conversion of sulfatides and cerebrosides. There is retardation of development, speech disorder, bulbar paralysis and dementia. Death usually occurs in the third to sixth years of life.

Refsum's Syndrome

Refsum's syndrome is associated with the appearance of tapetoretinal degeneration with a concentric visual field loss and extinguished ERG. Refsum's syndrome (heredopathia atactica polyneuritiformis) is a heredity disorder in the metabolism of phytanic acid to pristanic acid. The recessively inherited disorder leads to polyneuritis, paresis, muscle atrophy, myocarditis and deafness.

Glycosphingolipid Lipidosis (Fabry)

Fabry's disease (angiokeratoma corporis diffusum universale) (see page 167) leads to cornea verticillata (Fig. 13.41) similar to that of chloroquine. Conjunctival and retinal veins are irregular and tortuous with aneurysmal dilatation.

Similar to Gaucher's disease, there is a disturbance of metabolism of a single lipid in Fabry's disease. Heredity is sex-linked recessive with some clinical expression in female carriers.

Angiokeratoma occurs in the skin and mucous membranes. Renal, cardiac, and brain damage develop.

Hand-Schüller-Christian-Syndrome

(see page 336)

Other Hereditary Metabolic Disorders

Wilson's Disease

The so-called Kayser-Fleischer ring (see page 173) occurs in Wilson's disease. This is a green-brown or yellow-blue, ring-shaped deposit in the corneal periphery (Plate XI, Fig. 4, page 192 c) at the level of Descemet's membrane. Rarely, a second ring is seen located more centrally. This is due to the deposition of copper, occasionally with some silver. Very rarely, a sunflower cataract (chalcosis lentis) occurs. The disease begins in school-aged children with extrapyramidal signs (similar to parkinsonism), debility, hepatosplenomegaly and cirrhosis of the liver.

Lowe's Syndrome

(see page 246)

Porphyria

Congenital porphyria results in marked photophobia. As elsewhere, the skin on the lids develops pigmentation and blisters. Blisters, ulcers and symblepharon occur in the conjunctiva. Keratoconjunctivitis sicca with punctate staining is common. Keratoscleromalacia with loss of the eye may occur (rare). Fundus changes (optic atrophy) are seen. Recessively inherited congenital porphyria results in hemolytic anemia with tumors of the spleen. There is a red discoloration of the teeth and urine. The *chronic cutaneous form* and *porphyria variegata* usually begin during adulthood. Both lead to photodermatitis and conjunctival inflammation. Abdominal symptoms occur in the latter. *Intermittent acute porphyria* has a dominant heredity and appears in late childhood. Ocular findings are limited primarily to the fundus: papillitis, a picture resembling grade IV hypertensive retinopathy, choroiditis. Disturbances of extraocular muscles and exophthalmos may develop. Colic, vomiting, psychoses and constipation are rare findings.

Hypophosphatasia, Hypoparathyroidism (Pseudo-)

Hypocalcemia is the primary finding with hypophosphatasia and hypoparathyroidism. This can lead to congenital cataracts when the hypocalcemia is present during pregnancy (see page 245), or cause acquired permeability cataracts in adults (see page 241).

References

Bickel, H.: Augenveränderungen bei hereditären Stoffwechselerkrankungen im Kindesalter. Ber. dtsch. ophthal. Ges. 69 (1969) 14–16

Cotlier, E.: Biochemical detection of inborn errors of metabolism affecting the eye. Trans. Amer. Acad. Ophthal. Otolaryng. 76 (1972) 1165–1192

François, J.: Maculabefunde bei Speicherkrankheiten. 73. Ber. dtsch. Ophthal. Ges. Heidelberg 1975, 223–265

Goldberg, M. F.: Genetic and metabolic eye disease. Little, Brown & Co., Boston 73–138

Kenyon, K. R., H. A. Quigley, I. E. Hussels, R. G. Wyllie: The systemic mucopolysaccharidoses. Amer. J. Ophthal. 73 (1972) 811–833

Rodger, F. C., H. M. Sinclair: Metabolic and nutritional eye diseases. Thomas, Springfield, Ill., 1969

Warburg, M.: Diagnosis of metabolic eye disease. Munksgaard, Copenhagen 1972

Wollensak, J.: Das Auge und die angeborenen Stoffwechselstörungen des Bindegewebes. Klin. Mbl. Augenheilk. 154 (1969) 473–486

Index

Italicized numbers refer to figure legends.

B

C

D

E

F

O

P